"The 4th edition of *Animal-Assisted Therapy in Counseling* is
and provides the reader with strong practical suggestions fc
is a great asset for any mental health practitioner interestec
interventions to their practice."

Aubrey H. Fine, EdD, *professor, California State Polytechnic University,*
editor of Handbook on Animal-Assisted Therapy

"This is a foundational resource for practitioners who want to include AAT in counseling
practice. It is very well written, thorough, and approachable for novice and experienced AAT
practitioners alike. Of particular value is Chandler's HART theory and SHARM concepts.
From my perspective, HART is the first tool of its kind to translate this highly nuanced
approach into concrete and descriptive elements that are irreplaceable for teaching and
learning the complex nature of AAT-C. Chandler's strategies for including AAT-C into well-
established counseling theoretical orientations are highly specific to mental health providers
and essential to developing one's own professionalized approach in AAT-C. It is the first
book I recommend to my AAT students in my own program."

Leslie A. Stewart, PhD, LCPC, C-AAIS, *professor of counseling,*
Idaho State University, lead author of
Animal-Assisted Therapy in Counseling Competencies

"This volume is comprehensive and well-written. I am most excited by the attention paid
to understanding the variety of species who may be involved in counseling and how these
species offer a unique contribution that is different from one another and different from
their human counterparts. I think this beautifully nuanced book will offer a very useful
perspective for any therapist interested in including animals in clinical practice."

Leif Hallberg, MA, LCP, LCPC, *author of* Walking the
Way of the Horse: The Clinical Practice of
Equine-Assisted Therapy *and* The Equine-Assisted Therapy Workbook

Animal-Assisted Therapy in Counseling

The fourth edition of *Animal-Assisted Therapy in Counseling* is the most comprehensive book available dedicated to training mental health practitioners in the performance of animal-assisted therapy in counseling.

This edition includes material on real-world animal-assisted interventions featuring counselor–client dialogues and sample therapeutic opportunities. Each chapter includes the most recent research and practice, and a wide variety of case examples present animal-assisted interventions in different settings with different types of animals.

This unique resource is an indispensable guide for any counselor or psychotherapist looking to develop and implement animal-assisted therapy techniques in practice.

Cynthia K. Chandler, EdD, has been involved with animal-assisted therapy for more than 20 years and has been a professor at the University of North Texas and a licensed mental health therapist and supervisor for more than 30 years.

Animal-Assisted Therapy in Counseling

Fourth Edition

Cynthia K. Chandler

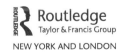

Routledge
Taylor & Francis Group

NEW YORK AND LONDON

Designed cover image: Images created by Cynthia Chandler, Hallie Sheade, and Kristen Watson

Fourth edition published 2024
by Routledge
605 Third Avenue, New York, NY 10158

and by Routledge
4 Park Square, Milton Park, Abingdon, Oxon, OX14 4RN

Routledge is an imprint of the Taylor & Francis Group, an informa business

First edition published by Routledge 2005
Third edition published by Routledge 2017

Library of Congress Cataloging-in-Publication Data
Names: Chandler, Cynthia K., author.
Title: Animal-assisted therapy in counseling / Cynthia K. Chandler.
Description: Fourth edition. | New York, NY : Routledge, 2024. | Includes bibliographical references and index.
Identifiers: LCCN 2023051174 (print) | LCCN 2023051175 (ebook) | ISBN 9781032193519 (hardback) | ISBN 9781032193465 (paperback) | ISBN 9781003260448 (ebook)
Subjects: LCSH: Animals—Therapeutic use.
Classification: LCC RC489.P47 C48 2024 (print) | LCC RC489.P47 (ebook) | DDC 615.8/5158—dc23/eng/20231116
LC record available at https://lccn.loc.gov/2023051174
LC ebook record available at https://lccn.loc.gov/2023051175

ISBN: 978-1-032-19351-9 (hbk)
ISBN: 978-1-032-19346-5 (pbk)
ISBN: 978-1-003-26044-8 (ebk)

DOI: 10.4324/9781003260448

Typeset in Minion Pro
by Apex CoVantage, LLC

This book is dedicated to my pets, Rusty, Dolly, Snowflake, and Jesse, who have been my companions, friends, and co-therapists.

Contents

List of Figures

Acknowledgments

I express sincere gratitude for the many persons who contributed photographs and stories for use in this book.

Preface

Humans are designed to thrive through relationships. Our emotional, physical, and spiritual essence craves connection with others, not only so that we may have our needs met but also so that we may experience purpose and meaning in the time that we dwell on this earth. The human journey is a relationship journey. Some relationships provide love, nurturance, and companionship. Some relationships present hardship and pain. Some relationships endure through time, while others can be ever so brief. Even terse encounters can leave a lasting impact on us, for better or for worse. We journey along, affecting and being affected by our interactions with one another. We need, we desire, we flourish, and we flounder because of the types of relationships we have or strive for in our life. Humans thrive best in comforting relationships and struggle greatest when alone, neglected, or abused. The nature of relationships can determine the state of the human condition. Humans have great capacity to give support, encouragement, and love to one another. Yet they also can and often do hurt one another. When someone feels abandoned, betrayed, hindered, or attacked, the ability to form and sustain relationships with those who may provide love, support, or healing may be compromised. When such instances occur, it can be a struggle to regain the capacity for healthy functioning within relationships, and one may require some assistance to do so.

The profession of counseling involves the facilitation of human growth and healing through the method of relationship. A facilitative relationship is one in which a client feels safe enough to lower self-defenses and expose emotional and social vulnerabilities so that growth and healing may occur via therapeutic intervention. That which enhances the therapeutic alliance between counselor and client increases the facilitative potential of counseling. Within the profession of counseling there is a therapeutic modality referred to as animal-assisted therapy (AAT) that contributes greatly to the healing dynamic of relationship in counseling. With human–animal interaction interwoven into the counseling process there are significantly more therapeutic opportunities to impact a client.

I am frequently asked why I decided to integrate AAT into my professional counseling practice. The prominent reason was so that I could share with others in my world the love and companionship my pets have to offer. As a result of a mutually nurturing relationship between me and my pets, they learned to love and trust humans and developed the confidence to extend their nurturing ways to those outside my family. They brought smiles and comfort to those they met. They provided occasions for interaction that enhanced the counseling process and facilitated the growth and healing of my clients. They increased the potency of the therapeutic alliance. They provided additional opportunities for therapeutic interventions.

Domesticated mammals such as dogs, cats, and horses share with the human mammal a similar internal social system designed such that thriving occurs by way of beneficial relationships. Such beneficial relationships may form both within and across species. Humans and certain types of animals have naturally partnered up as social companions throughout history, and as humans gained greater appreciation for this partnership, relationships became more formalized with animals being integrated as family members and referred to as pets. Humans' experience of pets is that they provide us with love, companionship, entertainment, nurturance, and support. The continuous genuine presentation by animals makes a relationship with a pet more easily formed and maintained than the more complex relationship with a human, who can disguise motive and reaction. Thus, pets provide us with opportunity to practice being in relationships and better prepare us for being in a relationship with another human. During lapses in our human relationships, pets provide us with the emotional support vital for thriving. Incorporating the therapeutic modality of AAT can significantly enhance the properties of counseling. Involving interactions with a therapy animal can increase a client's sense of safety and experience of nurturance during counseling as well as providing additional opportunities for insight, growth, and healing. Human relationships with domesticated animals are, for most people, more easily formed, understood, and maintained than relationships with people, who can hide their true feelings, thoughts, or intentions. Animals are by their nature more genuine and obvious about these things, making them ideal companions for humans to learn how to be more honest and functional in relationships. Thus, counselor-facilitated client interactions with a therapy animal can assist the counseling process.

Interest in AAT continues to grow in the mental health field and thus so does the need for information and training in this modality. This book is designed to provide information on AAT applications for mental health professionals and students as well as those who wish to instruct and supervise students in AAT. The book is ideal for individual self-study as well as group or classroom instruction. The information is organized around the author's recommended competencies and performance guidelines for AAT practice within the counseling arena. In-depth discussion is provided on how to integrate AAT into counseling practice in ways consistent with various counseling guiding theories. Much research is described, and many case scenarios are provided of AAT in a variety of environments including agencies, private practice, schools, hospitals, hospice, prisons, juvenile detention centers, and crisis and disaster response. Work with a variety of therapy animals is described including dogs, cats, horses, guinea pigs and other small animals, farm animals, and dolphins. Special attention is paid to ethical considerations and ways to perform AAT that promote and protect the safety and welfare of both humans and animals.

WHAT IS NEW IN THIS EDITION

The first edition of *Animal Assisted Therapy in Counseling*, published in 2005, was the first comprehensive book dedicated to training mental health therapists in the practice of AAT. From 2005 forward, the field of AAT grew significantly, attracting many more practitioners and researchers. This created a need for the second edition of the book, published in 2012. As the field continues to grow, so does the need for keeping up with new advances in practice and research. In my third (2017) and now this fourth edition, I describe research and material that has been published by various authors. I discuss culturally sensitive practice and work with special populations. Also, I discuss my ground-breaking theoretical model to facilitate understanding, practice, supervision, and research of AAT; the human–animal relational theory (HART). In my presentation of HART, I apply constructs to both practice and supervision of AAT, with true case examples provided to demonstrate application and the impact of application.

.

List of Abbreviations

AAA	animal-assisted activity
AAE	animal-assisted education
AAI	animal-assisted intervention
AAS-C	animal-assisted supervision of counseling
AAT	animal-assisted therapy
AAT-C	animal-assisted therapy in counseling
ADHD	attention-deficit hyperactivity disorder
ADLs	activities of daily living
ASD	autism spectrum disorder
E-HARP	external human–animal relational processing
EAA	equine-assisted activity
EAC	equine-assisted counseling
EAET	equine-assisted experiential therapy
EAI	equine-assisted intervention
EAL	equine-assisted learning
EAMH	equine-assisted mental health
EAP	equine-assisted psychotherapy
EFL	equine-facilitated learning
EFP	equine-facilitated psychotherapy
EFT	equine-facilitated therapy
E-HARP	external human–animal relational processing
EPPT	Equine-partnered play therapy
HARP	human–animal relational processing
HART	human–animal relational theory
HARTI	human–animal relational therapeutic impact
I-HARP	internal human–animal relational processing
PAPs	prison animal programs
PE	prolonged exposure
PTSD	post-traumatic stress disorder
REPC	Relational equine-partnered counseling
RM	relational moment
SHARM	significant human–animal relational moment

About the Author

Dr. Cynthia K. Chandler has been active in animal-assisted therapy since 1999. For her work in the field of animal-assisted therapy, Dr. Chandler received the 2016 Professional Development Award from the American Counseling Association and the 2009 Thelma Duffey Vision and Innovation Award from the Association for Creativity in Counseling, a division of the American Counseling Association. Additionally, she received in 2006 the Pet Partners Beyond Limits Award for Instructor and Evaluator along with her dogs Rusty and Dolly. Dr. Chandler is a 2006 recipient of the Texas Counseling Association Writer of the Year Award for the first edition of this book, published in 2005.

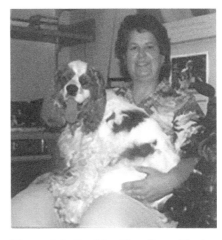

Figure 0.1 Cynthia Chandler with dog Rusty.

Dr. Chandler was born in Ft. Worth, Texas, on July 17, 1956. Her first 7 years of school were undertaken in El Paso, and then her family relocated to Muleshoe, Texas, where she graduated from Muleshoe High School in 1974 (I could not resist throwing in that fun piece of trivia). She received her doctoral degree in educational psychology with a counseling specialty in 1986 from Texas Tech University. Dr. Chandler has been working as a full-time professor since 1989 in the University of North Texas (UNT) counseling program in the Department of Counseling and Higher Education. She developed and directs the Consortium for Animal Assisted Therapy at the university. The Consortium for Animal Assisted Therapy provides continuing education training by sponsoring on-campus workshops and providing distance learning through the Animal Assisted Therapy Distance Learning Program. Dr. Chandler developed and teaches the graduate course Animal-Assisted Therapy, which was the first such course offered in this subject at the University of North Texas. Other graduate areas she teaches at UNT include women's emotional health, basic counseling techniques, assessment, and counseling supervision.

Dr. Chandler is a licensed professional counselor and a licensed marriage and family therapist in the State of Texas as well as an approved supervisor in each of these fields. She was nationally registered with Pet Partners as well as a licensed Pet Partners instructor, and handler–animal team evaluator for over 20 years. She has several publications in nationally refereed professional journals and has presented at professional venues across the United States and in Canada, Austria, Greece, South Korea, Hong Kong, Sweden, St. Maarten, India, and Spain. She created and led, for over 20 years, the annual state-wide training Institute in Counselor Supervision for the accreditation of approved supervisors. Also, for over 20 years, she presented community workshops every year to train volunteers in animal-assisted activities and professionals in AAT.

About the Author's Therapy Animals

I could not have engaged in any animal-assisted activity or therapy were it not for my trusted therapy partners Rusty, Dolly, Snowflake, and Jesse. They are first and foremost beloved family members, my companions, and my friends. Without their loyal and dutiful efforts I would not have written this book.

Rusty was my first therapy animal. He was born in Denton, Texas, on June 6, 1999 and passed away in December 2011. He was a red-on-white parti-color American Cocker Spaniel. He had an abundance of dark red freckles on his face and large red furry patches all over his body including over both eyes, with solid red, long, droopy ears. He had extraordinarily curly fur for an American Cocker. I brought Rusty home when he was 7½ weeks old and named him after a player on my favorite baseball team, Rusty Greer, who then played left field for the Texas Rangers. Rusty's full American Kennel Club (AKC) registered name was Chandler's Rusty Ranger. His personality was friendly, affectionate, and playful. He always had robust energy until old age slowed him down a little. He loved working as a therapy dog

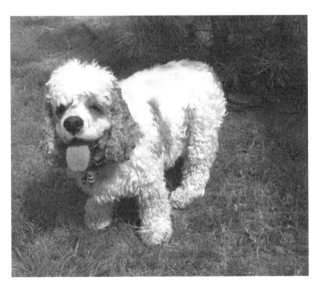

Figure 0.2 Rusty, therapy dog.

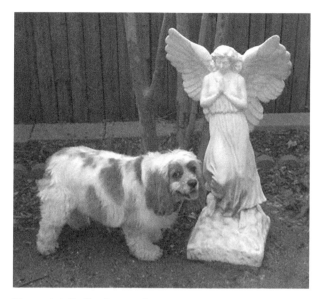

Figure 0.3 Dolly, therapy dog.

and served in this role for 9 years before he retired because of age-related health issues. He still loved to play fetch and go for walks. He shared his healing social gifts with many different people in a variety of situations. I learned so much about the comforting and healing capacity of animals by working with Rusty. He was a nurturing companion and my most valuable teacher. I was greatly blessed for having him as part of my family. The pain from his loss intensely lingers in my heart.

Dolly was born near Lubbock, Texas, on September 30, 2002, and she passed away in September 2011. She was an American Cocker Spaniel and looked almost like Rusty, only smaller, with straight, long, flowing fur. She joined my family when she was 7 weeks old. Her personality was friendly, affectionate, and playful, but she was quieter and more reserved than Rusty. She exhibited a hint of delicate, petite femininity in her demeanor and pranced along as if bouncing like a ballerina off the tips of her toes. Her AKC registered name was Chandler's China Doll. She engaged in therapy work for 7 years until she became ill. She was a sweet companion and loving therapy dog. She is greatly missed.

Snowflake was a solid white domestic American short-hair cat. His left eye was green, and his right eye was blue. His nose was a bright pink, as were the pads of his paws. He was large and husky with a very playful personality. He was a stray cat that, when a kitten, wandered up into my yard in Denton, Texas, and had no one to claim him, so he joined our family. He was named Snowflake because of his unique appearance. Snowflake's uniqueness was compounded by the fact that he was deaf, most likely from birth. The veterinarian estimated his age at about 8 to 9 weeks when he arrived at our home, and thus his approximate birth date is toward the end of February 2001. He accompanied me to the juvenile detention center where he enjoyed being petted and cuddled and playing with the adolescents in the post-adjudication program during group and individual therapy sessions. He lost interest in working after a little over 3 years and he retired from therapy work. For the remainder of his long life, he was healthy and mobile and enjoyed basking in the warmth of the sun and gazing out through the window at the birds and squirrels feeding in the backyard. He passed away March 2, 2020. As with Rusty and Dolly's passing, he is greatly missed.

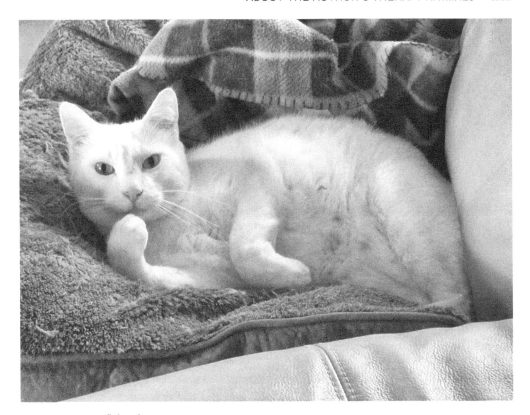

Figure 0.4 Snowflake, therapy cat.

Jesse was born on July 22, 2011 in South Carolina and came to live with my family when she was 8 weeks old. She is classified as a buff and white American Cocker Spaniel, but that does not fully describe her unique beauty. She has long, flowing fur that starts as a tan color on her back, lightens to a sandy color at her waist, and is a champagne color at her belly and legs. She has long tan-and-sandy ears, and a tan, sandy, and white face with deep red freckles laid across her nose. She also has a sprinkling of large red freckles laid against a white background on her forelegs, though this is not visible unless you move aside the long wisps of champagne-colored fur. People frequently call Jesse nicknames: "Miss Wiggle-butt" as a reflection of her excitement when greeting, or "Puff-ball" as a comment on her fluffy appearance. Consistently upon meeting Jesse for the first time, an initial comment from someone who touches her is, "Ooh, she is so soft!" While she is pure-bred, she is not registered with the AKC because she is a little shorter than a typical female Cocker Spaniel. Characteristics of Jesse's personality fall somewhere between the speedy robustness of Rusty and the subdued gentleness of Dolly. Jesse is very laid back and easy going, but ready to play or socially engage in an instant. She is excellent at assessing the emotions and attitudes of clients with whom we work. When she determines that nurturance is needed then she snuggles with the client. When the client is experiencing distress, she is excellent at alerting me and the client that something needs attention, even when the client's distress is not overtly obvious.

All of my pets that have worked with me as therapy animals have been excellent teachers regarding the power of AAT in benefiting a client. Rusty taught me the most because he was a great teacher and my first therapy animal, so I had very much to learn. Rusty gave me a strong foundation for practicing and teaching AAT. Working with Snowflake and Dolly furthered

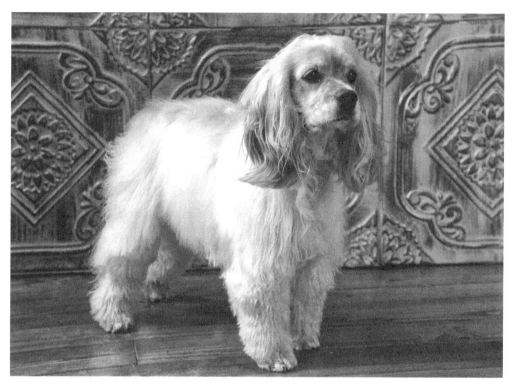

Figure 0.5 Jesse, therapy dog.

my knowledge and refined my skills; they taught me how pets with different personalities can serve different needs for different clients. My work with Jesse brought me to new heights of comprehension regarding the potency of AAT. Jesse's profound ability and willingness to detect, signal, and respond to the internal experience of the client, along with her persistence to keep signaling until I paid attention, led me to the other side of the rainbow regarding AAT, to a land of greater possibilities. It was from my work with Jesse that I gained insights that contributed to my development of a new theoretical model to facilitate understanding, practice, supervision, and research of AAT, the human–animal relational theory (HART). I honor the teachings of my therapy animals by sharing them with you in this book. I hope you are also inspired in the way they have inspired me.

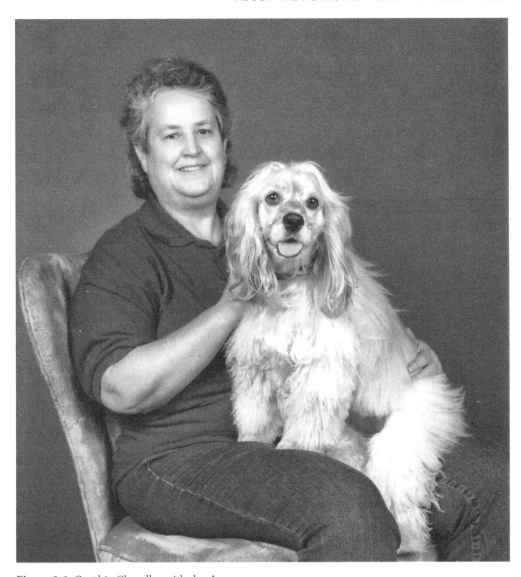

Figure 0.6 Cynthia Chandler with dog Jesse.

1

An Introduction to Animal-Assisted Therapy

Imagine you are 13 years old and poor decisions you have made mean you find yourself in a residential juvenile detention facility. On this first day of your confinement, your own clothes have been replaced by a drab set of brown coveralls, your street shoes have been taken, and you have to wear thick, institutional orange socks and flimsy slippers. You are escorted everywhere by stern-looking adults in security uniforms composed of black T-shirts and camouflage pants with large, black army boots. The cinderblock walls are painted pale gray and form long, cold corridors interrupted only by an occasional heavy metal door and interior window of thick glass with wires running through it in a crisscross pattern. The loud sounds you hear are the clicks and clangs from the security locks on the doors opening and then closing behind you as you travel deeper into the abyss of freedom lost. The order barked from the adult security escort to pass on through the door startles you, interrupting your concentrated yet futile thoughts to regain some sense of control over the situation. You are scared. No, it's more like you are petrified. You are no longer as sure of yourself as you thought you were a few days ago. Your mind is in a flurry. You ask yourself, "Should I run, but where would I run to and how would I get out? Should I act defiant, showing them how tough I am and that I am not going to give in to their attempts to dominate me? Or, should I just cry, because that is what I really want to do?" In desperation you resolve, "No, I must not show them how scared I am. I must not let them control me. I will . . . I will . . ." Then, all of a sudden, your spiraling thoughts are interrupted. "Wait a minute. What is that jingling noise? Is that—is that—a dog? Yes, it is a dog! Wow, it's a Cocker Spaniel, and he looks so happy!" Then you ask out loud, "Can I pet him? Is it a boy or a girl? What's his name?" You speak to the dog. "Hi Rusty! What are you doing here?" You say to the dog's handler, "Oh, look, he likes it when I scratch his ears. I think he really likes me. You know, I have a dog at home. His name is Scooter. He's just a mutt. But he is really smart. I have taught him some tricks. Can Rusty do tricks? Oh wow, that is so cool; he gave me a high five! You say Rusty is a counselor here? Wow, a dog counselor. So, can I have counseling with Rusty? Great! Thanks for letting me pet Rusty." Now you are not so scared. Maybe this place is not where you want to be, but maybe, just maybe, you can make it through this dark period of your life all right, especially since the people here bring dogs for you to pet and play with.

Sometimes life is painful. Sometimes we do not feel as safe and secure as we would like. Sometimes we need comfort and affection to help us through tough times. We need a broad

DOI: 10.4324/9781003260448-1

support system. We need people to help us. And yes, sometimes we really need a dog. Or we need a cat, or a horse, or some other animal to help us through our pain and to move us toward a better place in our life. Animal-assisted therapy (AAT) is one way animals can be very helpful to people, and working with therapy animals in the profession of counseling is what I want to talk to you about in this book. Animals that assist in the therapy process are referred to by a number of different and interchangeable titles including therapy animal, therapy pet, pet practitioner, and pet facilitator. Regardless of the variation in descriptive titles, each therapy pet serves the same basic purpose: working in partnership with a professional human therapist to provide compassionate and stimulating therapy designed to facilitate human client recovery.

Animal-assisted therapy in counseling (AAT-C) is the incorporation of pets as therapeutic agents into the counseling process. This can be done in a variety of ways and by using a variety of techniques. AAT-C is appropriate for numerous settings including schools, hospitals, agencies, and private practice. The most common and most preferred application model of AAT-C is for counselors to work in partnership with their own pet; a pet that has been evaluated as appropriate for such work. This model is preferred because a counselor is most familiar with his or her own pet and can best predict the pet's emotional and behavioral reactions. In addition, the strong and healthy bond demonstrated between counselor and pet can contribute greatly to the therapeutic process, especially by reassuring clients that the therapist can be trusted because they observe positive interactions between the pet and the therapist. Another application model of AAT-C is for a counselor to obtain the assistance of a trained animal handler who has a qualified therapy pet. This model requires the trained animal handler to facilitate interactions between the therapy pet and client under the counselor's guidance and supervision. This model allows counselors to provide AAT-C for clients without having their own pet serve in therapy. Also, trained animal handlers may be able to facilitate animal-related tasks that are outside of the counselor's skills, such as involving clients with animal training, grooming, and other appropriate animal-related activities. The disadvantages of this second AAT-C application model include the necessity of obtaining permission from clients to involve another person in the therapy process, securing a confidentiality agreement from the animal handler, and having confidence in both the animal handler and the therapy pet. A counselor who wishes to use the second model—to employ the assistance of an animal handler with a therapy pet—has the additional obstacle of finding such an animal therapy team located conveniently nearby. Some organizations provide training and evaluation for persons who wish to work with their therapy pets, most of which have a website that can assist in contacting a registered animal therapy team. The national organization that currently provides the most rigorous training, evaluation, and registration process for handler–animal teams for a variety of animal species is Pet Partners (www. petpartners.org). Another popular organization that registers handler–animal teams is Therapy Dogs International (www.tdi-dog.org).

AAT-C is one type of application in the broader field of AAT; thus, it is important to first briefly introduce the overall construct of AAT. AAT promotes positive human–animal interaction and incorporates the talents and traits of a therapy animal into a therapeutic setting to facilitate the recovery of patients seeking physical or mental health services. Under the careful guidance of a trained therapist, the animal contributes to clients' recovery process. Examples of AAT in physical therapy would be having a patient walk a dog down a hallway or pet or brush a cat; activities designed to increase muscle strength and control. One example of AAT in a mental health counseling session could involve a child victim of abuse gently petting and talking to a dog or cat to teach the concept of appropriate touch and gentle relations; the warm and caring attitude of the therapy pet and human therapist combined reinforces the child's positive experience.

Why involve pets in therapy?—because therapy pets can alter the dynamics of the therapy process in several productive ways:

- Clients may be more motivated to attend and participate in therapy because they desire to spend time with the therapy pet.
- Clients' focus may be temporarily shifted away from disabling pain due to the interaction with the therapy pet, to the extent that they can work harder and longer in therapy and potentially gain more benefit per session.
- Clients may receive healing nurturance and affection through physical contact with the therapy pet.
- Clients may experience soothing comfort from petting or holding the therapy pet.
- Clients may experience genuine acceptance by the therapy pet.
- Clients may experience enjoyment and entertainment from interaction with the therapy pet.
- Clients may be able to form a more trusting relationship with therapists who demonstrate that they can be trusted by the way they interact with the therapy animal.
- Clients' personal awareness may be enhanced from the way the animal interacts with or responds to them.
- In many instances, based on the unique characteristics of clients' conditions or needs, they may be able to perform activities and achieve goals that would not otherwise be possible without the assistance of a therapy pet.

As a result of the unique dynamics presented, participation of a therapy pet in the therapy process may reduce the stress of therapy for clients and may allow for quicker and greater recovery.

While it is true that professionals in the field of counseling have been facilitating clients' recovery quite well without the assistance of animals, it is important to consider what greatly significant benefits might be gained with the addition of a therapy animal. Two of the greatest assets a therapy animal brings to a counseling setting are: (1) the animal's capacity and desire to nurture people and, (2) the animal's ability to detect and signal emotional distress it perceives occurring in a person. The animal species that excel at this are horses and dogs because they are designed to interact in a family-like social system; horses are biologically designed to be herd animals and dogs are designed to be pack animals. There are numerous other species that work effectively as therapy animals, most of which are domesticated mammals. Each animal species varies in its desire and ability to nurture people and in its ability to detect and signal emotional distress in people. Additionally, any individual animal within a species, depending on its personality, may not demonstrate a desire to nurture people or to signal distress it perceives in a person. Many types of animals might serve as a therapy animal, but dogs and horses are the most common and I believe they offer some of the greatest benefits in the role of assistant in counseling. It is with dysfunctional or resistant clients that counselors are seeing the most dramatic positive effects of working with a therapy animal compared with the same work without a therapy animal. Yet highly functional and less resistant clients can also benefit greatly from the work of a therapy animal, in that they can have significant and important insights brought to conscious awareness.

The psychosocial and psychophysiological benefits of animals have been well documented (Fine, 2000a; Wilkes, Shalko, and Trahan, 1989). In a qualitative research study, interviewed pet owners reported that their pets enhanced their life in eight domains of personal wellness: emotional and physical nurturance, sense of family, sense of responsibility and purpose, friendship and/or companionship, social interaction and connections, personal values and/or spiritual meaning, fun and play, and physical health (Chandler et al., 2015). Studies have reported quicker recovery and increased longevity for cardiac patients who owned a pet (Friedmann et al., 1980; Friedmann and Thomas, 1995). Reductions in levels of blood pressure, stress, and anxiety in children occurred when a researcher was accompanied by a pet (Friedmann et al., 1983). Decreased depression and increased socialization occurred in elderly persons interacting with residential or visiting therapy pets (Holcomb et al., 1997; Perelle and Granville, 1993). More socially appropriate behaviors occurred for children with developmental disorders who interacted with a therapy pet (Redefer and Goodman, 1989). Also, fewer behavior problems occurred in children with emotional and developmental disorders when they interacted with a therapy pet (Kogan et al., 1999).

AAT has been incorporated into numerous healthcare professions including nursing, counseling and psychology, physical rehabilitation, therapeutic recreation, and speech therapy (Gammonley, et al., 1997). It has been shown to be beneficial in a variety of settings, such as schools, counseling agencies, hospitals, nursing homes, hospice care, developmental disability facilities, juvenile detention centers, and prisons (Burch, 1996, 2003; Chandler, 2005a; Delta Society, 1997). Much has been written on the subject of AAT, yet more controlled research studies are needed to support and expand on existing clinical findings.

DEFINITION AND DESCRIPTION OF AAT

It is important to comprehend the difference between animal-assisted activity (AAA) and AAT. Most people tend to lump AAA and AAT into one category called "animal-assisted therapy." However, technically speaking, AAA involves mostly social visits with a therapy animal, whereas AAT strategically incorporates human–animal interactions into a formal therapeutic process.

AAA involves goal-directed activities designed to improve patients' quality of life through use of the human–animal bond (Gammonley et al., 1997). Animals and their handlers must be screened and trained. Activities may be therapeutic but typically are not guided by a credentialed therapist. AAA usually involves such tasks as visiting with persons and friendly petting with some playful activity. It may also include education about or related to the animal itself. However, AAA is a less formal human–animal interaction when compared with AAT.

AAT uses the human–animal bond in goal-directed interventions as an integral part of the treatment process. Working animals and their handlers must be screened, be trained, and meet specific criteria. A credentialed therapist, working within the scope of a professional practice, sets therapeutic goals, guides the interaction between patient and animal, measures progress toward meeting therapy goals, and evaluates the process. AAT may be billed to third-party payers just as any other kind of reimbursable therapy (Gammonley et al., 1997).

A taskforce for the International Association of Human–Animal Interaction Organizations (IAHAIO, 2014) produced their White Paper in 2014, presenting definitions, descriptions, and guidelines for animal-assisted interventions (AAI):

> An Animal-Assisted Intervention is a goal oriented and structured intervention that intentionally includes or incorporates animals in health, education and human service (e.g., social work) for the purpose of therapeutic gains in humans. It involves people with knowledge of the people and animals involved. Animal-assisted interventions incorporate human-animal teams in formal human service such as Animal-Assisted Therapy (AAT), Animal-Assisted Education (AAE) or under certain conditions Animal-Assisted Activity (AAA).
>
> (p. 5)

IAHAIO (2014, pp. 5–6) recognizes AAT and AAE as planned, structured, goal-oriented, professional activities that are to be performed by credentialed professionals within the respective fields; and AAA as "planned and goal-oriented informal interaction and visitation" performed by handler–animal teams with at least appropriate introductory training, preparation, and assessment. The White Paper presents detailed definitions and descriptions for the various AAIs. The IAHAIO White Paper 2014 is an attempt to increase clarity of differences between interventions, as well as to provide what the task force hopes will be universally accepted definitions and descriptions to be used by all research scholars and practitioners. Readers may obtain, via a search of the organization's website, the IAHAIO White Paper 2014: The IAHAIO Definitions for Animal-Assisted Intervention and Guidelines for Wellness of Animals Involved.

AAT is considered an adjunct to existing therapy. A therapist can incorporate the animal into whatever professional style of therapy the therapist already enacts. AAT therapy can be directive or nondirective in its approach. AAT sessions can be integrated into individual or group therapy and used with a very wide range of age groups and persons with varying ability. AAT is a practice modality and not an independent profession. Persons guiding AAT must have the proper training and credentials for their professional practice, such as those for a licensed professional counselor.

A therapy animal should not be confused with an animal designated as an emotional support animal. "Emotional support animal" is a designation by the U.S. Department of Housing and Urban Development that an individual can assign to a personal pet when the individual procures a letter from a health or mental health provider, while under the provider's care, that states the individual has a physical or psychiatric disability and could directly benefit from having a pet live with them (Chandler, 2015, Chandler, 2019). An emotional support animal is not given legal rights to accompany an individual outside of the home to any other facility; the designation of emotional support animal is to guarantee the right of an individual to have a pet live with them at no financial penalty even in housing designated as not allowing pets. A therapy animal should also not be confused with a service animal. A therapy animal does not have the same recognition or protection as a service or disability assistance animal. Service or disability assistance animals are specially trained to assist the disabled and must be allowed, by law, to accompany their owner, handler, or trainer into just about any facility. Some states in the United States have passed laws formally recognizing and protecting therapy animals, but the status of a therapy animal still does not match the unimpeded stature of a service or disability assistance animal. A credentialed therapy animal may be invited into many places barred to a nonworking animal due to its status as a professional working animal, but the key words are "by invitation only." A professional vest or neck scarf worn by the therapy animal identifying it as a working professional goes far in gaining acceptance into many places. I do not mean to be confusing, but some organizations, such as Pet Partners, allow service animals and emotional support animals to serve on a handler–animal team that provides AAA or AAT. So, while service animal, emotional support animal, and therapy animal are three different and separate roles, an animal can serve in more than one of these roles. For instance, an animal trained and designated as a service animal may be able to work as a therapy animal if it meets the qualifications for a therapy animal; and a pet properly designated as an emotional support animal might also meet the qualifications to work as a therapy animal. The fact that an animal might qualify to serve in more than one role makes it easy to see why there is some public confusion about these three roles that animals can serve.

NEUROBIOLOGY OF THE HUMAN–ANIMAL SOCIAL CONNECTION

There seems to be a natural tendency for humans and pets to form a relationship with one another, even if the animal is not that person's pet. This natural tendency is what fosters such quick rapport and empathy between clients and therapy pets. The pet practitioner does little but be itself and has clients' trust well before they trust the human therapist. The typical relationship between a therapy pet and clients can be rapidly formed and easily terminated, although some issues may need to be addressed around saying goodbye to the therapy animal. The therapy animal–client relationship does not have the depth of attachment that a bond between a pet and its owner may have, but it can still be a strong and positive relationship.

Some have referred to the therapeutic benefit of AAT as based on the concept of a basic human–animal bond (Kaminski, Pellino, and Wish, 2002). However, in *Veterinary Ethics* Tannenbaum (1995, p. 184) raises questions about the use of the term and suggests that a true bond possesses the following characteristics:

It must involve a continuous, ongoing relationship rather than one that is sporadic or accidental.

It must produce not just a benefit but a *significant* benefit to both, and that benefit must be a *central* aspect of the lives of each.

It must involve a relationship that is, in some sense, voluntary.

It must be bidirectional.

It must entitle each being in the bond to respect and benefit in their own right rather than simply as a means to an end.

Based on these conditions, it is clear that the relationship between clients and therapy animals does not meet the elements described by Tannenbaum that are needed for the type of bond more likely to be formed between a pet and its owner. It is more likely that the benefits gained by clients in therapy with a therapy animal are a result of a different type of relationship between them and the pet than that of an owner and a pet. The client–therapy animal relationship is likely formed on the basis of a shared connection that is situational and based on a desire for nurturing interaction. While pet owners typically form a permanent attachment or bond with their pet, the relationship between a therapy pet and client is less about the formation of a permanent attachment. It is more about a desire for affiliation with a nurturing being, a desire that is present at the initiation and early stages of an attachment or bonding process. Clients may perceive a therapy animal as a potential source of nurturance for a number of reasons. Clients initially find a therapy pet easier to trust than a human therapist, in that the pet characteristically does not deceive; and in seeking affection and interaction, the therapy pet displays that it desires and provides a nurturing association, much like clients may desire in a therapeutic situation. Clients trust the genuine presentation of the therapy pet and affiliate with the pet's desire for, and provision of, nurturance; this may expedite the formation of a strong relationship between the therapy animal and the client. There is certainly a human–animal bond at play in AAT; that of the bond between the therapy animal and the therapist or the animal's handler. The mutual enduring trust, affection, and communication between the therapy animal and the animal's handler are what allow for this relationship to be therapeutic for clients. The bond between the handler and therapy animal is a vital component of effective AAT. I agree with the concept presented in *Veterinary Ethics* (Tannenbaum, 1995) that the client–therapy animal relationship does not meet the conditions necessary for a human–animal bond, which is the strong attachment the animal and owner have to one another.

The strength of the social connection that is formed between a therapy animal and a client is not as strong as the social connection formed between a pet and its owner. However, both types of social connections do involve similar biological bonding or attachment processes, and the difference in the connection formed is a matter of strength. Thus, I think it is more correct to speak of the client–therapy animal relationship as a social connection having been formed through the human–animal bonding process, or in similar terms, through the human–animal attachment process. Yet, the client–therapy animal relationship will not be as strong a connection as a pet–owner relationship. Even without a client's having a strong bond or attachment to the therapy pet, interaction with the animal can still facilitate the client's exploration of interpersonal relational dynamics and move the client toward greater functionality in relationships. Zilcha-Mano, Mikulincer, and Shaver (2011) share a similar opinion:

> Positive experiences with a pet could pave the way, with the empathetic mediation and guidance of a therapist, to creating more secure interpersonal attachments and re-evaluating and modifying maladaptive working models and attachment orientations.
>
> While empirical findings show that people can form an attachment relationship with their own pet, it can be questionable whether a pet in the therapy room could fulfill the role of an attachment figure in its full manner. In fact, unlike the relationship with one's own pet, the relationship with a therapy pet is restricted to the therapy sessions and therefore is time-limited. In this context, it might be hard for some clients to form a full-blown attachment relationship with the pet in the same way that it might be hard for them to form a full-blown attachment with the therapist. However, we don't intend to say that the relationship with the therapy pet meets the strict criteria used to define full-blown attachments . . . or that the therapy pet would become the client's primary attachment figure. We are only arguing that the therapy pet can potentially become one of the figures in a client's attachment hierarchy and that this pet can provide some sort of safe haven and secure base to the client during therapy sessions.
>
> (p. 545)

It is important to note that a client may also benefit from the human–animal bond that exists between the therapist and the therapist's therapy animal because that relationship can demonstrate the mutual trust and nurturance potential in both the human therapist and the therapy animal. This demonstration, when observed by a client, can assist the client to build trust in the therapeutic duo, and the client can be stimulated to form a social connection to each, thereby creating and reinforcing a therapeutic alliance.

All mammals have similar capacity to form social connections and social attachments. Mammals can even form social connections with mammals from a different species. One of the most extraordinary examples of a cross-species social connection is demonstrated by the interactions between polar bears and sled dogs observed in the arctic region. One normally thinks of dogs and polar bears as natural enemies. Indeed, polar bears are very dangerous carnivorous animals with a diet favoring seals. Yet numerous video clips have been taken showing sled dogs and wild polar bears interacting socially with no aggression (Firstscience TV, 2007). The polar bears could easily maim or kill the sled dogs, but instead they play together. Another example of cross-species bonding is the cheetah and companion dog program at various zoos. Cheetahs are by their nature very nervous animals, but zoo staff have found that when paired with a canine companion the cheetah is calmed by its presence. A baby cheetah and puppy are paired and socialized together during frequent supervised visits and they become familiar friends. The cheetah will read the body language of its canine companion to determine its own sense of safety. When the cheetah travels, its canine companion comes along. This allows the cheetahs to participate in ambassador educational programs. As long as the dog is expressing a sense of safety and calm, then so does the cheetah (Attractions Magazine, 2012; Pamer and Manning, 2013).

Understanding mammals' capacity and desire to form within- and cross-species social connections is very useful in more fully comprehending the potential benefits of AAT. Let's examine what science has discovered about the biology of the bonding (or attachment) process in mammals and how this contributes to a desire for social connectedness.

Making and maintaining social connections is a biological necessity to survive and thrive for mammals. Mammals are animals of the highest class of vertebrates, and humans are included in this group (encyclopedia.com, n.d.). Mammals give birth to live young that are relatively helpless at birth. The female has mammary glands that secrete milk for the nourishment of the young after birth. Young mammals require lots of attention from a parent to survive and thrive. Thus, a biological process must be in place to promote caregiving. This biological caregiving system is rather complex. It includes a mechanism for a young one to signal that it is, for example, hungry, cold, or frightened. But why should a parent respond to a young one signaling a need? A parent responds because it receives a benefit in doing so. So, the caregiving process also includes a mechanism that rewards a parent for responding to a young one signaling a need.

Let's examine the mechanism that drives a young mammal to call for need gratification. In the brain of mammals there is a neural network for seeking that drives movement toward something for investigation (e.g., sniffing, exploring) to obtain need gratification, such as food or shelter (Panksepp, 1998). This "seeking" network has close neural connections with the neural network for panic, which produces distress vocalizations signaling a desire for social contact. So, when a young one is in need, it seeks gratification of that need by signaling a desire for social contact. When a parent responds to the young mammal's need, the young one's existing neural networks and close neural connections are reinforced. So, a young mammal has a capacity to seek nurturance through social contact, and this capacity strengthens with each act of need gratification by the caregiver. Nurturing social contact memories form in the young and strengthen with reinforcement. Thus, social seeking and social gratification capacities can grow and can be generalized beyond a parent and even beyond its species as the animal matures. This explains why mammals have the ability and desire to seek social contact that is rewarding (Panksepp, 1998). The reward that a mammalian young one receives from parental engagement goes beyond the provision of food, protection, and warmth. Close positive social contact, and especially nurturing physical contact, is soothing and calming for the young mammal. This same type of effect occurs within the parent that provides the positive, nurturing contact. Thus, the parent is rewarded by acts of providing for its young. When a mammal makes positive social contact with its child, especially physical contact, then a hormone called oxytocin is released in the brain of both the parent and child (Panksepp, 2005). This hormone creates internal positive feelings. Oxytocin has been shown to be more effective than brain opioids in reducing separation distress in animals. It is critical for facilitating mother–infant bonding (attachment). Oxytocin is also very effective at facilitating pair bonding between mates (Panksepp, 2005).

THE SCIENCE OF HUMAN–ANIMAL INTERACTION

Within a few minutes of positive interaction between a dog and a human, levels of oxytocin, endorphins, and dopamine in both the person and the dog rise significantly (Odendaal, 2000; Odendaal and Meintjes, 2003); though one study showed the increase in oxytocin to be more significant for women than for men (Miller et al., 2009). Dopamine helps control the brain's reward and pleasure centers, while endorphins help relieve pain and induce feelings of pleasure or euphoria. Oxytocin has numerous positive effects including the experience of pleasure, soothing and calming moods, and stress reduction (Uvnäs-Moberg, 2010, 1998a, 1998b; Uvnäs-Moberg, Arn, and Magnusson, 2005). Oxytocin also contributes to social connection and pair bonding (MacGill, 2015).

Females have much higher levels of oxytocin than males, though both sexes have significant amounts. Also of note, estrogen perpetuates the effects of oxytocin in females. Oxytocin is a powerful player in reproduction. It is released in high levels during sexual intercourse and thus contributes to pair bonding (oxytocin is often referred to as a "cuddle hormone"). Oxytocin is released in the female during birthing to help shrink the uterus, to diminish the painful memories of birthing, and to help produce milk for breastfeeding. During breastfeeding, additional oxytocin is released into the mother's system that stimulates emotional bonding (attachment) with the child. Research with new mothers has shown that breastfeeding has the following effects on the mother: decreased blood pressure, increased social interaction, and reduced anxiety. In fact, mothers who breastfed their child longer stayed healthier over the 10-year period post-breastfeeding, with lower incidence of stroke and diabetes and lower blood pressure. Thus, increased exposure to oxytocin over time can have significant long-term health benefits (Uvnäs-Moberg, 2010).

As mentioned, positive social contact between the child and either parent, especially nurturing physical touch, releases oxytocin into the system of both the parents and the child. Oxytocin is a hormone that stimulates social attachment because it has special properties that increase sensitivity of brain opioid systems, that is, pleasure stimulants. So, oxytocin is a prime mover in the construction and maintenance of social bonds (attachments) and social connections in mammals because positive social contact is rewarded by the experience of pleasure from oxytocin release. Research confirms that the oxytocin molecule and its effects are the same in all mammals (Uvnäs-Moberg, 2010); thus, mammals are drawn to make contact with other beings perceived as sources for nurturance. This is a biologically based social system. This aspect of mammals' thrive biology is an extension of the biological social bonding (or attachment) process, which is initiated in the parent-to-child caregiving process. This explains why a client desires to pet a therapy animal: the client perceives the therapy animal as a potential source of nurturance. A client who does not perceive a therapy animal as a potential source of nurturance will likely not be drawn to pet a therapy animal.

Most of us are familiar with the fight–flight–freeze response system in animals. When a human or animal is in distress, stress response hormones such as cortisol, aldosterone, and adrenalin are secreted into the system (Uvnäs-Moberg, 2010). The fight–flight–freeze response system, also known as the stress response system, is a self-preservation system that is a reaction to threat, danger, or harm. The "stress response system" interacts with the "social system." One such interaction is when the stress response system stimulates a signal call for help.

Although the stress response system and the social system communicate with one another, the social system is a very different biological system and is where the hormone oxytocin plays a major role (Uvnäs-Moberg, 2010). The social system is a quieter system than the stress response system, yet it is just as active. When the stress response system is activated, the social system secretes oxytocin to rebound from stress. The social system assists in calming and soothing and is also activated at times other than stress, such as from positive social contact of the emotional or physical type. With physical contact, sensory nerves in the skin will trigger a release of oxytocin after positive touch. The social system contributes to social bonding (attachment) and assists with caring and with saving energy for growth and restoration. If you give small amounts of oxytocin to rats, the result is reduced aggression, increased social interaction, decreased fear responses, and decreased pulse rate and blood pressure. Multiple doses of oxytocin over several days result in blood pressure staying low for days and weeks afterward. Oxytocin helps to activate the parasympathetic nervous system, which is linked to growth and restoration. The oxytocin brain network involves the hypothalamus and extends to the amygdala and brain stem. In fact, oxytocin nerve fibers project to all major areas of the brain; thus, oxytocin can have multiple effects. It is secreted from individual cells and cell bodies so enormous amounts can be available. It combines noradrenergic and dopaminergic systems for a pattern of effects. Animal research has shown that long-term effects of oxytocin exposure can increase the pain threshold, lower blood pressure, lower cortisol levels, increase vagal tone, decrease inflammation, increase wound healing, facilitate learning, and have anxiolytic-like effects (anti-anxiety). Research with humans taking doses of oxytocin via nasal spray resulted in increased social interaction, increased ability to interpret social cues, anxiolytic-like effects, increased trust in other individuals, increased sense of wellbeing, decreased cortisol, and decreased sensitivity to pain. Since one of the ways oxytocin is released is through skin-to-skin contact, and since the skin is the biggest sensory organ, one of the easiest ways to increase oxytocin levels is through positive physical touch. In summary, petting an animal is not only soothing and calming but also has a number of long-term health benefits, both for the human and the animal (Uvnäs-Moberg, 2010).

Remember, when we pet a therapy animal, not only are we experiencing an oxytocin release but so is the animal. Petting is pleasurable for both humans and animals. When I went home at night and my dogs Rusty and Dolly bounded happily up to greet me, I responded by giving them each a good petting, and sometimes when I did so, just for fun, I would say in a pleasant, playful tone, "Do you want some oxytocin? Do you? Do you want some oxytocin? Here's some oxytocin. Good dogs. Here's some oxytocin." And they would wag their tails and wiggle like they knew exactly what I was talking about. The skin has countless sensory nerves, and gentle nurturing touch stimulates A-beta-type nerve fibers (Daley Olmert, 2009). These fibers relay pleasant touch sensations to the brain whereby there is a release of oxytocin that produces a sense of pleasure, calm, and connection. This works for both humans and animals for both within- and cross-species contact.

The powerful role that oxytocin plays in our wellbeing is further demonstrated by what we understand about the detriment of oxytocin deficit (Daley Olmert, 2009). Oxytocin deficit results in less buffering of our stress response, and the result is increased stress, anxiety and depression, and less satisfying relationships. People suffering from depression have significantly lower levels of oxytocin. Oxytocin deficit allows the physiological stress response to become hyperactive—a state that exacerbates a range of disorders from depression to bipolar disorder. The deficiency is thought to contribute to the rise of sensory defensive disorders (e.g., lights are too bright, smells are overpowering, and noises too loud). Oxytocin deficiency may contribute to the rise in autism because it has been linked to physical behaviors and social isolation associated with autism. Postmortem examinations of autistic human brains show that the amygdala has a deficit of neurons in the areas that should be rich in oxytocin receptors. Today, various antidepressant and antipsychotic drugs are prescribed to treat certain symptoms of autism. These drugs also happen to raise oxytocin levels. Research is directed at developing a chemical that will improve the pattern and sensitivity of oxytocin receptors in the brain (Daley Olmert, 2009).

The ability of a dog to assist a child with autism to function better in social situations has been recognized by the medical community. Dogs are being trained and placed as service animals to assist children with autism (Burrows, Adams, and Spiers, 2008). Doctors have begun recommending that families with a child who has autism should get a service dog for the child because autistic children seem to make a social connection with a dog more easily than with humans and because dogs assist an autistic child to engage in social interactions with people. Therapists who work with autistic children often incorporate a therapy dog into their work because interactions with a therapy dog assist with decreasing behaviors associated with autism and increasing prosocial behaviors (Redefer and Goodman, 1989). So, if therapy animals can be helpful to people who are oxytocin deficient, then therapy animals can certainly be helpful to those who are not oxytocin deficient.

It is also important to explore the possible contribution of mirror neurons to the potential therapeutic impact of human–animal interaction. Mirror neurons allow humans to have vicarious experience from observations of other social beings, such as other humans with animals; for instance, a person smiling in response to seeing a happy dog wagging its tail or a person feeling nervous when seeing a horse acting nervously. Just from observation of other humans or animals, mirror neurons in humans can stimulate activation of the social response system or stress response system and the hormonal releases that accompany activation of those systems, such as adrenalin, cortisol, and aldosterone for stress responses and endorphins, dopamine, and oxytocin for social responses.

> [Pets] are almost always happier to see us than our human companions are, rushing toward us with a greeting that cannot help but make us smile. And just like that, they are already soothing [us]. When we see a smiling face, our own smile muscles are activated involuntarily. The mirror neurons that perform this internal response release oxytocin and its calming, socializing sensations.
>
> (Daley Olmert, 2009, pp. 228–229)

Mirror neurons in humans are a type of brain cell that responds both when we perform an action and when we witness someone else perform the action (Winerman, 2005; Marcus, 2013). The discovery of mirror neurons in macaque monkeys was reported in the 1980s by Italian researcher Giacomo Rizzolatti and colleagues at the University of Parma (Rizzolatti et al., 1981, 1988). The discovery that mirror neurons occur in humans was reported in 1995 by Luciano Fadiga and colleagues (Fadiga et al., 1995). They recorded motor-evoked potentials—a signal that a muscle is ready to move—from human participants' hand muscles as the participants watched the experimenter grasp objects. They found that these potentials matched the potentials recorded when the human participants actually grasped objects themselves.

> The concept might be simple, but its implications are far-reaching. Over the past decade, more research has suggested that mirror neurons might help explain not only empathy but also autism and the evolution of language . . . Other researchers are interested in whether mirror neurons respond not only to other people's actions or emotions, but also to the *intent* behind those actions.
>
> . . . According to neuroscientist Vittorio Gallese, a colleague of Rizzolatti, "This neural mechanism is involuntary and automatic," he says—with it we don't have to *think* about what other people are doing or feeling, we simply know . . . "It seems we're wired to see other people as similar to us, rather than different . . . At the root, as humans we identify the person we're facing as someone like ourselves."
>
> (Winerman, 2005, p. 48)

Taking a leap from the research regarding mirror neurons in humans, we might assume that humans could generalize a mirror neuron response and view a socially engaging animal as somewhat similar to ourselves. When a human interacts with a social animal, such as a dog or a horse, it is likely the mirror neurons of the human play a role in the experience with the animal.

I have presented the idea that both observation of (via mirror neurons), and social or physical interaction with (via engagement or skin sensory stimulation), other social beings— humans and, most likely, some animals—can activate the social response system and the stress response system of humans. Comprehension regarding the activation of these systems in relation to human–human interaction also contributes to scientific understanding of the potential impact of human–animal interaction. The potential benefits of working with therapy animals have not yet been fully explored, but everything discovered so far is highly promising. Hormone release in humans, from social interaction with animals, is very important to the idea of therapeutic impact from AAT.

ANIMALS ARE POSITIVELY NOSEY

From what we currently understand, animals use their senses to examine social cues in their interactions with humans. Much like human therapists, therapy animals rely a great deal on their senses to perceive and ultimately evaluate clients with whom they engage in therapy sessions. A well-developed capacity to sense cues is an innate thrive-and-survive trait in animals. Unlike most human therapists, therapy animals also have available to them their sense of touch to evaluate client–therapy animal interactions. This is because human therapists are often discouraged from touching clients or being touched by clients to avoid sending the wrong message to a client or from concern over making a client feel violated. Therapy animals also have available to them their superior sense of smell, which they may use to discern social cues in client–therapy animal interactions, whereas human therapists, having a much less developed olfactory sense, can make significantly less use of their sense of smell in therapy sessions. In a physical sense, therapy animals are much more "nosey" than human therapists. What animals can and cannot discern with their sense of smell is still under investigation by animal researchers, but some fascinating discoveries have been made suggesting that animals may be able to use their sense of smell to assist with detecting emotions in humans.

Research involving pet dogs demonstrated some behavioral variability of olfactory (smell) exploration in relation to human adults (Filiatre, Millot, and Eckerlin, 1991). Sixty different pet dogs were studied, and each dog was used in only one series of trials to avoid the dog becoming accustomed to the environment. Each series consisted of two 5-minute trials: olfactory exploration of the dog's owner and olfactory exploration of a person unknown to the dog. "Sniffing" was defined as motor movements of the dog's muzzle directed toward the human subject, either touching the human or within 20 cm of the subject. The order of presentation, which human was sniffed first, was randomized. During the "sniffing," the human adult entered the experimental room, lay down on the floor, and remained motionless with eyes closed during the duration of the trial. Three types of data were obtained: (1) movements of the dog's muzzle sniffing the areas of the human's body; (2) the sniffing sequence from one area of the human's body to another; and (3) the time from the beginning to the end of sniffing of one area (i.e., the duration of sniffing).

The results showed that the dogs always sniffed more body parts of the known person than the unknown person, but the duration of total overall sniffing did not differ for the known and unknown person. The researchers (Filiatre, Millot, and Eckerlin, 1991) speculated that since the dog was already familiar with certain chemical smells of its owner, the dog did not need to focus on those for the purpose of identity and instead could focus on gathering additional chemical information about its owner. Regarding the human body areas explored by the dogs, the head, stomach, forearms, hands, legs, and feet were always of interest in the sniffing of both the known and unknown subjects. At the beginning of the observations, dogs who were in the presence of an unknown person insisted more on exploring the ano-genital area and thighs than dogs in the presence of their owner. It was suggested that the more frequent sniffing of this area of unknown persons was because the dogs were seeking chemical information provided by these areas before exploring other body areas.

> Various studies concerning social communication in mammals have suggested that the head could be the major area emitting chemical signals related to the emotional state of the animal, whereas the ano-genital area transmits mainly chemical substances concerning identity of the subject.
>
> (Filiatre, Millot, and Eckerlin, 1991, p. 349)

The researchers thought that, since the dogs most likely recognized their owner using visual cues, they did not need to spend the time necessary to recognize the owner through smell identification and could then search other areas of the body for different types of information. Finally, whatever the identity of the human subject, the head and upper limbs were always major areas explored by the dog. The researchers suggested that the behavior of the dogs with the human subjects was consistent with previous studies between animals, in that the current study showed the sniffing exploration of the human's ano-genital area was always the initial and greater focus of the dogs for unknown persons but not for known persons, and that the head and upper limb areas were the areas explored most for the known persons and second most for the unknown persons. The researchers believed this study may support the conjecture that chemical smells for emotion are more readily identified in the head and upper limbs and that the chemical smells for identification are more readily identified in the ano-genital and thigh areas (Filiatre, Millot, and Eckerlin, 1991). It has been determined that dogs, as well as other animals, do rely on their olfactory sense for identification of familiar smells, so it may be possible that they also rely on their olfactory sense for recognition of various emotions as well. The researchers (Filiatre, Millot, and Eckerlin, 1991) concluded:

> Analysis of the olfactory exploratory behaviour of dogs shows that behavioural mechanisms help the dog to acquire information concerning the identity and the emotional states of human beings. The pet dog can integrate this information and adjust its behaviour accordingly. . . . The emission of chemical signals by man and their reception by the pet dog can also be assumed to be major factors in the elaboration of the animal's behaviour and thus take part in the regulations of the relations between man and his pet dog.
>
> (pp. 349–350)

A canine's sense of smell is many times superior to that of humans. A dog's nose is designed to enhance scent (Smith, 2002). A human has relatively small oval-shaped nostrils, but a dog has apostrophe-shaped nostrils that set up a swirling effect when it inhales, distributing molecules around the nasal passages. A dog exhales through slits on the side of the nose so it can continue to take in fresh air and scent through the nostrils (PBS Deep Look, 2019). A dog can also flare its nostrils broadly to pick up more scent. A dog's moist nasal passages dissolve scent particles to release odors much more effectively than the drier noses of humans. It is estimated that humans have 5 million olfactory cells in their noses, whereas dogs have significantly more, depending on the breed—Dachshunds have about 125 million cells, a Fox Terrier has about 147 million, German Shepherds have approximately 220 million, and the estimate for Bloodhounds is nearly 300 million (PBS Nature, 2008; Smith, 2002). Each olfactory cell terminates in fine, hair-like strands coated with mucous; these strands are called cilia. Humans have about six cilia to each olfactory cell, whereas dogs have 100 or more. The olfactory lobe of the human brain is about the size of a pea, but the dog's olfactory lobe is about the size of a walnut within the dog's overall smaller-sized brain (Smith, 2002). While the human brain is dominated by a large visual cortex, the dog brain is dominated by an olfactory cortex (Smith, 2002). The canine nose is a remarkable organ. Much more sensitive than a human's nose, a dog's nose "can sniff out illegal drugs, track fugitives, [and] even find rot spots in wooden structures" (PBS Deep Look, 2019; Reisen, 2020). Dogs are also very effective at locating forensic cadaver material and disaster survivors (Correa, 2011).

A dog is so capable of discerning smell that it can even do so underwater (Smith, 2002). This capacity is due to the vomeronasal organ, or Jacobson's organ, which, in a dog, involves two holes in the roof of the mouth between the canine teeth. Nerves run from these holes, which are covered by skin, along the roof of the mouth, directly to the olfactory lobe.

> It's this mechanism that is at work when we throw a rock in water and the dog brings back the same rock. He's picking up several rocks and slushing the water in his mouth. Somehow he can pull the scent molecules up through these holes. Dogs obviously can't breathe [under] water.
>
> (Smith, 2002, p. 46)

The olfactory receptors in the dog's nasal cavity are anatomically distinct from the olfactory receptors in the dog's vomeronasal organ (Correa, 2011).

When humans smell something, it habituates, and the sensation of what they are smelling diminishes quickly, making it difficult for them to follow the scent for very long (Smith, 2002). Dogs do not habituate to smells as humans do. A dog can track and trail the same scent for hours without any sign of decreased perception. Dogs can also block out any unpleasant or unwanted smells to better enable them to focus on the smell they are tracking, but "No one knows exactly how dogs accomplish this individualisation and selection of smells" (Smith, 2002, p. 46).

> When a bloodhound sniffs a scent article (a piece of clothing or item touched only by the subject), air rushes through its nasal cavity and chemical vapors—or odors—lodge in the mucus and bombard the dog's sense receptors. Chemical signals are then sent to the olfactory bulb, the part of the brain that analyzes smells, and an "odor image" is created. For the dog, this image is far more detailed than a photograph is for a human. Using the odor image as a reference, the bloodhound is able to locate a subject's trail, which is made up of a chemical cocktail of scents including breath, sweat vapor, and skin cells. Once the bloodhound identifies the trail, it will not divert its attention despite being assailed by a multitude of other odors. Only when the dog finds the source of the scent or reaches the end of the trail will it relent. So potent is the drive to track, bloodhounds have been known to stick to a trail for more than 130 miles.
>
> (PBS Nature, 2008, p. 1)

Animals also use their tongues to enhance their sense of smell. By licking a surface, molecules are transferred via the tongue to the olfactory receptors in the nose and in the vomeronasal organ. Dogs also use licking to taste, to clean themselves, and to show affection among themselves or to humans by licking their faces (Horowitz, 2009).

Animals' superior capacity to smell is demonstrated by their ability to sniff out illness in humans. A research study published in March 2006 in the journal *Integrative Cancer Therapies* described how five household dogs were trained within a short 3-week period to detect lung or breast cancer by sniffing the breath of cancer patients (McCulloch et al., 2006). A research study published in September 2004 in *BMJ*, a leading medical journal in Britain, described the results of the first-ever meticulously controlled, double-blind, peer-reviewed study of dogs detecting bladder cancer by sniffing urine samples of human cancer patients (Willis et al., 2004). A team of French researchers, led by Dr. Jean-Nicolas Cornu, reported on June 1, 2010, at a San Francisco meeting of the American Urological Association, that they had successfully trained a Belgian Malinois—a Shepherd breed that has already been used for detecting bombs and in other cancer tests—to identify, through sniffing, urine from patients with confirmed cancer of the prostate and differentiate those from samples of healthy patients (Cornu et al., 2011). Italian researchers reported dogs sniffing urine detected prostate cancer with an accuracy of 98 percent (Taverna et al., 2015).

No one knows exactly what an epilepsy seizure detection dog is detecting, whether it is the scent of an oncoming seizure, feeling the acceleration in electrical impulses of the human's brain, or picking up on visual changes people fail to observe. Yet it is clear through demonstration that dogs do detect seizures in time to warn their human handlers to get into a safe position before the human is ever aware that the seizure is imminent (Green, 2000). Dr. Roger Reep, a physiological sciences professor at the University of Florida, worked with scientific researcher Deb Dalziel to study how dogs detect seizures and reported that:

> [O]f all the theories, it is most plausible that some dogs can smell a seizure coming. "Dogs are incredibly better at olfactory detection than we are, and in some [anecdotal] reports, the olfactory odor [of a seizure] rises to the threshold of human detection." He added that patients with epilepsy have reported that their dogs were able to detect seizures from other rooms in the house—behavior that could not, of course, depend upon visual or electrical cues.
>
> (Green, 2000, p. 1)

Michael Goehring, executive program director of the Great Plains Assistance Dog Foundation in Jud, North Dakota, where seizure-alert dogs are trained, explains that while every dog can alert for an oncoming seizure, not every dog cares to do so. To be a seizure-alert dog, the dog must have the right type of personality. According to Goehring:

> A very "independent" dog may pick up on a seizure, but won't feel any innate obligation towards helping the person. In contrast, a "super-submissive" dog will act very dramatically by stressing and panting, but they are doing that out of concern for themselves, and we don't want a dog to feel stress every time there's a seizure. Dogs that have a "middle-of-the-road cool temperament" make the best alert dogs.
>
> (Green, 2000, p. 1)

According to the Epilepsy Foundation (2007), dogs cannot be "trained to alert" for a seizure; rather the research reviewed shows dogs who do alert and attend to their handlers before, during, and after a seizure do so as a matter of their natural behaviors and tendencies, though the exact mechanism for how dogs detect and signal a seizure is still a mystery. Thus, research has demonstrated that dogs do have the capacity to detect illness in humans. Perhaps this same ability allows them to detect and differentiate human emotions, but this has not yet been proven.

Cats have about 200 million odor-sensitive cells in their nose, which make their olfactory capability much greater than humans' (Commings, n.d.). In 2007, it was widely reported that a cat residing at a Providence, Rhode Island, nursing home for humans could consistently predict when nursing home patients were going to die by curling up next to them in their final hours: "When Oscar curls up on a patient's bed and stays there, the staff knows it's time to call the family. It usually means the patient has less than four hours to live" (Henry, 2007).

Could it be that Oscar heard the slowing of the patient's heart, or did he smell the chemical reactions in the failing body, or both? A cat's sense of smell is:

> one of the most important ways in which he receives feedback about his environment. Sense of smell helps him communicate with others of his own kind and assess potential risks and pleasures. . . . Because of astonishing olfactory acuity, your cat can detect the presence of other cats even outside the home and can identify any strange animals you've contacted simply by smelling your clothing.
>
> (Commings, n.d.)

There is currently not much known about the horse's sense of smell, but it is generally agreed that it is well developed (Gore et al., 2008). The horse's smell receptors are located in the upper nasal cavity, and due to the length of the nasal cavity, there is a large area of receptors. The horse therefore has a better ability to smell than a human. The horse can also pick up pheromones and other scents when it gives the flehmen response, which forces air through the slits in the nasal cavity and into the vomeronasal organ. Unlike many other animals, the horse's Jacobson's organ doesn't open into the oral cavity (Gore et al., 2008).

> Most of us, at one time or another, have seen a horse tilt up his head and curl his upper lip in a "horse laugh." Although the expression is amusing, it actually has a practical purpose. The posture is called "flehmen" (roughly translated it means "testing"), and it appears to help horses trap pheromone scents in the vomeronasal organs (VNOs) so they can be analyzed more closely [pheromones are the chemical signals emanating from other horses, and on occasion from humans]. After a horse draws in the organic odor (by several seconds of olfactory investigation), he curls up his lip to temporarily close the nasal passages and hold the particles inside. Then an upward head tilt seems to help the airborne molecules linger in the VNOs, which are located under the floor of the horse's nasal cavity. A horse performing a flehmen is giving you an outward demonstration of a stimulated vomeronasal organ.
>
> Flehmen is not a uniquely equine behavior. Many ungulates (hooved mammals) exhibit very close variations of the same lip curl—cattle, deer, sheep, antelope, and goats, just to name a few. And it's not even exclusively a behavior of herbivores: many species of cat also flehmen.
>
> (Briggs, 2013)

Some evidence does exist to suggest that horses may rely on their sense of smell to assist with assessing social situations:

> Horses have apparently learned to associate certain odors with specific conditions considered to be friendly or life threatening. Horses use smell to locate feed and to identify each other as well as humans. They are frequently able to associate a medicinal smell with veterinarians and their function. When certain odors are associated with unpleasant or threatening conditions, horses may become nervous and difficult to control.
>
> (Cirelli and Cloud, n.d.)

Thus, horses most likely integrate information they smell with information they see and hear to more fully discern situations:

> It's generally agreed that dogs are the domestic animals with the most sensitive noses, but horses aren't far behind. As prey animals, it behooves them to be able to

detect even the slightest scent of danger on the wind. They're also quick to detect the "smell of fear" in other animals and in humans (probably an emanation of chemical signals we cannot detect). Many trainers over the centuries have agreed that horses also seem to be able to recognize the smell of death, sometimes reacting suspiciously to a spot where another horse has died, sometimes for months or years after the animal perished. . . . It's even suspected that the famous ability horses have to find their way home from unfamiliar territory stems largely from their talent for retracing their steps by sniffing out their own footprints and manure markers along the trail.

(Briggs, 2013)

Can animals use smell to discern emotions? Scientists do not know for certain. But since emotions are internal chemical reactions and chemical reactions are known to produce odors that are detectable, it is possible that animals can smell and discern emotions in each other and in humans. An animal's combined senses do make them capable discerners of social cues, so therapy animals' reactions to clients can be meaningful in ways that assist a therapist in evaluating the emotional state, attitude, and behavior of a client regardless of whether we understand where or how the animals are getting their information.

Understanding the sensory abilities of therapy animals and their implications for behavior is central to facilitation of AAT as this is key to more fully realizing what an animal's behavior is contributing to a session.

Vision, hearing, olfaction, taste, and touch comprise the sensory modalities of most vertebrates. With these senses, the animal receives information about its environment. How this information is organized, interpreted, and experienced is known as perception. . . . Sensory ability, perception, and behavior are closely linked.

(Rørvang, Nielsen, and McLean, 2020, p. 1)

Horses, dogs, and humans share the five most common sensory modalities; however, their ranges and capacities differ, so that humans, horses, and dogs are unlikely to perceive their surroundings in a similar manner. As a demonstration, consider how the sensory abilities of horses differ from those of humans in a number of aspects.

Equine vision is similar to that of red-green color-blind humans and horses see better in low light than humans. Horses can see almost a full circle around themselves and have a broad rather than a centralized focus. They can hear sound frequencies that humans cannot, but unlike most other large land mammals, they hear higher but not lower frequency sounds compared with humans. In addition, horses have a highly developed sense of smell, which is often overlooked, both in equine research as well as training. Horses are very sensitive to touch, but their tactile sensitivity has been very sparsely studied, despite it being used extensively in horse training and handling. The sensory abilities of individual horses may be a stable personality trait, with equine perception affected also by breed, age and in some cases even coat color, highlighting the need to differentiate the care and management of individual horses.

(Rørvang, Nielsen, and McLean, 2020, p. 12)

Unlike humans, horses have a well-developed olfactory epithelium and a vomeronasal organ, suggesting an extensive role of the sense of smell (Rørvang, Nielsen, and McLean, 2020). The vomeronasal organ of horses is receptive to non-volatile and poorly volatile molecules, often found in body secretions. When a horse gets into contact with a substance of interest, the associated molecules activate the vomeronasal organ which triggers a flehmen response, i.e., where the horse curls its upper lip back and inhales, often with closed nostrils. The adaptive advantage of the flehmen response is that it enables the horse to analyze poorly volatile compounds with far greater accuracy. During the flehmen response the nostrils are closed thereby reducing the escape of air and increasing the air pressure within the nasal cavity. This allows molecules from the compounds to be detected by the vomeronasal organ.

(Rørvang, Nielsen, and McLean, 2020, p. 7)

Understanding equine perceptual abilities and their differences is important when horses and humans interact, as these abilities are pivotal for the response of the horse to any changes in its surroundings.

(Rørvang, Nielsen, and McLean, 2020, p. 1)

When working with dogs during facilitation of AAT, it is important to understand how they perceive the world. In some ways canine hearing is superior to humans' (Singletary and Lazarowski, 2021). Dogs can hear sounds from approximately 65 to 45,000 Hz, whereas humans can hear sounds from approximately 20 to 20,000 Hz. Dogs can hear sounds that are too high-pitched for humans. In addition, at high frequencies dogs can detect much softer sounds than humans can. That means dogs can hear sounds that are not loud enough for human ears. Sensitivity to higher-pitched sounds likely explains several phenomena involving dogs, such as an ability to predict somebody's arrival at your door before you can hear it. Also, dogs can be distressed by everyday noises, like a vacuum cleaner or power drill, because they sound louder to dogs than to humans. And dogs can hear high-pitched noises from these devices that humans cannot detect. Dogs have an amazing ability to detect differences between frequencies. However, humans can generally locate sounds better than dogs (Singletary and Lazarowski, 2021).

Dogs are reported to be capable of detecting sounds much farther than the distance of human detection. Dogs also are capable of using sound to equate additional qualities, such as size, with regard to conspecifics and other animals. Erect ears of dogs are assumed to be especially good at localizing sound at longer distances due to their orientation and accessible funnel-like anatomic properties, but generally this difference from floppy-eared dogs is negligible. Any alteration of the ear through injury (e.g., lacerations and aural hematoma) or surgery (e.g., ear cropping) may impair the normal function of sound localization. The muscle attachments allow for fine pinna movement and control for orientation and improved hearing sensitivity, especially at higher frequencies. . . . The auditory system is important to directing attention and providing key awareness for spatial orientation responses, although, especially in working dogs, there likely is a task-based prioritization that occurs with use of olfactory and visual cues for these responses as well. . . . The auditory system is important especially to performance of working dogs and suitability for work. This could reference ability to respond to verbal cues or detect the sound of an approaching object. Although not representative for all dogs, some reports suggest hearing loss may be associated with behaviors in dogs that are of concern in relation to performance, such as aggression, increased startle and stress-related responses, and training difficulties. A loss of hearing or impairment of hearing may result in a working dog being unsuitable for continued service and considered for retirement. Severity of hearing loss and task-specific requirements of the working dog may allow for continued service through use of hand gestures or limited service with clearly outlined protocols for limitations of use.

(Singletary and Lazarowski, 2021, pp. 847–849)

Canine vision is considered poor in comparison to human vision, although there are instances where specialized features allow for task-specific enhancements. Vision in the canine is thought to be less specialized for acuity and more for motion detection, with an increased function under low light conditions.

(Singletary and Lazarowski, 2021, p. 844)

This means dogs can see in low light better than humans. Due to eye placement, dogs have a 60- to 70-degree greater field of vision; this may mean that, compared with humans, dogs have a larger horizontal scanning vantage but with reduced depth perception due to the decreased degree of binocular vision.

Dogs exhibit dichromatic vision expressing 2 forms of light-sensitive photo pigments in the retinal cells pertaining to color vision in comparison to humans, who have tri-chromatic vision and express 3 forms. Although this is likened to human red/green color blindness, dogs are capable of discriminating colors by brightness intensities and distinguish red and green from gray. The visual spectrum in dogs allows for differentiation of hues in the blue spectrum and yellow spectrum . . . dogs likely are able to appreciate UV light as a blue-violet color.

(Singletary and Lazarowski, 2021, pp. 845–846)

The olfactory system, that is the sense of smell, is superior in canines over humans in many ways (Singletary and Lazarowski, 2021; Jenkins, DeChant, and Perry, 2018; Tyson, 2012).

Dogs' sense of smell overpowers our own by orders of magnitude – it's 10,000 to 100,000 times as acute, scientists say . . . they possess up to 300 million olfactory receptors in their noses, compared to about six million in us. And the part of a dog's brain that is devoted to analyzing smells is about 40 times greater than ours.

(Tyson, 2012, p. 1)

Canine olfactory detection of emotion has support from clinical controlled study of canine olfactory behavior with humans that led researchers to conclude dogs sniff the breath and hands of humans in order to detect emotional state and sniff the genital area to acquire information about identification, disease, and sexual reproduction (Filiatre, Millot, and Eckerlin, 1991). Additionally, there has been speculation that dogs can predict epileptic seizures in humans by being alerted to subtle pre-ictal human behavior changes or by being sensitive to heart rate or olfactory cues (Brown and Goldstein, 2011). Also of interest is a clinically controlled study that observed canine ability to accurately smell cancer cells (Willis et al., 2004).

Dogs' noses function very differently from those of humans (Filiatre, Millot, and Eckerlin, 1991; Tyson, 2012). Unlike humans, when dogs inhale, a fold of tissue just inside their nostrils separates airflow into two pathways, one for olfaction and one for respiration. While most of the inhale travels down the pharynx and into the lungs, about 12 percent of every breath a dog takes travels to a recessed area in the back of the nose where odor molecules are made accessible for analysis by the brain. Furthermore, when we exhale through our nose, we send the spent air out the way it came in, forcing out any incoming odors. When dogs exhale, the spent air exits through the slits in the sides of their noses. The manner in which the exhaled air swirls out actually helps usher new odors into the dog's nose. More importantly, it allows dogs to sniff more or less continuously. . . . On top of all this, dogs have a second olfactory capability that we don't have, made possible by an organ we don't possess: the vomeronasal organ, also known as Jacobson's organ.

(Tyson, 2012, p. 1)

The vomeronasal organ (VNO) is located in the bottom of a dog's nasal passage.

VNO sensory neurons detect chemical signals that stimulate behavioral and/or physiological changes, provides alternate neuronal pathway to the hypothalamus, and is very slow to adapt to odors. The VNO functions in the detection of non-volatile odorants, especially pheromones, and is believed to play a role in social behavior and reproduction.

(Jenkins, DeChant, and Perry, 2018, p. 2)

While we cannot always know if an animal is behaving based on what odors it is detecting, we can presume that some behaviors are based on what an animal is smelling. Thus, during AAT attention to how a canine or other animal participant behaves, possibly as a response to detection of smells emitted by humans, may provide useful information to a facilitator about the state of the person in the session. Research has shown odors to play a major role in learned behavior of animals.

Once an animal has successfully learned the association between [an] odorant and a reward, it will consider this odorant as a rewarded stimulus irrespective of its concentration. Biologically, this makes perfect sense as odors that are behaviorally relevant for an animal hardly ever change their significance as a function of concentration: a food odor will always be attractive, whether detected at high or low concentrations, and a predator odor will be always avoided, whether at high or low concentrations. Thus, it takes an animal extensive training to overcome this perseverance with regard to the learned reward value of odorants.

(Fleischer, Breer, and Strotmann, 2009, p. 683)

What a dog sees and hears also contributes to its social-behavioral understanding and response to persons with whom it interacts. It has been demonstrated that via visual and auditory pathways dogs can recognize emotions in both humans and dogs and discriminate between positive and negative emotions in both (Albuquerque, Guo, Wilkinson, Savalli, Otta, and Mills, 2016). The combination of visual and auditory cues to categorize others' emotions facilitates information processing and indicates high level cognitive representations. The perception of emotional expressions by animals enables them to evaluate the social intentions and motivations of each other as well as humans (Albuquerque et al., 2016). From a human point of view, there is evidence supporting how humans tend to assign complex emotions to animals, such as anger, happiness, fear, surprise, sadness, disappointment, compassion, to name a few (Konok, Nagy, and Miklósi, 2015; Martens, Enders-Slegers, and Walker, 2016). Clients' speculations about emotions animals may have might reveal important information about the state or attitude of a client who projects their own internal experience onto the experience of the animal; clients may do this consciously (aware), subconsciously (semi-aware), or perhaps even unconsciously (unaware).

Animals rely on sensory perception and processing to gather and interpret thrive-and-survive stimuli in the environment presented by humans and other animals that are present. If an animal detects stimuli associated with a positive experience (i.e., safety, food, comfort, petting, play, satisfying curiosity, etc.), it may likely seek out the source. Contrarily, if an animal detects stimuli associated with a negative experience (anxiety, fear, anger, threat, danger, etc.), then it may communicate distress and exhibit calming signals, alerting behavior, posture displacement, or another corollary behavior. An animal may respond by moving more slowly around or toward a stressed being, in an attempt to calm or comfort the stressed one. Or an animal may move away from the stressor source for self-preservation. Also, an animal that perceives a stressor or experiences distress may move closer to a familiar being in order to receive comfort or to feel safer. Interpreting behavioral communications by an animal after it detects stimuli during human–animal interaction can be valuable during AAT sessions. This is where an AAT facilitator's familiarity with animal behaviors is quite valuable. Facilitators may be provided with additional information about a person with whom they are working based on an animal's sensory perceptions and resulting behaviors. Familiarity with a species, and also an individual animal, allows an AAT facilitator to recognize patterns of animal behavior presented in the context of various associated human stimuli. The additional information presented from the animal can contribute much to how a session is facilitated.

It is highly likely that an animal utilizes its various senses to detect emotional states in humans. The ability of the animal to detect an emotional state in a human client, even when the client shows no outward signs of experiencing that emotion, in combination with the animal's ability to signal its perception of a client's emotion to a counselor, is incredibly valuable. A counselor should watch for and identify signals sent by a therapy animal that reflect internal emotional experiences of a client. Using these signals as a guide for consideration or for exploration, a counselor can assist a client in gaining important awareness and insight that might not otherwise be addressed. Through various senses, an animal may perceive emotional distress in a client and may relay to a counselor through verbal and nonverbal signals that a significant emotional state has been detected and needs to be attended to. A counselor must be knowledgeable regarding animal communication to fully value the contribution the therapy animal makes to the psychodynamics of a counseling session. Various additional animal communications are described in Chapter 6.

GENERAL BENEFITS OF AAT

There are numerous benefits to incorporating pets into the therapy process. These benefits extend to the client, the therapy animal, and the human therapist. The benefits of AAT to the client include a strong entertainment and relaxation component. A dog fetching a ball and performing tricks or a cat chasing a feather toy across the floor evoke a smile in the client. Opportunities to interact with a social animal that seeks and outwardly displays pleasure with contact, such as a purring cat in a lap or a dog displaying its tummy for petting, can facilitate personal and social development in a client. Petting an animal can also create a soothing and calming effect for the client. A dog's or horse's ability to be attentive to commands and training cues can facilitate skill development in a client as well as strengthening a client's self-concept and self-esteem. AAT is a multisensory experience for the client that may enhance attention to tasks and integration of therapeutic experiences. The presence of an animal adds significant kinesthetic, tactile, auditory, visual, and olfactory stimulation to an environment, and a more alert individual may integrate information to a deeper, more meaningful level.

The benefits for the pet practitioner are based largely on the animal's innate needs. The therapy work provides a stimulating activity for a highly intelligent creature. The therapy pet spends more time with its owner/handler, avoiding being left at home alone and getting bored. The therapy animal is often a healthier and happier animal due to the amount of time it spends with its owner/handler and the rigorous health and training requirements for the therapy animal.

There can be multiple benefits of AAT to the human therapist. The handler gets to spend more quality time with the pet. The handler gets to share with others the affection, gifts, and talents of the pet. The therapy animal contributes to a warm and friendly work atmosphere. Some clients will respond better to therapeutic intervention that involves a therapy animal than to therapy without an animal. Some basic therapeutic goals and interventions can actually be better achieved with therapy animal participation. When word gets out about the pet practitioner, many clients will prefer going to the therapist with the animal rather than to other therapists who do not work with an animal. Another potential benefit may be that the care and training costs associated directly with a professional therapy animal may be tax deductible as a business expense.

GENERAL RISKS INVOLVED WITH AAT

There are some risks involved in practicing AAT for the client, the therapy animal, and the therapist. However, a counselor may prevent these risks by following proper risk management procedures. Specific methods for risk management are covered in Chapter 6. One type of risk is injury to a client. Examples of how injury may occur to a client who interacts with a therapy pet include a horse stepping on a client's foot during mounting, a cat scratching a client during play, and a large dog knocking a client down while running to fetch a ball. Therapy animals are trained and screened for proper temperament, so although injury to a client by a pet practitioner would most likely be inadvertent, it is still a possibility. Another risk is that the client can become attached to the therapy animal, and thus grief and loss issues may have to be addressed upon termination of services. Also, the client may be allergic to or afraid of the therapy animal. Thus, careful screening and evaluation of clients is necessary. In addition, some clients having had little or no contact with a pet before may prefer not to be around animals.

The risks to the pet practitioner are largely due to threat from the pet's clients. A more fragile animal, such as a bird or a small dog, is at greater risk of injury from being dropped, squeezed, or hit by a client. A therapy animal can also experience stress and overwork. The pet practitioner must rely on the counselor for prevention of injury and management of stress.

The counselor has the responsibility to ensure the safety and welfare of the client and the pet practitioner. In addition, the counselor must allow ample time in the schedule for caring for the therapy pet. This includes training, feeding, exercising, playtime, rest, and healthcare. Also, the time it takes a counselor to get to a destination can increase significantly when accompanied by a therapy animal because many people met along the way may approach and initiate conversations about the therapy animal or their own pet at home. However, the advantage to this is that it increases the opportunity for counselors to interact with persons they might not otherwise have had an opportunity to meet.

HISTORICAL HIGHLIGHTS OF AAT

Significant historical events have contributed to a greater understanding of the emotionally therapeutic value of human–animal social interaction. In many instances, the specifics of these events hold educational value, so I have included much detail when describing these events. For those who enjoy reading about the happenstance of history, I think you will enjoy this section very much.

York Retreat, England

It is believed that the York Retreat, founded in 1792 in York, England, was the first instance of emotional therapy involving animals. During this period of history, so-called lunatic hospitals and asylums treated their patients badly, often with cruelty or neglect, and thus the Society of Friends, a Quaker group, started the York Retreat for such persons to be treated with kindness. The York Retreat was neither a hospital nor a private asylum; it was organized on a nonprofit basis and treatment was based on "Christianity and common sense" (Jones, 1955, p. 57). The York Retreat was the brainchild of William Tuke, a tea and coffee merchant and head of a Quaker family that had resided in York for several generations. He came up with the idea for the retreat when a patient named Hannah Mills was sent to the existing York Asylum, which was founded in 1777, and her relatives recommended her to the care of the Society of Friends. Yet when members of the Society attempted to visit her in the York Asylum,

> [they] were refused admission on the grounds that she was "not in a suitable state to be seen by strangers," and she subsequently died under circumstances which aroused suspicions of ill-treatment or neglect. . . . Tuke saw that time was not yet ripe for a full-scale public inquiry at the Asylum [and believed that] reform was impossible until some system of treatment other than that in operation at the Asylum had been tried and found successful.
>
> (Jones, 1955, pp. 57–58)

At first, Tuke's project for a retreat met with opposition from within the Society of Friends:

> Some members thought that the incidence of mental disorder was too low to warrant the construction of a special institution for Quakers. Some were "averse to the concentration of the instances of this disease amongst us," and others thought that York was not a suitable site for such an institution, being "not central to the Nation." . . . A man of outstanding personality and considerable administrative gifts, Tuke overrode all objections . . . His project was approved at the Quarterly Meeting of the Society in March, 1792 . . . The Friends proceeded to buy eleven acres of land . . . and to approve a building . . . sums were raised by private donation and covenant from members of the Society by the end of 1797.
>
> (Jones, 1955, p. 58)

The retreat concept was suggested to William Tuke by his daughter-in-law "to convey the idea of what such an institution should be, namely . . . a quiet haven in which the shattered bark might find the means of reparation or of safety" (Jones, 1955, p. 58). The Tuke family felt that many patients would be rational and could be controlled if they were not aggravated by cruelty, harsh methods of restraint, and hostility:

> The Retreat was built to accommodate thirty patients, who were to be either members of the Society of Friends, or recommended by members. . . . The patients were never punished for failure to control their behavior, but certain amenities were given to them in order to foster self-control by a show of trust. The female superintendent gave tea-parties, to which the patients were invited, and for which they were encouraged to wear their best clothes. There was an airing-court in the grounds for each class of patients, and each court was supplied with a number of small animals—rabbits, poultry, and others—so that the patients might learn self-control by having dependent upon them

creatures weaker than themselves. "These creatures are generally very familiar with the patients, and it is believed that they are not only the means of innocent pleasure, but that the intercourse with them sometimes tends to awaken the social and benevolent feelings," commented Samuel Tuke. . . . Every attempt was made to occupy the patients suitably. Some cared for the animals, some helped in the garden, the women knitted or sewed. Writing materials were provided, and books were carefully chosen to form a patients' library.

(Jones, 1955, pp. 59, 61)

As a side note, both William and his grandson, Samuel Tuke, were among the body of citizens who finally achieved the reform of the old York Asylum in 1814–1815 (Jones, 1955); this suggests that the York Retreat had been a significant success.

Bethel Center, Bielefeld, Germany

The next instance when animals were involved in emotional recovery is thought to be with the founding of Bethel in Bielefeld, Germany, in 1867 (Bustad, 1980). The center was originally begun as a home for epileptics but evolved into

an extensive center of healing for disadvantaged people, with over five thousand patients and more than five thousand staff members. . . . Birds, cats, dogs and horses are evident in many of the residences and work sites, in addition to farm animals and a wild game park.

(Bustad, 1980, p. 118)

Leo Bustad, dean of the College of Veterinary Medicine at Washington State University, visited Bethel in 1977 and inquired to his host as to "how long pets had been utilized with their patients," and his host replied that they "had only recently began using horses, but he thought they had kept other pets since the very early years. They realize that using pets to help people is natural, just common sense" (Bustad, 1980, p. 118).

Saint Elizabeths Hospital, Washington, D.C.

It is believed that human–animal interaction as emotional therapy first began in the United States in 1919 after U.S. Secretary of the Interior, Franklin K. Lane, suggested the use of dogs to socialize with patients at Saint Elizabeths Hospital in Washington, D.C. (it was previously known as the Government Hospital for the Insane and was renamed Saint Elizabeths Hospital in 1916) (D'Amore, 1976). This facility was the dominant psychiatric institution on the federal scene. Since peacetime, military services were small and their psychiatric services even smaller, so soldiers with mental health problems were sent to Saint Elizabeths Hospital. The Veterans Bureau (renamed the Veterans Administration in July 1930) also sent its "insane veterans" to Saint Elizabeths Hospital (D'Amore, 1976). Dr. William Alanson White (1870–1937) was appointed superintendent of the Government Hospital for the Insane in 1903 by President Theodore Roosevelt. On August 12, 1919, Secretary Lane wrote to Saint Elizabeths Hospital superintendent, Dr. William Alanson White (who was thought of at the time as the "Chief Psychiatrist of the United States"):

Would it not be practicable for you to have some dogs over there that the men could play with and chum with? If you could find friendly fellows like bulldogs, who look fierce and are gentle, or big noble fellows like Newfoundlands, I should think they would be a great entertainment for the men. A poor insane chap naturally reaches out for companionship and finds himself barred by the various limitations of his unfortunate associates, but he could develop great friendship with a dog. The lonesome boys in France found their dogs great comforts, and men with shell shock recover their balance sometimes getting close to a dog with his limited mind but his unequalled capacity for affection. Has this thing been tried in any of our institutions?

(D'Amore, 1976, p. 2)

To which Dr. White replied on August 18:

I have your letter of the 12th instant, suggesting the use of dogs at this Hospital as chums and playmates for the patients. Such an experiment, so far as I know, has never been systematically tried out, but I see no reason why it should not be. . . . You speak in your letter of the loneliness of the insane. This is the outward feature of what within is a serious withdrawal of interests from the world of reality and a turning within to the unreal world of psychosis. It is one of the very difficult symptoms to meet and when pronounced may make the patient wholly inaccessible; he may refuse to speak, or even to eat or move. . . . At all times, however, the patient has sane and normal people about him who represent possible social contacts, but he lacks the initiation to respond, and the problem is, how to help him out of the unreal world of his psychosis and back to reality. The hospital is at present utilizing various means to this end—walks, rides, calisthenics, music, games, athletics, theatrical entertainments, excursions, moving pictures, picnics, etc., etc. and is developing a comprehensive program of amusements, entertainments, diversional and vocational occupations with which to supplement the more specific therapeutic approach to the individual problems. The procedure is largely empiric and no one can foretell what may be the experience which may finally attract the patient's interest, wake him, so to speak, from his morbid phantasies and be the beginning of the re-socialization of his instincts. In this general scheme, animals, and particularly dogs, because of their peculiarly friendly relations with humans, may well be fitted to serve useful ends. In addition to the dogs you mention it occurs to me that the police dog might also be useful and I should think that it might be well to have one attached, so to speak, to a ward or building as a mascot much as the sailors use animal mascots on battle ships. I shall be very glad to try it.

(D'Amore, 1976, p. 2)

Secretary Lane responded in a one-sentence note on August 19:

I am glad to get your letter regarding the dogs and to know that you look so favorably upon the experiment.

(D'Amore, 1976, p. 3)

Sigmund Freud, Vienna, Austria

Sigmund Freud of Vienna, Austria, is the founder of psychoanalysis. The first dog known to be in the family of Sigmund Freud was an Alsatian (also known as a German Shepherd) called Wolf, acquired in the 1920s for his daughter Anna so she could go for walks on her own in Vienna (Freud, 1983, pp. 190–192; Freud, 1992, p. 61; Gay, 1988, p. 540). Dorothy Burlingham, an American who had come to Vienna in 1925, became a good friend of Anna

Freud and she gave Sigmund Freud his first dog, a Chow named Lun Yug (or Lin Yug) who was with Freud for only 15 months before she was run over and killed in August 1929 (Freud, 1992, p. 61; Gay, 1988, p. 540). Lun Yug's sister, Jofi (or Jo-Fi), arrived at the Freud household in March 1930 (Freud, 1992, p. 61). Freud wrote frequently and fondly in his diary and letters of Jofi and other dogs in the Freud family (Freud, 1992). Freud often had his Chow Jofi in his office with him during psychoanalytic sessions in the early 1930s (Freud, 1983, p. 190).

> Freud and a succession of chows, especially his Jo-Fi, were inseparable. The dog would sit quietly at the foot of the couch during the analytic hour.
>
> (Gay, 1988, p. 540)

Hilda Doolittle, American poet, and a patient of Sigmund Freud in 1933–1934, described her initial encounter with Freud that occurred during her first psychoanalytic session with him at his Vienna apartment office. Freud's dog Jofi made a strong impression on Doolittle, one that reflected Doolittle was initially more comfortable with Freud's dog than with Professor Freud himself:

> But waiting and finding that I would not or could not speak, he uttered. What he said—and I thought a little sadly—was, "You are the only person who has ever come into this room and looked at the things in the room before looking at me."
> But worse was to come. A little lion-like creature came padding toward me—a lioness, as it happened. She had emerged from the inner sanctum or manifested from under or behind the couch; anyhow, she continued her course across the carpet. Embarrassed, shy, overwhelmed, I bend down to greet this creature. But the professor says, "Do not touch her—she snaps—she is very difficult with strangers." *Strangers?* Is the Soul crossing the threshold, a stranger to the Door-Keeper? It appears so. But, though no accredited dog-lover, I like dogs and they oddly and sometimes unexpectedly "take" to me. If this is an exception I am ready to take the risk. Unintimidated but distressed by the Professor's somewhat forbidding manner, I not only continue my gesture toward the little chow, but crouch on the floor so that she can snap better if she wants to. Yofi—her name is Yofi—snuggles her nose into my hand and nuzzles her head, in delicate sympathy, against my shoulder . . . My intuition challenges the Professor, though not in words. That intuition cannot really be translated into words, but if it could be it would go, roughly, something like this: "Why should I look at you? You are contained in the things you love, and if you accuse me of looking at the things in the room before looking at you, well, I will go on looking at the things in the room. One of them is this little golden dog. She snaps, does she? You call me a stranger, do you? Well, I will show you two things: one, I am not a stranger; even if I were, two seconds ago, I am now no longer one. And moreover I never was a stranger to this little golden Yofi."
>
> (Doolittle, 1956, pp. 148–149)

From her initial experience with Dr. Freud, Ms. Doolittle offers the following conclusion:

> The wordless challenge goes on, "You are a very great man. I am overwhelmed with embarrassment, I am shy and frightened and gauche as an over-grown school-girl. But listen. You are a man. Yofi is a dog. I am a woman. If this dog and this woman "take" to one another, it will prove that beyond your caustic implied criticism—if criticism it is—there is another region of cause and effect, another region of question and answer."
>
> (Doolittle, 1956, p. 150)

It is intriguing how Doolittle found comfort in the greeting by Freud's dog Jofi during her anxious first meeting with Freud. She found herself accepted and liked by the dog, which provided assurance of her worth in the presence of Freud by whom she, at first, felt judged.

American psychiatrist Dr. Roy Grinker, Sr. was one of Freud's patients in 1932 while Grinker was on fellowship in Vienna, and during his psychoanalytic sessions Freud would occasionally speak to Grinker through Jofi. Grinker recalls his impressions of the dog after first being greeted at the door by Anna's dog Wolf:

> In Freud's own office there was also another dog, a Chinese chow named Jofi. Jofi would sit alongside the couch, and after a while got up and scratch at the door to be let out. The Professor would get up, let the dog out, and come back and say, "Jofi doesn't approve of what you're saying." Then, after a while, the dog would scratch at the other side of the door, and the Professor would get up, open the door, and say, "Jofi wants to give you another chance." . . . Once, when I was emoting with a great deal of vigor, the dog jumped on top of me, and Freud said, "You see, Jofi is so excited that you've been able to discover the source of your anxiety!" But I wasn't paying the dog!
>
> (Grinker, Sr., 1979, p. 10)

The Freud family held in high regard the ability of their dogs to judge a person's character. Such is depicted from the following recollection written in 1958 by eldest son Martin Freud:

> Our dogs had the freedom of the flat and met everybody who came, being quite selective, even judicious, in the receptions they offered. The whole family, including Paula, our faithful maid, showed considerable respect for this canine sensibility. When the dogs condescended to be stroked, the visitor enjoyed the best possible introduction. If, Jofi for instance, sniffed somewhat haughtily around the legs of a caller and then stalked off with a touch of ostentation, there was at once a strong suspicion that there was something wrong with that caller's character. Contemplating Jofi's selective qualities at this distance of years, I feel bound to admit that her judgment was most reliable.
>
> (Freud, 1983, pp. 191–192)

Martin Freud recalls how his father, Sigmund, valued his dog Jofi:

> Jofi was father's favourite and never left him, not even when he treated patients. Then she would lie motionless near his desk, that desk adorned with its Greek and Egyptian antique statuettes, while he concentrated on the treatment of patients. He always claimed, and we must accept him at his word since there were never witnesses during analytical treatment, that he never had to look at his watch to decide when the hour's treatment should end. When Jofi got up and yawned, he knew the hour was up: she was never late in announcing the end of a session, although father did admit that she was capable of an error of perhaps a minute, at the expense of the patient.
>
> (Freud, 1983, pp. 190–191)

Although Sigmund Freud never formally addressed the concept of AAT, in the context of history it is important to acknowledge that he recognized value in the presence of his dog during psychoanalytic sessions, for both himself and his patients. In the current age of counseling, more than 85 years after Jofi joined Freud in psychoanalytic practice, we think of a dog's presence in a session as being central to therapy in many ways.

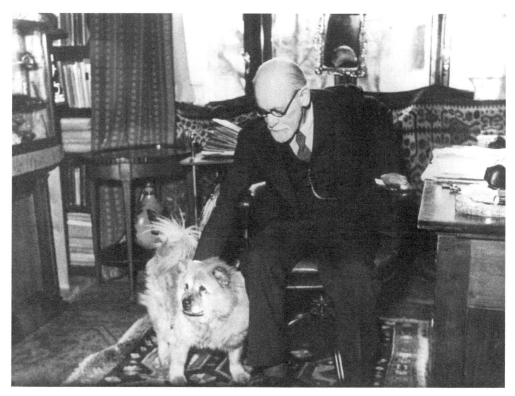

Figure 1.1 Sigmund Freud with his dog Jofi, a Chow, in his office in Vienna, Austria, 1937.

(*Source:* used with permission of Associated Press.)

Pawling Hospital, New York

No application of human–animal interaction as emotional therapy is known to have occurred again in the United States until the 1940s, and this was at the Pawling Air Force Convalescent Hospital in Pawling, New York, a comprehensive rehabilitation facility conceived and developed by Howard Archibald Rusk (1901–1989). The program incorporated patients working with farm animals and caring for pet dogs (Blum and Fee, 2008). Rusk closed his private practice of internal medicine in St. Louis and joined the Air Force as a medical service major in August 1942; he was instrumental in starting the comprehensive rehabilitation program for disabled servicemen in 1944 at the Pawling Air Force Convalescent Hospital, the first of its kind (Rusk, 1972). In his autobiography, Rusk (1972) discussed the plight of disabled servicemen of this period. As of early 1943, wounded and disabled veterans had no provision for proper care, and when they were turned over to the Veterans Administration it was "like sending them into limbo":

> They would simply lie around getting custodial care, with nothing to do, bored to distraction, helpless, hopeless, waiting for some kind of infection or disease to carry them off.
>
> (Rusk, 1972, p. 58)

Gradually the concept of rehabilitation came to Rusk, but he knew it could not be accomplished at current regional Air Force hospitals (Rusk, 1972, pp. 58–59). The Air Force already had hospitals to treat specific illnesses such as the facility at Davis-Monthan Field in Tucson, Arizona, which specialized in treating patients for rheumatic fever. One of the patients treated successfully there was Lowell Thomas Jr., son of the famous news commentator. Owing to his son's recovery, Lowell Thomas Sr. became interested in the convalescent program and went to Washington, D.C. to meet with Rusk. During the meeting, Rusk told Lowell of his dreams of rehabilitation, whereupon Lowell suggested that Pawling, New York, where he lived, would be a good place for Rusk's rehabilitation hospital. It had a "wonderful school" that had been closed and next to it was a "fine recreation area," and besides Pawling was a "wonderful community" with "very interesting people" (Rusk, 1972, pp. 59–62). Rusk went to Pawling accompanied by his commander, General Grant, and found they agreed with everything Lowell Thomas had said about Pawling. They then set to work refurbishing the school and grounds to become the first comprehensive rehabilitation center for servicemen. They officially opened the first Air Force rehabilitation center at Pawling on "a bitter cold day" in early 1944 with about 90 patients. The Pawling center was described by Rusk (1972) as:

> A combination of a hospital, a country club, a school, a farm, a vocational training center, a resort and a little bit of home as well. The discipline was minimal and the program informal . . . Pawling was the first of twelve such centers the Air Force opened during World War II. Some of the boys there had physical disabilities; others had psychological disabilities. Many had combinations of the two. . . . A lot of men in combat did reach the breaking point and needed a place like Pawling. Eventually, we had between four and five hundred patients there, beat-up boys from battlefronts all over the world. About one third of these boys had purely psychological problems from flying fatigue, while the other two thirds had severe physical disabilities, which, of course, were often coupled with psychological problems.
>
> (Rusk, 1972, pp. 68–72)

In addition to educational courses and vocational training, the Pawling Hospital rehabilitation program included a working farm with livestock, horses, and poultry. It also included extensive parkland, where the patients could encounter animals in a natural setting. The purpose of the work with the farm animals was to help divert attention to constructive therapy efforts. The idea to incorporate dogs as part of the emotional recovery program at Pawling transpired in response to a patient who was not responding to rehabilitation, as outlined by Rusk in his autobiography (1972):

> There were some boys, though, who had become so withdrawn as a result of the battle experience that it was difficult to get through to them. I remember one in particular. He wasn't hostile or aggressive. He just wouldn't talk to anybody—not the doctors, the nurses, or his fellow patients. It seemed as if no one up there could get through to him. One day, a Red Cross Gray Lady, who had a very nice way about her, decided she would give him a try.
> "Hello," she said. "Hello," he said. "How are you?" she said. He shrugged and turned away.
> The next day she tried again, and the next day and the next day, until she began to get as discouraged as everyone else who had tried. Finally one day, in exasperation, she said to him, "Isn't there anything in the world you want?" He looked up at her and said, "Why should I tell you? I can't have it anyway." "You can at least tell me what it is." "All right. There's only one thing I want. A dog." "A dog!" she said. "In a place like this? Why?" "Because I've always liked dogs. I like to work with them and train

them. I could take a dog for a walk in the woods and he wouldn't ask me a lot of silly questions."

The poor woman may have been somewhat bewildered, and she may have felt unwanted, but the one additional question she asked him went straight to the heart of the matter. "What kind of dog do you want?" "I'd take any kind," he said, "but I'd prefer a Cocker Spaniel about two or three months old."

Before nightfall the boy had his dog, and it was the key to his whole rehabilitation. He trained it, and all the other boys became interested in it. He began to talk and to open up in general. Soon he was just one of the boys.

(p. 76)

A cocker spaniel was essential to this young veteran's recovery. And from his experience sprung the addition of a new approach to rehabilitation, the integration of dogs into therapy.

This created an amusing complication. Before long everyone wanted a dog, and we had to make a decision ... Major Todd, the commanding officer, called the boys together and said, "All right, anyone who wants a dog can have one. We'll even get it for you, provided you're responsible for it. You've got to train it and housebreak it, and make sure it doesn't become a nuisance."

From them on, we had almost as many dogs as people. Outside the mess hall at noon there was always an absolute pack of dogs, from Great Danes to fox terriers, but all tied up to trees or chairs or benches, waiting for their masters to come out. And before long we had added one more course to our curriculum: dog training.

(pp. 76–77)

The great experiment at Pawling, first dubbed "Rusk's folly" by the medical establishment, was a landmark program that spawned rehabilitation medicine becoming a new medical specialty (Pelka, 1997, pp. 271–272, 344). Howard Rusk is generally recognized as the father of comprehensive rehabilitation medicine (Blum and Fee, 2008; NYU Langone Medical Center, 2013; Yanes-Hoffman, 1981).

While the Saint Elizabeths Hospital and the Pawling Convalescent Hospital human–animal interaction programs were important historical predecessors of today's more formalized animal-assisted mental health programs, neither of these hospital programs was known to have collected data or performed research studies on the therapeutic benefits of patients' interactions with animals.

Boris Levinson, New York

In the 1960s, American child psychologist Boris M. Levinson (1907–1984) became the first professionally trained clinician to formally introduce and document the way that companion animals could hasten the development of a rapport between therapist and patient, thereby increasing the likelihood of patient motivation and hastening recovery. Levinson's psychotherapy work with his dog Jingles started quite by accident one day in 1953 when a mother and her child arrived several hours early for the child's first appointment. The event is described in the words of Levinson as follows:

Early one morning, Jingles was lying at my feet while I was busily writing at my desk when the doorbell rang. Jingles was never permitted into my office when I expected patients, but this day no one was due until several hours later. Jingles followed me to the door where we were greeted by a very distraught parent and child—several hours early for their appointment. This child had already been exposed to a long stretch of unsuccessful therapy. Hospitalization had been recommended. The appointment with me had been set up for a diagnostic interview, at which time I would decide whether or not to take on as a patient this boy who showed increasing symptoms of withdrawal. While I greeted the mother, Jingles ran right up to the child and began to lick him. Much to my surprise, the child showed no fright but instead cuddled up to the dog and began to pet him. When the mother wanted to separate the boy and dog, I signaled her to leave them alone. Before the end of the interview with the parent, the child expressed the desire to return and play with the dog. With such auspicious beginnings, the treatment of Johnny commenced. For several subsequent sessions he played with the dog, seemingly unaware of my presence. However, we held many conversations during which he was so intent upon the dog that he seemed not to be listening to me although his replies were coherent. Eventually, some of the affection elicited by the dog spilled over onto me and I was consciously included in the play. Slowly, we came to the establishment of a sound rapport which made it possible to work out Johnny's problems. Some of the credit for the eventual rehabilitation of Johnny must go to Jingles who was a most willing cotherapist.

(Levinson, 1969, pp. 41–42)

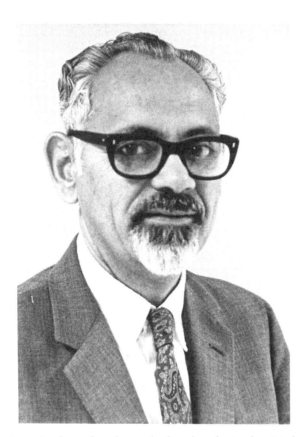

Figure 1.2 Boris Levinson is often referred to as the founder of animal-assisted psychotherapy.

(*Source:* photo courtesy of Yeshiva University Archives, New York, NY.)

Levinson went on to find that many child clients who were withdrawn and uncommunicative would interact positively with the dog. The pet served as a transitional object to aid in facilitating a relationship between the patient and the human therapist. Levinson published his first work on pet-oriented psychotherapy in the journal *Mental Hygiene* in 1962, "The dog as a 'co-therapist,'" and published his book *Pet-Oriented Child Psychotherapy* in 1969.

Professional Association for Therapeutic Horsemanship, International, Colorado

The Professional Association for Therapeutic Horsemanship, International (PATH, Intl.) was the newly adopted name in 2011 for the North American Riding for the Handicapped Association (NARHA). NARHA was established in 1969 in Denver, Colorado, and by the year 2003 had over 700 affiliated centers across the United States and Canada (M. Kaufman, personal communication, September 2003). NARHA began as a membership organization to foster safe, professional, ethical, and therapeutic equine activities through education, communication, standards, and research for people with and without disabilities (NARHA, n.d.). NARHA evolved to incorporate mental health intervention. The NARHA special interest section that set standards for equine-assisted counseling was the Equine Facilitated Mental Health Association (EFMHA). When NARHA became PATH, Intl., it developed new structure for the organization, including dropping EFMHA and integrating a mental health focus into its general mission. PATH, Intl. is recognized as a leading organization for the certification and accreditation of equine programs. It hosts an international conference and helps members to establish equine-assisted therapy programs. PATH-accredited centers offer a wide range of therapeutic equine activities, such as hippotherapy, mental health counseling, growth and development, leadership training, team building, life skills enhancement, driving, interactive vaulting, competition, groundwork, and stable management. According to PATH, Intl., in 2016 there were more than 55,000 volunteers, 4,666 instructors, and 7,672 equines associated with the organization (PATH, Intl., n.d.a, n.d.b). For more information, see their website at www.pathintl.org.

Green Chimneys, New York

Green Chimneys initially began as a school where children could learn surrounded by and involved with nature, and it eventually evolved to add mental health services. The founder of Green Chimneys was Samuel B. Ross, Jr. (1928–2018), known to his friends as "Rollo." He was only 19 years of age when he started the school. His wife of 63 years, Myra M. Ross (1930–2019), was with him the whole way, since their marriage in 1954, as they ran Green Chimneys together well into their later years, eventually turning direction over to their foundation. To this day Green Chimneys continues to have great success with children who face mental health issues and associated emotional and behavioral problems. As a sanctuary for both animals and children, Green Chimneys is a place where farm animals not only provide companionship to the children but also motivate and facilitate recovery.

Green Chimneys had its beginnings on October 27, 1947, when the Ross family purchased and then converted a 75-acre dairy farm to house a private boarding and day school and summer camp where children could interact with farm animals. The Ross family purchased the farm, which was located in Putnam County of New York, from the widow of New York State Senator Ward Tolbert of Pelham Manor. The farm was renovated and opened as a private school on June 15, 1948; it was named "The Green Chimneys Farm for Little Folk" and was designated for children between the ages of 3 and 6 years and "designed to be a place where children and animals could grow up together" (Green Chimneys, n.d.).

Over the years the program grew in numbers and expanded to include preschool through to eighth grade. In the 1960s it was operating 24 hours a day, 365 days a year (with no separate summer camp), and the population shifted to serve children who needed a more specialized program. By this time, it was serving children not only from the United States but also from Canada, Central and South America, and other countries. In 1974, Green Chimneys obtained a license from the New York State Department of Social Services to assist children who were emotionally disturbed and learning disabled. At this time the program's focus shifted to an around-the-clock residential treatment center with comprehensive education and mental health services for children referred from social services and schools:

> An emphasis was placed on the integration of the children with farm animals, nature and the environment.
>
> (Green Chimneys, n.d.)

Over the following decades, Green Chimneys continued to expand and to offer a variety of services to a diverse population. In the 1970s, Green Chimneys added the 50-acre Hillside Outdoor Education Center, located less than a mile from the main campus in Brewster, New York. The Green Chimneys farm expanded to include a wildlife conservation and rehabilitation program that houses a large collection of permanently disabled birds of prey and other assorted wildlife. In 2000, Green Chimneys opened a new multimillion dollar day school with state-of-the-art classrooms for both residential and day students. The Brewster campus has several structures including classrooms, gymnasium, playground, learning center, dining hall, residence halls, greenhouses, wildlife center with several aviaries, dog kennels, barns with indoor and outdoor pens, horse stables, small and large corrals, and large fenced pastures. There are also small and large gardens. In residence, there are dogs, camels, llamas, sheep, goats, chickens, rabbits, pigs, cows, horses, donkeys, and a peacock. Today, Green Chimneys serves a multistate area (Green Chimneys, n.d.).

Green Chimneys is an internationally recognized program that also provides internships for a few lucky students from around the world who want to benefit first-hand from the vast training opportunities offered by this program. Human–animal interaction is a major focus of the internship program. One of my university students was fortunate enough to be accepted into the Green Chimneys internship program where she worked with children interacting with animals, and she considered it one of her most valuable learning experiences. In the spring of 2015, I was able to attend a conference meeting held at Green Chimneys, satisfying a long-held desire to see for myself the wonderful facility and services there. It is an incredible place with dedicated staff assisting many children. The many types of animals receive great care from paid and volunteer staff. While there, I was fortunate to attend one of the more meaningful activities of Green Chimneys: releasing a rehabilitated hawk back into the wild. Before leaving, I had the honor and pleasure of interviewing the founders of Green Chimneys, Samuel and Myra Ross (see the published interview in my 2018 book, *Animal-Assisted Interventions for Emotional and Mental Health: Conversations with Pioneers of the Field*). I obtained an autographed copy of Sam's book which I highly recommend, *The Extraordinary Spirit of Green Chimneys* (2011). For more information, see the website www.greenchimneys.org/.

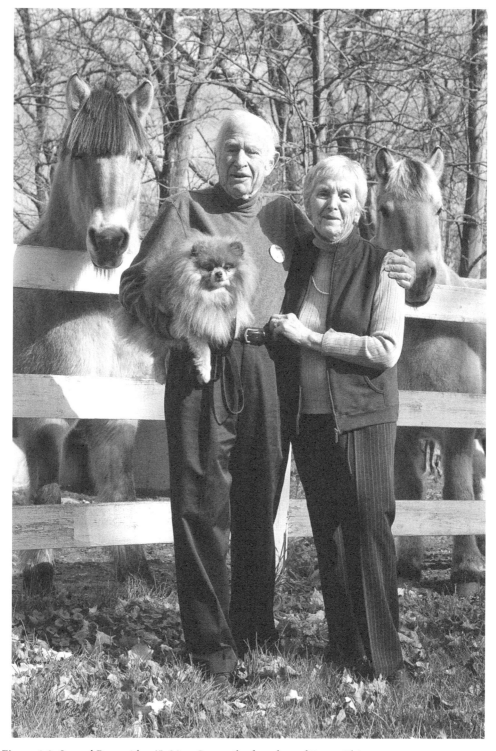

Figure 1.3 Samuel Ross with wife Myra Ross—the founders of Green Chimneys.

(*Source:* photo courtesy of Green Chimneys.)

Samuel Corson and Elizabeth O'Leary Corson, Ohio

Samuel Corson and Elizabeth O'Leary Corson, along with their associates at the Ohio State University, were the first to conduct a systematic study on the incorporation of pet dogs in psychotherapy in a hospital setting. They published their work in the 1970s (Corson et al., 1975). Samuel Abraham Corson (1909–1998) was born in a small village, Dobryanka, 200 miles from Odessa, Ukraine, and died in Granger, Indiana, according to his daughter Olivia Corson (personal communication, November 6, 2010). His wife Elizabeth O'Leary Corson (1920–2004) was born in St. Paul, Minnesota, and died in Oakland, California. The Corsons became interested in pet-facilitated psychotherapy by accident. They kept a colony of dogs in the hospital for use in their longitudinal experiments on "the interaction of genetic and psychosocial factors in reactions to emotional stress and in social interactions" (Corson et al., 1975, pp. 278–279). The kennel for the dogs, known as the "dog ward," was located one floor below the day room of the psychiatric ward, and the dogs could occasionally be heard barking:

> Some of the patients, especially the adolescents, many of whom had been uncommunicative throughout their hospital stay, broke their self-imposed silence and began to inquire whether they could play and interact with the dogs or help take care of them. Our initial experience with the patient–dog interactions encouraged us and the patients sufficiently to warrant the initiation of a pilot research project to determine the efficacy of pet-facilitated psychotherapy.
>
> (Corson et al., 1975, p. 279)

The colony of 20 helping dogs involved in the pet facilitation project included Wirehair Fox Terriers, Border Collies, Beagles, a Labrador Retriever, a German Shepherd/Husky cross, and several mixed breeds. The patients selected to participate in the pet-facilitated psychotherapy investigations "were chiefly those who failed to respond favorably to traditional forms of therapy" (i.e., drugs and electroconvulsive shock therapy) (Corson et al., 1975, p. 278). These patients were withdrawn, self-centered, and uncommunicative (some of them almost mute); they lacked self-esteem and exhibited infantile helplessness and dependence. The patients were introduced to the dogs (in some cases also cats) in the kennels ("dog ward"), on the patient ward, or on the bed of patients who spent most of their time in bed. In some cases, the patient would first interact with different dogs in the kennels so the patient could "choose a dog to suit his temperament or his particular needs, at the particular time" (Corson et al., 1975, p. 278).

> A good deal of insight into the patient's feelings may be obtained by ascertaining what type of dog a patient chooses and by considering the reasons he gives for the choice. Whenever possible, video recordings were made of patient–therapist interactions, patient–dog interactions, patient–dog–therapist interactions, and patient–patient interactions.
>
> (Corson et al., 1975, p. 278)

The pet-facilitated psychotherapy involved the same therapy as other patients, with the addition of interactions with a dog (or sometimes a cat). The number and type of interactions varied somewhat based on the preferences of the patients and included social visits, grooming the dogs and other care responsibilities, walking the dog indoors and later outdoors, and running with the dogs outdoors for greater exercise.

This assumption of responsibility for the safety and care of the dogs served to develop self-confidence in the patients and gradually transformed them from irresponsible, dependent psychological invalids into self-respecting responsible individuals.

(Corson et al., 1975, p. 280)

The potency of the Corsons' pet-facilitated psychotherapy approach is demonstrated in the following abbreviated description of one of their patients:

Sonny was a 19-year-old psychotic who spent most of his time in bed. The staff tried unsuccessfully to get him to move about and interact. Nothing seemed to interest him; he would not participate in occupational therapy, recreational therapy, or group therapy. In individual therapy he remained withdrawn and uncommunicative. His drug regimen (haloperidol and other drugs) did not improve him. A work-up for electroshock therapy (EST) was begun. A token system was introduced, but again Sonny showed little response.

   Before starting the electroshock therapy, we decided to use a dog as a component of the token reward system. . . . When the psychiatrist brought the dog Arwyn, a wirehair fox terrier, to Sonny's bed, Sonny raised himself on one elbow and gave a big smile in response to the dog's wildly friendly greeting. The dog jumped on Sonny, licking his face and ears. Sonny tumbled the dog about joyously. He volunteered his first question, "Where can I keep him?" Then to everyone's amazement, he got out of bed and followed the dog when she jumped to the floor. In the first few days after being introduced to the dog, Sonny became active in working for tokens. . . . He began to notice other patients on the unit . . . began to go to group therapy, and asked that he be given ECT [since he was still psychotic] . . . and he was later discharged much improved. The psychiatrist judged the introduction of the dog as the turning point in the course of Sonny's recovery.

(Corson et al., 1975, p. 284)

Once they had accidentally discovered the benefits for psychiatric patients of social interaction with dogs, the Corsons' work evolved from inhumane experimentation on dogs to measure psychophysiological stress responses, to much more humane study of the social and relational value of dogs that provided company to psychiatric patients. As an interesting historical side note, see the reflections by Olivia Corson on her parents' work in the section "Moral Implications of AAT" in Chapter 6.

Lima State Hospital, Ohio

Another interesting accident occurred in the 1970s that resulted in the establishment of the first formal AAT program at a maximum security mental hospital in the United States (Lee, 1983). One day, in about 1975, staff of the Lima State Hospital in Ohio discovered that a patient had found an injured sparrow in the large prison courtyard and had carried the small bird to a ward housing the hospital's most depressed, noncommunicative patients. No animals, wildlife, or even plants were permitted in wards at that time. However, attendants and patients joined in the conspiracy to keep this bird regardless of rules:

Patients adopted the bird—and the results were remarkable. Despondent and noncommunicative men began catching insects for the small sparrow and caring for it. For the first time in this ward for the severely disturbed, patients began acting as a group and relating openly with staff.

(Lee, 1983, p. 24)

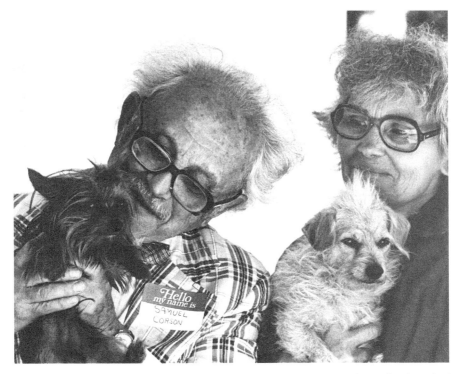

Figure 1.4 Samuel Corson and Elizabeth O'Leary Corson were pioneers in the study of pet-facilitated psychotherapy in the 1970s.

(*Source:* photo courtesy of Olivia Corson.)

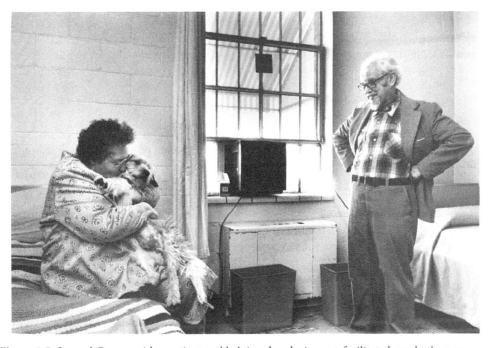

Figure 1.5 Samuel Corson with a patient and helping dog during pet-facilitated psychotherapy.

(*Source:* photo courtesy of Olivia Corson.)

Convinced by this experience that interaction with animals could be effective in therapy, hospital personnel proposed a formal pet therapy program involving careful documentation of progress, guidelines to ensure animal care, and an overall system of monitoring. The program was introduced with three parakeets and one aquarium. Many years later, the AAT program had evolved to include five of ten wards and various other areas within the hospital: the dentist's office, the education section, and recreation areas. Since its origin:

> The pet program has produced outstanding results, especially in the treatment of patients suffering from depression or suicidal impulses. . . . A comparison study between two wards, identical except that one had pets and one didn't, demonstrated statistically what the staff already knew. The medication level was double in the ward without pets, as was the incidence of violence and suicide attempts.
>
> (Lee, 1983, pp. 24–25)

Since the patients at Lima State Hospital could be violent at times, strict regulations were applied in the pet therapy program to monitor the welfare of the animals. Additionally, patients were taught about humane treatment and animal care and were provided with all necessary support and supplies for these purposes (Lee, 1983).

Therapy Dogs International, New Jersey

A significant event in the history of AAT was the founding of Therapy Dogs International (TDI, 2023a) in New Jersey in 1976 by Elaine Smith (1930–2012). Smith was born in Newark, New Jersey and nursing became her profession. While she was in England, she got the idea for TDI after observing the positive impact a visiting Chaplain's golden retriever had on patients. Smith brought her concept of therapy dog visits back to the United States:

> Using her German Shepherd, Phila, and her Shetland Sheepdog, Genny, in therapy sessions, Smith got a woman to talk who hadn't spoken in years.
>
> (Burch, 2003, p. 11)

TDI is described on the website as:

> a volunteer organization dedicated to regulating testing and registration of therapy dogs and their volunteer handlers for the purpose of visiting nursing homes, hospitals, other institutions and wherever else therapy dogs are needed.
>
> (Therapy Dogs International, 2023a, p. 1)

TDI describes their dog organization as the oldest in the United States and has registered handler-dog teams in all 50 states and in Canada (Therapy Dogs International, 2023a). For more information, see their website at www.tdi-dog.org/.

Pet Partners, Washington

The Pet Partners organization is located in Bellevue, Washington. According to their website, "Pet Partners is the national leader in demonstrating and promoting positive human–animal interactions to improve the physical, emotional and psychological lives of those [they] serve" (Pet Partners, 2023a, p. 1). Indeed:

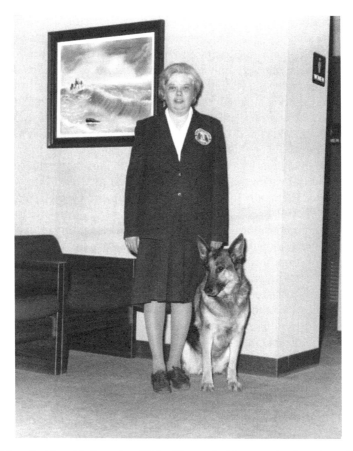

Figure 1.6 Elaine Smith with her dog Phila. Elaine Smith was the founder of Therapy Dogs International.

(*Source:* photo courtesy of Therapy Dogs International.)

> Pet Partners is the nation's largest and most prestigious nonprofit registering handlers of multiple species as volunteer teams providing animal-assisted interventions.
>
> (Pet Partners, 2023b, p. 1)

The earliest history of Pet Partners is in 1977 when the Delta Foundation was formed in Portland, Oregon with Michael J. McCulloch, MD as the president. In 1981 the organization's name was changed to Delta Society to "symbolize an expanding group of interested researchers and medical practitioners in both human and animal fields" (Pet Partners, 2023a, p. 1). At this time Leo K. Bustad became president. Bustad is widely credited with introducing the term "human–animal bond." Bustad's work is still recognized today through the Bustad Companion Animal Veterinarian of the Year Award. This is awarded each year by the American Veterinary Medical Association. Dr. Leo K. Bustad died on September 19, 1998 (Kay, 2011, p. 4). He was an outstanding educator, scientist, and humanitarian. He co-founded Delta Society while serving as dean of the veterinary school at Washington State University.

By 2003, Delta Society had over 6,400 therapy animal teams in its Pet Partners program, servicing individuals in all 50 states of the United States (Delta Society, 2003). In 2012, the name of the organization changed from Delta Society's Pet Partners to simply Pet Partners. By 2016, there were almost 14,000 Pet Partners therapy animal teams in 50 states; the previous year, Pet Partners teams made more than 1 million visits to people in need; nearly 50,000 teams have been registered since the program's inception (Pet Partners, 2023b, p. 1). Pet Partners promotes the work of therapy dogs, cats, birds, small animals (i.e., rabbits, rats, guinea pigs), horses, llamas and alpacas, and pigs. Pet Partners handler–animal teams volunteer in a variety of settings, such as schools, colleges and universities, libraries, nursing homes, hospitals and other healthcare facilities, and prisons and detention centers. Many facilities will not allow a handler–therapy animal team to enter unless it has a national registration credential, such as that from Pet Partners, which reflects that the handler and pet have adequate training and preparation for volunteer therapy work. Pet Partners is recognized nationally for its rigorous training and evaluation requirements for animal–handler teams.

Pet Partners is an organization for training and registering human handler teams who wish to provide nonprofessional, volunteer animal-assisted applications and interventions. Pet Partners does not train for professional practice nor does it provide a registration credential for professional practice. However, I recommend the Pet Partners training and registration program as introductory-level training for those who wish to perform professional animal-assisted applications and interventions. Of course, professionals will need additional specific and advanced training from other sources. Also, as the Pet Partners membership includes practice liability insurance for nonprofessional volunteer services only, then anyone practicing with a pet as a professional service would need to obtain their own professional

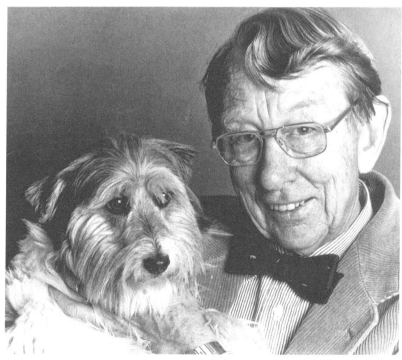

Figure 1.7 Leo K. Bustad with his dog Brigid. Leo Bustad is a co-founder of the foundation organization for Pet Partners and he is widely credited with introducing the term "human–animal bond."

(*Source:* photo courtesy of Pet Partners.)

practice liability insurance through affiliation with a professional practice organization. For more information, see their website at www.petpartners.org.

Center for the Human-Animal Bond, Indiana

The Center for the Human-Animal Bond (CHAB) began as the Center for Applied Ethology and Human-Animal Interaction that was established in 1982 at Purdue University. The original purpose was to study human–animal relationships and to communicate findings to scientists and the public. In 1997, the name was changed to Center for the Human-Animal Bond "to reflect the relationship that exists between people and the animals that share this earth" (Center for the Human-Animal Bond, n.d., p. 1). While CHAB attends to a wide variety of human–animal interaction and relationship issues, it includes attention to the study and practice of animal-assisted counseling and psychotherapy. CHAB provides a valuable resource called HABRI Central, which is:

> an online platform for open research and collaboration into the relationships between humans and animals, specifically companion animals. HABRI Central uses a combination of library resources to facilitate the discovery, access, production, and preservation of human–animal interaction research. A bibliography of references to human-animal interaction literature helps you to discover existing research while a full-text repository allows you to freely access a wide-array of materials and tools.
>
> (HABRI Central, n.d., p. 1)

HABRI Central is a combined collaborative effort of Purdue University's College of Veterinary Medicine and Purdue University Libraries. For more information, see their website at www.vet.purdue.edu/chab/.

Contributions by Nursing and Other Healthcare Professions in the 1980s

The nursing profession has significantly contributed to the acceptance of AAT into mainstream medicine and healthcare. Professional nursing practice journals began to publish on the area of AAT in the 1980s (Hooker, Freeman, and Stewart, 2002). In the beginning, most of these were descriptive works on how animals fulfilled the desire of patients to be needed and how the animals reduced the stress levels of patients, visiting family members, and staff. Over the next few years, more scientific investigations began to appear in nursing and other healthcare journals. These documented the physiological benefits of pets, such as lowered blood pressure and greater 1-year survival rates for patients in cardiac recovery after experiencing a myocardial infarction or angina (Friedmann et al., 1980, 1983).

William Thomas, the Eden Alternative, New York

Another historical milestone in the application of human–animal interaction as a form of emotional healthcare was the formation of the concept of the "Eden Alternative." William Thomas, a Harvard Medical School graduate, was a reluctant new physician at a nursing home—that is, until summer 1991 when he and his associates at Chase Memorial Nursing Home in New Berlin, New York, began "to toy with a radically unscientific, nonmedical approach to life" for the 80 residents of the nursing home (Thomas, 1994, p. 28). The Eden Alternative was based on the premise that human beings need variety in their surroundings. At this period of time the status quo of nursing homes was that of a sterile, cold environment where elderly people were treated with medical practices until they died. Thomas, frustrated by this idea, wanted to transform nursing homes from a place of only medical treatment into a place for caring:

> We began to think of our nursing home not as a nursing home in need of improvement, but as a human habitat.
>
> (Thomas, 1994, p. 30)

The three principles of the Eden Alternative are that (1) "biological diversity is as good for human habitats as it is for natural habitats" (Thomas, 1994, p. 31); (2) "social diversity is as important to the nursing home as it is to true human community" (Thomas, 1994, p. 32); and (3) "human habitats must be driven by the same devotion to harmony that enlivens music and nature" (Thomas, 1994, p. 32). The Eden Alternative approach was to integrate into the nursing home care program: entertaining and educational interaction with adults and children; indoor plants; lush outdoor flower and vegetable gardens; and lots of pets for social interaction.

Visiting dogs and their handlers provided pet therapy:

> This is good and it certainly beats having no contact at all with dogs. It is easy to see that residents enjoy these visits and, from the Eden Alternative point of view, it is easy to see what ought to be done: all nursing homes should have dogs living in them.
>
> (Thomas, 1994, p. 115)

Thus, residential dogs were also incorporated into the nursing home care program. In addition, Thomas wrote:

> Cats are an essential part of Edenized nursing homes. These animals are so inexpensive, require such little care, and give so much in so many different ways that it is a sin for a nursing home to be without them.
>
> (Thomas, 1994, p. 127)

Another species favored for the program was birds:

> Birds are relatively inexpensive to buy and feed, and they require little space. Birds are fairly well suited to the temperature and humidity of the average nursing home, and can flourish there. Best of all, birds can become true personal pets and companions for the people with whom they live.
>
> (Thomas, 1994, p. 133)

Other animal species recommended include a large tank of fish, rabbits (which can be kept outside or inside as they can be trained to use a litter box), and chickens. The chickens serve additional purpose by providing fresh eggs for the residents and rich manure for the gardens (Thomas, 1994).

International Association of Human–Animal Interaction Organizations, Washington

The International Association of Human–Animal Interaction Organizations (IAHAIO) was founded in 1990 and is located in the state of Washington. According to their website, "IAHAIO is a global umbrella organization drawing together many associations doing exciting work in the human–animal interaction (HAI) field" (IAHAIO, n.d., p. 1). Their mission is to provide international leadership for those who are working in research, education, and practice of human–animal interaction. IAHAIO is incorporated as a not-for-profit entity. IAHIAO sponsors an international conference for networking and research presentations on human–animal interaction. IAHAIO is also known for its leadership in bringing together experts in the field of human–animal interaction from all over the world and publishing findings from these meetings. For more information, see their website at www.iahaio.org/new/.

International Society for Anthrozoology, Pennsylvania

The International Society for Anthrozoology (ISAZ) was founded in 1991 as a "supportive organization for the scientific and scholarly study of human–animal interaction" (ISAZ, n.d., p. 1). It was based originally in Europe but was registered in 2004 as a nonprofit organization in Pennsylvania. As of 2016, ISAZ had over 300 members representing nearly 30 countries. It is a nonpolitical organization of professionals, students, and scholars of many disciplines. The organization sponsors a regular conference for networking and research presentations. ISAZ publishes the journal *Anthrozoös* for scholarly works on human–animal interaction. For more information, see their website at www.isaz.net/isaz/.

Equine Assisted Growth and Learning Association, Utah

The Equine Assisted Growth and Learning Association (EAGALA) was established in 1999 in Utah to promote equine-assisted therapy in education and mental health (EAGALA, n.d.a, n.d.b). EAGALA is a leading organization for the training and certification of professionals worldwide in the performance of educational and therapeutic equine-assisted activities. The association sponsors an annual national conference for exchange of research and educational information. In 2016, EAGALA reported there were over 700 EAGALA programs and 4,500 members in 50 countries (EAGALA, n.d.a). For more information, see their website at www.eagala.org.

Contributions by Healthcare Professions in the 1990s and Early 2000s

In the 1990s and early 2000s, healthcare journals published several experimental research articles documenting the benefits of AAT in a variety of healthcare settings (Hooker, Freeman, and Stewart, 2002). For example, AAT was found to be beneficial in home healthcare settings as it was used to divert patients' attention during painful procedures as well as to create more enjoyable nurse visits. It was determined that AAT reduced the strain and stress for patients and visitors in hospice settings (and home nursing care for the terminally ill). AAT was found to be helpful for patients with Alzheimer's disease, resulting in increased socialization and social activity, and decreased agitation. Research has also demonstrated decreased anxiety and depression and increased socialization for hospitalized psychiatric patients with a variety of mental health diagnoses (Barker and Dawson, 1998; Marr et al., 2000; McVarish, 1995). Research in AAT continues today in both mental and physical health fields. While existing studies already demonstrate many benefits of AAT, additional studies are needed to both replicate existing work and elaborate on potential benefits that have yet to be discovered.

AAT Grows in Popularity Near the Turn of the Century

AAT grew much more popular in the United States in the late 1990s and early 2000s partly because the public received greater exposure to it through stories published by mainstream newspapers, magazines, and television broadcasts. As a result of these media stories, an abundance of schoolteachers and counselors across the nation began seeking out AAT training so they could share the benefits of pet therapy with the populations they served. Following are some examples of these media stories.

Cindy Ehlers of Eugene, Oregon, took her Husky, Bear, to visit with students and others traumatized by the 1998 shootings at Thurston High School in Springfield, Oregon, and the violence in 1999 at Columbine High School in Littleton, Colorado (Rea, 2000). Tracy Roberts brought her two Australian Shepherds, Lucy and Dottie, to school to act as teachers' aides in the fourth- and fifth-grade classes at the Canterbury Episcopal School in DeSoto, Texas (Tarrant, 2000). Lucy and Dottie were reported to be a comfort to the children and a welcome relief from the stress of school. Dena Carselowey and her Labrador Retriever, Buggs, served as co-therapists at Minneha Core Knowledge Magnet Elementary School in Wichita, Kansas (Associated Press, 1999). Buggs provided positive acceptance the moment a student entered the counselor's office. Often the children came in to see the dog and stayed a while to talk to the counselor while they petted and played with Buggs. Therapy dog teams volunteered counseling services through the Red Cross in New York, providing comfort and stress relief to victims and families affected by the World Trade Center terrorist attack of September 11, 2001 (Teal, 2002). *Time* magazine published an article on new dog-assisted reading programs popping up across the United States. Reading-assistance dogs provided a fun atmosphere for reading practice for reading-challenged children (Barol, 2002). Stories about animal-assisted reading programs initiated the development of an abundance of these types of programs across the United States in schools and public libraries as well as in community bookstores.

Consortium for Animal Assisted Therapy, Texas

I founded the Consortium for Animal Assisted Therapy (CAAT) in 2000 at the University of North Texas in Denton, Texas, within the Counseling Program of the College of Education (CAAT, n.d.). CAAT provides research support, graduate training, internships, community workshops, and distance learning for students and mental health professionals aspiring to practice and study AAT in counseling and psychotherapy.

People throughout the United States and across the globe have benefited from the distance learning program that advances knowledge to distant regions of the world. The University of North Texas Counseling Program was the first CACREP-accredited counseling program to provide training in AAT; CACREP is the acronym for the national accrediting body for counselor training programs (Council for the Accreditation of Counseling and Related Educational Programs). Students pursuing a doctorate or master's degree in counseling at our Counseling Program can receive concurrent training and supervision in AAT clinical practice.

Through CAAT, I have evaluated well over 500 handler–animal teams and trained many more persons through community workshops and my distance learning program. This book is central to the training I provide. CAAT is an identified resource for international networking and information provision. Additionally, I have traveled across the United States and internationally to train others in AAT. For more information, see the website at www.coe. unt.edu/consortium-animal-assisted-therapy.

Institute for Human–Animal Connection, Colorado

The Institute for Human–Animal Connection (IHAC) was founded in 2005 by Philip Tedeschi and Jennifer Fitchett at the University of Denver within the Social Work Program.

IHAC provides training and research opportunities for those who wish to work or study in the field of human–animal interaction.

> The Institute for Human–Animal Connection (IHAC) is leading the way in animal-assisted social work and human–animal interaction education and professional development. University of Denver's Graduate School of Social Work remains one of the only programs in the world to offer specialization in human–animal interactions alongside a graduate level social science degree.
>
> (IHAC, n.d., p. 1)

For more information, see their website at www.du.edu/humananimalconnection/.

AAT Formally Recognized by Professional Mental Health Organizations

Two prominent U.S. national mental health organizations formally recognized the field of AAT in the first decade of the twenty-first century. In 2008, the American Psychological Association's Division 17, Society of Counseling and Psychology, formed a new section addressing AAT called Human–Animal Interaction, and they launched a new journal, the *Human–Animal Interaction Bulletin*. This new section and journal are dedicated to professional and scholarly activities that advance the understanding of human–animal interactions as they relate to counseling psychology, including AAT (Human–Animal Interaction, n.d., p. 1). The American Counseling Association (ACA) Governing Council approved the establishment of the Animal-Assisted Therapy in Mental Health (AATMH) Interest Network in November 2009. The primary goals of the AATMH Interest Network include promoting safe and effective AAT research and practice in mental health, providing a medium for counselors to share research and practice ideas related to AAT, and promoting publication of AAT research in ACA and mental health journals (Chandler and Johnson, 2009). The AATMH interest network evolved into the Human–Animal Interactions in Counseling (HAIC) interest network, part of the ACA Community, ACA Connect, available to ACA Members (ACA, n.d.), "The mission of the HAIC is to promote understanding of human-animal interactions (HAI) and ethical practice of animal-assisted interventions (AAI) in counseling by attending to issues relevant to provider competence, animal advocacy, and empirical research."

In 2016, the American Counseling Association first presented their competencies for the practice of AAT in counseling. These competencies were based on the work of Stewart, Chang, and Rice (2013), who explored the theoretical underpinnings of mental health providers of AAT. They performed semi-structured interviews with 14 professionals who practice AAT in a counseling setting. From analyses of these interviews, four categories emerged describing providers' philosophical framework and approach to AAT: (1) possessing unique skills and competencies, (2) utilizing a highly developed relationship with a therapy animal, (3) impacting the therapeutic process, and (4) enhancing the scope of traditional counselor-client relationships (Stewart, Chang, and Rice, 2013, p. 329). The work of Stewart, Chang, and Rice (2013) provided the framework for the eventual publication, on June 21, 2016, of the first ACA-recommended competencies for the practice of AAT-C, which was a major acknowledgment of AAT-C as an accepted method within the field of professional counseling (Stewart et al., 2016). The ACA AAT-C competencies delineate nine different areas under three domains: Domain 1, Knowledge: (1) AAT-C training, assessment, and supervision, (2) in-depth animal knowledge, and (3) integrated ethics; Domain 2, Skills: (1) mastery of general counseling competence, (2) intentional incorporation, and (3) specialized skill set; and Domain 3, Attitudes: (1) animal advocacy, (2) advocacy to the profession of AAT-C, and (3) professional values (Stewart et al., 2016).

Animal Assisted Intervention International

Animal Assisted Intervention International (AAII) was established in 2013, "to promote animal-assisted interventions and to act as a focus for all of those who work, or have an interest, in the field of animal-assisted interventions" (AAII, n.d.). AAII was formally registered in the Netherlands in 2013. A message on its website in 2016 from the president, Melissa Winkle (of Albuquerque, New Mexico), states:

> We visualize AAII as being a coalition of qualified practitioners and organizations working in the field of animal-assisted intervention. Membership of AAII is planned to be open to individuals and organizations that are actively involved in selecting, training and supporting human–animal teams to work in the field of AAI and who agree to abide by, and meet the minimum standards agreed by the members of AAII. Our objectives include the establishment of a high level standard of practice for AAI healthcare and social service providers, to facilitate communication and education amongst members, and to disseminate information to the public about the benefits of AAI.
>
> (AAII, n.d.)

AAII has published Standards for Practice and Competencies for AAA, AAE, and AAT. For more information, see their website at www.aai-int.org/.

Association of Animal-Assisted Intervention Professionals, Bellevue, Washington

The Association of Animal-Assisted Intervention Professionals (AAAIP) was founded in 2022 as an outgrowth of the well-established volunteer organization for nonprofessionals, Pet Partners. The mission of AAAIP "is to empower professionals to responsibly integrate the healing power of therapy animals into their practice while advancing the field of animal-assisted interventions (AAI). We envision a future where AAI is practiced widely, ethically, and successfully" (AAAIP, n.d., p. 1). AAAIP offers training and certification courses for the practice of AAT and presents a code of ethics for practice.

A RELATIVELY NEW FRONTIER THERAPY

Despite a lengthy history in the United States, AAT in the counseling field is still considered a relatively new frontier therapy for promoting client welfare, growth, and development. To date, few universities in the United States offer training for counselors in AAT, even though child psychologist Boris Levinson empirically demonstrated in the early 1960s that pets help to form a strong connection between client and therapist. Pet practitioners can be especially helpful when working with populations who might be discouraged, unmotivated, resistant, or defiant, or who have poor self-insight, deficits in social skills, or barriers to developing relationships. The pets involved with AAT-C can enhance the motivation, encouragement, inspiration, and insight properties of therapy. Those professionals who choose to explore the new frontier of AAT-C may face resistance and criticism from their peers. Levinson was ridiculed and laughed at when he presented his findings in 1961:

> When presented at the Annual Convention of the American Psychological Association in 1961, my findings met with a mixed reception. While most of the auditors were enthusiastic, some guffawed and a few others asked whether my dog shared in the fees. This reaction was commented on by Carl Rogers (1963) who felt that it was

symptomatic resistance to new psychotherapeutic techniques. I feel, however, that the reason some therapists objected to the use of the dog in a psychotherapeutic relationship was because of the anxiety which clinicians "possess along with other human beings, generally, concerning our relatedness with the nonhuman environment."

(Levinson, 1969, p. 42)

Unfortunately, collegial rejection regarding the consideration of nontraditional treatment modalities does occur. A nontraditional modality typically refers to a relatively new intervention focus compared with more established therapeutic modalities with a long history of research and application. While it is important to examine, assess, and otherwise thoroughly scrutinize any new type of therapy, we must not use the need for rigorous scrutiny as a justification for premature dismissal of a potentially beneficial treatment approach. The potential benefits to engaging in responsible practice and research of AAT-C would seem to make up for the potential obstacles that this engagement presents. Those who do become involved in AAT-C will be included among other pioneers who lay the foundation for a therapy that continues to grow in popularity. Furthermore, it is important to consider the truly wonderful benefit that it is a lot of fun to take your pet to work.

The purpose of this book is to help further the interest of AAT in the counseling field. It is primarily designed for beginners in AAT-C. It has drawn from a number of worthwhile resources in an effort to consolidate information into one succinct and valuable guide. In previous years, I had to pull information from a number of different places, including my own experience and training, to provide students with the knowledge they needed to practice AAT-C. Placing that information in one source will now make it much more convenient to teach these important training concepts. I have incorporated real-life stories into the book chapters to enhance the subject matter. Some of these stories were shared with me by colleagues and students, and many are from my own experience working in the field.

I sincerely hope you enjoy reading this book as much as I enjoyed writing it. If the book fails to meet your needs or expectations, then I would be happy to hear from you and will endeavor to include that information in a possible future edition. If you are satisfied with aspects of the book, then I would also very much like to hear what you liked about it so I may retain and reinforce that information for the future. In any case, if you are reading this book, you must have an interest in AAT-C, and that makes us colleagues who share a mutual interest in a highly valuable profession; for this, I salute you. Thank you very much for reading my book. Here's wishing you and your pet "Happy Tails!" By the way, you can reach me at the University of North Texas, Counseling Program, in the College of Education.

AAT READING RESOURCES

A handful of books have been written that are useful in regard to animal-assisted mental health applications, including the following:

- *Animal-Assisted Psychotherapy: Theory, issues and practice* (Parish-Plass, 2013).
- *Handbook on Animal-Assisted Therapy: Theoretical foundations and guidelines for practice, 5th ed.* (Fine [Ed.], 2019).
- *Animal Assisted Play Therapy* (VanFleet and Faa-Thompson, 2017).
- *Animal-Assisted Brief Therapy: A solution-focused approach, 2nd ed.* (Pichot, 2011).

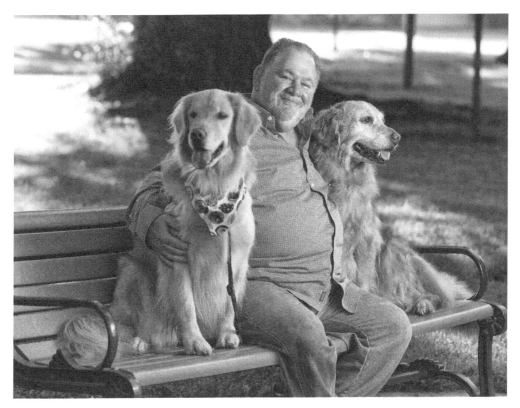

Figure 1.8 Aubrey Fine with his dogs. He is a leader in the field of AAT and editor and author of the landmark book *Handbook on Animal-Assisted Therapy: Foundations and Guidelines for Animal-Assisted Interventions.* I interviewed Dr. Fine in 2015 and this interview can be found in my 2018 book, *Animal-Assisted Interventions for Emotional and Mental Health: Conversations with Pioneers of the Field* (Chandler and Otting, 2018).

(*Source:* photo courtesy of Aubrey Fine.)

RECOMMENDED COMPETENCY AREAS FOR AAT IN THE COUNSELING FIELD

The most important first step toward achieving competency to practice AAT in counseling and psychotherapy in the United States is obtaining a mental health license to practice as a professional counselor, psychologist, marriage and family therapist, clinical social worker and so forth. As a prerequisite to obtaining such a license to practice, one needs to complete a college/university graduate degree associated with the license. Some countries other than the United States do not have or require licensure for mental health professionals to practice. In that case an individual should at least obtain an appropriate college/university degree in a mental health field (counseling, psychotherapy, psychology, social work, and so forth). In addition to training and licensure in a mental health field, an individual who desires to practice animal-assisted counseling and/or psychotherapy needs advanced training and supervision in incorporating AAI in ways that are respectful and safe for both humans and animals. Such training is often difficult to find, but reading this book is an excellent method of furthering your knowledge.

AAT is not a standalone profession and should not be practiced as such. AAT is a modality integrated into clinical practice by properly trained and credentialed health and mental health providers. Obtaining some type of credential in AAT does not by itself qualify one to actually professionally practice AAT. There is no current requirement in any state in the United States that I am aware of that requires a person to have "certification" to practice AAT. According to most state licensing boards, what is required is an appropriate state license in a health or mental health field, and then some type of associated training in AAT: the type and amount of AAT training required is usually not described. Training for professional AAT practice is still difficult to find. That is why a resource such as this book is considered so valuable today for those wishing to practice professionally.

Practice standards provide guidelines for establishing and maintaining quality and safety of therapeutic applications. Based on my knowledge and experience in the field of AAT-C, I provide my recommendations for competencies needed to practice AAT-C. Additionally, I direct the reader to areas of this book where detailed information can be found on each competency area and accompanying performance guidelines. I recommend the following umbrella goal statement for the practice of AAT-C:

> The professional AAT counselor or psychotherapist is able to effectively incorporate an animal as a therapeutic change agent into the counseling process in a manner that protects the safety and welfare of both humans and animals.

Consistent with this goal statement, recommended competency areas for the practice of AAT in counseling and psychotherapy are the ability to do the following:

- Describe the history, evolution, and current status of AAT applications, training, and credentialing related to counseling.
- Understand and explain the benefits, role, and function of AAT in counseling.
- Integrate AAT in a manner consistent with the counseling process.
- Comply with ethical and professional standards and guidelines related to AAT applications in counseling.
- Work as a team with a therapy animal in a counseling facility, practice, or program.
- Serve as an advocate for the therapy animal.

See Table 1.1 for the location of information on each competency area and accompanying performance guidelines in this book. Also, see Appendix A for a description of the recommended competency areas and accompanying performance guidelines.

Table 1.1 Primary Location in This Book of Information on Recommended Competency Areas

Competency Area	Book Chapters
AAT Applications	Chapters 1, 2
AAT Training and Credentialing	Chapter 5
Benefits, Role, and Function of AAT	Chapter 7
Integrate AAT into the Counseling Process	Chapter 7
Ethical and Professional Issues in AAT	Chapter 6
Diversity and Cultural Issues in AAT	Chapters 11, 14
AAT in a Facility, Practice, or Program	Chapters 8, 9, 10, 11, 12, 13, 14
Advocate for the Therapy Animal	Chapters 3, 4, 6

Information on recommended competency areas and accompanying performance guidelines for AAT-C applications serve to guide the education and supervision processes for AAT-C practice. Counselor education curricula for AAT-C training, and counselor supervisors of AAT-C practitioners, should strive to attend to all six areas, and counselors who practice AAT-C should adhere closely to these recommended competencies and performance guidelines. Given that the frequency of practice of AAT-C is increasing, the provision of recommended practice competencies and accompanying performance guidelines provides a valuable service to the field.

2

Research in Animal-Assisted Counseling and Related Areas

With any relatively new treatment modality, it is important to establish a base of research to validate its value. Although many more experimentally based clinical trials in AAT in a counseling setting are needed, we shall examine in this chapter some existing research as a baseline for future research endeavors. The literature presented in this chapter is not meant to be all-inclusive, but rather serves to describe research that supports the efficacy of AAT in the field of counseling and related areas.

Let us begin by describing a meta-analysis of AAT performed by Nimer and Lundahl (2007). These researchers conducted a comprehensive search of articles on AAT. Three strategies were used to identify studies investigating the effectiveness of the outcomes after an animal was introduced into the study. First, a computer search of 11 databases was conducted in 2004 using 19 keywords. Second, hand searches were conducted on three journals that tend to publish studies on AAT from the years 1973–2004; these were *Anthrozoös*, *Applied Animal Behavior*, and *Society and Animals*. Third, there was a search through all the reference sections of all retrieved articles for additional studies. These search strategies resulted in the review of 250 studies, 49 of which met inclusion criteria and were submitted to meta-analytic procedures.

> Studies were included if they a) reported on AAT and not AAA or pet ownership, b) included at least five participants in a treatment group, c) were written in English, and d) provided sufficient data to compute an effect size.
>
> (Nimer and Lundahl, 2007, p. 227)

The overall results determined that:

> AAT was associated with moderate effect sizes in improving outcomes in four areas: Autism-spectrum symptoms, medical difficulties, behavioral problems, and emotional well-being. Contrary to expectations, characteristics of participants and studies did not produce differential outcomes.
>
> (Nimer and Lundahl, 2007, p. 225)

The researchers concluded:

> AAT shows promise as an additive to established interventions and future research should investigate the conditions under which AAT can be most helpful.
>
> (Nimer and Lundahl, 2007, p. 225)

DOI: 10.4324/9781003260448-2

BIOPHILIA CONSTRUCT OF HUMAN INTEREST IN ANIMALS AND NATURE

The concept of biophilia is frequently used to provide at least a partial explanation of the beneficial effects associated with human–animal interaction. In his book, Wilson (1984) described biophilia as humans' "innate tendency to focus on life and lifelike processes" (p. 1). Wilson states,

> I will make the case that to explore and affiliate with life is a deep and complicated process in mental development. To an extent still undervalued in philosophy and religion, our existence depends on this propensity, our spirit is woven from it, hope rises from its currents . . . . The conclusion I draw is optimistic: to the degree that we come to understand other organisms, we will place a greater value on them, and ourselves.
>
> (Wilson, 1984, pp. 1–2)

The innate tendency of humans to be drawn to explore and understand nature and animals suggests why and how animal-assisted therapy can be effective in counseling and psychotherapy. Biophilia construct may explain enhanced motivation to participate in treatment as well as the comforting tendencies of animal-assisted therapy for clients.

BIOPSYCHOSOCIAL THEORY OF THE HEALTH BENEFITS OF HUMAN–ANIMAL INTERACTION

The biopsychosocial theory addresses the impact on human health of biological, psychological, and social factors (Engel, 1980). This theory has been used by some to explain the positive impact of human–animal interaction, such as humans and companion animals. Biological influences include effects on heart rate, blood pressure, endocrinology, and so forth. Psychological influences include mood, personality, and emotions. Social influences relate to social relationships, relational dynamics, culture, and so on. Following a review of related literature, Gee et al. (2021) concluded that the biopsychosocial model is appropriately applied to human–animal interaction research and an affective avenue to promote future theoretically grounded research in the field. They proposed that "the psychological, biological, and social domains can be used to elucidate the mechanisms that both impact and are impacted by interactions between humans and animals" (p. 8).

PSYCHOPHYSIOLOGICAL HEALTH

Psychophysiological health can be enhanced by positive human–animal interactions. Odendaal (2000) measured significant changes in blood plasma levels of various neurochemicals after subjects engaged in a positive interaction with an unfamiliar dog. Neurochemicals associated with a decrease in blood pressure increased; in humans and dogs, endorphin, oxytocin, prolactin, phenylectic acid, and dopamine levels increased significantly. Cortisol, a hormone associated with increased stress levels, decreased significantly in humans, but in dogs the decrease was nonsignificant. This nonsignificant result might be because the dogs found the novel situation initially very exciting. As Odendaal (2000) states:

> The results of this experiment support the theory of attentionis egens in human–dog affiliation. Once the physiology is known, i.e., the role that neurochemicals and

hormones might play during positive interaction, it is possible to use this information as a rationale for using animals in animal-assisted therapy.

(p. 279)

From the results, Odendaal (2000) drew these conclusions:

- The greatest psychophysiological benefit of the human–animal interaction occurred between 5 and 24 minutes after the start of the interaction, and thus interactions shorter or longer than this may offer no additional benefit.
- "(A)ttentionis egens needs (affiliation behavior, positive interaction) are described on the neurochemical level and on an interspecies basis . . . The dog experiences the same physiological effects as the patient" (p. 279).
- Neurochemical changes occurred that are associated with decreases in blood pressure; thus, if biochemistry measures are not available for a future study, the much simpler blood pressure measure could be a valid indicator of whether the interaction has the desired physiological effects.
- The six neurochemical changes measured in this study can be used as a profile for affiliative behavior.
- The physiological parameters "are regarded as effects of a complex biological interaction, and in a sense, the physiological changes are results of the phenomenon of human–dog interaction" (p. 279).

Odendaal and Meintjes (2003) discovered that concentrations of beta-endorphin, oxytocin, prolactin, beta-phenylethylamine, and dopamine increased in both dogs and humans after positive interspecies interaction, while that of cortisol decreased in the humans only. The researchers speculated that indicators of mutual physiological changes during positive interaction between dog lovers and dogs may contribute to a better understanding of the human–animal bond.

Barker et al. (2010) explored the stress-buffering response patterns from interaction with a therapy dog. Participants in group one were five dog owners interacting with their own therapy dog and in group two were five dog owners interacting with an unfamiliar therapy dog under similar conditions. Following a 30-minute baseline period, participants completed a stress task followed by a 30-minute dog interaction and then watched a neutral video for 60 minutes. The outcome variable was the biobehavioral stress response, measured by systolic and diastolic blood pressure, heart rate, salivary cortisol, salivary alpha-amylase, and self-report. Results showed moderate increases with the stressor and decreases from baseline following the animal interaction for salivary cortisol, systolic and diastolic blood pressure, heart rate, and self-reported anxiety. Both groups showed physiological benefits from interacting with a therapy dog, their own or the unfamiliar dog. Although the participants interacting with their own therapy dog tended to perceive less stress and anxiety during the intervention than those visiting with the unfamiliar therapy dog, greater reductions in physiological measures were observed in the group visiting with the unfamiliar therapy dog (Barker et al., 2010).

Cole et al. (2007) examined the benefits of AAT visits in patients hospitalized with heart failure. A total of 76 patients were randomly assigned to one of three groups: the treatment group received a 12-minute visit from a volunteer with a therapy dog; the comparison group received a 12-minute visit from a volunteer (with no dog); and the control group received usual care (at rest). Specific guidelines were given to volunteers for the therapy dog visit that included introducing self and dog, patient hand washing before and after the visit, having the dog lie on the patient's bed on a clean sheet barrier, and inviting the patient to pet and talk with the dog and volunteer. No attempt was made to control the content of the conversation during the visit. Data were collected at baseline, at 8 minutes, and at 16 minutes. Compared with controls, the volunteer-dog group had significantly greater decreases in systolic pulmonary artery pressure and in pulmonary capillary wedge pressure during and after the intervention. Compared with the volunteer-only group, the volunteer-dog group had significantly greater decreases in epinephrine levels and in norepinephrine levels during and after the intervention. After the intervention, the volunteer-dog group had the greatest decrease from baseline in state anxiety sum score on the Spielberger State-Trait Anxiety Inventory compared with the volunteer-only and the control groups. The researchers concluded that AAT improves cardiopulmonary pressures, neurohormone levels, and anxiety in patients hospitalized with heart failure (Cole et al., 2007).

Friedmann et al. (2007) investigated the impact of the presence of a friendly dog on cardiovascular response to speech in cognitively intact, older hypertensives. The conditions were: sitting silently without the dog; talking; sitting silently again with no dog; and sitting quietly with a dog present. Each session was 2 minutes in length, and the order of sessions with and without the dog were randomized. The results showed that during speech, blood pressure was lower when the dog was present than when it was not present. Blood pressure while sitting quietly did not differ according to the presence of a dog. The researchers concluded that pets might provide a viable means of decreasing blood pressure surges during stressful activities in older hypertensives (Friedmann et al., 2007).

Barker et al. (2005) investigated the optimal time for measuring stress and immune function in 20 healthcare professionals following interaction with a therapy dog for 5 and 20 minutes. Serum cortisol, epinephrine, and norepinephrine were collected at baseline, and at 5, 15, 30, 45, and 60 minutes post-condition. Salivary cortisol and blood for lymphocytes were collected at baseline, and at 30, 45, and 60 minutes post condition. Analysis indicated significant reductions in serum and salivary cortisol. The optimal time for measuring was 45 minutes post condition. Results also indicated that participants benefited from interaction with a therapy dog within 5 minutes of interaction (Barker et al., 2005).

Wu et al. (2002) evaluated the effectiveness of a pet visitation program in helping 30 children (10 girls and 20 boys) and their families (28 mothers and 17 fathers) adjust to hospitalization on a pediatric cardiology ward. A total of 31 pet visits were observed and followed by interviews with patients and parents. The dogs and their handlers were already participants in the hospital's Pets at Work Program. The dogs in the program had been previously trained to come and sit still on command, to fetch a small thrown toy, to climb onto beds and chairs only on command, to remain calm and relaxed in the presence of several human beings, and not to bark or bite under any circumstance. Three dogs were used in the project: Blue, a 9-year-old Golden Retriever; Bertie, a 7-year-old Shih Tzu; and Gioia, a 7-year-old mixed breed. The dogs would visit in pairs, an arrangement that allowed for flexibility and variety for patients and their parents. For the visitation, dogs were brought to visit patients and their families privately in their rooms once a week. During the visit, both the patient and parent were free to interact creatively with the dogs in any manner they wished under the supervision of the trained dog handler.

To assess milieu impact, the patients and parents were asked to describe what they thought and felt about the hospital environment and what kind of impact the pet visit had on these opinions and feelings, if any. They were then asked to choose which of five levels, 1 (low) to 5 (high), most accurately described how the pet visit affected their perception of the hospital milieu. Patient and parent satisfaction with the pet visitation program was also assessed. Both patients and parents were asked whether they felt that they benefited from the visitations and, if so, to identify in which way they felt they gained the most benefit. Physiologic parameters were gathered from monitors already connected to the patient, and these measures included beginning and ending notations of heart rate, respiratory rate, and oxygen saturation. Significant positive differences were found in comparing beginning and ending physiologic measures of respiratory and heart rates. Regarding results for activity, rapport, and feelings, all 30 children had interactions with the dogs that included physical contact (observed activity levels of 3, 4, and 5); 24 established rapport that was observed to be at positive levels (levels 3 and 4); and 26 children reported positive feelings generated by and during the pet visitations (levels 4 and 5). A significant correlation was found between level of rapport and the degree of positive feelings reported by the patients.

Further, an even stronger significant correlation was found between level of activity and the establishment of rapport and the generation of positive feelings. Regarding results for milieu impact, 35 percent of the children and 48 percent of the parents reported that the presence of the dogs helped normalize their hospitalization experience, and 61 percent of the children and 40 percent of their parents thought that the pet visitations were a pleasant distraction from the reality of hospitalization. Regarding benefits and satisfaction, most patients (73 percent) considered relief the most important benefit of the pet visits, 19 percent chose the giving of unconditional love, and the remaining 8 percent said it was the motivation to get better or to stay optimistic. Among the parents, 52 percent identified relief as the most important benefit, 16 percent said it was the giving and receiving of unconditional love, 16 percent felt that they personally received no benefit, 12 percent felt that the most important benefit was the facilitation of social interaction, and 4 percent identified having the pet as an object for the projection of feelings was the most important benefit. From their analysis of all of the data, the researchers concluded that the pet visits relieved stress, normalized the hospital milieu, and improved patient and parent morale. Also, the benefit received by the participants correlated with the amount of physical contact and rapport developed with the visiting animal (Wu et al., 2002).

Coakley and Mahoney (2009) utilized a single group pre-, post-, quasi-experimental design with mixed methods to evaluate the effect of an existing pet therapy program on hospitalized patient outcomes and experience. A convenience sample of 61 patients, 18 years of age and over, was recruited for the study. Physiologic measures such as vital signs, including blood pressure, pulse, and respirations were used as noninvasive indices of physiological stress. Pain and energy level were measured using separate visual analog scales (VAS) rating pain or energy from "0" (none) to "10" (as much as possible). Mood was measured with the Profile of Mood States survey (POMS) (McNair, Lorr, and Droppleman, 1992), which is a self-report assessment using a Likert scale of 1 to 5 to rate six transient mood states: tension-anxiety, depression-dejection, anger-hostility, vigor-activity, fatigue-inertia, and confusion-bewilderment.

Immediately prior to the visit with the dog, the research nurse collected baseline measures of vital signs, and pain and energy VAS levels at the bedside, and all participants completed the short version POMS. The research nurse waited outside the room as the volunteer handler and the dog entered the room. After the handler and dog left the room, the research nurses returned to obtain post-visit measures of vital signs, pain and energy VAS, and POMS immediately following the intervention. Additionally, all subjects were asked to answer predetermined open-ended questions about their perception of the pet therapy experience. For the pet therapy intervention, the volunteers introduced themselves to the patient and then the pet therapy intervention was conducted in an individualized manner within the standard protocol based on patient preference. Some patients preferred to talk with the handler about the dog, their own dogs, or other pets from their childhood. Other patients wished to visit quietly with the dog while the handler stood nearby. The pet therapy interventions lasted an average of 10 minutes with each subject. Results of data analysis showed that, compared with baseline, patients had significant decreases in pain, respiratory rate, and negative mood state and a significant increase in perceived energy level. Researchers concluded that the quantitative and qualitative findings provide support for decreased tension/anxiety and fatigue/inertia, and improved overall mood in hospitalized patients after visiting with a therapy dog (Coakley and Mahoney, 2009).

Kaminski, Pellino, and Wish (2002) compared AAT with play therapy for hospitalized children. Five variables were tested: (1) mood (child self-report); (2) mood (parent report); (3) affect (assessed by a video recording observation panel); (4) stress levels (measured by salivary cortisol levels); and (5) physiology (heart rate and blood pressure). They found that affect and happy mood were greater in the children during AAT than play therapy, and that heart rate was higher in AAT, most likely due to anticipatory excitement of being with the animals (Kaminski, Pellino, and Wish, 2002).

Sobo, Eng, and Kassity-Krich (2006) investigated the effectiveness of canine visitation therapy (CVT) in pediatric pain management in a children's hospital. A convenience sample of 25 English-speaking children ages 5 to 18 years who underwent surgery and experienced acute postoperative pain participated in a standard, one-time CVT intervention. All children completed a pre–post survey and a postintervention interview. The therapy dog was a 9-year-old West Highland white Terrier female named Lizzy. She and her handler had both been registered with Delta Society. In the CVT intervention patients decided what level of interaction (passive, low, high) they preferred. In passive interaction, the dog would sit or lie quietly with the children; in low, the dog would do an occasional pet trick; in high, there was active play and going for walks with the children.

Paired *t*-tests were used to examine the significance of before and after differences on the pre–post assessments. Despite the small sample size, significant differences were found for both physical and emotional pain, meaning the children perceived significantly reduced pain after the CVT intervention. From the postintervention interviews, eight themes were identified: (1) the dog provided "distraction" from the pain or situation; (2) the dog brought "pleasure/happiness"; (3) the dog was "fun/entertaining" (for active CVT); (4) the dog reminded the children of "home"; (5) the children enjoyed "snuggling/contact" with the dog; (6) the dog provided "company"; (7) the dog was "calming"; and (8) and the dog "eased pain." The researchers concluded that CVT may be a useful adjunct to traditional pain management for children and that nurses may better serve their patients when CVT is an option (Sobo, Eng, and Kassity-Krich, 2006).

DeCourcey, Russell, and Keister (2010) evaluated five previous studies on AAT in healthcare settings:

- Baun et al. (1984)
- Cole et al. (2007)
- Kaminski et al. (2002)
- Sobo et al. (2006)
- Wu et al. (2002).

From their evaluation of these studies, DeCourcey, Russell, and Keister (2010) concluded that:

animal-assisted therapy is invaluable on a critical care unit, as it enables the nurse to affordably treat the patient's body in a holistic manner, and may be the only available complementary therapy to offer therapeutic touch to socially and emotionally isolated people . . . AAT provides several physiological and emotional benefits for many people.

Animals offer a unique kind of support and unconditional love that human companions often cannot. They offer comfort on demand, in a quantity tailored to the patient's need, without bargaining or expectations of gaining something in return.

(p. 213)

ANXIETY AND DISTRESS

Barker and Dawson (1998) reported a successful use of a single AAT session in the reduction of anxiety with hospitalized psychiatric patients with psychotic disorders, mood disorders, and other disorders. A comparison group, a single session of therapeutic recreation, experienced a reduction in anxiety only for patients with mood disorders. Thus, AAT was determined to be effective in the reduction of state anxiety levels for psychiatric patients with a variety of psychiatric diagnoses.

The presence of a qualified therapy dog, a 9-year-old Golden Retriever, was found to significantly alleviate distress in children undergoing a standard pediatric physical examination (Hansen et al., 1999). A total of 34 children aged 2 to 6 years participated in the study. A two-group repeated-measures design was used to examine rating scores of videotaped sessions using the Observation Scale of Behavioral Distress. Although distress scores increased for both groups over time regardless of the dog's presence, when the dog was in the examination room fewer behaviors indicative of distress were exhibited, so these children had significantly lower distress scores.

Tsai, Friedmann, and Thomas (2010) examined the effects of AAT on cardiovascular responses, state anxiety, and medical fear in hospitalized children using a quasi-experimental, repeated-measures design with two intervention conditions: an AAT group and a comparison group. Participants were eight girls and seven boys, aged 7 to 17 years. The comparison condition was a research assistant completing an age-appropriate puzzle with each child for 6 to 10 minutes. The AAT condition was a 6- to 10-minute social visit with a therapy dog where the children were allowed to pet, touch, and brush the dog. Both conditions took place in the children's hospital room. Each child participated once in each of the two intervention conditions that were presented on 2 consecutive days with the order of presentation of each condition alternated between participants. Participants' systolic blood pressure (SBP), diastolic blood pressure (DBP), and heart rate (HR) were measured 18 times: three pre-, during, and post-visit measurements for each condition. State anxiety and medical fear were measured after each visit. The Child Medical Fear Scale (CMFS) (Broome et al., 1992) was used to measure medical fear. Level of state anxiety was measured by the State-Anxiety scale of the State-Trait Anxiety Inventory for Children (Spielberger, 1970). Repeated-measure analysis of variances (ANOVAs) was used for data analysis. In AAT, SBP decreased throughout—before, during, and after the intervention. The decreases in SBP after AAT continued after the intervention was over. In contrast, SBP decreased from before to during the comparison intervention, but then increased from during to after the comparison intervention. Children's anxiety and medical fear measures did not differ after the AAT visit compared with the comparison intervention. The researchers suggested that this exploratory study indicated that AAT can decrease physiological arousal in hospitalized children and therefore may be useful in helping them cope better in a hospital setting (Tsai, Friedmann, and Thomas, 2010).

Tahan and collegues (2022) assessed the effectiveness of animal-assisted therapy on alleviation of anxiety in pre-school children. A total of 20 children (ages 5–7 years) with above average anxiety levels participated. The study was carried out as a randomized controlled trial with pre-test and post-test design with treatment ($n = 10$) and control groups ($n = 10$).

The treatment group received eight sessions of AAT. Sessions included introduction of the animals, sharing information about feeding and care of the animals, playing with the animals, washing and feeding the animals. The results showed that AAT had a significant effect on general anxiety after adjusting for post-test assessments ($f = 32.49$ and $p = 0.001$) with the effect equal to 0.70. Additionally, the effect of AAT on anxiety of separation ($f = 5.63$, $p = 0.03$), generalized anxiety disorder ($f = 8.56$, $p = 0.01$), social phobia ($f = 14.58$, $p = 0.002$) and specific anxiety ($f = 11.63$, $p = 0.005$) was significant with effects equal to 0.30, 0.40, 0.53, and 0.47, respectively. Researchers concluded AAT was effective in alleviating anxiety in preschool children and suggested these results support the inclusion of AAT in therapeutic practice with children having anxiety (Tahan et al., 2022).

Adamle, Riley, and Carlson (2009) investigated the perceived potential benefits of pet therapy visitation as a social support to help relieve stress in college freshmen. College freshmen participants ($n = 246$) completed a questionnaire followed by a 20-minute presentation about pet therapy that ended with a pet therapy visitation by six dogs and their six handlers. Approximately 50 participants were in each session. During the pet therapy visitation, the six pet therapy teams mingled among the participants so participants could have physical contact with the therapy dogs. The Pet Therapy Program Questionnaire was developed for the purpose of this study and included 13 questions designed to elicit information about (1) having a family pet or perceived value of pets, (2) previous knowledge of pet therapy programs, (3) their opinions about receiving a visit from pet therapy teams while living on the college campus, and (4) any perceived benefits after receiving a visit from pet therapy teams. Of the participants who had pets at home, a majority considered them an integral part of their lives (92.5 percent, $n = 221$) and indicated receiving support and comfort during stressful times when interacting with their pets (90.3 percent, $n = 214$). Some of the participants had previous knowledge of pet therapy programs (41 percent, $n = 100$), and of those who had heard about pet therapy the majority also reported some experience with pet therapy ($n = 84$). A large majority of participants (96 percent, $n = 239$) expressed positive student interest in the possibility of introducing a pet therapy program on their campus (Adamle, Riley, and Carlson, 2009).

McCullough and colleagues (2018) demonstrated the effects of animal-assisted intervention in the reduction of anxiety in child oncology patients and reduced stress for their parents. They used a multicenter, parallel-group, randomized trial design. Data was collected on patients ages 3 to 17 years, over a 4-month course of treatment. Children received visits from a handler-therapy dog team that lasted 10–20 minutes. Therapy dog sessions were not structured to allow for the handler team and parents to decide what type of interaction would be most appropriate for each child. The researchers concluded that animal-assisted interventions provide certain benefits for parents and children during the initial stages of cancer treatment (McCullough et al., 2018).

Coto et al. (2022) performed a correlational study exploring nurse work anxiety and animal-assisted therapy. Animal-assisted therapy interventions were performed for both day and night shifts. Beck's Anxiety Inventory (BAI) tool was used pre and post intervention. Each nurse interacted with the therapy dog for at least 10 minutes. Pet-assisted therapy as an intervention for nurses during work reduced work-related anxiety ($t = 5.878$, $P < 0.05$). A Pearson's correlational study displayed a strong positive correlation between the animal-assisted therapy and reduction in BAI scores ($r = 0.7717$, $R^2 = 0.5955$). The researchers concluded the study results show that nurse work anxiety significantly decreased during worked hours of active bedside care when the nurses actively engaged with a therapy dog (Coto et al., 2022).

Anderson and colleagues (2021) evaluated the influence of dogs in decreasing student anxiety at a nursing program prior to a medication dosage calculation exam. This study used a convenience sample that randomly assigned to a control and intervention group with a pre-pre, pre, post and post-post-test using the Spielberger State-Trait Anxiety Inventory. The intervention group experienced a brief therapy dog intervention prior to the medication dosage calculation exam. Using a repeated measures one-way MANOVA (multivariate analysis of variance), there was a statistically significant difference between the intervention and the control groups: Wilks' $\Lambda = 0.761$, $F(8, 79) = 3.103$, p < 0.01. The results reflect that a brief interaction with therapy dogs prior to a medication calculation exam decreased anxiety in a convenience sample of nursing students. The researchers concluded the study adds empirical knowledge to the field of animal-assisted therapy and nursing student anxiety-coping methods (Anderson et al., 2021).

In a two-part systematic review of literature (Holder et al., 2020a, 2020b), AAIs were shown to reduce stress and anxiety and provide a distraction from pain and distress in oncology patients, and to relieve stress in family members and medical staff. Cognitive stress relief from positive social interaction with a therapy animal and neuroendocrine mood enhancement from nuturing physical touch of the animal were believed to be primary mechanisms for positive impact of AAIs in oncology (Holder et al., 2020a, 2020b).

Gee and colleagues (2019) examined how observing live fish improves perceptions of mood, relaxation, and anxiety, but does not consistently alter heart rate or heart rate variability. Data were collected and used from 35 undergraduate students (31 female, 3 male, and 1 gender nonidentified) currently enrolled in a state university. In two separate experiments, participants were asked to watch identically equipped fish tanks for 5 minutes in each of three conditions: (1) live fish, (2) plants and water, and (3) empty tank. Linear mixed models used across both experiments revealed similar results: greater perceptions of relaxation and mood, and less anxiety during or after viewing the live fish condition, compared with the other conditions.

DEMENTIA

A "pets as therapy" program was found to be beneficial with persons with dementia in a psychiatric ward (Walsh et al., 1995). Seven participants who were over 65 years of age and who were diagnosed as having some form of dementia, usually of the Alzheimer's type, served as the experimental group. The study was conducted over a 12-week period. The intervention involved an equal amount of supervised visitation time for each subject over a 3-hour period twice per week. The pet therapist was a trained public relations Labrador for the Guide Dog Association that was very experienced with people, of a quiet temperament, and not likely to become excited. The handler was a qualified obedience instructor of 8 years who owned and trained the dog. Measures included ratings on the London Psycho-Geriatric Rating Scale (LPRS; for the measurement of mental disorganization or confusion), the Brighton Clinic Adaptive Behaviour Scale (BCABS; to assess daily functioning), diastolic blood pressure, heart rate, and ward noise levels. Results indicated significant experimental group changes in reduction in heart rate and a substantial drop in noise levels during the presence of the dog. No significant differences in pre- and post-test comparisons between the experimental and control group were found on the LPRS or the BCABS. Although no significant differences were found between the experimental and control group in blood pressure change, there was a slight drop in mean diastolic blood pressure for the experimental group (Walsh et al., 1995).

The presence of a therapy dog visiting with residents at three long-term care facilities increased socialization for participants with Alzheimer's disease (Batson et al., 1998). The mean age of participants was 77.9 years. The therapy animal was a miniature Schnauzer certified as a therapy dog. Patients participated in 10-minute sessions on two different days: one day with the dog present and one day without the dog present. The conditions were randomly presented based on a random numbers table. Sessions were videotaped for later coding. Dependent *t*-tests analysis revealed significant increases when the dog was present for the following socialization variables: smiles, tactile contact, looks, physical warmth, praise, and duration of leans toward. The researchers also examined several physiological parameters, but no significant difference was found for blood pressure, pulse, or peripheral skin temperature (Batson et al., 1998).

Greer et al. (2001) performed research to compare the effects of toy cats versus live cats as stimuli for verbal communication in six female elderly nursing home residents with moderate dementia of the Alzheimer's type. Verbal communication was analyzed for three measurements: total number of words, meaningful information units, and initiations. Measurements were recorded for three conditions: without stimuli, in the presence of two toy cats, and in the presence of two live cats. Each condition consisted of three 10-minute phases (total of 30 minutes per condition) during which participants were videotaped. Results indicated that live cats had the greatest influence on average subject performance across all three measurements (Greer et al., 2001).

In a study performed in Italy by Mossello et al. (2011), ten patients attending an Alzheimer Day Care Center participated in a repeated measures study, which included: 2 weeks' pre-intervention, 3 weeks' control activity with plush dogs, and 3 weeks' AAA. The AAA operator and the two dogs used for the intervention (one 15-month-old male Poodle, and one 3-year-old female Golden Retriever) were highly experienced in AAA and AAT. Both AAA and the control activity were provided to the whole group for approximately 100 minutes three times a week, from 10 a.m. to about 12 noon. The results showed that AAA was associated with a decrease in anxiety and sadness and an increase in positive emotions and motor activity in comparison with a control activity (Mossello et al., 2011).

Nordgren and Engström (2014) evaluated the effects of an AAI program on the quality of life of persons with dementia in four Swedish nursing homes. Participants were 12 women and eight men between the ages of 58 and 88 years; but only nine people completed the intervention. The AAI was ten training sessions, 45 to 60 minutes in length, once or twice per week, with a certified therapy dog team. Target behaviors addressed were cognitive, physical, and psychosocial and were documented and evaluated by the therapy dog team and by an occupational therapist who set the goals. A pre–post-test measure design was incorporated using the Swedish version of the Quality of Life in Late-Stage Dementia (QUALID). Results of the study showed that quality of life improved for participants after the AAI (Nordgren and Engström, 2014).

Tournier, Vives, and Postal (2017) assessed the efficacy of an animal-assisted therapy (AAT) program in the reduction of neuropsychiatric symptoms in older adults with medium to severe dementia. The study was performed in an Alzheimer's disease/dementia care unit. The intervention included 11 elderly residents aged 71 to 93 years (mean age = 82.91 years; mean Mini-Mental State Examination score = 7.8/30). Behaviors during the AAT sessions as well as pre/post intervention neuropsychiatric symptoms were examined during this 5-month weekly intervention conducted by an AAT-certified psychologist along with her dog. It was determined AAT had a positive effect on total score and caregiver distress score for several neuropsychiatric symptoms (i.e., delusion, depression, disinhibition, euphoria, and aberrant motor activity). Moreover, the ratings of the various behaviors during each session suggested that the beneficial effects of AAT appeared during the first few sessions. The researchers concluded the results supported the notion that regular and long-term AAT sessions were an effective alternative to pharmacological interventions for the reduction of neuropsychiatric symptoms (Tournier, Vives, and Postal, 2017, p. 51).

DEPRESSION

Souter and Miller (2007) conducted a meta-analysis to determine the effectiveness of AAA and AAT for reducing depressive symptoms in humans. Criteria for inclusion required studies to demonstrate random assignment, to include a comparison or control group, to use AAA or AAT, to use a self-report measure of depression, and to report sufficient information to calculate effect sizes, a statistical standardization of the strength of a treatment effect. Five studies were identified for analysis: Brickel (1984), Struckus (1989), McVarish (1995), Wall (1994), and Panzer-Koplow (2000). Following analysis, the researchers concluded that the aggregate effect size for these studies was of medium magnitude and statistically significant, indicating that AAA and AAT are associated with fewer depressive symptoms (Souter and Miller, 2007).

McFalls-Steger, Patterson, and Thompson (2021) conducted a systematic review of animal-assisted interventions in treatment of adults with depressive symptoms in articles published from 2010 to 2020. Only journal articles that used an empirically established depression evaluation tool were chosen for review. A total of ten articles met the criteria for review. The researchers discovered that results were moderately favorable, with statistically significant effect on outcomes in most studies.

Exposure to an aviary was reported to be effective in reducing depression in elderly males at a veteran's hospital (Holcomb et al., 1997). The aviary was $10 \times 8 \times 4$ feet and contained 20 songbirds representing about 10 different breeds. The walls of the aviary were Plexiglas to allow for easy viewing. It was well lit and clearly visible from any point in the activity room. A video camera taped interactions of hospital residents with the aviary, and judges viewed and rated the videotaped interactions on a six-point scale. Interactions rated included length of time focused on the aviary, intensity of aviary observation, ignoring the aviary, glancing at the aviary, talking to the birds, and talking with others about the birds. Statistical covariance analysis demonstrated a significant relationship between improvements in depression, as measured by the Geriatric Depression Index, and greater use of the aviary (Holcomb et al., 1997).

AAT with a therapy dog was shown to be effective in reducing depression in adult college students (Folse et al., 1994). Students were selected for participation based on their scores on the Beck Depression Inventory (BDI) and placed into one of three groups: AAT with directive group psychotherapy; nondirective group AAT without psychotherapy; and a control group. The greatest differences were discovered between the AAT-only group and the control group, with BDI scores reducing significantly for the AAT-only group. Nonsignificant mixed results were found between the AAT psychotherapy group and the control group. It was thought that the nondirective interactions with the therapy dog in the AAT-only group uplifted the mood of the group members, whereas the directive psychotherapy with AAT focused clients on painful issues and thus mediated the results of this combined therapy approach. It is important to note that six out of the nine participants in the AAT and psychotherapy combined group did show reductions in BDI scores (Folse et al., 1994). However, the statistics applied to the study compared the statistical significance of pre- and post-test scores and failed to investigate the possibility of clinical significance or effect size. It is possible that, if it had been used, the more sensitive effect-size statistic may have demonstrated some clinically significant impact for the AAT and psychotherapy combined group.

The positive effects of pet-facilitated therapy to impact depression seem to be based on more than just an opportunity for patients to socialize in the presence of novel stimuli. McVarish (1995) demonstrated that patients shown photographs of pets did not show the decrease in depression that patients did who interacted briefly with an animal. Participants consisted of 74 inpatients recruited from two psychiatric hospitals. The photograph group included one 40-minute visit with trained volunteers who shared 250 photographs of pets. The pet therapy group consisted of one 40-minute visit of the same trained volunteers who introduced dogs and kittens to the group. It was found that (1) the pet-facilitated therapy group showed a significantly greater decrease in depressive symptoms than inpatients who received the animal photograph session, and (2) the animal photograph group showed a significantly greater decrease in depressive symptoms than inpatients who did not receive any treatment as evidenced by a decrease in total mean scores of the BDI and the Brief Psychiatric Rating Scale. Thus, although social visitation that centers on novel inanimate stimuli (animal photographs) does seem to positively impact depression, what is most important is that social visitation that centers on the presentation of animals has a significantly greater positive effect (McVarish, 1995).

Sockalingam et al. (2008) describe a single-case study of an AAI to treat the depression of a 43-year-old single male with disability. The patient had a history of bipolar affective disorder and had been stabilized on lithium for more than 6 years. Following an assault, the patient became depressed and sought additional treatment:

> [He] presented with an atypical depression consisting of low mood, hopelessness, persistent tearfulness, rejection sensitivity, reduced spontaneous speech, worsening of self-esteem, and significant lack of motivation. He also was experiencing significant residual anxiety related to his assault and demonstrated psychomotor agitation, irritability, insomnia, and difficulty concentrating and settling. He did not meet criteria for mania, nor did he have psychotic symptoms.
>
> (Sockalingam et al., 2008, p. 77)

The medication the patient was taking included the mood stabilizer lithium (900 mg daily), which was augmented with desipramine (200 mg daily), but with no significant response. The treatment team included a trial of pet therapy that was thought to add some benefit to the patient's treatment. The patient spent several hours a day with a therapy dog named Ruby, a Golden Retriever, over a 3-week period in the treatment facility. The time with Ruby was relatively unstructured, but the patient was instructed to care for the therapy dog, including taking her for walks. Emphasis was placed on the idea that Ruby was the patient's responsibility during their time together at the facility. The treatment team concluded that this pet therapy resulted in improvement in the patient,

> over a multitude of areas, including improved mood, improved outlook on life, and increased spontaneous speech. He displayed decreased anxiety and psychomotor agitation and had improvements in quality of sleep and ability to concentrate .... The patient developed increased self-esteem [and] reported improvements in physical health and wellbeing as a result of the extra exercise he obtained from walking the dog. His social isolation from women decreased as the dog helped him attract female attention. His overall self-control was now a focus as he realized that the dog was dependent upon him during their interactions.
>
> (Sockalingam et al., 2008, p. 78)

Even with these many improvements, the patient still exhibited a lack of confidence that contributed to discharge-related difficulties: he was unable to search for an apartment, contact old friends, obtain his possessions, and perform daily duties without other people present. Thus, the treatment team decided to incorporate Ruby into this aspect of the patient's treatment. Through the benefits of AAT the patient then,

accomplished these tasks with improved confidence and motivation, enhanced decision making ability, and less dependence on others for approval and reassurance. He
was then discharged and was scheduled to receive follow-up care from his previous
outpatient psychiatrist and intermittent social visits, during which he would spend
time with Ruby, over the next year.

(Sockalingam et al., 2008, p. 79)

The researchers concluded that this clinical case study demonstrated the effectiveness of
AAT in the psychiatric rehabilitation of an assault victim with a concurrent mood disorder
(Sockalingam et al., 2008).

Pedersen et al. (2011) studied the effects on depression of working with farm animals in
Norway. Fourteen adults with clinical depression participated twice a week for 12 weeks in
a farm animal-assisted intervention consisting of work and contact with dairy cattle. Each
intervention lasted between 1.5 and 3 hours. Each participant was videotaped twice during the intervention and the recordings were categorized with respect to various work tasks
and animal and human contact. Assessments included the BDI (Beck and Steer, 1987), the
State-Trait Anxiety Inventory-State Subscale (STAI-SS; Spielberger, Gorsuch, and Lushene,
1983), and the Generalized Self-Efficacy Scale (GSE; Schwarzer and Jerusalem, 1995). The
researchers found that levels of anxiety and depression decreased and self-efficacy increased
during the intervention (Pedersen et al., 2011).

NEUROREHABILITATION

Künzi and colleagues (2022) examined the effects of animal-assisted psychotherapy incorporating mindfulness and self-compassion group intervention (MSCBI) with patients with
acquired brain injury utilizing a randomized controlled feasibility trial design. Patients were
randomly assigned to a 6-week intervention with ($n = 14$) or without animal assistance
($n = 17$). Psychological distress significantly decreased in both groups from pre- to follow-up
treatment with no difference between groups. However, patients in the animal-assisted
MSCBI group reported significantly higher increases in feeling secure, accepted, comforted,
grateful, motivated and at ease during the session compared with patients in the MSCBI
group without animal assistance. Adherence to sessions was significantly higher in the
animal-assisted MSCBI group.

Hediger and colleagues (2019) studied the effects of animal-assisted therapy on social
behavior in patients with acquired brain injury. The results of their randomized, controlled
trial design included examination of 222 AAT and 219 control sessions of 19 patients.
Patients showed a significantly higher amount of social behavior during AAT. Additionally, for AAT sessions, patients' positive emotions, verbal and nonverbal communication,
mood, treatment motivation, and satisfaction were increased. Researchers concluded that
AAT increased aspects of social competence and led to higher emotional involvement of
patients with acquired brain injury, reflected in higher social engagement, motivation, and
satisfaction during a therapy session.

WELLBEING

Binfet, Green, and Draper (2022) explored the importance of client–canine contact in
canine-assisted interventions to enhance wellbeing in 284 undergraduate college students.
The researchers used a randomized, controlled trial design to compare the effects of sessions
with positive touching of animals versus sessions where there was no touching of the animals.
Wellbeing of clients was reflected by measures for: flourishing, happiness, positive affect, and

social connectedness. Results indicated that participants across all conditions experienced enhanced wellbeing on several measures; however, only those in the direct canine contact condition reported significant improvements on all measures of wellbeing. Additionally, direct interactions with therapy dogs through touch elicited greater wellbeing benefits than did no touch/indirect interactions or interactions with only a dog handler.

Kivlen and colleagues (2022) examined canine-assisted intervention effects on the wellbeing of health science graduate students using a randomized controlled trial design. A total of 104 college student participants were randomly assigned to either the treatment ($n = 53$) or control ($n = 51$) condition. An analysis of covariance revealed that, compared with participants in the control condition, participants who interacted with therapy dogs had significantly higher self-reports of quality of life ($p < .001$) and decreased anxiety scores ($p < .045$). Within-subject paired t tests confirmed significant stress reductions for participants in the treatment condition ($p < .000$). No significant differences in self-reports of occupational performance or in adjustment to the graduate college student role were found. The researchers concluded that canine-assisted intervention may be a valuable tool for students and young adults experiencing mental health challenges such as stress, anxiety, and decreased quality of life.

A Pets as Therapy program was initiated in a women's prison in Australia to train companion dogs for the elderly and individuals with disabilities (Walsh and Mertin, 1994). The prisoners who participated in the program were rated as needing low security, and the dogs were kept in an area with this same rating for the dogs' safety. The inmates built kennels for the dogs and were responsible for the complete care and training of three dogs each, including dog grooming, dog obedience, and guide dog training. In addition, the women engaged in play and exercise activities with the dogs. Pre- and post-assessment score comparisons revealed significant improvement in the women participants of the AAT program on the Coopersmith Inventory (for measuring self-esteem) and the IPAT Depression Scale (Walsh and Mertin, 1994).

CHILDREN WITH DEVELOPMENTAL DISORDERS

AAT has been effective in helping children with developmental disorders. Redefer and Goodman (1989) have reported that a dog, when used as a component in therapy, can have a strong impact on the behavior of seriously withdrawn children. A repeated-measures analysis of variance of AAI with 12 children with autism demonstrated significant improvements in behaviors, with fewer autistic behaviors (e.g., hand posturing, humming and clicking noises, spinning objects, and repetitive jumping and roaming), and more socially appropriate behaviors (e.g., joining the therapist in games, initiating activities by giving the therapist balloons to blow up or balls to throw, reaching up for hugs, and frequently imitating the therapist's actions). Redefer and Goodman (1989) caution that it was not the mere presence of the dog that made the difference, but rather therapist-orchestrated child–dog and child–therapist interactions. The types of child–dog activities started with simple ones and gradually increased to more complex tasks over several sessions. Example activities were modeling and verbally encouraging approaching and exploring the dog through touching, holding, and petting activities; engaging the child to pet and touch the dog while identifying body parts; feeding; ball throwing; bubble blowing; and grooming.

In an attempt to determine if interaction with a live animal is more effective for children with pervasive developmental disorders than interaction with an inanimate object, a repeated-measures analysis of variance was used in a study of ten children to compare three conditions: (1) a nonsocial toy (ball); (2) a stuffed dog; and (3) a live therapy dog (Martin and Farnum, 2002). Researchers reported that when these children were in the presence of the live therapy dog, they exhibited a more playful mood, were more focused, and were more aware of their social environments.

Fung and Leung (2014) investigated the effects of interaction with a dog during play therapy for children (aged 7 to 10 years) with autism in Hong Kong. Researchers utilized a group-comparison design comparing two interventions: an experimental group, which was animal-assisted play therapy with a therapy dog; and a comparison group, with identical play therapy procedures using a doll as the dog surrogate. A total of ten participants were randomly assigned to either the experimental or comparison group. The magnitude in the increase of verbal social behavior in the experimental group increased significantly, but this increase was not significantly larger than in the comparison group. However, the researchers concluded that the interactions with the therapy dog in the experimental group suggested that the therapy dog had a positive impact on language output and that a therapy dog plays a positive role as a "speech elicitor" for children with autism (Fung and Leung, 2014, p. 253).

Grigore and Rusu (2014) explored the effects of a combination of two methods to enhance the social abilities of three children in Romania with autism—Social Story and AAT. The presence of the therapy dog while reading the social story increased the frequency of social initiations of the children with autism and decreased the level of social prompt needed to elicit social responses from these children.

Interactions with a therapy dog have been demonstrated to positively impact children with learning disabilities. A repeated-measures control group design was used to observe eight children (six girls and two boys) with Down syndrome (Limond, Bradshaw, and Cormack, 1997). The children's ages ranged from 7 to 12 years. The experimental session consisted of adult-supervised interaction with a real dog for a 7-minute period, while the control group consisted of adult-supervised interaction with a toy dog for the same length of time. Significant differences were found for the real-dog group over the imitation-dog group. Subjects in the real-dog interaction group showed more visual attending and verbal and nonverbal initiation and response behaviors. Thus, the real dog provided a more sustained focus for positive and cooperative interactions between both the children and the dog and the children and the adult (Limond, Bradshaw, and Cormack, 1997).

Sams, Fortney, and Willenbring (2006) demonstrated the efficacy of AAT incorporated with school-based occupational therapy for 22 children with autism between the ages of 7 and 13. Each child received one session of standard occupational therapy per week and one session of occupational therapy incorporating animals per week, over a period of 15 weeks. However, as a result of situational factors, such as school absences and school holidays, children varied in the number of sessions of therapy they received (between 2 and 12 sessions of each form of therapy). Yet the number of standard versus animal-assisted sessions was kept proportional for each child. The length of standard occupational therapy sessions was 26.3 minutes, and the average length of animal-assisted occupational therapy sessions was 28.5 minutes. Therapeutic activities for standard and animal-assisted sessions were geared toward facilitating sensory integration, language use, sensory skills, and motor skills. In the standard occupational therapy sessions, the techniques and tools included: teeter-totters and swings for proprioceptive and vestibular input; stretchy play clay, mechanical toys, sensory balls, creative artwork, and puzzles for sensory and motor skills development; and letter magnets for language training. In the animal-assisted occupational therapy sessions, the techniques and tools included: riding in wagons drawn by llamas, riding on the backs of llamas, and guiding llamas through an obstacle course including hoops and tunnels for proprioceptive and vestibular input; brushing and feeding llamas, petting or stroking dogs and rabbits, carding llama wool, throwing balls for dogs, and loading and unloading llamas for sensory input and motor skills development; and responding to and issuing directions in training llamas for competition, asking to interact with specific animals, and talking about animals for language training (Sams, Fortney, and Willenbring, 2006).

Research assistants observed children and recorded each instance of language use and social interaction on a behavioral rating form with categories for prompted or spontaneous, and subcategories for signing, sound, word, sentence, and interaction. A paired-sample *t*-test was used to analyze results and demonstrated that children engaged in greater use of language and significantly greater social interaction in the animal-assisted occupational therapy sessions than in the standard occupational therapy sessions. The researchers concluded that occupational therapy incorporating animals in the treatment of children with autism is an effective approach that warrants further study (Sams, Fortney, and Willenbring, 2006).

Prothmann, Ettrich, and Prothmann (2009) examined the preference for people, dogs, and objects displayed by children with autism. In this study, 14 children with autism (3 females and 11 males with a mean age of 11.4 years) participated. The children were observed when given the choice to interact with a person, a therapy dog, or objects (e.g., toys). The children did not know, or were not familiar with, any of the three stimuli prior to the study. The three stimuli were presented to each child simultaneously over a period of 20 minutes, during which time each participant was allowed to freely interact with the three stimuli. Each participant was tested three times. The researchers found that the children interacted most frequently and for longest with the dog, followed by the person, and then the objects. The researchers suggested,

> that animals, specifically dogs, communicate their intentions in a way more readily understandable to people with autism … [and that] autism affects predominantly interpersonal interactions.
>
> (Prothmann, Ettrich, and Prothmann, 2009, p. 161)

The finding of this study—that children on the spectrum for autism have a preference for a therapy dog over a person or an object (toy)—contributes to understanding why children with autism respond more favorably to therapy and educational activities that involve a therapy dog in comparison with these activities without a therapy dog present.

Schuck et al. (2015) performed a randomized clinical trial using a canine-assisted intervention with 24 children with attention deficit hyperactivity disorder (ADHD). Children were randomly assigned to cognitive-behavioral group therapy with or without canine-assisted intervention across 12 weeks. Both groups also participated in weekly group therapy sessions with parents. While parents reported improvements for children in both groups, the canine-assisted intervention group exhibited greater reductions in the severity of ADHD symptoms than children in the cognitive-behavioral therapy without canine-assisted interventions. Improvements were reported in children's social skills, prosocial behaviors, and problematic behaviors (Schuck et al., 2015).

Kršková, Talarovičová, and Olexová (2010) investigated the effects of a small therapeutic animal, a guinea pig, on the social behavior of nine autistic children (four girls and five boys, ranging in age from 6 to 13 years). The researchers compared the number and type of social contacts by the autistic children made with their acquaintances (1) when in the presence of an unfamiliar person, and (2) when in the presence of a guinea pig. The researchers found that when in the presence of the guinea pig the quantity and quality of the social contacts of the autistic children were significantly enhanced compared with when just in the presence of the comparison stimulus, the unfamiliar person (Kršková, Talarovičová, and Olexová, 2010).

Kern et al. (2011) performed a study to examine the effects of equine-assisted activities (EAA) on the overall severity of autism symptoms using the Childhood Autism Rating Scale

(CARS), and the quality of parent–child interactions using the Timberlawn Parent–Child Interaction Scale. Children with autism spectrum disorder were evaluated at four time points: (1) before beginning a 3–6 month waiting period, (2) before starting the riding treatment, and (3) after 3 months and (4) 6 months of riding. Twenty-four participants completed the waiting list period and began the riding program, and 20 participants completed the entire 6 months of riding. Pretreatment was compared with post-treatment, with each child acting as his or her own control. Results indicated a reduction in the severity of autism symptoms that occurred with the therapeutic riding treatment (Kern et al., 2011).

Lanning et al. (2014) used quality of life assessments to determine the behavioral changes of children diagnosed with autism spectrum disorder who participated in EAA. Ten children were in the EAA group and eight children were in a nonequine intervention comparison group. The EAA group participated in weekly 1-hour riding sessions for 12 weeks; the main focus was to improve riding and horsemanship skills.

> Parents noted significant improvements in their child's physical, emotional and social functioning following the first 6 weeks of EAA. The children participating in the non-equine program also demonstrated improvement in behavior, but to a lesser degree.
> (Lanning et al., 2014, p. 1897)

CHILDREN AND ADOLESCENTS WITH EMOTIONAL AND BEHAVIORAL PROBLEMS

Balluerka et al. (2014) studied the influence of AAT on the attachment representations of a group of adolescents in residential care who had suffered traumatic childhood experiences and exhibited mental health problems. Forty-six teenagers (between the ages of 12 and 17 years) participated; 21 in the treatment group and 25 in the control group. The AAT intervention took place at a farm over 12 weeks. The teenagers spent two consecutive days each week staying overnight at a "caserío" (a typical farm in the Basque region of northern Spain). The intervention consisted of 34 sessions in which group therapy (23 sessions) and individual therapy (11 sessions) were combined. A dog and nine horses (five adults and four colts) were used as therapy animals. Additionally, guided interactions were developed using cats and farm animals such as sheep, goats, chickens, and pigs. Animal-assisted psychotherapy and attachment-based psychotherapy models were considered in the design of the AAT intervention. The measurement instrument was a reduced version of the CaMir questionnaire for the evaluation of attachment. Results showed the teenagers displayed significantly more secure attachment after undergoing AAT (Balluerka et al., 2014).

Beetz et al. (2011) investigated whether boys (aged 7–12 years) with insecure/disorganized attachment would benefit more from the presence of a therapy dog, than from a friendly human or a toy dog, as social support during a stressful situation. Salivary cortisol in the boys was found to be significantly lower in the real dog condition than in the other two conditions. Thus, the presence of a therapy dog helped the boys manage their stress levels (Beetz et al., 2011).

A case study of AAT with two emotionally disturbed children was conducted using change measures: the ADD-H Comprehensive Teacher Rating Scale and direct observation, as well as video recordings of therapy sessions with the therapy dogs (Kogan et al., 1999). Each participant took part in weekly AAT sessions that were 45 to 60 minutes in duration. The AAT intervention sessions consisted of two main segments: rapport-building time and animal training time. Rapport-building time included brushing and petting the dog and child-initiated discussions with the dog's handler. Then the children worked with the dog and used a variety of commands and training techniques with the dog.

Improvements were demonstrated in most of the identified goal areas for the two children, including decreased negative comments, decreased self-talk related to the fantasy world, decreased distractibility, decreased learned helplessness, decreased pouting and tantrums, improved relationships with peers, and increased eye contact with other humans (Kogan et al., 1999).

Mallon (1994a) assessed the effects of visiting farm animals on children with behavior and emotional problems at the Green Chimneys Children's Services residential treatment facility. Qualitative findings indicated the children visited the farm animals with a high rate of frequency and went to see the farm animals more frequently when they were sad or angry because visiting the farm animals made them feel better (Mallon, 1994a).

Also, at the residential childcare program at the Green Chimneys Children's Services, Mallon (1994b) used a combination of quantitative and qualitative methods to examine the benefits and drawbacks of placing therapy dogs in residential dormitories with children who had conduct disorder. Methods entailed questionnaires, observations, and interviews. The results of the study revealed that the primary therapeutic benefits of this program were that the dogs provided the children with opportunities for love, companionship, and affection. Three primary drawbacks were also detected: (1) some of the children abused the dogs by hitting them; (2) caring for the dogs and cleaning up after them was labor intensive; and (3) not all of the therapeutic staff members were supportive of the program. Although concerns were expressed about placing the therapy dogs with the children, it was felt that the benefits to the children outweighed the difficulties. It was recommended that the program have greater supervision to prevent the abuse of the dogs. Also, staff members reported that they could have been more supportive if they had had greater input into the design of the program and more participation in interventions involving the dogs (Mallon, 1994b).

Heindl (1996) demonstrated how pet therapy could be useful as an intervention in a community-based children's day treatment program. A randomized control group pretest versus post-test design was used. Two separate one-way analyses of covariance were used to test for differences. The experimental group participated in a 1-hour-per-week pet therapy intervention for 6 weeks. No significant differences were found in self-concept, as measured by the Joseph Pre-School and Primary Self-Concept Screening Test. However, significant differences were found for behavior problems, as measured by the Woodcock–Johnson Scales of Independent Behavior: Problem Behaviors Scale, with a decrease in such behaviors being the result (Heindl, 1996).

The efficacy of equine-assisted counseling (EAC) was demonstrated with 164 elementary and middle school children at risk for academic and social failure (Trotter et al., 2008). This study compared EAC with a well-respected classroom-based counseling curriculum called Kids' Connection, an award-winning program of Rainbow Days, Inc. (1998, n.d.). Students identified as being at high risk for academic or social failure participated in 12 weekly counseling sessions. Using a paired-sample t-test, a comparison was made of within-groups pre- and post-treatment scores on the Basic Assessment System for Children (Reynolds and Kamphaus, 1992) for externalizing, internalizing, maladaptive, and adaptive behaviors. This analysis showed that the EAC group made statistically significant improvements in 17 behavior areas:

- BASC Self-Report:

  — Emotional symptom index ($p = 0.027$)
  — Clinical maladjustment composite ($p = 0.030$)
  — Atypical behaviors ($p = 0.002$)

— Sense of inadequacy *(p = 0.004)*
— Relations with parents *(p = 0.018).*

- BASC Parent Report:

    — Behavioral symptom index *(p = 0.000)*
    — Externalizing problems composite *(p = 0.000)*
    — Internalizing problems composite *(p = 0.000)*
    — Adaptive skills composite *(p = 0.003)*
    — Hyperactivity *(p = 0.000)*
    — Aggression *(p = 0.000)*
    — Conduct problems *(p = 0.001)*
    — Anxiety *(p = 0.000)*
    — Depression *(p = 0.001)*
    — Somatization *(p = 0.036)*
    — Adaptability *(p = 0.003)*
    — Social skills *(p = 0.010).*

In contrast, the classroom-based group showed statistically significant improvement in only five areas:

- BASC Self-Report:

    — Emotional symptom index *(p = 0.026)*
    — Personal adjustment composite *(p = 0.026)*
    — Social stress *(p = 0.028)*
    — Self-esteem *(p = 0.012).*

- BASC Parent Report:

    — Depression *(p = 0.016).*

The only common improved behavior area for both treatment groups was emotional symptom index. Thus, the children and adolescents in each modality, as well as their parents, found both treatments to be effective, but for the most part each treatment modality affected different behaviors and the EAC affected more behaviors than the classroom-based counseling. Results from a between-groups analysis of covariance of pre- and post-test scores additionally indicated the EAC treatment to be superior by showing more statistically significant improvement in six areas $(p < 0.05)$, and near significance in a seventh area $(p = 0.05)$, when compared directly with the classroom-based counseling comparison group:

- BASC Self-Report:

    — Social stress $(p = 0.039)$
    — Self-esteem $(p = 0.024).$

- BASC Parent Report:

    — Behavioral symptom index $(p = 0.050)$
    — Externalizing problem composite $(p = 0.007)$
    — Hyperactivity $(p = 0.018)$
    — Aggression $(p = 0.001)$
    — Conduct problems $(p = 0.031).$

Using analysis of variance, a 12-point repeated-measures trend analysis of the EAC participants' social behavior ratings was performed on the Psychosocial Session Form (Chandler, 2005b), and this showed statistically significant improvement with increases in positive behaviors and decreases in negative behaviors across the 12 treatment sessions. Results from analysis of the BASC and the Psychosocial Session Form provide evidence that EAC is very effective with children in reducing emotional and behavior problems and in this respect was found to be superior to a well-respected classroom-based counseling curriculum (Trotter et al., 2008). Details about the techniques used in this equine-assisted intervention are provided in Chapter 9 (Equine-Assisted Counseling).

Rabbitt, Kazdin, and Hong (2014) compared the acceptability of four different treatment options (AAT, medication, psychotherapy, and no active treatment) for common externalizing behaviors in children. After reading sample vignettes representing each treatment option, participants (N=189) who were parents rated AAT as a highly acceptable form of treatment and more acceptable than no active treatment and medication. Experiences with animals (both positive and negative) were unrelated to the acceptability of the AAT treatment option. The researchers concluded that, because AAT was so highly rated by participants, this modality should be more systematically investigated as a treatment for children's mental health problems (Rabbitt, Kazdin, and Hong, 2014).

Burger et al. (2009) investigated the effectiveness of an animal-assisted group training technique called MTI (Multiprofessionelle Tiergestützte Intervention) that is designed to assist adolescents in the regulation and recognition of emotion. This concept of dog-assisted group therapy or training was developed by clinical psychologist Birgit Stetina, educational expert Ursula Handlos, and cognitive-behavioral therapist Ilse Kryspin-Exner (Karoline Turner, personal communication, September 27, 2010). The core principle of the training is respectful interaction with a therapy dog that is specifically trained to communicate effectively. The program consists of basic and special modules with the dog as an integral part of the training and therapy, acting as a co-trainer and co-therapist. The dogs (mostly two) work with the participants by playing a part in role-playing sequences as well as group exercises that enhance the dogs' health, such as grooming. Participants work with the dogs in teams, conducting diverse actions such as agility sequences, playing, and basic tasks (come, sit, lie down)—all without leash and collar (Karoline Turner, personal communication, September 27, 2010). The researchers (Burger et al., 2009) used a pre–post design where the intervention group was evaluated in comparison with a control group. Participants were 27 students, 11 to 14 years of age. The animal-assisted training took place in school on a weekly basis and was conducted by a multiprofessional team. Pre- and post-measures were obtained using (1) a questionnaire designed to analyze how people perceive and deal with their own emotions (the *Skalen zum Erleben von Emotionen*), and (2) an instrument designed to measure self-esteem and wellbeing (the Self-Perception Profile for Children). Analysis was performed using *t*-tests to determine the significant differences, and Cohen's *d* was used to measure effect size of the outcome, independent of sample size. Significant differences were found for the AAI versus the control group (no intervention). Participants in the intervention group developed greatly in their regulation of emotions. They also learned how to better accept their own emotions and not be ashamed of them. Regarding emotion recognition, they were able to reduce the instances of lack of emotions and establish an improved interpretation of body-related signals. Self-esteem and wellbeing of the participants also underwent significant positive changes during the training (Burger et al., 2009).

Turner et al. (2009) investigated whether MTI can influence the use of emotion regulation strategies and the ability to recognize emotions in children in first grade. The researchers used a pre–post design where the intervention group was evaluated in comparison with a control group. Participants were 19 first-graders, aged 5 to 7 years. The intervention group participated in a dog-assisted competence training session, and the control group received no training. The instruments used were the Questionnaire Emotion Regulation and Vienna Emotion Recognition Tasks. Analysis was performed using t-tests to determine the significant differences, and Cohen's d was used to measure effect size of the outcome, independent of sample size. The results for the intervention group demonstrated significantly larger improvements in adaptive strategies than the control group. Significant and relevant results were found regarding the use of problem-oriented action and reappraisal. In addition, the intervention group significantly enhanced the strategy "activation of social support." The intervention group members also increased their skills in emotion recognition regarding neutral facial expressions. They needed less time to recognize joy and sadness. The researchers concluded that the dog-assisted training improved emotional competence and seemed to be a promising way to develop essential life skills and personal resources (Turner et al., 2009).

TRAUMA AND ADVERSE EXPERIENCES

Research using dog-assisted therapy in Israel was conducted to reduce the psychological distress of teenage girls who were exposed to the traumatic event of physical or sexual abuse (Hamama et al., 2011). The study was a mix of cross-sectional design (contrasting the intervention group and comparison group at the beginning and at the end of the intervention) and longitudinal design (measuring the intervention group before and after and applying the same timeframe to the comparison group). Participants were 18 high school girls, aged 14–16 years, Hebrew speaking, having a history of abuse (3 to 4 years prior to the study), with low achievements in a school setting, and having interpersonal difficulties. Nine girls agreed to be in the intervention group and nine in the comparison group. Participants completed assessments that measured trauma symptoms, subjective wellbeing, and depressive symptoms. The 12-session group intervention included the following types of activities: acquaintance with the canine's world and pairing a canine with a participant, building trust with the canine, training the canine to obey orders, talking to the canine about feelings, and farewell to the canines. Results of the AAI versus comparison (cross-sectional matching) groups were not conclusive, showing elevated symptom levels in the intervention group at first that became nonsignificant by the end of the intervention. However, the longitudinal results of the intervention group were promising. Findings from the longitudinal perspective showed a rapid decline in the level of post-traumatic stress disorder (PTSD) symptoms in the AAI group, along with a significant reduction in the proportion of participants with elevated risk for PTSD (Hamama et al., 2011).

Dietz, Davis, and Pennings (2012) evaluated and compared the effectiveness of three group interventions on trauma symptoms for children who had been sexually abused. A total of 153 children (aged 7–17 years), who were already in group therapy at a Child Advocacy Center in north Texas, participated in the study. The three conditions were: no dogs, dogs with no therapeutic stories, and dogs with therapeutic stories. Groups had six to ten children each. Condition one was 12 sessions of treatment as usual group therapy with no dogs present. Condition two followed the same format but added to the group therapy visits of a handler with a therapy dog one time per month for an average of four visits during each child's treatment. Condition three followed the same format as condition two but added to the group therapy presentations by dog handlers of stories written about the dogs by the agency's clinical director. The stories addressed session topics and helped clarify the purpose for the dog's visit. Assessment of symptoms was measured using the Trauma Symptom Checklist for Children (TSCC: Briere, 1996). The results of the study indicated:

that children in the groups that included therapy dogs showed significant decreases in trauma symptoms including anxiety, depression, anger, post-traumatic stress disorder, dissociation, and sexual concerns. In addition, results show that children who participated in the group with therapeutic stories showed significantly more change than the other groups.

(Dietz, Davis, and Pennings, 2012, p. 665)

Flynn and collegues (2018) examined the effects of animal-assisted therapy delivered as an adjunct to standard-of-care intensive family preservation services, compared with usual care alone. They utilized a randomized controlled trial design. Participants were families referred to Child Protective Services and randomly selected for treatment (with AAT, $n = 14$) or control intervention (non-AAT, $n = 14$). Family functioning outcomes were measured using the North Carolina Family Assessment Scale for Reunification. The results showed all four targeted family functioning outcomes were significantly increased for participants who received animal-assisted therapy as an adjunct to intensive family preservation services ($n = 14$) with medium to large effect sizes. These improvements were sustained in two of the subscales through discharge. The researchers concluded that adding animal-assisted therapy as an adjunct can improve evidence based clinical interventions aimed at enhancing the caregiving contexts of children.

Earles, Vernon, and Yetz (2015) examined the efficacy of equine-assisted therapy for treating anxiety and PTSD symptoms. Participants ($N = 16$, aged 33–62 years) engaged in activities with horses for six weekly two-hour sessions. Activities included: meeting the horses, learning about horse body language and nonverbal interaction, haltering, leading and backing up, safety issues, setting boundaries, staying focused in the midst of distraction, and increasing inner stillness and stability. Immediately following the final session, participants reported significantly reduced PTSD symptoms, less severe emotional responses to trauma, less generalized anxiety, fewer symptoms of depression, decreased alcohol use, and increased mindfulness strategies (Earles, Vernon, and Yetz, 2015).

Craig (2020) performed a qualitative study of equine-assisted psychotherapy that included observations and interviews with 11 female adolescents (ages 13–17) with adverse childhood experiences (ACEs). The adolescents were receiving treatment at an established horse therapy farm that had ten horses of varying size and breed. Farm staff included the program director/equine specialist, program assistant, psychotherapist, barn manager, education coordinator, and a variety of volunteers for care and feeding of the horses, and performing some other tasks. The researcher received permission from the farm and the adolescents (and their guardians/parents) to perform semi-structured interviews that lasted 30–45 minutes and took place in a quiet facility on the farm. The following were examined: (a) equine communication as a mechanism for client awareness and emotion regulation, (b) the development of communication competencies for adolescents, and (c) the transference of communication competencies in other relational contexts. Analysis of data reflected:

adolescents cultivated altercentrism (e.g., ability to decode communication, to focus consciously on the other), communication composure (e.g., ability to deal with psychological stress, while engaging assertiveness), communication coordination (e.g., ability to effectively communicate, manage misunderstandings), and expressiveness (e.g., provide clarity and emotional control in one's own communication). Finally, adolescents described how these communication competencies transferred to other relationships (e.g., family, peers, and teachers).

(Craig, 2020, p. 643)

ELDERLY, ASSISTED LIVING, AND NURSING HOME RESIDENTS

Older individuals often experience a decreased quality of life and increased stress due to age-related life transitions. AAA and AAT have been reported to provide a number of positive benefits for the elderly. A review of several studies involving AAA with residential geriatric patients reported several positive findings: decreased blood pressure and heart rate, decreased depression, and increased life satisfaction (Steed and Smith, 2002).

Researchers examined the effects of a structured 12-week, bi-weekly, pet-assisted living (PAL) intervention involving assisted-living residents ($n = 22$) in four facilities with mild to moderate cognitive impairment (Friedmann et al., 2019). Physical activities included looking at, talking to, touching, giving treats to, brushing, and walking the dog. The (PAL) intervention led to improved physical activity and mood. In linear mixed models, the more participants walked the dog the more their physical activities level changed, and the more participants looked at the dog the more their moods changed (Friedmann et al., 2019).

The presence of a dog in a therapy group significantly increased verbal interactions for elderly residents in the nursing home care unit of the Veterans Administration Medical Center (Fick, 1993). Participants attended a therapy group designed to improve social interactions. Analysis of variance comparisons of videotaped session segments showing when the dog was present for 15-minute intervals, and when the dog was not present, over a 4-week period demonstrated that, while the dog was present, twice the number of verbal interactions occurred (Fick, 1993).

A 10-week pet visitation program demonstrated increases in social interaction in nursing home residents ranging in age from 35 to 95 years with a mean age of 75.39 years (Perelle and Granville, 1993). Pet visitation volunteers were students at a nearby veterinary college with training in animal handling. Animals consisted of four cats, two small dogs, and one rabbit. Six of the animals were brought to the facility each week for 2 hours. Nursing home residents were encouraged by the volunteers to stroke or handle the animals. Volunteers also talked with participants about animals and the residents' former pets and answered participants' questions. Analysis of variance comparisons of pre- and post-test scores on the Patient Social Behavior Scale showed a significant increase in social behaviors. After termination of the visitation program, 6-week follow-up scores showed a significant decline; however, these follow-up scores were still significantly higher than the original pretest scores (Perelle and Granville, 1993).

AAT was reported to reduce loneliness in elderly residents of a long-term care facility (Banks and Banks, 2002). The 6-week program involved a pet attendant accompanying a dog to residents' rooms at the facility for a 30-minute session that included such activities as holding, stroking, grooming, walking, talking to, and playing with the animal. To circumvent the socialization between the attendant and the resident participant, the attendant's interaction with the participant was limited to a script read at the beginning of each session. The attendant did not interact with the dog or the participant during the visit. The dog was always kept on a leash, and the same dog was used for the same resident for the entire 6 weeks. Analysis of covariance comparisons of pre- and post-test scores on the University of California at Los Angeles (UCLA) Loneliness Scale demonstrated significant improvement for participants in a once-per-week AAT group as well as a three-times-per-week AAT group, but no significant improvement was found for the no-AAT group. The once-per-week AAT group did not significantly differ from the three-times-per-week AAT group. This study provides strong evidence for the social benefits of AAT (Banks and Banks, 2002).

Banks and Banks (2005) examined the phenomenon of loneliness and social interaction in a sample of 33 older persons residing in a long-term care facility. They used a quantitative method to compare the effectiveness of AAT administered one-on-one to residents (without other residents present), with AAT administered in a group of residents. A total of 6 weeks of AAT, one 30-minute session per week, in an individual or group setting, was performed, with post-testing during week 5. A total of 17 participants received individual AAT, and 16 participants were in the group AAT condition. AAT sessions consisted of bringing a registered therapy dog into the facility accompanied by the principal investigator of the study. The same dog was used for all participants throughout the study. The therapy dog always remained on a leash. To avoid possible inadvertent effects of conversing with the principal investigator (the dog's handler), for both individual AAT and group AAT sessions a script was read to each resident informing them of the need to avoid talking to the principal investigator during the AAT session. For the individual AAT sessions, residents were allowed to interact with the dog, talk to the dog, and groom and pet the dog whenever they wanted; participants sat on a chair while the dog sat on another chair facing them. For the group AAT sessions, the participants sat in a semicircle that consisted of two to four participants, while the dog sat on a chair facing them; the participants were allowed to interact with each other and interact with the dog (pet, groom, talk to), without any interference or input from the principal investigator. Following a two-way ANOVA of results comparing pre- and post-tests scores on the UCLA Loneliness Scale (Version 3), researchers concluded that AAT was more effective in improving loneliness when provided individually to residents in a long-term care facility than when applied in a group situation. Another interesting finding from the study was that lonelier individuals benefited more from AAT (Banks and Banks, 2005).

An analysis of variance repeated-measures comparison between AAT and no-AAT with elderly residents at a long-term care facility was performed by Bernstein, Friedmann, and Malaspina (2000). The study was undertaken at two facilities. Observations were made of 33 patients, both alert and semi-alert to nonalert, during regular recreational therapy sessions. Most patients were women (with four men participants) and geriatric (in their seventies and eighties). Nonanimal therapy sessions included arts and crafts and snack bingo. AAT therapy sessions involved animals from local animal shelters being brought by volunteers to group sessions. Overall, during AAT sessions residents were involved in as much or more conversation with others, including the animals, as residents in nonanimal therapy and were more likely to initiate and participate in longer conversations. The researchers concluded:

> The finding that different kinds of therapies seem to encourage different kinds of conversation might be an important consideration when investigating health benefits.
> (Bernstein, Friedmann, and Malaspina, 2000, p. 213)

It was reported that the most dramatic differences between the two groups was that the touching of the animals added significantly to resident engagement in and initiation of touching social behavior. The researchers suggested that:

> since touch is considered an important part of social stimulation and therapy, the enhancement of this social behavior by the animals is an important, and perhaps undervalued effect [and in addition,] since touch between people or between people and animals has been shown by others to have beneficial health effects, this source of tactile contact may have some health value for this population, and this aspect should perhaps be studied more directly.
> (Bernstein, Friedmann, and Malaspina, 2000, pp. 213, 223)

Kawamura, Niiyama, and Niiyama (2009) demonstrated AAA to be effective in positively impacting interactive relationships in eight institutionalized elderly Japanese women. The women resided in a private nursing home in northern Japan and ranged in age from

67 to 94 years. All were in various stages of dementia but were still capable of stating their opinions themselves and giving consent to participate in the study. The women attended AAA in the nursing home two times per month for 2 years prior to the study's data collection. The same therapy dogs participated in the AAA during the 2-year period: two Papillons, one miniature Dachshund, and one Yorkshire Terrier. On each occasion, three or four dogs were taken to the nursing home. Each dog was placed on a separate table, and the residents were able to freely feed, hold, and play with the dogs for 30 minutes with the assistance of the AAA volunteers and nursing home staff. Following the 2-year period of participation in AAT, semi-structured interviews were conducted with the elderly participants, and data were analyzed using phenomenological procedures.

Following analysis, 41 significant statements and phrases were extracted and determined to be clear in meaning. Six themes concerning the interactive relationships between the participants and the dogs emerged in the interviews: positive feelings about the dogs, confidence in oneself from being able to connect with the dogs, recalling fond memories about dogs, a break from the daily routine, greater interest in interacting with other residents through the dogs, and enhanced communication with the AAA volunteers. The researchers noted that it appeared that participants bonded with the dogs and became comfortable with the AAA experience, which differed from their daily life when the dogs were not present in the nursing home. The researchers concluded that AAA positively influenced participants by awakening their interest in themselves, their fellow residents, and their surroundings; creating a pathway for the participants to express themselves; providing participants with a positive change from their usual routine; and helping them feel refreshed by providing contact with people from outside the nursing home (Kawamura, Niiyama, and Niiyama, 2009).

PHYSICALLY DISABLED PERSONS

AAT has been shown to be effective in increasing self-efficacy and self-confidence for the physically disabled (Farias-Tomaszewski, Jenkins, and Keller, 2001). A total of 22 adults with physical disabilities participated in a 12-week therapeutic horseback-riding program. The physical disabilities included multiple sclerosis, closed-head injury with concomitant physical impairments, spinal cord injury, cerebral palsy, and scoliosis. Comparisons of pre- and post-test scores demonstrated increased physical self-efficacy, as measured by the Physical Self-Efficacy Scale, and increased behavioral self-confidence, as measured by a behavioral rating scale. This study provided evidence in support of the psychological value of this type of intervention for adults with physical impairments (Farias-Tomaszewski, Jenkins, and Keller, 2001). However, it is important to note that the behavioral rating scale was developed for the purposes of the study and has limited validity and reliability.

Demiralay and Keser (2022) examined the effects of pet therapy on the stress and social anxiety levels of physically disabled children. The study was a single-blind randomized controlled experimental study with a pre-test, post-test, and follow-up design. It was carried out in two separate special education and rehabilitation centers with a total of 44 physically disabled children, 23 in the control and 21 in the intervention group, who met the inclusion criteria. Measures included the Perceived Stress Scale (PSS) and the Social Anxiety in Children Scale-Revised Version (SACS-R). A 7-week pet therapy program lasting between 45 and 60 minutes per week was applied to the intervention (pet therapy) group. Apart from the standard training given in the rehabilitation center, no intervention was made on the control group. After the pet therapy program intervention, it was found that there was a decrease in the mean PSS and SACS-R scores of the children in the intervention group, and this decrease was significant compared with the scores of the individuals in the control group ($p < 0.05$).

Researchers concluded that the pet therapy program was an effective intervention in reducing the stress and social anxiety levels of the physically disabled children.

SUBSTANCE ABUSE

Wesley, Minatrea, and Watson (2009) evaluated the effect of AAT group therapy on an adult, residential, substance abuse population. Participants numbered 231 and were randomly assigned to treatment or control groups, with 96 in the control group (no therapy dog) and 135 in the experimental group (with therapy dog). Each group session for this study lasted approximately 1 hour. The Helping Alliance Questionnaire (HAQ-II) was completed by participants (treatment and control groups) at the end of each group session. The professional therapy dog (registered with the Delta Society) was a Beagle cross named Mitzi Ann who weighed 27 pounds, stood 17 inches high at the shoulder, and was estimated at 7 years of age (she was rescued from an animal shelter when she was young so her exact age was unknown). The dog's owner and handler was a doctoral-level therapist who conducted the group therapy sessions for the study. Prior to this study, Mitzi Ann and her handler had provided approximately 157 hours of service work integrating counseling with AAT. A total of 26 group sessions were conducted over a period of 3 weeks. The therapeutic philosophy of the group therapist was Glasser's (1999) choice theory and reality therapy to assist clients in achieving personal goals for positive change. The specific AAT techniques included various social interaction activities, such as petting, and tricks performed by the therapy dog that were integrated as psychoeducational tools by the therapist. The results of the study indicated that, overall, the therapeutic alliance was enhanced with the addition of the therapy dog. The AAT group had a significantly more positive opinion of the therapeutic alliance, as measured by the HAQ-II, than the control group. Males, females, pet owners, court-ordered clients, and clients seeking treatment for polysubstance, cannabis, and methamphetamine dependence were all more positive about the therapeutic alliance if they were in the AAT group than if they were in the control group. The researchers concluded, "This study demonstrates that addiction professionals could increase treatment success by adding this complementary, evidence-based practice" (Wesley, Minatrea, and Watson, 2009, p. 137).

Prior to the previously described research, Minatrea and Wesley (2008) performed an initial study comparing AAT (involving therapy dog Mitzi Ann) with non-AAT when using Glasser's (1999) choice theory and reality therapy with 24 individuals experiencing a history of substance abuse or addiction. The data yielded results showing that AAT positively influenced the counselor–client relationship; and the group using AAT appeared more attached to the counseling process, placed a higher value on the counseling experience, and exhibited less stress during the process (Minatrea and Wesley, 2008).

Coetzee, Beukes, and Lynch (2013) found the experience of AAT to be beneficial to substance abuse inpatients at a residential treatment center in South Africa. AAT consisted of two 1-hour-long activities at a local animal park. During the first hour, participants viewed a number of wild animals (e.g., lions, tigers, wild dogs, and cheetahs) and interacted with a number of tame animals (e.g., giraffe, impala, donkey, rabbits, goats, ostriches, and a mongoose). The second hour was dedicated to group therapy promoted by the treatment facilitator. During the group therapy, patients were asked to provide general feedback with regards to their experiences with the animals. The resulting discussions from the group therapy were later examined for themes. Data were thematically analyzed utilizing independent judges over multiple phases of coding and confirmation. Three themes emerged: (1) participants focused more on positive talk when describing their experience of the animals; (2) participants found particular significance in the self-awareness that was gained as a result of the experience of the animals; (3) animals served as a catalyst for social interaction because the animals tended to stimulate conversation through their presence, character traits, unscripted behavior, and provision of a neutral, external focus (Coetzee, Beukes, and Lynch, 2013).

PSYCHIATRIC PATIENTS

AAT has been demonstrated to be effective in increasing prosocial behaviors in psychiatric patients being treated for chemical dependency and abuse. An experimental versus control group comparison using a repeated-measures analysis of variance was performed with 69 subjects in a psychiatric rehabilitation facility; subjects had a mental illness diagnosis as well as a history of chemical abuse or dependency (Marr et al., 2000). The most frequent diagnoses were schizophrenia (48 percent), bipolar disorder (27 percent), unspecified psychosis (18 percent), and depression (7 percent). By the fourth week of AAT, patients in the AAT group were significantly more interactive with other patients, scored higher on measures of smiles and pleasure, were more sociable and helpful with others, and were more active and responsive to surroundings. The experimental group and the control group were identical except that the experimental group had animals to visit each day for the entire group time. Both groups were designed to build a foundation that aids in the development and maintenance of coping skills necessary to resist social pressures to experiment with alcohol or street drugs, or to initiate a recovery process if usage had already begun. The animals that participated included dogs, rabbits, ferrets, and guinea pigs: "Patients were allowed to observe the animals or interact with the animals—hold them, pet them, and/or play with them as long as they did not disrupt the group" (Marr et al., 2000, p. 44). Patients were not required to participate—participation was voluntary; however, only one patient out of all the AAT subjects elected not to interact directly with the animals (Marr et al., 2000).

Monfort et al. (2022) evaluated the efficacy of an animal-assisted therapy (AAT) program in patients diagnosed with schizophrenia-spectrum disorders and substance-use disorders (dual diagnosis) in residential treatment in order to intervene in the remission of negative and positive symptoms and improve quality of life and adherence to treatment. This was a quasi-experimental prospective study with intersubject and intrasubject factors. The sample comprised 36 patients (21 in the experimental group and 15 in the control group) who were evaluated at three time points (in the third, sixth, and tenth sessions). The program lasted 3 months and consisted of ten sessions that were implemented once a week, with a maximum participation of ten patients per group. The participants were evaluated with the *Positive and Negative Syndrome Scale* (PANSS) for schizophrenia and the *Life Skills Profile-20* (LSP-20) questionnaire. Researchers observed a decrease in the positive symptoms of psychosis (F: 27.80, $p = 0.001$) and an improvement in functionality (F: 26.70, $p < 0.001$) as the sessions progressed. Regarding the intervention, one session lasting 45 minutes was delivered per week in groups of a maximum of ten patients. A therapy dog, social educator, psychologist, AAT technician, and dog trainer all participated in delivering the sessions. Each therapy session started with the presentation and greeting to the patients, animal, and therapist, who made up the therapy group. The greeting consisted of introducing oneself to the dog and petting it at the beginning of the session. The warm-up exercise continued with a very specific objective: focus the attention of the patient and the animal on the initiated group. The exercises were simple: introduction, greeting, brushing, and caressing specific areas. After the warm-up, the specific exercise of the session was given, and dog–patient interaction occurred to achieve the objectives set for the session. Before the end of the session, a time of sharing experiences, sensations, and emotions was shared, and the session concluded with the farewell of the dog and therapist patients, and a call for the next session. In the session, patients were informed of different aspects of canine behavior, such as their care, feeding, and the learning or extinction of behaviors through positive reinforcement (prizes in the form of food, caresses, or congratulations), and the behavior that should be observed. The researchers concluded that AAT seemed to be valid as a coadjuvant therapy as part of the rehabilitation processes of patients diagnosed with schizophrenia and addiction-spectrum disorders (dual diagnosis) (Monfort et al., 2022, p. 1).

Researchers evaluated, in a blind, controlled study, the effects of AAT in a closed psychogeriatric ward over 1 year. Participants were ten elderly schizophrenic patients and ten matched patients with a mean age of 79.1 years (Barak et al., 2001). AAT was conducted in weekly 3-hour sessions, and treatment encouraged mobility, interpersonal contact and communication, and reinforced activities for daily living, including personal hygiene and independent self-care, through the use of dogs and cats as modeling companions. AAT activities included petting, feeding, grooming, bathing, and walking the animals on a leash inside and outside the facility around the grounds. AAT participants were provided with their own dog or cat. Control group patients were assembled for reading and discussion of current news for a similar duration on the same days that AAT was undertaken. Pre- and post-test comparisons on the Scale for Social Adaptive Functioning Evaluation were significantly better for the AAT group than the control group. The researchers concluded that AAT proved to be a successful tool for enhancing socialization, activities of daily living, and general wellbeing for this population (Barak et al., 2001).

Berget, Ekeberg, and Braastad (2008a) explored attitudes to AAT with farm animals among psychiatric therapists and farmers in Norway. Questionnaires were sent to 60 therapists and 15 farmers. In answer to the question as to whether animals in general can contribute positively to therapy, significant gender differences between therapists were found, with 28 percent ($n = 14$) of the female therapists believing that "animals in general" to a very large extent could contribute positively to therapy, while none of the male therapists was that positive. The attitude to AAT in general was positive among both the therapists and farmers, with farmers being significantly more positive than therapists. Regarding the question specifically about whether "farm animals" could contribute positively to therapy, a great majority of the therapists believed that farm animals could have positive effects additional to those provided by pets: there were significant gender differences also for this question, with 86 percent of female therapists believing to a large or a very large extent, and 40 percent of the males being less positive. The opinions among the farmers generally agreed with those of the therapists. Regarding the question as to whether AAT with farm animals to a large extent could contribute to better mental health than other types of occupational therapy, a majority (64 percent) of the therapists believed this, while 30 percent believed it to some extent. In answer to the question as to whether AAT with farm animals could contribute to increased skills interactions with other humans, 30 percent of the therapists thought this to some extent, and 65 percent believed it to a large extent: female therapists were more optimistic about this than males. The researchers concluded that the study confirmed the marked potential of offering AAT services with farm animals for psychiatric patients by documenting positive attitudes to this type of therapy among psychiatric therapists (Berget, Ekeberg, and Braastad, 2008a).

Berget, Ekeberg, and Braastad (2008b) performed a study in Norway that demonstrated beneficial effects of AAT with farm animals for persons with psychiatric disorders in schizophrenia, affective disorders, anxiety, and personality disorders. A total of 90 patients (59 women and 31 men) participated in the study; 60 participated in the AAT with farm animals, and 30 participants were in a control group. Both the AAT treatment group and the control group received standard therapy as usual (individual or group) with the AAT treatment group receiving the additional AAT treatment. In the AAT intervention, patients visited a farm for 3 hours twice a week for 12 weeks to work with the farm animals. One or two patients visited the farm at each time. The patients worked only with the animals and were not allowed to do other kinds of farm work. The type of work with the farm animals depended on the patient's coping ability, and farmers remained in proximity to patients during the therapy. Three different inventories were used to obtain participants' scores before the intervention, at the end of intervention, and 6 months after the end of the intervention. The Generalized Self-Efficacy Scale (GSE) was used to measure self-efficacy; the Coping Strategies Scale of the Pressure Management Indicator was used to measure coping; and a Norwegian version of the Quality of Life Scale (QOLS-N) was used to reflect relations to other humans, work, and leisure. ANOVA showed a significant increase in self-efficacy in the ATT treatment group but not in the control group from before intervention to 6 months follow-up. There was also a significant increase in coping ability within the ATT treatment group between before intervention to 6 months follow-up. No changes in quality of life were found. The researchers concluded that AAT with farm animals may have positive influences on self-efficacy and coping ability among psychiatric patients with long-lasting psychiatric symptoms (Berget, Ekeberg, and Braastad, 2008b).

Iwahashi, Waga, and Ohta (2007) explored the expectations and preferences for AAT as a day-care program for Japanese schizophrenic patients. Inpatient ($n = 311$) and outpatient ($n = 170$) individuals aged 14–80 years old (273 male, 208 female) diagnosed with schizophrenia completed a questionnaire inquiring about their favorite animals and impression of hopes for AAT (82.5 percent of the patients had experience with keeping animals). A total of 397 patients (82.7 percent) said they "like animals"; favorite animals were identified as dogs (312 patients), cats (206 patients), birds (150 patients), horses (86 patients), and dolphins (51 patients). Other favorite animals mentioned were rabbits, hamsters, and goldfish. Some patients mentioned animals they disliked: cats (113 patients), dogs (86 patients), horses (62 patients), birds (58 patients), and dolphins (51 patients). Many patients said they disliked snakes. Of the total participants, 56.7 percent (273) said they wanted contact with animals, and 49.1 percent (236) thought that contact with animals was useful as a therapy for a change. The researchers concluded that, though there were currently few hospitals in which AAT was performed as a psychiatric therapy in Japan, it was shown by the results of this study that many psychiatric patients like animals, do not mind animals coming into the hospital, and think AAT may be useful as a therapy for change (Iwahashi, Waga, and Ohta, 2007).

Kovács et al. (2004) examined the benefits of AAT for middle-aged schizophrenic patients living in a social institution in Budapest, Hungary. Seven patients (four women and three men) diagnosed with schizophrenia participated in weekly 50-minute sessions of ATT for a 9-month period. The therapy team consisted of a psychiatrist, a social worker, a therapy dog, and its owner. At the beginning of each session the therapy dog went around to patients for petting, thereby enhancing social interactions. In this phase the patients could share their feelings and thoughts with the therapeutic staff. As the treatment progressed, various simple and complex exercises with the dog were integrated into the sessions, such as feeding and grooming the dog, which were useful for learning how to care for the needs of another living being. The researchers described patients as relaxed and positive during the sessions and reported that they enjoyed the activities with the dog and became more and more spontaneous as sessions progressed. The outcome measure for the AAT was a comparison of the Independent Living Skills Survey (ILSS) completed 7–10 days prior to the first AAT session and 7–10 days after the last AAT session. The ILSS measures the living skills of chronic psychiatric patients, living with caregivers or in institutes, in eight areas—eating, grooming, domestic activities, health, money management, transportation, leisure, job-seeking or job-related skills—as rated by significant others or facility staff. A paired-sample t-test procedure was used to compare means of the pre- and post-assessment. Results showed that the group's ILSS scores improved after the completion of the AAT, and in the areas of domestic activities and health the social skills improved significantly. The researchers concluded that AAT seemed to be helpful in the rehabilitation of schizophrenic patients living in a social situation (Kovács et al., 2004).

Kovács et al. (2006) performed an exploratory study of the effect of animal-assisted group therapy on nonverbal communication in three severely disabled schizophrenic patients. Working with the patients were one therapist, one co-therapist, and the owners of two therapy dogs (a 5-year-old female Boxer and a 2-year-old female Bichon Frise). The therapy was designed to improve nonspecific (general wellbeing) and specific (communication patterns) areas of patients' daily activities. The therapy took place weekly over a 6-month period, with each session lasting 50 minutes. In a typical therapy session the first part was a loosely structured warm-up phase, where the therapy dog made contact with each patient; the main goals of this part were: "to elevate the level of patient motivation; to enhance the general well-being of patients, and to let them speak freely about their problems or good experiences in a comfortable and pleasant environment" (p. 356). The next part of the session was more goal oriented toward enhancing "both verbal and nonverbal communication, psychomotor functions, and concentration ability by having the patients groom and feed the dog, and by introducing some specific exercises" (p. 356). Patients were asked to communicate with staff and with other patients during the session. Role-playing situations were used, with the help and presence of the therapy dog, "in order to help the development of adaptive verbal and non-verbal communication and gestures, and as a consequence, the adaptive behavior in certain situations" (p. 356). The assessment tool was a rating scale of 109 items related to anatomy of movement, space usage, dynamics, touch, and type of gesture.

> All three patients improved in the usage of space during communication, while partial improvement in other domains of nonverbal communication (anatomy of movements, dynamics of gestures, regulator gestures) was also observed.
>
> (Kovács et al., 2006, p. 353)

The researchers concluded that AAT can improve certain aspects of nonverbal communication in schizophrenic patients. They also suggested a need for further research in this area of study (Kovács et al., 2006).

Prothmann, Bienert, and Ettrich (2006) investigated the effects of dogs on the "state of mind" of children and adolescents undergoing inpatient psychiatric treatment. All patients were asked by their therapists if they wanted to participate in AAT using dogs. A total of 100 children and adolescents, aged 11 to 20 years, participated in the study. A total of 61 children and adolescents participated in AAT during their inpatient stay in a maximum of five separately conducted and videotaped therapeutic sessions with a registered therapy dog. A total of 39 children and adolescents were put in a comparison group without AAT. The dog therapy was conducted as nondirected, free-play therapy. The five sessions took place in the video studio of the clinic, which measures about 30 meters square. In the AAT sessions, a dog was made available to each participant for 30 minutes of individual–dog interaction, once a week over a period of 5 weeks. There were no direct instructions regulating the course of therapy; the participants were free to choose the kind of interaction they had with the dog (playing, stroking, cuddling, or feeding), and the same toys were made available to each participant to play with the dog. Every participant was motivated to interact with the dog—nobody ignored the animal. The assessment instrument was the Basler Befindlichkeits-Skala (BBS), a self-rating method to measure changes in state of mind over time that is "especially suitable in investigations which evaluate the progress of psychiatric therapy, and it can be used to measure the state of mind in four dimensions" (p. 269). For the AAT, participants were asked individually 5 minutes before the start and again after the end of each session to assess their current mood using the BBS. For the non-AAT comparison group, participants completed the BBS pre- and post-test around one 30-minute therapy session, because there was only one comparison therapy session provided for the study. A paired *t*-test was used to ascertain differences in the mean values of participants in each group. For the AAT group, patients showed highly significant increases in all dimensions of the BBS. These changes were not found in the non-AAT group. The researchers concluded, "Incorporating a dog could catalyze psychotherapeutic work with children and adolescents" (Prothmann, Bienert, and Ettrich, 2006, p. 265).

Nathans-Barel et al. (2005) investigated the effect of AAT on anhedonia, a component of the negative symptom dimension and a core phenomenon in schizophrenia that is associated with poor social functioning and is resistant to treatment. The hedonic tone of ten chronic schizophrenia patients who participated in ten weekly interactive sessions of AAT was compared with a control group, also ten participants, treated without animal assistance. The treatment sessions were 1 hour each week with the same therapist, and the content of each session was pre-planned. The therapy dog was a well-trained Golden Retriever. In each treatment session participants were invited to choose among several possibilities: talking, making contact with the dog, petting the dog, feeding, cleaning the dog, and taking the dog for a walk on a lead. The control group followed the same procedures with the exception of the dog-related activities. Results were analyzed using analysis of variance. The AAT group showed a significant improvement in the hedonic tone compared with controls. They also showed an improvement in the use of leisure time and a trend toward improvement in motivation (Nathans-Barel et al., 2005).

Beck, Seraydarian, and Hunter (1986) investigated the impact of the presence of animals on therapy and activity groups on two matched groups of eight and nine psychiatric inpatients. Over 11 weeks, daily sessions of the groups were held in identical rooms except for the presence of four caged finches in one of the rooms. Comparison of pre- and post-evaluations showed that the group that met in the room containing the caged birds had significantly better attendance and participation, and had also significantly improved in the area of hostility, as assessed by the Psychiatric Rating Scale (Beck, Seraydarian, and Hunter, 1986).

Nepps, Stewart, and Bruckno (2014) performed a study with 218 participants who were patients hospitalized in a mental health unit of a community hospital where the average stay was 7.13 days. Half of the research participants attended a 1-hour AAA session and the other half attended a 1-hour traditional stress management session. For the AAA condition, participants met in a large room with the therapy dog and its owner. The dog was Jesse, a female Border Collie, and Jesse's owner was an experienced volunteer at the hospital, who used specific AAT strategies in the session. To improve social interaction skills, the owner encouraged participants to ask questions about the dog and to speak about their own experiences with pets and animals. The dog's feelings and responses to human emotions were discussed to encourage emotional expression. Patients were asked to try commands such as "sit" and "fetch" with the dog in order to enhance their self-efficacy. The comparison group (with no animal present) watched a video-based stress management program using a DVD presentation called *The Joy of Stress*, which was designed to teach coping through cognitive restructuring and humor. A trained facilitator managed the program, although no effort was made to encourage discussion, and this design controlled treatment consistency across all participants. Self-report ratings of depression, anxiety, and pain were collected before and after treatment sessions, and blood pressure, pulse, and salivary cortisol were measured. There were significant decreases in depression, anxiety, pain, and pulse after the AAA program, comparable to those in the more traditional stress management group (Nepps, Stewart, and Bruckno, 2014). While both the AAA intervention and the no-animal-present intervention were brief (a single 1-hour session), it is important to note that significant desired effects were still obtained. However, without the incorporation of a control group in the study, it is difficult to ascertain whether either the experimental or comparison intervention would have produced better results than no intervention at all.

Chen and colleagues (2022) studied functional outcomes in a randomized controlled trial of animal-assisted therapy on middled-aged and older adults with schizophrenia. The AAT group participated in a 1-hour session with dog-assisted group activities once a week for 12 weeks. The control group participated in dose-matched, nonanimal-related recreational activities. The AAT group showed a greater increase in lower extremity strength and social skills, but no improvement in cognitive function, agility, or mobility (Chen et al., 2022).

Holcomb and Meacham (1989) reported AAT served as a source of motivation for psychiatric clients' participation in therapy. Over the course of 2 years, an animal-assisted occupational therapy (OT) group attracted the highest percentage of psychiatric inpatients voluntarily choosing to attend an OT group. The types of OT groups offered included Hug-a-Pet (the AAT group), living skills, clinic, communication, assertiveness, special topics, chemical dependency, and exercise. In addition, it was found that AAT was the most effective of all of the various types of OT groups offered in attracting isolated individuals to participate regardless of diagnosis (Holcomb and Meacham, 1989).

CHALLENGES AND RECOMMENDATIONS IN AAT RESEARCH

As demonstrated in this chapter, a variety of empirical research supports the psychophysiological and psychosocial benefits of animal-assisted intervention. However, more empirical research is needed to more firmly establish the clinical efficacy of including therapy animals in counseling and related areas.

> On first glance it seems surprising that the potential benefits of therapeutic interventions incorporating non-human animals have not been more extensively researched and utilized. Reasons for such neglect possibly include the lack of available empirical evidence to support proposed benefits. A general bias against the value of non-human animal interactions for human psychological wellbeing may further explain the lack of empirical interest in the area. Thus, one bias perpetuates the other, as in: there are no empirical data so the relationship must not be important, and the relationship is only anecdotally supported so is probably not worthy of empirical investigation. . . . And given the enormous potential therapeutic benefits to be gained from the incorporation of non-human animals into therapeutic interventions, it is to the detriment of our science and practice that we continue to neglect such opportunities.
>
> (Fawcett and Gullone, 2001, pp. 130–131)

According to Serpell and colleagues (2017),

> Practical challenges to AAI research include issues of study design and methodology, the heterogeneity of both AAI recipients and the animals participating in these interventions, the welfare of these animals, and the unusual pressure from the public and media to report and publish positive findings. Such challenges need to be carefully considered in designing and implementing future studies in the field.
>
> (p. 1)

Furthermore, according to Rodriguez and colleagues (2018),

> there is a scarcity of valid and reliable assessment tools specific to measuring constructs directly related to HAI [human-animal interaction]. As the field continues to develop, there is a critical need for the consistent use of standardized, well-validated, and appropriate assessment tools.
>
> (cited in Serpell et al., 2017, p. 1)

AAT practice continues to rise in popularity, yet greater acceptance as a treatment requires the field to undergo more quality investigation. Many existing studies lack sufficient quality because they have significant methodological flaws (Stern and Chur-Hansen, 2013). Kazdin (2011) points out that many studies in AAT lack rigor and have methodological problems that dilute the legitimacy of findings. Common methodological problems he describes include: utilization of a single group; pre- to post-test design only; failure to properly address intentionality for change; use of heterogeneous samples; use of ambiguous samples and treatment foci; questionable or unsupported assumptions; use of a single therapist or single animal; failure to properly codify or describe key procedures; and utilization of only one measure for assessment or using a measure that has insufficient validity or reliability. He encourages greater utilization of randomized controlled trials (RCTs) in AAT research as this is considered the "gold standard" in scientific research. However, he also recognizes the validity of single-case experimental designs as well as qualitative research. He recommends AAT-C researchers strive for quality in their investigations, which includes but is not limited to:

> Random assignment of participants to conditions.
> Careful specification of the client sample and the inclusion and exclusion criteria required for participation.
> Use of strong control or comparison groups (e.g., treatment as usual or another variable treatment).
> Use of treatment manuals to codify procedures and practices to permit replication of treatment.
> Assessment of treatment integrity (i.e., the extent to which the intervention was carried out as intended).
> Use of multiple outcome measures with multiple assessment methods (e.g., self-report, parent report, direct observation) and measures of multiple domains of functioning (e.g., symptoms, prosocial functioning).
> Evaluation of the clinical significance of change (i.e., whether the changes at the end of treatment make a difference in returning individuals to adaptive functioning).
> Evaluation of follow-up weeks, months, or years after post-treatment assessment of functioning.
>
> (Kazdin, 2011, pp. 36–37)

Rodriguez, Herzog, and Gee (2021) describe human–animal interaction research as being "plagued with mixed results" that are "likely due to the wide variety of methodologies implemented, intermittent use of standardized measures and manualized protocols, variability in human and animal participants, and limited quantification of human-animal interactions" (p. 1). Due to the complexity of dynamics in human–animal interaction, they conclude that research in this field "requires a broad spectrum of theoretical and methodological considerations to improve rigor while ensuring the validity and reliability of conclusions drawn from study results" (p. 1). Rodriguez et al. (2023) discuss complexities, considerations, and recommendations surrounding conducting an RCT of an AAI program in regard to study planning, conceptualization, design, implementation, and dissemination.

> Recommendations pertain to such unique issues as ethical considerations, theory, control and comparison groups, sampling, implementation fidelity, and transparent reporting of findings. These considerations and recommendations seek to aid HAI researchers in the design, implementation, and dissemination of future RCTs to continue to advance the rigor of the field.
>
> (Rodriguez, Herzog, and Gee, 2021, p. 1)

3

Selecting an Animal for Therapy Work

A most important decision you will make as part of your AAT career is the selection of a therapy animal. Your hopes are high that your pet dog, cat, or horse will have the "right stuff" to be a pet practitioner, and beginning your career in AAT depends on it. However, you do not have to delay your own AAT training until you find the "right" pet. In fact, the earlier you start your own training in AAT, the better prepared you will be to select and train a pet for therapy work. Thus, I tell my students that they do not have to have a therapy pet before they take my training course. The training material provided creates a more in-depth understanding of what you will need from a therapy pet so you will be better able to judge a pet's appropriateness or preparedness for work in counseling. For information on understanding what your pet is communicating, see Chapter 6. For information on evaluating a pet for therapy work, see Chapter 5.

If for some reason the pet you select does not work well as a therapy pet, the news is still good. You still have a loving, cuddly family member—and you can always try again with another pet. Like many of us animal lovers, I have often had more than one pet around at any given time. Some are pets that have worked with me as professional pet practitioners, such as my cat Snowflake, and my dogs Rusty, Dolly, and Jesse, and some are pets that do not work as therapy animals. Like me, you may end up with more than one therapy pet, although having only one therapy pet can be quite sufficient for your work.

The most common pet practitioners in a counseling setting are dogs, followed closely by horses, cats, tame small animals such as rabbits and gerbils, and aquarium fish. Typically, reptiles are frowned upon in a therapy setting as a result of their high risk for carrying or being receptive to disease and causing injury to the client and because it is difficult to provide proper care and a safe environment for the reptile. Farm animals can be beneficial as therapy animals, the most common of these being llamas, alpacas, and pot-bellied pigs, but there are also therapy chickens, cows, sheep, and goats. There is even a therapy camel (L. Norvell, personal communication, November 6, 2004). Now let us look at some of these potential therapy animals a little more closely. Often, farm animals are not formally evaluated for therapy work using a standard evaluation, as is done for dogs, horses, cats, and small animals (i.e., rabbits and guinea pigs). But the Pet Partners organization does provide a formal, standardized evaluation for farm animals such as llamas and alpacas, as well as pigs.

DOI: 10.4324/9781003260448-3

THERAPY DOGS

There is no special breed of dog for work in a counseling setting. Some breeds are better known for their ease of training, friendliness toward people and other dogs, tendencies toward affection, calm temperament, and desire and tolerance for high-energy activity (Coile, 1998). However, any breed of dog or a mixed breed can be a successful therapy dog if it meets the necessary criteria. In selecting a candidate for therapy work, it is not so much about the breed as it is the breeding. A dog bred from a line that has tendencies toward, for example, aggression, fear, hyperactivity, shyness, or oversensitivity increases the chances that it may inherit some of these negative traits and so make it inappropriate for therapy work. Knowing as much as possible about a dog's biological parents and even grandparents will make it easier to predict potential characteristics in a dog. However, even dogs born from the same litter can have different personalities.

My preference for a therapy dog is the American Cocker Spaniel because this is my favorite breed and I have had American Cocker Spaniels as pets for most of my adult life. Cocker Spaniels are generally known for their friendly and affectionate attitude. As a sporting breed, they have a history of being very intelligent and very trainable. They have a great deal of energy and are very playful. You might occasionally come across an atypical Cocker Spaniel with a bad attitude that would not be appropriate for therapy, but most Cocker Spaniels are very sweet and lovable.

A very common breed for a therapy dog is a Labrador Retriever. Labradors do not usually calm down until they are 2 to 3 years old but after that are typically calm dogs. As a sporting breed, Labradors are very intelligent and easily trained. This is why you see a large number of Labradors as service dogs for the disabled. Labradors are friendly and well mannered, and that makes them a popular choice as a therapy dog. They are also very strong dogs, quite hardy, and can cope well with stress. Golden Retrievers are also very popular as therapy dogs for many of the same reasons listed for Labradors.

As a Pet Partners evaluator of over 500 handler–animal teams, I have evaluated and passed dogs of a variety of breeds and many mixed-breed dogs, large, medium, and small. There truly is no breed that is not potentially appropriate as a therapy dog. A therapy dog must have the right temperament for therapy work. It must be affectionate, friendly, and sociable with persons of all ages and ethnicities and both sexes. It must tolerate high levels of noise and activity. The dog must not be aggressive toward other dogs, and it is most helpful if the dog is well behaved around other dogs. The dog must be relatively calm. It is imperative that the dog be obedient and easy to control. A therapy dog needs to be comfortable with traveling in a car. It must be comfortable away from home when visiting unfamiliar places and greeting unfamiliar persons. Most importantly, the dog needs to have a fairly good tolerance for stress. Aggressive or fearful dogs are not appropriate for therapy work. Dogs that bark or whine frequently or continuously when away from home are also not appropriate for therapy work.

Sometimes it is important to match a dog's personality with the population with which it will work. Most professional therapy dogs are versatile enough to serve just about any group; however, certain characteristics of the dog may suggest a better fit between the pet practitioner and a certain clientele. For example, a younger and more playful dog might be more appropriate for work with high-energy adolescents, whereas a more mature and calmer dog may be more appropriate with elderly clients or very small children.

There are a variety of advantages and disadvantages to working with a dog in therapy (Burch, 1996, 2003). One of the more favorable advantages is that most people really like dogs. Most dogs are very extroverted, friendly, and sociable, and they outwardly demonstrate their emotions, especially with their tails. It is easy to predict how a dog feels about being approached or interacted with because it tends not to hide its feelings. Thus, people can feel more comfortable being able to understand the animal's behavior when around them. Dogs enjoy engaging in activity with humans. Therapy dogs like just about everyone, so clients can feel immediate, genuine acceptance the moment they enter the counseling room. Dogs are a very trainable species. They can learn various obedience commands and fun tricks useful in therapy work. Except for the very small breeds, dogs don't get sick easily and are fairly sturdy, and this minimizes the risk of injury to them. Dogs can make and maintain good eye contact with people, and they are fun and playful. Dogs may remind clients of a dog they have or had at one time, and this may stimulate the sharing process (Burch, 1996, 2003).

There are potential disadvantages to working with a dog in therapy (Burch, 1996, 2003). Some people are allergic to dogs. Some have the opinion that dogs belong outside in the yard. Dogs require a certain amount of grooming and training. Food and water must be made available to dogs as needed. Time must be taken to exercise dogs outside so they may relieve themselves and stretch their muscles. You must pick up and properly dispose of excrement after dogs relieve themselves. Some facility staff members or clients may be afraid of dogs. Some dogs have the potential to have behavior problems. Dogs have a shorter lifespan than humans and must be retired from therapy when age-related ailments create too much discomfort for the dog to get around. Thus, a dog that you have relied on as your co-therapist can assist you at most for only about 10 years, or less depending on its age when it began and its breed and health. Finally, the termination process with clients is more complicated as clients are most likely to miss the dog when treatment is complete (Burch 1996, 2003).

Selecting a Dog that Comes from a Rescue Situation or a Shelter

A dog that has been rescued or that comes from a shelter can find a new lease on life providing therapy services. If you are considering a dog that has been rescued or comes from a shelter, before you select it ask if the dog's temperament can be evaluated for its potential as a working therapy dog. Many shelters have this capacity or can point you to an animal evaluator or animal behavior specialist in your area. In the absence of a trained professional animal evaluator, your local veterinarian may be able to evaluate the dog's temperament and attitude. The reason it is vital to have the temperament of a rescued or shelter dog evaluated is because the dog's history is usually unknown. Many rescued or shelter dogs were neglected or abused by previous owners, and this history may impair the dog's ability to work as a therapy dog. Another important consideration is whether you feel a strong connection to the dog because, after all, it is first and foremost a member of your family and you will have a relationship with it that potentially will last for many years.

Following are suggestions for performing an evaluation of a dog that comes from a rescue situation or a shelter to determine its potential to be a therapy dog. Also, there are some obvious characteristics you can check for in a rescued or shelter dog to see if the animal will potentially make a good therapy pet. For instance, a test for sociability is to observe if and how a dog will come to you when called when you are in both a standing and a squatting position. A dog that has enthusiasm and friendliness would be a good candidate. If the dog does not happily move toward you while you are standing or moves toward you only when you make yourself smaller by squatting down, then the dog is fearful and not likely to be a good candidate for a therapy dog. Another test is to clap your hands loudly and see if the dog is afraid of loud noises coming from you; if it is then, again, it may not be a good candidate for a therapy dog. Dogs that are obviously aggressive, shy, or fearful are less likely to be good candidates for therapy work even with socialization and training. A dog that is fearful and shy may or may not be able to overcome the shyness enough to be a therapy animal. If a rescued or shelter dog has shown no aggressive tendencies during this brief testing, then it is safe to check whether it is hand shy by quickly moving a flat hand toward the dog's face and stopping about a foot from the dog's nose to see if the dog cowers away from your hand. Alternatively, wave your hand back and forth in front of the dog's face about a foot away from its nose. A dog that is afraid of quick hand movements has likely had a poor history with aggressive or neglectful interactions and may not be a good candidate for a therapy dog.

Volhard and Volhard (2001) recommended three tests that give a good indication of what to look for when evaluating a shelter dog (p. 153):

- *Restraint:* Place the dog in a down position with food and then gently roll the dog over on its back and hold it there with just enough pressure to keep the dog on its back. If the dog struggles a lot then ease up on the pressure. If the dog struggles too much, jumps up immediately, or is aggressive, then it is not a likely candidate to be friendly and sociable. A better response would be for a dog to turn over readily, even if the dog squirms around a little bit. Intermittent squirming is okay; constant squirming is not okay.
- *Social dominance:* Directly after the restraint test, if the dog did not struggle too much and if you think it is safe, try sitting with the dog and just stroking it, getting your face relatively close to the dog while talking to it softly, to see if the dog licks you and forgives you for the upside down experience. A dog that wants to get away from you is probably not a good candidate.
- *Retrieving:* Crumple up a small piece of paper and show it to the dog. Have the dog on your left side with your arm around it and throw the paper with your right hand about 6 feet, encouraging the dog to get it and bring it back. You are looking for a dog that brings the paper back to you. "Guide dog trainers have the greatest faith in this last test . . . . They know that if a dog brings back the object, they can train him to do almost anything" (Volhard and Volhard, 2001, p. 153).

Lucidi et al. (2005) tested a model to identify shelter dogs' skills to be potential service animals, therapy animals, or adoptable pets. They used 23 cross-breed dogs (from any mix) from two shelters. The subjects were all older than 1 year of age; fifteen were sterilized females, and eight were males, six of which were neutered. A three-step evaluation grid was created to select the animals that had suitable characteristics based on authoritative publications. Test A examined aggressiveness and temperament (any aggressive tendency eliminated the dog for further consideration): to the presence of an unknown dog (assessing aggressiveness); and toward the presence of people (assessing aggressiveness), stroking (assessing temperament), and rough handling (restraining the dog and pushing it to the ground as an additional test for temperament). Test B was used to select those dogs showing behavioral features consistent with the role of co-therapist and measured dogs' responses to: people approaching the dogs' fenced environment and standing outside the closed fence for 5 minutes (assessing the dog's initiative to approach people); people outside an opened gate of the fence (assessing the dog's initiative to approach people through the gate); people calling the dog while in the dog's enclosed area (assessing the dog's sociability); and the introduction of a strong stimulus (making a loud noise to assess fearfulness). Test C assessed dogs' trainability and measured their willingness and responses when: entering a new room first with and then without a leash, going upstairs, walking on a leash, sitting down, laying down, standing up, playing, jumping on people during play, and socializing (going near and interacting with unknown people). The researchers applied weighted values to the dogs' responses (−1, 0, 1, 2, or 3). In conclusion, the researchers determined their model to be effective at selecting shelter dogs to be potential service dogs, AAA and AAT dogs, or adoptable pets (Lucidi et al., 2005).

Selecting a Puppy for Possible Therapy Work

If you do not have a dog, or your current family dog does not seem appropriate as a working dog, you may want to select a puppy that can grow up to work with you. A dog must be at least 1 year of age before it can work as a therapy dog. There is no guaranteeing what a dog will be like when it grows up, but there are ways to put the odds more in favor of it being a suitable dog for AAT. Get a puppy from a highly reputable breeder with many years of experience who is familiar with the genetic line for several generations back of the puppy you are considering. If you get the opportunity, meet the canine mother and father of the puppy and examine whether they are friendly and sociable.

When you are shopping for a puppy, you can present certain tasks to it to test its temperament and social capacity. Puppy testing has several versions today, but a brief version consists of five basic exercises that all together take only about 20 or 30 minutes. The puppy test can be performed on a puppy that is as young as 7 weeks old (49 days). The puppies should have some identifying characteristics or different-colored collars or bow ties so that you can tell them apart and make notes in your head or on paper.

The first exercise is to observe the puppy as it interacts with the other pups in the litter. You are looking for a pup that plays well with others—one that seeks interaction with the other pups in the litter but is neither overly rough and aggressive nor overly submissive and fearful. The remaining four tasks involve seeing the puppies one at a time in an area large enough for you to play and interact with each puppy but out of sight and sound of other dogs, if possible. There are two tasks to determine if the puppy is sociable. See if the puppy comes to you when you clap your hands and call it to you. As it walks away, call it back again. A puppy that comes back to you again and again is one that seeks and enjoys social interaction. Another exercise for social interaction as well as affection is to see how the puppy responds to you when you hold it and play with it. A puppy that seeks to cuddle next to you or lick your face and likes to be near you and held by you is an affectionate puppy. This is a fine quality in a therapy dog. A puppy that does not like to be held and does not care to play with you is not a good therapy dog candidate. The next exercise is a test for dominance, a characteristic not good for a therapy dog. Gently place the puppy on its back and pet its chest for just a moment. The longer it stays on its back willingly, the more likely it will have a personality that will submit to your will. A puppy that immediately fights to turn back over is a willful pup that may try to boss you around. A bossy dog does not make a good therapy dog. The next exercise is a test for fearfulness. Take a soda can and put a few pebbles or pennies in it and tape up the top. This device should make a nice loud sound when you rattle it. Gently toss the noisemaker about 2 or 3 feet from the puppy, being careful not to get too close to the puppy or to hit it with the can. It is natural and normal for the puppy to be startled by the loud object and jump a few feet away. What you are looking for is a puppy that recovers quickly from the startle and then walks back close to the can or sniffs it out of curiosity. This type of reaction demonstrates a dog that is not overly fearful and deals well with the unexpected. On the other hand, if after you toss the noisemaker the puppy runs away or will not approach the can, you may have a pup that does not deal well with surprises. These five basic exercises can tell you a great deal about a puppy even if the puppy is only 7 weeks old.

For a more professional approach to puppy testing, Clothier (1996) wrote a booklet, *Understanding Puppy Testing*, with standardized guidelines and exercises. She recommends that the puppy be tested no earlier than 49 days after birth. The tester should be someone who is not familiar to the puppies. The test should be performed at a location that is unfamiliar to the puppies and as free of distractions as possible. It should be performed out of sight and sound of littermates, other dogs, and other people. If the results of the test are inconclusive, the puppy can be retested 24 to 48 hours later. The exercises Clothier suggests are briefly described as:

- *Social attraction:* to determine the pup's willingness to approach a stranger.
- *Following:* to examine the pup's posture and behavior when getting it to follow you.
- *Elevation:* to determine the pup's response to being held off the ground with all feet off the floor.
- *Restraint:* to test the pup's willingness to be held.
- *Social dominance:* to test the pup's willingness to be placed in and maintain a subordinate position on its side or back.
- *Retrieve:* to test the pup's willingness to work with a human by engaging in a fetch game.
- *Sound sensitivity:* to evaluate the pup's response to a sudden sharp noise (e.g., banging a metal dog dish against a concrete floor about 6 to 10 feet from the pup and looking for a quick recovery by the pup after the initial normal startle response).
- *Sight sensitivity:* to test the pup's reaction to a sudden visual stimuli (e.g., quickly opening an umbrella near the pup and looking for a quick recovery by the pup after the initial normal startle response).
- *Stability:* to test the pup's reaction to a large, unstable, and unfamiliar object (e.g., rolling a chair a few feet away from the pup).
- *Touch sensitivity:* to test the pup's response to unpleasant physical stimuli by gently squeezing the webbing between the pup's toes.
- *Energy levels:* to observe the pup's energy level from the moment all testing begins.

A similar test for measuring puppy aptitude, the *Puppy Aptitude Test* (Volhard, 2003), may assist with choosing a puppy.

THERAPY CATS

There is no particular breed of cat that is preferred for therapy. To be a feline facilitator in a counseling setting, a therapy cat must be calm and well mannered. It must have a relatively high tolerance for stress. It must feel comfortable with greeting unfamiliar people. It does not need to know any basic obedience commands, but it must be willing to sit quietly in a lap while being petted even by someone it has met for the first time.

There are some advantages and disadvantages to working with a cat in a counseling setting (Burch, 1996, 2003). Many people prefer cats to other therapy animals due to their personalities. Cats are smaller and less threatening than many other animals, so most people are not afraid of them. Cats are active and playful and therefore entertaining to play with and watch. A lap cat provides nurturing and affection. Cats will lie in a lap and provide companionship for long periods of time without requiring activity. Short-haired cats do not require as much grooming as dogs, but long-haired cats may need grooming attention. Cats may remind clients of a cat they have, or had at one time, and this may stimulate the sharing process. A common disadvantage to working with a therapy cat is that many persons are allergic to cats. Cats can be trained but are not as trainable as dogs and cannot perform a wide range of skills. Cats can be more introverted and may require more breaks or quiet time. Food and water must be accessible to the cat as needed. A cat needs a litter box to relieve itself. Though cats require less care than a dog, they do require more care than small, confined therapy animals, such as hamsters or aquarium fish. Some cats can have behavior problems (Burch, 1996, 2003).

Lee et al. (1983) developed the Feline Temperament Profile (FTP), a testing procedure for evaluating a cat's general levels of sociability, aggressiveness, and adaptability to new situations. The FTP has nine tasks to perform with a feline. The tester must be unknown to the cat. The tester marks the cat's responses to each testing task as either "acceptable" or "questionable" (Lee et al., pp. 23a–24a). The tester is encouraged to be patient to allow the cat sufficient time to make a response. Before the test begins, the cat should be taken from its cage (if caged) and placed in the testing room (of average size) for several minutes to allow it time to become accustomed to the unfamiliar environment. The tasks assess responses of the cat in relation to sociability, friendliness, willingness to engage, and tolerance for or response to visual and auditory stimuli. The tasks are basically: (1) calling the cat from 5 to 6 feet away; (2) extending one's hand toward and beneath the cat's head; (3) talking to the cat while gently stroking its head, back, and sides; (4) moving a piece of string along the floor to initiate play; (5) picking the cat up gently and cradling it against one's chest; (6) gently stroking the cat while it is in one's lap; (7) placing the cat back on the floor and motioning toward it in a manner that is inviting the cat to re-engage; (8) grabbing the cat's tail firmly and applying pressure, but not enough to hurt the cat; and (9) making a loud noise several feet behind the cat to check for quick startle recovery. A cat's responses to these nine tasks of the FTP should assist in determining the cat's appropriateness for work as a therapy animal (Lee et al., 1983).

Siegford et al. (2003) evaluated the validity and reliability of the FTP with cats before and after their adoption as pets. They rated the cats' responses to both familiar and unfamiliar persons before adoption, after adoption, and over time (across 8 months after adoption). Their data indicated that, for adult cats, the FTP preadoption ratings of the cats accurately predicted their behavior and was relatively stable over time.

THERAPY HORSES

Therapy work is most often a second career for a horse. Horses of good temperament and that are still in good health after retiring from their first career are commonly donated to work at equestrian therapy centers. For a helping horse to work in a counseling setting it must be well trained, calm, and friendly toward people and other horses. A therapy horse must not startle easily to noises or unfamiliar objects.

There can be both advantages and disadvantages to working with a horse in a counseling setting (Burch, 1996, 2003). A common advantage is that many people love horses but have no or little occasion to interact with them. The opportunity to be around or work with a horse can be a very motivating force for participation and cooperation. The client can gain self-confidence from being able to control such a large and powerful animal. Horses are very trainable. Horses are sturdy and durable. People can ride a horse, so horses provide opportunities for clients to work on skills in a way not possible with other animals. A disadvantage to working with a horse in a counseling setting is that a good therapy horse that fits all the necessary temperament and health requirements is often hard to find. Some clients may be afraid of horses. Some family members of clients may be nervous about the client getting near or on such a big animal. Some people are allergic to horses. A large space is required to work with a therapy horse. A great deal of manure cleanup is required. Client transportation to the facility where the therapy horse is located may be a problem. For the safety of the rider, work with a therapy horse usually requires a counseling team as opposed to just the one handler; other team members may serve as side-walkers or may be needed to lead the horse while the rider is in the saddle. Special equipment is required for working with a therapy horse. Horses need a great deal of time and expensive care. The potential injury from working with a therapy horse could be more severe than an injury incurred from working with a cat or dog (Burch 1996, 2003).

SMALL THERAPY ANIMALS

Small therapy animals are considered to be rabbits, pocket pets (e.g., guinea pigs, gerbils, and hamsters), birds, and aquarium fish. These petite pet practitioners are very common in school classrooms but can also be very therapeutic in a counselor's office. A counselor who wishes to work with a small therapy animal must ensure that the animal is tame and free of disease. It is best to acquire such an animal from a pet store that can guarantee its stock is from a reputable source. A small therapy animal must be comfortable being picked up and handled, with the exception of aquarium fish, of course. As with other therapy animals, the small therapy animal must be relatively calm and have a good tolerance for stress.

There are certain advantages and disadvantages to working with a small therapy animal in a counseling setting (Burch, 1996, 2003). A very favorable advantage is that small animals are kept in, and presented in, cages or small baskets and thus do not move around much. Small therapy animals are easy to transport. They are easier and smaller to handle compared with other therapy animals. They often require less care and attention. Smaller animals are less expensive to purchase and care for. Small animals are especially good for a more subdued or passive approach to therapy. It is practical to have more than one small therapy animal since they take up little space and require less care. Small therapy animals are different from the more common cat or dog, and thus may be more interesting. A key disadvantage to working with small therapy animals is that they are more fragile and susceptible to injury. Small therapy animals cannot be handled as readily as the larger and sturdier therapy animals. Small therapy animals are not as stress-tolerant as the larger therapy animals. Most small therapy animals, with the exception of some birds, do not have very long lifespans. Smaller therapy animals cannot be trained as easily as dogs, cats, or horses, nor are they as affectionate, or as responsive to interactions with humans as are dogs, cats, and horses (Burch 1996, 2003).

THERAPY FARM ANIMALS

A counseling setting that incorporates farm animals typically involves a working therapy farm. Some therapy farms are self-described as an animal sanctuary, meaning the farm has a no-kill policy for its farm animals. Most farm animals are not formally evaluated for candidacy as a therapy animal. However, there are exceptions to this; farm animals that can be formally evaluated include pigs, llamas, and alpacas (Pet Partners, 2014). Pot-bellied pigs are very smart and easy to train. Pigs can learn obedience commands, perform fun pet tricks, and be taught to use a litter box or a doggy door. Any farm animal is appropriate for therapy work as long as it is healthy and not aggressive.

There are some advantages as well as disadvantages to working with farm animals in a counseling scenario (Burch, 1996, 2003). One major advantage is that most people do not have much opportunity to interact with farm animals so they hold one's attention. Farm animals can give a client a sense of competence when working on a farm. Farm tasks lend a sense of accomplishment, and many farm tasks can teach vocational skills. Farm animals do not require intense interaction as do dogs. Farm animals are fun to be around with all of their funny noises and shapes. Farm therapy animals do not require training. A major disadvantage to choosing to work with farm animals in a counseling scenario is that working therapy farms are hard to find. Transportation of a client to a working therapy farm can be problematic. If you own a farm animal as a pet it may be difficult to transport that farm animal to the counseling setting. Most farm animals are large, and injuries incurred from interaction with a therapy farm animal can be more severe compared with smaller therapy animals like dogs or cats. Farm animals are difficult to train and can be unpredictable. Work with therapy farm animals usually requires an adequate number of trained staff members. Finally, a person has to be willing to get dirty when working with a therapy farm animal (Burch 1996, 2003).

4

Training a Pet for Therapy Work

The animals we choose to work with are first and foremost our beloved pets and family members. It is our obligation to ensure their happiness, safety, and health. This requires provision of proper nurturance, nutrition, socialization, preventive as well as reactive healthcare, recreation and physical exercise, and positive training techniques. In addition, there are areas that require attention if your pet is to be a working animal in AAT. This chapter delineates the training process you need to perform with your therapy pet to prepare it for therapy work.

The training a therapy pet needs to work in AAT requires proper socialization, touch desensitization, species-appropriate behavior training (e.g., obedience training for dogs), and, ideally, some special skills and trick training. It is a common misconception that AAT workshops or training courses involve animal training, when in fact the AAT courses and workshops offered are specifically designed to train the human, not the pet. The pet's training is performed by the pet's owner. While workshops and courses are useful in explaining what type of training the pet requires, it is up to the owner to train the animal. This is why most AAT workshops and courses ask participants not to bring their animal.

The training of a pet by the pet's owner for therapy work is really not much different from the training any pet should receive to be a well-behaved citizen of the community. Even special skills and tricks that are helpful for a therapy pet to know to enhance AAT work are simple commands easily taught by the pet's owner. AAT pets do not require the highly structured and standardized training regime that service animals require. Training a pet for AAT work is a relatively simple process. However, make no mistake: proper training for a pet that is to be a pet practitioner is vitally important.

SOCIALIZATION

Any pet that is going to go out and work in the community needs to be well mannered. The best way to provide for this is to socialize the pet; that is, to expose it to a variety of stimuli starting early in the pet's life while it is still very young. The pet should meet and be petted by a number of different types of persons varying in age range, ethnicity, ability/disability, and both sexes. Include those with whom the pet is not familiar; that is, persons other than just family members or friends. The pet should be taken out into the community to meet and greet lots of different folks. A pet that stays at home most of the time is not going to be comfortable meeting people when away from home. The pet should be exposed to a variety of

DOI: 10.4324/9781003260448-4

different types of clothing and accessories that people may wear or accompany; for instance, coats, hats, backpacks, briefcases, purses, crutches, canes, walkers, and wheelchairs. The pet should become comfortable with being transported, for example riding in the car. Start by going short distances at first, and then gradually extend the time and distance of the trip until the pet is very comfortable with travel.

When I get a new puppy, I spend a few minutes several times a week training my dog to get into the car and go for a ride. If the pup is still too small to get in by itself, then I gently lift it into the car. I use lots of praise and, in the beginning, some very small dog treats. My dogs travel in a crate secured in the back of the car, or sometimes they sit in the back seat wearing a canine seat belt. Rusty never had a problem with riding in the car and would run to the car with exuberance when I suggested a trip. However, Dolly experienced bad car sickness when she was a puppy. Consequently, she had to be medicated with prescription medication for motion sickness at least 1 hour before any car trip and carried to the car against her will. It was important that I never got angry with her at these times and that I provided as much loving assurance as possible during her car-sickness episodes. I also had to carry material to clean up an almost certain mess when the medicine did not work as well as it should. At about 6 months of age, Dolly grew out of being car sick, but she had a very good memory of it. So I had to continue to carry her to the car and give loving reassurance during the trips. By the age of 9 months, Dolly's behavior began to change, and she began following Rusty to the car of her own free will, albeit without his enthusiasm. Her behavior suggested that she was feeling, "Okay, I want to go on a trip with Rusty and my mom, but I am not really excited about having to go in a moving vehicle." Finally, at 11 months of age Dolly began happily trotting to the car behind Rusty when I suggested a trip.

If you have more than one pet, such as two dogs, practice taking them out separately at times so that they become comfortable spending time away from one another. To exemplify the need for this, I share the following story of an evaluation I performed. The initial evaluation exercise allowed the handler with her dog on a leash to walk around the designated evaluation area briefly to become familiar with the sights and smells. During this exercise the dog acted so frightened when just walking around the evaluation room beforehand that I chose not to continue on with the evaluation. The handler was shocked to see her normally confident, friendly, and outgoing Labrador Retriever act very shy and afraid during the initial evaluation exercise. In a discussion with the handler, it was revealed that this was the first time this dog had ever gone anywhere without the family's other Labrador Retriever. The dog showed confidence and friendliness when out and about in the community with the family's other dog, but without the company of his familiar companion this dog was very frightened. I recommended that the handler spend several weeks to months taking each dog out separately at times so the dogs could become comfortable with being apart from one another. Then, when she thought he was ready, she could take the dog for another evaluation.

The potential therapy pet should be exposed to different types of places with a variety of activity and noises. Pet stores, hardware stores, and garden stores usually allow you to bring your pet inside. In the pet store, walk by the birdcages and aquariums and by any other animals so that you can expose the pet to a variety of species. Make sure your pet does not upset the pet store stock, however. In a hardware store or garden store, be careful not to allow the pet to consume any poisonous or hazardous material. Walk the pet around large moving equipment and loud noises, such as loud saws cutting lumber and construction equipment, while keeping a safe distance. However, do not force your animal to approach any loud noise or moving object. Allow your animal to become accustomed to loud noises and moving objects from a distance at first and gradually reduce the distance as the animal is comfortable.

When Rusty was less than 1 year old, we would go walking in a city park that was being re-landscaped by large, noisy bulldozers and big hauling trucks. I walked Rusty in a safe area of the park, but only about 15 yards from the equipment. I watched him carefully to make sure that the loud noises were not too stressful. If they had been, I would have done the training at a farther distance to start and then would have gradually moved in closer as his comfort level allowed. I also walked Rusty several times near a construction site on the campus where I work with large, looming cranes that were lifting steel beams and sections of concrete wall into place. This type of training really paid off: Rusty remained calm around large and loud vehicles including motorcycles, large trucks, buses, and speeding fire trucks and ambulances with their sirens blaring. This type of exposure is imperative for your pet if you ever want to provide animal-assisted counseling services in response to a crisis, disaster, or other emergency situation.

It is important for a dog to be comfortable around other dogs. Give your puppy many opportunities to play with other friendly dogs of various sizes in the neighborhood or in a dog park to allow for adequate social interaction with other dogs. Be careful that your puppy has the necessary vaccinations before exposing it to unfamiliar dogs. It is also important that a dog be exposed at an early age to other types of animals such as cats, horses, and farm animals. Both Rusty and Dolly were comfortable around cats since they were raised around two playful cats at home. I was fortunate that this transferred to their behavior of showing only a polite, casual interest toward cats they would see away from home or on therapy visits.

When Dolly was 6 months old, I obtained permission to take her with me to an equine therapy center where I occasionally volunteered. I made special trips out there just for the purpose of exposing her a little at a time. The first visit to the ranch was only 15 minutes long so as not to overstress Dolly. I started with a large, well-trained, friendly, and calm horse that was in a small corral. I kept Dolly on a leash, and we stayed outside of the corral. We started about 25 feet away, and we approached the corralled horse gradually until Dolly began to show some visible signs of discomfort, such as slowed walking, hesitation, looking away from the horse or back at me, growling, and barking. I would pet and reassure Dolly, and then we would casually walk away to a distance that was comfortable for her. We gradually approached the horse in the same way two more times and then moved on. We used the same technique with the other ranch critters: miniature horses, goats, sheep, a donkey, a mule, pigs, rabbits, chickens, and ducks. On the next visit, I followed the same regime but spent a little more time with each animal. Each time we visited the ranch critters, Dolly showed fewer signs of discomfort, and we could walk closer to the animal. By the fourth visit, Dolly could be led within only a few feet of each of the ranch critters with no visible signs of discomfort and showing no more than casual interest in each. Dolly was a small dog, so I watched her carefully when she went to the ranch with me to prevent injury to her. She was very comfortable with the horses and even touched noses with them. I also watched the behavior of the horses toward Dolly to make sure they did not injure her. Dolly really enjoyed her visits to the ranch, and I enjoyed having her there with me. The teens who received therapy services at the ranch nicknamed her "Daring Dolly" due to her fearless nature around the large horses. We heard the occasional comment from the kids who were initially afraid to get near the horses: "If Dolly can do it, then I can," followed by their moving closer to pet the horse. During the group process portion of the therapy at the horse ranch, adolescents were comforted when they held and petted Dolly while sharing feelings. I am glad Dolly was socialized to go just about anywhere with me because her therapeutic skills came in very handy for a variety of AAT settings. Dolly was a very versatile therapy dog, getting along with every person and every creature she met, with the exception of squirrels, which she chased from tree to tree in our backyard.

I trained my therapy dog Jesse to be comfortable with being around horses, thus she has served in the "neutral dog" role during my evaluation of horses.

It is important to socialize a therapy animal in the setting in which the animal is going to work. Some simulated, brief practice sessions with your animal is useful training. Ask various volunteers of different ages to play the role of a client with you working as a therapist and your pet as a pet practitioner in the actual therapy room. This assists an animal to become familiar with the therapeutic environment. The volunteers who pretend to be a client for you should be relatively unknown to the therapy animal. With this practice, the therapy session experience becomes familiar and comfortable to the pet. The more familiar a pet is with a particular atmosphere and routine, the more comfortable it will be in that situation while working.

TOUCH DESENSITIZATION

From the time the pet is very young, it should be handled gently and frequently. It is important for a young pet to become desensitized to human touch so that it may be handled by you and by unfamiliar persons. A good approach for this is to incorporate a daily gentle massage into the pet's routine care. This gives you and the young pet some special time together for bonding and trust building while at the same time teaching the pet that it is safe to be touched by humans. Massaging your pet also gives it added health benefits.

One animal massage technique was designed specifically for touch desensitization training and was taught to me by an obedience trainer who was working with me when I was training Dolly. When massaging your pet, position yourself and your pet on the floor or on a couch and make sure the pet is comfortable and well supported so it feels safe enough to relax. Make sure you have good back support so you are comfortable during the exercise. Gently and slowly massage all parts of the pet's body by making small circles on the surface of the skin with the tips of your fingers. For dogs and cats, massage the mouth, the head, ears, neck, shoulders, torso, hips, legs, paws, toes, chest, stomach, and tail. For the ears, start at the base of the ear and make gentle kneading motions all the way out to the tips (some animal behaviorists have said that the quickest way to calm a dog is to rub its ears in this manner). During the pet's massage, use a simple calming word or phrase that the animal can associate with relaxing. As you massage, say in a calm quiet voice, "Just relax." This same phrase can come in handy at other times when you want or need the animal to relax. Even if your pet is tense the first few times you try the massage, it will gradually get used to the routine and respond more positively each time you do it. It is important for you to be relaxed while doing the pet's massage; otherwise, the animal may pick up on your tension, which would prevent the pet from relaxing. Frequent massage for my pets helps to alleviate the stress that may build up in their bodies.

From the time Dolly was a puppy, she was very uncomfortable with anyone touching her tail, and she would pull away and sometimes even growl if you did so. Her dislike got worse as she grew older. It was going to be very important that she stop this reaction if she was going to be a candidate for working as a therapy dog. Incorporating the touch desensitization massage technique with a relaxing anchor phrase, "Just relax," eventually desensitized Dolly to having her tail touched by the time she was several months old. Dolly became comfortable with being touched all over her body, even by persons with whom she was not familiar. I have also used the anchor phrase, "Just relax," when the veterinarian needed my dog to lie still for a procedure or when I needed to calm my dog.

Another good massage technique is called Tellington touch, or T-touch, developed by Linda Tellington-Jones (Tellington-Jones and Taylor, 1995). T-touch is designed for use with a variety of species including dogs, cats, and horses.

OBEDIENCE TRAINING

Every therapy animal must be well mannered, but horses and dogs require special training. Horses may be trained for riding, pulling, vaulting, or other appropriate equine activities, and dogs must at least be trained in basic obedience. At a minimum, a therapy dog must be able to respond to the commands of sit, down (lie down), stay in place, come when called, and walk politely on a leash. Obedience training can begin when the dog is just a few months old in a low-stress puppy class. As the dog gets older, it can take basic obedience and even advanced obedience. The dog must be able to perform obedience commands at home and away from home in the presence of many distractions. Check with your local pet store or veterinarian for an obedience training group near you. I will warn you that some of the pet store-sponsored obedience trainers do not have much experience or knowledge. Check the background and experience of your dog trainer, and use only those who have several years of training experience and who come highly recommended by persons you trust. Only use positive training techniques with your pet—toys, healthy food treats, and petting for motivation. Group obedience training is preferable to individual obedience training because the addition of the other dogs is good for socialization of your animal and effective training around distractions. Also, I highly recommend that you work with your dog in the obedience classes; in other words, do not send your dog away to dog school to be trained by someone else. The high level of mutual communication and understanding that you and your dog form during the shared obedience training process is priceless and will serve much better when you and your dog work together as co-therapists. A good obedience trainer will teach you what you need to know to train your dog; however, my many years of training and working with dogs have provided me with some additional tips that I would like to share with you.

You will need to practice a great many times with your dog all of the commands you learn in group obedience class. Practice at home, in the park, in the pet store, and so forth, so the dog learns to generalize its training outside of the obedience class. Use only positive training methods when training your dog. Positive training methods include lots of praise and treats. Treats can be the reward of a favorite toy, or very small food pieces that are healthy and not fattening, given to the dog after the completion of a command. Training must be fun for your dog and for you. During a training session, never get angry or frustrated with your animal. Also, never yell at your dog or hit your dog. Use encouraging techniques. Be patient, kind, and understanding. Your dog will eventually learn if you are dedicated to working with it and you maintain a positive attitude during the training. Dogs are very intelligent and will look forward to a training session when you make it a fun and playful experience.

When training your dog, teach it to respond to both verbal commands and hand signals. Hand signals are especially useful when you and your dog are working in a loud area or when you need to command your dog from a distance. You can design your own hand signals or have an obedience trainer teach you some common hand signals used by trainers in the field. Hand signals can be associated with any number of verbal commands, but the most common hand signals are taught for the commands of *sit*, *down*, *stay*, *come*, *wait*, *heel*, *let's go*, and *get back* (sit close to me at my side).

When you want your dog to stop what it is doing, such as barking, or you want to teach a young pup not to bite, then you should attach a command name to the word "no," such as *no bark* or *no bite*. If you simply say "no" all the time without differentiating between behaviors, the dog may not understand what you want from it. Also be careful not to use the same word for different intentions. For example, you should not use the word "down" for both a lie down command and to tell the dog to get off the furniture or to stop jumping up on a person. I use *down* for the lie down command and the word *off* to mean get off something or stop jumping up on someone. You will need a correction command for obedience training, but I recommend you do not use "no" as an obedience training correction command because too frequent use of the word "no" in training could dilute its usefulness when you really need it to mean other things. Instead of using the word "no" when a dog fails to fulfill a training command, use a negative vocalization sound; if the dog is supposed to be in a stay position and starts to get up and walk, then you can use the negative vocalization sound that the dog comes to understand as "Oops, I'd better not do that." For example, if my dog has been told to sit and stay and she starts to get up and move without my permission, then I make a loud sound deep in my throat that sounds like *eh, eh*. From training, she has learned that this means to stop her intended behavior and remain with what she was doing before. By having *eh, eh* as a useful and commonly used training correction sound, the use of the word "no," such as in *no bark*, is reserved for meaning other more direct behavior cessation.

Outside of the obedience class, keep your training sessions to only 10 minutes, or at the most 15 minutes, with a built-in break in the middle. You should aspire to have up to two short training periods per day with your pet for at least 5 days a week. A dog's attention span is short, and it will start to lose interest in training after just a few minutes. Positive reinforcement with food rewards, praise rewards, and interspersed playtime with the dog's favorite toy will help to keep the dog's interest in training. You will have to repeat each training exercise many times before a dog learns it well enough to retain it. Some dogs learn faster than others, especially working breeds and sporting breeds. Just about any dog can learn obedience if you spend the time and effort necessary to train it and you make it a fun and enjoyable experience for the dog.

As you will learn in your basic obedience class, animal training requires trial-and-error training with you rewarding any behavior that slightly resembles the ultimate behavior goal for which you are striving. For instance, when training a dog to shake hands, you first make sure the dog knows you have a treat, such as a favorite toy or a small morsel of food, in your hand so the dog is interested in what you are doing and motivated to get that treat. Then you can start with touching the dog's paw and say *shake*. The dog will have no idea what you want so you will have to repeat the action. The dog will start getting excited because it wants the treat and it will eventually move its paw accidentally in its excitement, even though it may have moved its paw only ever so slightly. You immediately reward the dog because it moved its paw. You reward the dog by giving it a morsel of food or toy to play with as soon as the desired behavior is achieved. Pair the treat reward with the phrase *good dog*, and give the dog a friendly rub on the head or shoulder. Then keep touching the paw and saying *shake* until the dog moves the paw even more. Repeat this command, dog movement, and reward-the-dog interaction until the dog starts to consistently move the paw and even starts to raise the paw from the ground. So now you get the idea: you are gradually shaping the dog's behavior until it finally completes the task that you intended for it to complete. With continued praise and reward, you gradually shape the animal's behavior in the direction you want it to go until it successfully completes the command or trick you are trying to teach. Then you continue to reward it for the completed trick or command.

When the trick or command is new to the animal, it may be somewhat forgotten the next day. Thus, you may have to reshape the animal's behavior until it once again successfully completes the command or trick. In my experience with my American Cocker Spaniels, it takes about 2 to 3 days of brief training sessions twice a day to be able to successfully complete a newly learned trick upon my first request without the dog having to work up to it. It takes about 2 to 3 consecutive weeks of everyday practice, in 5- to 10-minute periods twice a day, before the dog thoroughly retains the newly learned command or trick. By always pairing the treat reward with praise, such as saying the words *good dog* and providing a friendly rub on the head or shoulder, the dog will eventually be willing to do the trick or command without the expectation of a treat and instead will do it for the gratitude expressed by you in the form of praise. Thereafter, only occasional practice of the trick or command with treats will be required to keep the animal's interest in maintaining the skill. Animal training is a lot of fun, but it does take time and patience. It is very rewarding for both you and your animal, so you will find it a very fulfilling accomplishment and the time it takes will be well-spent quality time with your animal.

When teaching a dog to perform a new command or a new trick, you may have to gently guide the dog into position the first few times to help it understand what you mean. For example, when training my dog to sit, I put a treat in my hand in a closed fist and move my hand over the dog's head from nose to neck just inches above the head, and the dog follows the treat with its nose and has to sit to keep looking at it as it passes backward. As soon as the dog sits I say *sit*. Then I immediately reward the dog with the treat and say *good dog* and pet it. Then I repeat the exercise. This is a natural way to train your dog. Sometimes you may have to gently fold the dog's legs beneath it in a "sit" position while saying *sit* to get the dog to perform the task. Since you need to repeat the exercise many times during training, you want to give tiny pieces of a treat so the dog does not get filled up fast. Also, train before the dog's mealtime so it is motivated to work for the treat.

Another training tip is to teach the dog commands separately and practice them with breaks in between the different types of commands. For example, practice *sit* with your dog, praising and rewarding after each successful try. Then take a brief 2-minute play break and then practice *down*. Then take a brief play break and then practice *stay*. Then take a brief play break and then practice *come*. This helps the dog to learn the commands separately and not fuse them together. If you always practice *sit* then immediately tell the dog *down* it may start lying down before you tell it to because it anticipates what is coming next. Or, if you always practice *stay* and then walk away and tell your dog to *come*, the dog may start breaking the *stay* prematurely because it anticipates that you will always call it to you soon after you say *stay*. So, *stay* has to be practiced separately from *come* many times in order to teach the dog each separate command.

Even though you intend to enroll in obedience class with your dog, it is important to supplement your dog training education with some selective reading. A good dog-training book is *Mother Knows Best* by Benjamin (1985). This book teaches you to communicate with and train your dog in ways that are more natural for the dog to comprehend. The training approach is positive and nurturing as well as effective. The book discusses housebreaking, crate training, leash training, and all of the basic obedience tasks. Another basic training book I recommend is *The Canine Good Citizen* by Volhard and Volhard (1997). The book is designed to help you train your dog to be a well-mannered dog and to pass the Canine Good Citizen Test sponsored by the American Kennel Club. Another popular training method is called clicker training, whereby a click sound quickly follows the successful implementation of a command by a dog and then the dog gets the treat. The click sound is made by a small handheld device, and because the click noise from a clicker device occurs faster than the action of getting and handing a treat to a dog, clicker training allows the dog to form associations faster between a behavior and a reward. There are several clicker training books and films available on the market.

Positive training methods will help you to avoid making mistakes that create a frustrating experience for both you and your dog. Positive training methods make the time training your dog very enjoyable and an experience that enhances the level of trust and communication between you and your canine.

TEACHING SPECIAL SKILLS AND TRICK TRAINING

It can be beneficial to teach your dog or cat some special skills and tricks that can come in handy in a therapeutic setting (Burch, 2003). In addition to basic obedience, special skills that are helpful for a therapy dog to know include:

- *Leave it:* to ignore food or some other object on the floor.
- *Take it:* to gently take an object you hand to the dog.
- *Drop it:* to drop an object the dog is carrying.
- *Hug:* to be receptive to getting a hug.
- *Say hello:* to approach and greet someone you point to or are facing.
- *Up:* to jump up on top of a sturdy surface to which you point.
- *Off:* to get off something or jump down from a higher surface.
- *Kennel:* to go into a crate or kennel.
- *Place:* to go to a designated mat or bed and lie down and be quiet.
- *Stand:* to stand up on all four feet.
- *Paws up:* to reach up and place the front paws on a designated surface, such as the edge of a sturdy chair or bed.
- *Heel:* to walk close in at your left side and at exactly your pace.
- *Wait:* to wait in the same place and position until you give another command. (This is especially helpful when going through doors or waiting at a street curb for traffic to pass.)
- *Let's go:* tells the dog to come with you.
- *Release:* to be released from an existing command and to relax at ease.
- *Watch:* to look at you, be attentive, and get ready for another command.
- *Get back:* to move in close to your left side, face the direction you are facing, and sit down and be quiet. (This prepares the dog for when you start walking with a *let's go* or *heel* command.)
- *Do it:* to relieve itself or go potty on command (if the animal needs to relieve itself).

Some fun tricks to teach a therapy dog are:

- *Shake:* shake hands.
- *High five:* while sitting, slap its paw up in the air against your palm.
- *Kiss:* give kisses on command.
- *Sit pretty:* sit back on its haunches with its front paws in the air.
- *Over:* roll over.
- *Dead* or *Bang:* roll over on its back and play dead.
- *Crawl:* crawl along the floor on its belly.
- *Fetch:* fetch a ball, Frisbee, or other object.
- *Catch:* catch a ball, Frisbee, or other appropriate object.
- *Through:* jump through a hoop.
- *Jump:* jump over an object.
- *Speak:* vocalize a sound such as a bark.
- *Find it:* find an object that was shown to the dog (and that the dog was allowed to smell) and then hidden for the dog to find.

There are several good dog trick training books on the market, but some I have found useful are *The Trick Is in the Training* by Taunton and Smith (1998) and *Dog Tricks* by Rombold Zeigenfuse and Walker (1997).

My dog Rusty just loved to train. He would train until I tired out. As a result, he knew most of these tricks and a few more to boot. He would jump high in the air and do a 360° twist and land back on his feet. He would go either direction depending on your hand motion. If you held a ball or Frisbee at the apex of the jump he would grasp it in the middle of his twist and come back down with it. Likewise, he was very good at catching a ball and Frisbee in the air, and he chose to do so, most of the time, by doing a half-twist in the air and then catching the ball or Frisbee over his shoulder. As you can probably guess, clients who engaged in play with Rusty got a big kick out of watching Rusty perform his acrobatics. To see a chunky fur ball like an American Cocker Spaniel perform this trick was very entertaining.

While a therapy cat is not required to know basic obedience commands of any kind, it can be helpful if the cat knows some special skills, such as:

- Walk on a leash attached to a harness.
- Travel quietly in the car.
- Be comfortable in a crate or kennel.
- Enjoy being held and petted by unfamiliar persons.
- Sit or lie quietly in a lap for prolonged periods of time.
- Sit or lie quietly next to someone while being petted.
- Tolerate being in a crowd of people.
- Play with a toy during therapy.
- Go to see another person when called.
- Tolerate being hugged.
- Give kisses on command.
- Retrieve a toy.
- Tolerate being brushed.
- Get off something on command.
- Respond to the *no* command.

It is also possible to teach a cat a few fun tricks if you are a patient type of person.

Evaluation of a Pet for Therapy Work

An animal must successfully complete a standardized evaluation before working in a therapy setting. Dogs and cats must be at least 1 year old before they can be evaluated. Other species can be evaluated once they reach maturity, whatever age that may be for that animal. There is more than one model for evaluating the fitness of a pet for therapy work. Well-known models are reviewed here. The American Kennel Club and Therapy Dogs International only recognize dogs as therapy animals. Pet Partners organization recognizes several different domesticated species as therapy animals.

AMERICAN KENNEL CLUB: CANINE GOOD CITIZEN TEST

The American Kennel Club (AKC) evaluation is referred to as the Canine Good Citizen (CGC) test and can be used to evaluate dogs for good behavior and temperament. The AKC CGC was first introduced in 1989 "to ensure that our favorite companion, the dog, can be a respected member of the community" (AKC, 2023a, p. 1). The CGC emphasizes the importance of training a dog to be well behaved and under control at all times, even if just a family pet. The CGC consists of ten exercises. During all ten exercises, the dog must be obedient and under the control of its handler (typically its owner), as well as friendly and cooperative with the evaluator, and not show aggression, shyness, or fear. The exercises are as follows:

- *Test 1:* Accepting a friendly stranger. The dog allows a stranger to approach its handler and shake hands with the handler.
- *Test 2:* Sitting politely for petting. The dog sits quietly while being petted by a stranger.
- *Test 3:* Appearance and grooming. The dog permits an examination for cleanliness and allows the evaluator to lightly brush it.
- *Test 4:* Out for a walk (walking on a loose lead). The handler walks the dog a short distance, and the dog must be able to walk with the leash hanging loosely, requiring no significant control efforts by its handler.
- *Test 5:* Walking through a crowd. The handler and dog walk around the room with several persons walking in close proximity.
- *Test 6:* Sit and down on cue and staying in place. The dog must respond to the handler's commands of *sit*, *down*, and *stay*.
- *Test 7:* Coming when called. The dog must stay in place while the handler walks about 10 feet away and then come to the handler when called.

- *Test 8:* Reaction to another dog. A second handler and dog walk past the handler and dog being tested, the handlers shake hands and then walk on past. The dogs must show little to no interest in one another.
- *Test 9:* Reaction to distraction. A dog may show curious interest to a loud noise or distraction made by the evaluator but should not react with great fear or aggression.
- *Test 10:* Supervised separation. A dog is left with a person other than its handler for a minute and should not whine, bark, or pull on the leash.

All of the tests must be performed on a leash. Owners or handlers may use praise and encouragement throughout the test and may pet the dog in between exercises. Any dog that eliminates during the test is marked as failed. A dog that growls, snaps, bites, attacks, or attempts to attack a person or another dog is not a good citizen and must be dismissed from the test.

Many therapy animal organizations use some form of the AKC CGC as part of their evaluation and screening tool. It is my opinion that although the AKC CGC is useful as a guide for pet owners to train their pets to be well behaved in the community, the AKC CGC by itself is not a sufficient credential for a volunteer or professional who desires to work with a pet to perform AAA or AAT. A more rigorous evaluation process is required to determine if a human–animal therapy team is ready to provide service to the community.

The AKC has a Therapy Dog Program, but the AKC does not certify therapy dogs or provide a therapy dog team credential (AKC, 2023b, p. 1). The AKC Therapy Dog Program provides recognition for accomplishment by an owner and dog. The AKC belief is that the certification or credentialing of a therapy dog or therapy dog team is done by qualified therapy dog organizations; "the certification organizations are the experts in this area and their efforts should be acknowledged and appreciated." The purpose of the AKC Therapy Dog Program is "to recognize AKC dogs and their owners who have given their time and helped people by volunteering as a therapy dog and owner team." Owners with their pets can earn various levels of achievement or "title" based on the number of visits they accrue, ranging from "Novice" which is ten visits, all the way to "Distinguished" which is 400 visits (AKC, 2023b, p. 1).

The leading AAT volunteer service organizations in the United States are Therapy Dogs International (TDI) and Pet Partners. The following evaluation procedures are designed specifically to determine the readiness and appropriateness of a handler–animal therapy team to provide AAT volunteer services as a representative of TDI.

THERAPY DOGS INTERNATIONAL: TESTING REQUIREMENTS

The TDI testing requirements incorporate 13 tests designed to simulate activities that might occur during a therapy visit (TDI, 2023b, p. 1), and are as follows:

- *Test 1:* TDI Entry Table (simulated as a Hospital Reception Desk). This part of the test is to simulate the arrival at a facility where the coordinator first greets the visiting dog team and instructs the handler on proper grooming before a therapy dog visit.
- *Test 2:* Check-in and out of sight (time: 1 minute). This part of the test is to observe if the dog is able to be left with someone while the handler has to be briefly absent.
- *Test 3:* Getting around people. This part of the test is to observe if the dog has been taught to heel properly on a leash without pulling or lagging, and at the same time is capable of interacting with multiple people in a friendly manner.
- *Test 4:* Group sit/stay. This part of the test is to observe if the dog is under control even if the handler is not very close to the dog and other dog–handler teams are close by.

- *Test 5:* Group down/stay. The same procedure as in the sit/stay test.
- *Test 6:* Recall on a 20 ft. leash. This part of the text is to evaluate how close the working relationship is between the dog–handler team. Does the dog come willingly and happily if recalled on a 20 ft. lead? It will demonstrate if the dog is under the control of the handler.
- *Test 7:* Visiting with a patient. The dog should show willingness to visit a person and demonstrate that it can be made readily accessible for petting (i.e., small dogs will be placed on a person's lap or held; medium dogs will sit on a chair or stand close to the patient to be easily reached; and larger dogs will be standing). Shyness, aggressiveness, jumping up, or not wanting to visit is an automatic failure.
- *Test 8:* Testing of reactions. (The dog must walk in a straight line, respond to commands, and make turns during tasks of visiting with a variety of people.) The dog must visit with a person on crutches, in a wheelchair, or using a walker, and people will be shuffling, moaning, coughing, and also talking loudly.
- *Test 9:* Leave-it; part one. (The dog must not take a treat offered by a person in a wheelchair.) The leave-it exercises are extremely important. A treat from a stranger could be potentially lethal, as could medicine dropped on the floor of a healthcare institution. Drinking or licking up water or liquids from a floor could also be dangerous. The dog must be trained to avoid all of these situations.
- *Test 10:* Leave-it; part two. (The dog must not consume food and water in its path.)
- *Test 11:* Meeting another dog. This part of the test demonstrates whether a dog is well behaved around other dogs.
- *Test 12:* Entering through a door to visit at the facility. A person should be able to go through the entrance ahead of the dog–handler team.
- *Test 13:* Reaction to children. This part of the test can only assess reactions to the presence of children since physical contact with the unregistered dog is not permitted.

For more information or updates and revisions on this test, see the TDI website: www.tdi-dog. org. The TDI evaluation is performed by a TDI-certified evaluator. To locate a TDI evaluator near you, contact TDI or visit their website.

The following evaluation procedures are designed specifically to determine the readiness and appropriateness of a handler–animal therapy team to provide AAA/AAT nonprofessional volunteer services as a representative of Pet Partners.

PET PARTNERS: HANDLER–ANIMAL TEAM EVALUATION

Pet Partners has a rigorous evaluation that is based partially on the AKC CGC but is also designed to simulate the therapeutic environment. There is a strong emphasis on evaluating the pet, the handler, and the interaction between the two. The Pet Partners evaluation was designed to determine the fitness for handlers and their pets to receive registration as a handler–animal team in the Partners Program (Pet Partners, 2023a). A unique aspect of Pet Partners is that it considers a variety of animals, including dogs, cats, horses, llamas and alpacas, birds, rabbits, pigs, and certain small animals (i.e., guinea pigs and rats). There is a Pet Partners team evaluation format appropriate for each species. A therapy team's evaluation must be performed by a Pet Partners licensed team evaluator. Occasionally, an alternative evaluator, such as a veterinarian or animal behavior specialist, may be approved by Pet Partners if no licensed Pet Partners evaluator is available in a region. Alternative evaluators must use the same guidelines as a Pet Partners licensed evaluator. To locate a Pet Partners evaluator near you, visit their website: www.petpartners.org.

The Pet Partners team evaluation has variations specific to the species of the animal being evaluated, but here I will only present the evaluation for dogs (Pet Partners, 2019). The evaluation takes place in an area large enough for the exercises to be performed. The location must be one the pet is unfamiliar with, and the evaluator must be someone who is unfamiliar to the pet being evaluated. Both the handler and the animal are being evaluated. The handler is evaluated on appropriateness of interaction with the animal and ability to be proactive with the animal. The evaluator is looking for positive and affirming interactions between the handler and the pet during the entire evaluation. A small dog may be carried in the arms of the handler during some of the evaluation exercises. In place of the *sit* and *down* evaluation exercises, a small dog is required only to sit quietly while being held by three different strangers who are sitting down. Following is an abbreviated description for each of the Pet Partners' evaluation exercises for a dog (Pet Partners, 2019, pp. 59–85).

Pet Partners Skills and Aptitude Test (PPSAT)

Part One is the Pet Partners Skills Test (PPST) (Pet Partners, 2019, pp. 59–85), with exercises as follows:

- *Exercise 1:* Review the Handler's Questionnaire form. The evaluator reviews the form provided by the handler that describes the animal's preferences and behaviors. This is done while the handler and animal become accustomed to the evaluation area.
- *Exercise 2:* Accepting a friendly stranger. This exercise demonstrates that the team can greet strangers appropriately.
- *Exercise 3:* Accepting petting. This exercise demonstrates that the team has suitable social skills and control for visits.
- *Exercise 4:* Appearance and grooming. This exercise demonstrates that: (1) the team's appearance is suitable for visits; and (2) the animal welcomes being groomed and handled, and permits a stranger to do so.
- *Exercise 5:* Out for a walk. This exercise demonstrates that: (1) the handler is in control of the animal; and (2) the animal is comfortable being moved by the handler.
- *Exercise 6:* Walk through a crowd. This exercise simulates a crowded corridor and demonstrates that the team can move about politely in pedestrian traffic and remain under control in public places.
- *Exercise 7:* Reaction to distractions (both auditory and visual). This exercise demonstrates that the animal remains confident when faced with common distracting situations.
- *Exercise 8:* Sit on command. This exercise demonstrates that the dog has training and will sit at the handler's command.
- *Exercise 9:* Down on command. This exercise demonstrates that the dog has training and will lie down at the handler's command.
- *Exercise 10:* Stay in place. This exercise demonstrates that the dog has training and will stay at the handler's request.
- *Exercise 11:* Come when called. This exercise demonstrates that the dog will leave pleasant distractions to go to the handler and allow him or her to attach a leash.
- *Exercise 12:* Reaction to a neutral dog. This exercise demonstrates that the animal can behave politely around another dog, as well as the handler's awareness of the animal's potential response, and thus can help the dog to succeed.

Part Two is the Pet Partners Aptitude Test (PPAT) (Pet Partners, 2019, pp. 59–85), with exercises as follows:

- *Exercise A:* Overall handling. This exercise demonstrates that: (1) the animal will accept and is comfortable being physically handled by a stranger; and (2) the handler knows how to present the animal on a visit, and how to help the animal accept and welcome being touched all over.
- *Exercise B:* Exuberant and clumsy petting. This exercise demonstrates that: (1) the animal will maintain self-control and tolerate clumsy petting by people who have differing physical abilities or have no knowledge of proper animal etiquette; and (2) the handler can support the animal and be their animal's advocate.
- *Exercise C:* Restraining hug. This exercise demonstrates that: (1) the animal will accept or welcome restraint; and (2) the handler can support the animal and be their animal's advocate.
- *Exercise D:* Staggering and gesturing individual. This exercise demonstrates that: (1) the animal will exhibit confidence when a person who is acting in an unusual manner approaches and invites interaction; and (2) the handler has the handling skills to interact with such a person while supporting their animal.
- *Exercise E:* Angry yelling. This exercise demonstrates that: (1) the animal will not become overstressed when someone exhibits angry emotions; and (2) the handler can support the animal through such a situation.
- *Exercise F:* Two-fingered tap. This exercise demonstrates that: (1) the animal is able to recover when a person bumps or taps it unexpectedly; and (2) the handler can not only tolerate having his or her animal bumped (or tapped), but also helps the animal recover.
- *Exercise G:* Crowded and petted by several people. This exercise demonstrates that: (1) the animal will tolerate crowding and petting by several people at once; and (2) the handler has the skills to visit with a group of people.
- *Exercise H:* Leave it. This exercise demonstrates that the animal will ignore a toy when directed.
- *Exercise I:* Offered a treat. This exercise demonstrates that: (1) when permitted, the animal will politely take a treat; and (2) when not permitted, the animal will remain calm and under control in the presence of treats.

There are four possible ratings a therapy team (handler and animal) may receive from the Pet Partners team evaluation (Pet Partners, 2019, pp. 51–53), as follows:

- *Not suitable for therapy.* A pet may receive this rating if it is aggressive or overly fearful. These pets do not pass the evaluation, and it is recommended that they do not retest.
- *Not ready.* A therapy team does not pass the evaluation but shows some good potential and may retest at a later date.
- *Predictable.* The therapy team passes the evaluation, but it is recommended that they work only in environments where activity and circumstances are consistent and predictable and where there are additional staff members to assist if necessary.
- *Complex.* The therapy team passes the evaluation and is suitable to work in environments with high and potentially unpredictable activity, with no additional staff presence required.

When my dog Rusty was 17 months old, he and I were evaluated by a Pet Partners licensed evaluator for our first time. His playful attitude during the evaluation resulted in a passing rating called "Intermediate," now referred to as "Predictable," as opposed to the highest possible team rating we could have received, an "Advanced" rating, now referred to as "Complex." Rusty calmed down considerably after turning 2 years old and even more when he turned 3 years of age. When we were evaluated together a second time 2 years later, we received the highest possible rating of "Complex." My dog Dolly and I were evaluated for the first time when she was a little older and more mature than Rusty was his first time. Dolly and I were first evaluated when she was 23 months of age and we received the Pet Partners rating of "Complex" our very first time. After Dolly passed away at the age of 9 years, I got a puppy and named her Jesse. Jesse was evaluated for the first time at about 17 months of age and we received a "Predictable" rating as a team. After we had been practicing together for 2 years and were re-evaluated, we received a "Complex" rating as a team.

Pet Partners also requires handlers to complete a 1-day training course where no pets are present. The training can be accomplished by attending a workshop or by taking it online at the Pet Partners website. Look on the Pet Partners website to locate a workshop near you. The handler training must be completed before the therapy team can be evaluated. Pet Partners training workshops are led by a licensed Pet Partners instructor. Instructors are available across the United States. The handler–animal team evaluation is typically scheduled within a few days or a few weeks after the workshop, and the evaluation itself lasts only about 30–40 minutes for each team.

Pet Partners Registration

Advantages to registration as a team with Pet Partners include liability insurance for volunteer, nonprofessional service and the Pet Partners' periodical, *Interactions Magazine*. Handlers have to attend only one Pet Partners handler training no matter how many pets they want to get registered. However, if too much time passes between a handler's training and registration with Pet Partners then one may be asked to complete the training again. Also, if one allows a registration with Pet Partners to lapse and significant time has passed since the last Pet Partners handler's training, then one may be asked to complete a recent version of the Pet Partners handler's training. With active membership, registration for additional pets requires only the handler–animal team evaluation. Pet Partners teams must be re-evaluated every 2 years. Every handler who wishes to volunteer with a pet must be evaluated with that pet, even if the pet holds a current Pet Partners registration with another handler. Rigorous handler training and handler–animal team evaluation requirements are reasons a Pet Partners registration is often preferred over other AAT registrations by many facilities. The Pet Partners registration process also requires a thorough health screening by the pet's veterinarian using Pet Partners' guidelines.

To register with Pet Partners, the handler sends to the Pet Partners organization: the completion certificate from the Pet Partners handler training, the results of the Pet Partners handler–animal team evaluation, the health report completed by the animal's veterinarian, and a registration fee along with the appropriate Pet Partners registration forms and a photo of the handler with his or her pet. The handler receives from Pet Partners a small tag for the pet's collar and an identification badge for the handler to wear with the photo of the handler and the pet. The badge includes the evaluation rating of the handler–animal team and an expiration date (2 years from the current registration). The pet's tag and the handler's badge make it easy for others to recognize the pair as a qualified, registered therapy team. With Pet Partner's registration the handler may also purchase from Pet Partners a vest or a neck scarf for the pet to wear that identifies it as a registered therapy animal with Pet Partners.

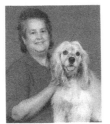

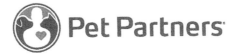

Handler since 1999
A New Leash on Life Therapy
Dogs
ID#   Exp. 9/30/17
Animal Name: Jesse

Qualification Rating:
Complex

Cynthia
Chandler

Pet Partners

Figure 5.1 This official badge identifies me with my dog Jesse as a registered handler–animal therapy team for Pet Partners. Also listed is the name of the local volunteer group of which I am a member, "A New Leash on Life Therapy Dogs."

(*Source:* Used with permission of the Pet Partners organization)

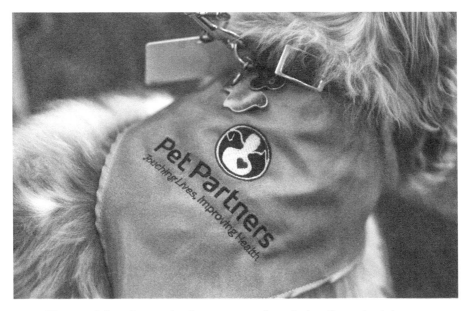

Figure 5.2 This scarf identifies my dog Jesse as a member of a handler–animal therapy team registered with Pet Partners.

(*Source:* Used with permission of the Pet Partners organization)

CONCLUSION

As you can see, the process of becoming a therapy team with your pet requires proper evaluation of you and your pet by qualified evaluators. It is important to obtain some type of registration credential with your pet as a quality control measure for providing non-professional, volunteer AAA services as well as professional AAT. Although TDI and Pet Partners registrations are specifically for nonprofessional volunteers, obtaining a registration credential by one of these organizations represents some measure of responsibility for preparation to practice professionally. By presenting yourself and your pet as a registered team, you are sending the message to your clients and colleagues that you are working within your competency area, meaning that you have met at least some minimal standard that demonstrates you are qualified to provide services that involve working with a therapy animal. I prefer Pet Partners registration over TDI registration for those who want to utilize AAT in their professional practice because Pet Partners requires a 1-day training course for the handler, whereas TDI does not. The Pet Partners handler training provides valuable introductory-level training for those who desire to become a professional practitioner of AAT. Following Pet Partners handler training, additional training and supervision are highly recommended for professional practice of AAT. Additional training for preparation to practice AAT within one's profession can be obtained from a university seminar course, an advanced training workshop, and through study of professional literature.

6

Animal Communication, Risk Management, and Ethics in Animal-Assisted Counseling

One of the best ways to minimize the risk of injury or accident while practicing AAT is to make sure one understands how to properly apply established techniques. AAT in the counseling field should be practiced only by a credentialed professional counselor or a student-in-training who is under proper supervision. Remember, AAT is not an independent profession, but rather it is a treatment modality used by professionals consistent with that professional's training and practice. In addition to being a credentialed counselor or supervised counseling student, the practitioner should have some standardized training in AAT. At a minimum, the counselor and therapy pet should have registration equivalent to Pet Partners training or Therapy Dogs International (TDI). In addition to obtaining an introductory-level training to practice AAT, such as that offered by Pet Partners, I highly recommend you obtain additional training to enhance your professional AAT skills. Although the entry-level credential is necessary and sufficient for volunteer AAA service, in my opinion it is not sufficient by itself for professional AAT work. Information presented throughout this book provides some advanced AAT training. This book provides a therapist with much information to determine which clients may or may not benefit from AAT and how to integrate various AAT techniques into the therapy process to achieve a variety of treatment goals. Brief workshops are also a good device for providing concentrated AAT training, but comprehensive AAT training is best provided via a college or university course format, though currently this type of semester-long training course is difficult to find. Hopefully, the popularity of AAT in a counseling setting will grow to the degree that more counselor education programs will offer an AAT training course.

The benefits of formal training in AAT include not only increasing the chances for therapeutic success but also reducing and managing risks that may be involved with this type of therapy. To minimize risks, a mental health professional who engages in AAT practice should:

- Provide proper socialization and behavior training for the animal.
- Obtain training in AAT.
- Establish and maintain a positive relationship with fellow staff.
- Assess the appropriateness of AAT with a particular client.
- Understand the basics of *zoonoses* (transmittable diseases) risk management, and injury prevention and response that includes attention to both client and therapy animal welfare.

DOI: 10.4324/9781003260448-6

- Be competent in establishing therapeutic or educational goals and applying AAT interventions.
- Assess therapeutic outcomes or client progress.

All counselors and counseling students practicing AAT should carry professional liability insurance for the practice of counseling and should inquire as to whether that insurance provider offers coverage for the practice of AAT. The American Counseling Association (ACA) performed a special committee review of this issue and in 2002 established a policy that the ACA insurance underwriter would cover the practice of AAT as long as the therapist and therapy pet held registration as a Pet Partners team, Therapy Dogs International team, or have American Kennel Club's Canine Good Citizen status or equivalent. I served as an outside consultant for this committee during its review process. Some organizations offer accesss to professional liability insurance for the professional practice of AAT; one such organization is the Association of Animal-Assisted Intervention Professionals (n.d.). Professional liability insurance providers are willing to cover incorporation of human–animal interaction into therapy because AAT is recognized by state and national professional counseling organizations as a legitimate form of therapy. Professional liability insurance may cover AAT counseling practice, but it does not cover physical injury that may occur from interaction with an animal. If you want coverage for physical injury that may occur during AAT you can ask your personal homeowner or renter insurance provider to write you a policy to cover it.

CLIENTS WITH ANIMAL FEARS OR PHOBIAS

If a client has no social familiarity with an animal species or has had a traumatic experience with an animal similar to the therapy animal, then a natural tendency to connect with a therapy animal can be impaired. Clients with severe impairment, such as a fear or phobia of dogs, should not be pressured to be around an animal of which they are fearful. However, if a client who is afraid of an animal requests to be near or around the animal, then those opportunities can be made available for the client. When a client desires to be near or have contact with a therapy animal, then the client should be allowed to set the distance parameters for that contact with the therapist's assistance. I have found that more often than not, those few clients who were initially afraid of my therapy dog and requested no interaction with the animal eventually requested the dog's presence during a therapy session and even initiated interaction with the animal before long. This process often took several weeks, but, observed from a comfortable distance, the dog's friendly demeanor and well-behaved manner won the client over. Until a client feels more comfortable with a therapy animal, arrangements must be made for a client to feel safe and comfortable in therapy. For example, a therapy dog may have to be placed in a corner of the therapy room, perhaps on the dog's bed or in a crate, or maybe placed in another room altogether. A therapist can from time to time offer the client opportunities to view the dog from a comfortable distance or even to watch the dog perform tricks.

At the juvenile detention center where I volunteered, adolescents who desired no interaction with a therapy dog were excused from group AAA and were allowed to sit at a comfortable distance at the other end of a long room or in an adjacent room with a glass wall dividing the rooms. In this way, they were able to observe the positive interactions of the other adolescents with the therapy dog while experiencing little to no anxiety associated with their animal phobia. Within a few sessions or less I usually began to see adolescents who were afraid of the therapy dog begin to lessen their anxiety reactions around the dog, such as walking more slowly away from the dog when the dog came in. Shortly thereafter, they began speaking to the dog with a friendly verbal greeting when the dog came in before walking away from the dog. Before long I noticed the adolescents started taking small risks in proximity to the dog such as choosing to stay in the same room as the dog or to sit closer in the same room to the group interacting with the dog. Within several weeks the once fearful adolescents would even join the group interacting with the dog, though it sometimes took a little more time for them to actually reach out and start touching or petting the dog. This type of recovery occurred with the majority of the dog-fearful adolescents at the detention center who had been given a chance to interact with the dog. At one detention center graduation ceremony I was attending with my therapy dog Rusty, a female adolescent who had overcome her extreme fear of dogs brought her parents over to meet Rusty. Her parents exclaimed how thankful they were that their daughter had the opportunity to overcome her fear of dogs and described how extreme the fear had been: before, the adolescent would cross streets to avoid a dog no matter how small the dog might be and would not walk in certain places in her neighborhood, limited by her fear of dogs, even though most of the dogs she was afraid of were very friendly toward other people. As the parents declared their appreciation for Rusty's assistance in helping their daughter overcome her fear of dogs, the adolescent was leaning over and petting Rusty on the head.

PROFESSIONAL DISCLOSURE AND INFORMED CONSENT TO PARTICIPATE IN AAT

Every practicing counselor must provide the client or the client's legal guardian with a professional disclosure of information statement describing the counseling service. A basic professional information statement and informed consent for services form should contain the following information (Bernstein and Hartsell, 1998):

- A description of the counselor and the counselor's credentials.
- A description of the services provided.
- Procedures for appointments.
- Length and number of sessions.
- The nature of the relationship between the therapist and client (i.e., it is a professional relationship and not a social one).
- Fees and payment information.
- Limits to confidentiality and the duty to warn.
- Addresses and phone numbers for communication with the client.
- Risks of therapy or counseling.
- After-hours emergency information.
- Disposition of client records in case of death of the therapist.
- Waiver of right to child's records and information.
- Signature lines for the client (or legal guardian) and the therapist.

A copy of the signed form should be given to the client and an original kept in the client's file. For AAT practice, it is recommended that the professional disclosure statement and informed consent for services form include the following additional information about AAT:

- The type of animal (e.g., dog, cat, bird).
- Any training or registration of the therapy animal.
- The relationship of the animal to the therapist.
- The types of activities a client can engage in with the therapy animal if the client chooses to do so.

The consent form should also inform clients of their right to request that the therapy animal not be present for counseling sessions.

CLIENT SCREENING FOR AAT

All clients should be screened before they participate in AAT for the protection of the client as well as for the pet. Clients with a tendency toward violence or history of animal abuse are unlikely candidates for participating in AAT. However, some programs with high supervision specialize in using AAT to help clients with an abusive or aggressive history develop empathy and rehabilitate their abusive and aggressive ways. Clients with diminished capacity who may not understand the consequences of their actions must be carefully supervised during therapy to protect the animal from injury. A colleague of mine performs animal-assisted play therapy with autistic children. On a first visit by one client, the child approached the therapy dog and in his excitement grabbed the dog's ear tightly and pulled hard. The dog let out several yelps before the therapist could get the grasp released. The dog was a bit shy around that child after that episode. Clients with specific animal phobias are unlikely candidates for therapy with an animal of which the client is afraid; however, if a client desires to work in a phobia desensitization program involving a therapy animal, then this can be designed. A therapist using AAT should always inquire about possible animal allergies of clients. If the allergy is severe and cannot be controlled by medication, then the client should not participate in AAT with that type of animal. See also the Client Screening Form for Animal-Assisted Therapy in Appendix B.

SERVING AS AN ADVOCATE FOR THE THERAPY ANIMAL

It is vital that an AAT practitioner serve as an advocate for the safety and welfare of the therapy animal. Therapy animal advocacy involves:

- Establishing and maintaining a healthy and functional owner or handler relationship with an animal that will be or is participating in the counseling process.
- Assessing an animal's ability to work as a therapy animal (therapeutic change agent).
- Providing a comfortable and safe environment for the animal to participate in AAT.
- Providing a comfortable, safe, and secure environment for the therapy animal when it is not participating in AAT.
- Acknowledging when an animal is experiencing fatigue, stress, distress, discomfort, or a lack of desire to participate in AAT, and providing for the animal's needs.
- Having knowledge of animal behavior and being able to interpret therapy animal vocal and nonvocal communications.

It is important from the first moment of contact with a potential or working therapy animal, and from that point forward, that an owner or handler be positive and nurturing with the therapy animal in all human–animal interactions. Mutual feelings of trust and safety between the therapist and the therapy animal are of paramount importance. All animal training regimens should be safe, fun, and positive and should consider the welfare of the animal. Therapy animals should be trained in accordance with their species (e.g., dog obedience) and socialized to be good citizens when interacting with people.

Therapy animals must be healthy and have good stamina to participate in AAT. Disabled animals may still participate if working does not cause undue stress for the animal (Pet Partners, 2014). The therapy animal should be able to pass a standardized evaluation for the provision of AAT that caters to the species of the animal. Therapy animals with their handlers should be re-evaluated periodically to determine if they are still qualified for AAT practice; every 2 years is recommended (Pet Partners, 2014). To be effective as a therapeutic change agent, therapy animals should demonstrate behaviors that depict them as confident, reliable, friendly, and with a visible desire to interact socially with humans in a positive manner.

The therapist should provide a safe and comfortable environment for the animal and client to participate in therapy sessions. Also, the handler should provide a place that the animal comes to know as its own space when it wants to rest during a session, such as a bed or crate in a corner of the office for a dog or a basket, crate, or cage for a cat or rabbit. The animal should be provided with food, water, rest, exercise, and recreation as needed. An animal should not be expected to work a long day with multiple consecutive clients. How much time a therapy animal can work with clients in a day, week, or month depends not only on the species but also on the individual animal. The therapy animal must be allowed time to rest between clients, and the handler must allow time and access for the animal's needs to be met. Therapy animals typically do not work on consecutive days, nor do they work long days. It is important for a handler to know a therapy animal's needs and to assist in providing for the animal. It is recommended that therapy animals work no longer than two consecutive hours per day, less if they are not comfortable working for that length of time (Pet Partners, 2014).

When a therapy animal is not working it should be provided with a comfortable and safe location in which to stay. Crate or cage training an animal can better protect the animal for when the handler is not able to supervise it, such as with having to move the animal to another room when working with a person with animal phobia or allergy, or when circumstances do not allow the therapy animal to accompany the handler for certain events or crisis situations. Comfortable crates or cages are also a safer way to travel with certain therapy animals since the crate or cage can be tied down or secured in the vehicle, adding additional protection to the therapy animal during transport.

RECOGNIZING STRESS IN THERAPY ANIMALS

As a therapist working with your pet, it is vital that you understand some of the basics of animal behavior. When an animal is experiencing stress or even perceiving stress in another animal or in a human, the animal may exhibit calming signals demonstrating its experience or perception of stress. These signals serve as useful information for the pet's handler who would then need to reassure the animal or remove it from the stressful situation (Gammonley et al., 2003). These signals from an animal are also useful for recognizing that stress may be present in a client or therapist. It is vital that a therapy pet handler be able to recognize signs of stress in a therapy pet. Some typical well-known signs of stress for animals are provided in Table 6.1. Each of these stress signals must be viewed in the context of the environment in which it occurs. For example, a dog panting can be a sign of stress, but if the animal is hot or thirsty then it will also pant. The key is to know your animal and be sensitive to its moods and needs. Be objective and receptive to what your pet may be trying to tell you.

When the signs of stress are recognized in a therapy animal, the animal's handler must take some type of action. An attempt to reduce the stress for the animal should be made. The handler could acknowledge and reassure the therapy animal. The animal could be given a break. If stress signals persist, the therapy animal may even need a vacation from therapy for a few days or weeks. If stress symptoms persist over the course of several therapy visits, the handler should reassess whether the therapy animal is appropriate for therapy work in a given environment, or appropriate for therapy at all. Also, when a therapy pet becomes too old or too ill to work, then the pet should be retired from therapy service.

Table 6.1 Signs of Stress in Animals

Animal	*Signs of Stress*
Dog	Body shaking
	Panting and salivating
	Dilated pupils
	Excessive blinking
	Sweating through the pads of the feet
	Restlessness, distraction, agitation
	Lack of eye contact
	Yawning
	Excessive shedding
	Excessive vocalizing
	Licking lips
	Hiding (behind handler)
	Turning away
	Attempts to leave
	Need for repeated commands
	Inappropriate defecation or urination
Cat	Restlessness, distraction, agitation
	Clinging
	Unusual passivity
	Defensive vocalizations
	Excessive shedding
	Dilated pupils
Rabbit or pocket pet (e.g., gerbil, guinea pig, hamster)	Body tense, with tail up
	Enlarged eyes with whites showing
	Ears laid back tightly
	Growling or squeaking noises
	Flinches when touched
	Rapid breathing
	Licking lips
	Lack of interest displayed
Bird	Ruffled feathers
	Lack of desire to socialize
	Increased elimination
	Increased pecking
	Looking away
	Abnormal vocalization
Horse	Eyes rolling
	Head up and pulled back
	Ears back
	Flared nostril (with or without blowing)
	Lips pulled back
	Tail tucked
	Hindquarters hunched
	Weight on hindquarters

Source: Pet Partners Team Training Course Manual, 5th ed. (Delta Society, 2000, pp. 68–69); *Pet Partners Team Training Course Manual*, 6th ed. (Delta Society, 2004, pp. 91–92); and *Interactions Magazine* (Lipin, 2009, p. 7).

One way to help an animal manage the stress that comes with working in therapy is to give the animal a massage before or after a day's work. One recommended technique that is very soothing for an animal is the Tellington touch, or T-touch, developed by internationally known horsetrainer and teacher of riding instructors and horse trainers, Linda Tellington-Jones (Tellington-Jones and Taylor, 1995). The T-touch technique is appropriate for many species of therapy animals.

An animal can work as a therapy pet if it has a long-term disability, but the handler must take precautions so that the disabled animal does not experience undue discomfort or stress from working with this disability. As a team evaluator for Pet Partners, I evaluated a dog that had only three legs; one front leg had been amputated as a result of being hit by a car. The dog could stand and walk by itself on three legs, but the owner would also position himself close to the dog so that it could lean slightly on him for balance when stopped. The handler allowed a little extra time for the pet to walk at a slower pace and for rest breaks. The dog did well on therapy visits and seemed to really enjoy interactions when it was visiting.

My therapy cat, Snowflake, was deaf from birth. While his visual startle reflex was a bit more heightened, his audio startle reflex was nonexistent. Despite his deafness, Snowflake acted calm and comfortable as well as sociable and playful on therapy visits. His hearing disability meant that I took special precautions at home and on visits to ensure his safety. At home, he was not allowed outside unless he was on a leash. On therapy visits, he primarily worked indoors, but on occasional therapy visits outdoors he wore a chest harness and a leash. I made sure those he visited were aware of his disability. If your animal has a disability, when you and your pet are ready for evaluation as a therapy team you should inform the animal evaluator of that disability before the evaluation begins so appropriate allowances may be made if necessary.

Most of us know our pets fairly well and can understand what their behaviors are conveying to us. However, some of us love our animals so much that we may be in denial about what they are communicating. If we lose our objectivity about our animal's behavior, then we place our pet and our clients in jeopardy. For example, one day I was evaluating a therapy team consisting of a teacher and her large mixed-breed dog that she had rescued from a shelter a little over a year before. She had already been taking the dog to her school and was so pleased with how the children were responding positively to the dog's presence that she had decided to start a reading practice program with her dog. She was even going to spearhead the recruitment of other volunteers to join in with their dogs. The whole venture was very exciting, and I was extremely pleased that she was interested in community service with her pet. She had decided that it was best to get some proper training and registration as a therapy team with her pet before continuing with her project, so she had completed the Pet Partners workshop the day before and now she and her pet were going to go through the animal team evaluation.

When she and the dog came into the evaluation room, I did not see the same enthusiasm in the pet that I saw in the pet's handler. The dog acted as if it was not very interested in its surroundings or in the people in the room. The pet's owner reassured me by saying that it was just a very calm dog and everything was all right. I had been an animal evaluator for only a brief period at the time, but still my training combined with my intuition about the dog led me to proceed with caution. The dog was very still and very quiet with an attitude of indifference. He quickly averted his head when I approached—this is called a "look away" calming signal—demonstrating his preference not to engage with me. I questioned the handler as to whether we should proceed because it did not seem to me that the dog really wanted to be a part of what was going on around it. The owner assured me that the dog was feeling just fine. I wrestled with the idea of terminating the evaluation, but, being fairly inexperienced at the time, I felt I did not have enough evidence to justify that position. The dog was not being friendly, but it was not aggressive either. The dog had been looking toward the exit door frequently as if plotting an escape route. I empathized with the dog's desire to leave and was watchful of additional signs that would support the termination of the evaluation. When we came to the part in the evaluation where I was to hug the dog, I moved forward and leisurely extended my reach. The dog lunged at me, targeting my left hand, snarling and baring all of his teeth. I moved quickly but still felt the outside of the dog's teeth brush against the tips of my fingers as I jumped back to get out of its way. After the initial lunge and snap, the dog did not pursue me further and immediately quieted back down. Fortunately, I was not bitten or injured by the dog despite its clear intention, but I put a stop to the evaluation at once.

The dog's owner was shocked by the dog's behavior. I consulted with the volunteers working with me in the room, and they had observed what I had: the dog had been uninterested and unhappy about participating in the evaluation, but had not shown signs of aggression until the moment I began to hug it. Obviously the dog did not pass the evaluation, and I gave it a "not suitable for therapy" rating. I informed the owner that she could not use the dog for therapy and should stop taking it to school because it was likely that someone was eventually going to get bitten by this dog. The owner erupted in tears and for the first few minutes exclaimed that she had never before seen any of that behavior in her dog and did not understand it. I sensed that this was a case where the owner was just not seeing what the dog was communicating. The owner, wanting desperately to work with this dog that she had rescued and she loved, saw only what she wanted to see in the dog's behavior. After a few minutes of inquiry, the owner began to acknowledge that she had seen certain similar behaviors of lack of interest and unhappiness in her dog when she took it to school but had not interpreted them to mean that the dog was uncomfortable. I conveyed two important considerations for the owner. First, the owner was not being as objective about the dog's behavior as she could be, and objectivity is extremely important for AAT work. Second, her dog is what I refer to as a "stealth dog": it gives clues but no real obvious warning that it is about to attack. You cannot see it coming unless you pay close attention and know what to look for. A stealth dog is a time bomb for biting someone.

The facts that owners are typically not objective about their own pet's behavior, and that some pets' negative behaviors and attitudes are not obvious to the untrained eye, make it very important that, before any pet works in therapy, it is evaluated to determine its appropriateness for that type of public activity. With more years of experience as an animal team evaluator since this incident, I now trust and follow my evaluator's intuitions much more quickly. Though I have been bitten during two evaluations, it must be taken into account that I have completed over 500 handler–animal team evaluations.

UNDERSTANDING YOUR PET'S COMMUNICATION

It is important to properly interpret animal behavior for the safety and welfare of animal and human participants in therapy. Also, it is important to interpret therapy animal behavior in order to achieve greater benefit for a client from human–animal interaction. Animals will perceive emotional states of other animals and humans through seeing, hearing, smelling, tasting, and feeling. If we can accurately interpret signals of an animal's perception of clients' emotional and attitudinal states, then we have significantly more information about our clients with which to understand them better and to assist them. All of the calming signals of animals described earlier in this chapter—signals of the experience or perception of stress— are useful for not only understanding the level of the animal's stress, but also in understanding the animal's perception of stress in someone with whom the animal is interacting.

My dog Jesse will signal a client's level of stress or distress through various signals even though the client is effectively masking or hiding emotions from me. I believe Jesse is responding to the smell of secretions from the client's body that reveal high levels of hormones associated with stress or distress in the client. After perceiving a client's stress or distress, Jesse may initially shift her body position (lift her head or sit up quickly from a resting position), briefly look away from a client, blink her eyes, or yawn. Further, if I or the client fail to see and acknowledge to her what she is signaling, she becomes more obvious in her communication, such as moving back and forth between me and the client, or jumping in the client's lap and licking the client's hand or face, or laying on her back in the client's lap and wriggling her paws in the air. She does this because she presents an attitude of care for clients she works with. Not all therapy animals have this attitude of care toward a human and will consistently respond to stress they perceive in a human by simply moving away. Jesse too may eventually move away from a client as a way of dealing with the stress that she is perceiving, but she most often makes several attempts to signal and attend to a client's stress while engaging with a client before she moves away. Her willingness and desire to stay engaged with a client when a client is stressed adds to Jesse's value in the role of a therapy animal. It is important that I or a client acknowledge to Jesse that we are receiving and trying to understand her signals by rewarding her with nurturing touch and vocal tone. Then we need to address in therapy with some immediacy what Jesse might be telling us. With this the client begins a catharsis, that is an emotional pressure release, that changes the hormonal secretions in the client's body and the animal, having perceived this change, settles back down and stops signaling perceptions of stress or distress. Consistently across my sessions and sessions I observed of my students where a therapy animal was participating, I saw that once a client moved past the fine line between holding back, from unawareness or resistance, and releasing, that is, delving into the most relevant or most distressing issues of concern, then a therapy animal no longer signaled it was perceiving stress or distress in a client by using a calming signal. An animal may have moved near a client or therapist during a client's catharsis, but it was now obvious the animal was satisfied that the stress or distress was being attended and the animal was calmer and more still than it was before the client's catharsis.

I will now describe some typical animal behaviors and accepted interpretations of those behaviors. Some of the behaviors I will describe, especially those of aggression and extreme shyness, would not necessarily come into play during a therapy session because the animal has been evaluated and prohibited from being a therapy animal if it is aggressive or too shy.

Dog Behavior

To learn more about a dog's communication behavior, I suggest you do some reading. A book I recommend for this is *Dogspeak* (Hoffman, 1999). Each dog has its own little behavior quirks, and you probably know your dog best. However, some universal facial patterns for dogs have been described that can be helpful in interpreting your dog's mood (Hoffman, 1999). A dog's eyes that are wide open can communicate surprise or fear. A frightened dog typically tightens its whole face, pulls its ears back, and pulls its lips down and back. A dog that is afraid may also lower its head and look away from the object that is causing concern. On the other hand, a long, hard, intense stare is usually a conveyed threat or warning by a dog. A slightly furrowed brow with a stare may convey intense interest, whereas a deeply furrowed brow with a stare may convey fear or extreme caution. Exaggerated eye blinking is a way for a dog to communicate that it is stressed and does not want to be seen as a threat, as is the averting of its gaze away from another dog or person. A blank stare and extremely limp ears can communicate boredom for a dog. Narrowed or half-closed eyes typically mean the dog is happy and relaxed. A keen, alert look with pricked-up ears may convey a dog is feeling happy and confident. A dog that is staring but trying not to show it, like staring out of the sides of its eyes, is probably planning something, usually something playful in nature (Hoffman, 1999).

Schaffer (1993), a veterinarian, classified and described six various canine postures that are helpful in interpreting a dog's communications. Negative behavior categories are aggressive, fearful, and passively submissive; acceptable or positive behavior categories are submissive, playful, and attentive:

- Aggressive Dog:

    — Will begin with its ears pointed forward and then pull the ears out and down as the aggression escalates, and will pull the ears all the way back when it actually attacks.
    — Eyes are fixed and staring.
    — Lips are raised with the mouth open and nose wrinkled.
    — Head is held high, and the body is stiff and tense and leans forward with the weight shifted to the front.
    — Tail is raised up and over the rump and toward the back of the neck.
    — Fur may be raised over the rump and neck; this is referred to as having the hackles raised.
    — Front leg may point at the object which is causing concern for the dog.
    — Typically vocalizing with a growl, snarl, and bark.

- Fearful Dog:

    — Lays the ears back and down against the head and has its eyes wide open and fixed.
    — Head is down and the mouth slightly open.
    — Fur is raised over the dog's neck.
    — Weight is shifted backward on its rear legs and tail tucked under its abdomen. (Note that some breeds of dog, such as the Greyhound, have a naturally tucked tail all of the time, and so this does not imply a negative expression.)
    — May tremble, urinate, or defecate.
    — May move in quick motions in an attempt to find an escape route and may whine.

- Passively Submissive Dog:

    — Ears are down, eyes down, lips down, hair flat, and head down.
    — Lying on its side or back with the tail tucked close to the body.
    — May urinate.

- Submissive Dog:

    — Ears and eyes are down.
    — Head is lowered with the lips down and pulled back horizontally.
    — Fur is down against a body that is leaning back with the weight shifted to the rear.
    — Tail may be wagging or hanging down or be tucked close to the body.
    — May whine.

- Playful Dog:

    — Ears are up and eyes are moving.
    — Fur is flat against a body that is leaning back with weight shifted to the rear.
    — Lips are relaxed.
    — A front paw may wave in the air.
    — Tail wags up high and fast in a broad motion.
    — May pant, bark, or whine.

- Attentive Dog:

    — Ears are up and eyes are moving.
    — Head is up with lips relaxed.
    — Fur lies flat against its body that has weight evenly distributed.
    — Tail is stiff and horizontal and moving slowly as aroused.
    — Typically the dog is not vocalizing.

Some simple illustrations of five dog postures are provided in Appendix D and may help to distinguish between different expressions.

Dogs have been shown to have a variety of communication patterns that convey complex messages; everything from demonstrations of feeling calm and relaxed, to feeling alert and engaged, to feeling anxious and distressed, or frightened. Dogs are also capable of a complex form of communication called referential communication:

> Referential communication occurs when a sender elaborates its gestures to direct the attention of a recipient to its role in the pursuit of the desired goal, e.g., by pointing or showing an object, thereby informing the recipient what it wants. If the gesture is successful, the sender and the recipient focus their attention simultaneously on a third entity, the target.
>
> (Malavasi and Huber, 2016, p. 1)

In an investigation of a dog's ability to perform referential communication, it was shown that dogs present intentional gaze alternation from an unobtainable target (food or toy) to an owner in an act of "showing" the location of what they desire (Miklósi et al., 2000).

Scientists have found evidence that dogs really understand some of what we are saying. Researchers in Hungary published a ground-breaking study that found dogs understand both the meaning of words and the intonation used to speak the words. To find out how dogs process human speech, Attila Andics, a neuroscientist at Eötvös Loránd University in Budapest, and his colleagues used brain scanners (fMRIs) and 13 willing family dogs from four breeds: Border Collies, Golden Retrievers, Chinese Crested Dogs, and German Shepherds (Andics et al., 2016). The dogs had been trained to lie motionless in the scanner while they listened to recordings of their trainer's voice. The dogs heard meaningful words ("well done!" in Hungarian) in a praising tone and in a neutral tone. They also heard meaningless words ("as if") in a neutral or praising tone of voice. When the scientists analyzed the brain scans, they saw that—regardless of the trainer's intonation—the dogs processed the meaningful words in the left hemisphere of the brain, just as humans do. But the dogs didn't do this for the meaningless words. According to the researchers, there is no acoustic reason for this difference; it shows that these words have meaning to dogs. The dogs also processed intonation in the right hemisphere of their brains, also like humans. And when they heard words of praise delivered in a praising tone, yet another part of their brain lit up: the reward area. Meaning and tone enhanced each other. They integrate the two types of information to interpret what they heard, just as we do (Andics et al., 2016).

These results add to scientists' knowledge of how canine brains process human speech. Dogs have brain areas dedicated to interpreting voices, distinguishing sounds (in the left hemisphere), and analyzing the sounds that convey emotions (in the right hemisphere) (Morell, 2014). This does not mean dogs understand everything that we say, although some dogs are known to recognize more than 1,000 human words—behavior that suggests they may attach meaning to human sounds. The research shows that it is indeed the words themselves—and not the tone in which they're spoken or the context in which they're used—that dogs comprehend (Andics et al., 2016).

Cat Behavior

Schaffer (1993) described six various cat postures that may help to interpret a cat's communications. Negative feline behavior categories are fearful, defensive aggressive, and offensive aggressive; positive feline expressive behaviors are submissive, friendly/relaxed, and attentive/playful:

- Fearful Cat:

  — Feels somewhat trapped.
  — Becomes very tense and crouches its body low against the ground.
  — Lays its ears flat, back, and down against the head.
  — Pupils are dilated, and stares intensely at the object of which it is afraid.
  — Whiskers point backward against the face.
  — Tail whips back and forth briskly.
  — Fur is up and bristled all over the body.
  — May make negative vocalizations like hissing or spitting.

- Defensive Aggressive Cat:

  — Afraid but feels it still has options open.
  — Lays its ears flat, back, and down.
  — Pupils are dilated and staring intensely.
  — Whiskers are pulled back against the face.
  — Fur is up and bristled all over the body.
  — Arches back up high, and lowers head.
  — Tail arches over the back and jerks briskly.
  — Leans away from and keeps its body at a right angle to the object of which it is afraid.
  — May slap its front paws.
  — Mouth is wide open, and nose curled into a snarl with teeth showing.
  — May hiss, growl, or spit.

- Offensive Aggressive Cat:

  — Intent on attack.
  — Ears are up, away from its head, but still point backward.
  — Head is held sideways and sways slowly.
  — Eyes are fixed on the target with constricted pupils.
  — Whiskers are spread out and point forward.
  — Fur is raised in a ridge down the back midline and on its entire tail.
  — Body is stretched and tense with the nails extended and a front paw raised.
  — Mouth is open with lips curled.
  — May make hissing, spitting, yowling, or growling noises.

- Submissive Cat:

  — Ears are flat, head down, and chin tucked.
  — Eyes are down with no eye contact and pupils dilated.
  — Eyelids are partly or totally closed.
  — Whiskers lie flat against the face.
  — Fur lies flat against a crouched body.
  — Tail is down and thumps the ground.
  — May mew or open its mouth and emit no sound.
  — Not aggressive but certainly not very comfortable.

- Friendly/Relaxed Cat:

  — Ears are up and pointed slightly forward.
  — Head is up with the eyes almost closed.
  — Pupil size will vary according to the light available in the room.
  — Whiskers are slightly fanned and point sideways.
  — Fur lies down against a body that is stretched out and relaxed.
  — May rub against a person or touch noses.
  — Tail is stiff, motionless, and vertical.
  — May purr, meow, or murmur.

- Attentive/Playful Cat:

  — Head is up with ears up and pointed forward.
  — Whiskers are spread out and point forward.
  — Eyes are moving with dilated pupils.
  — Fur lies down flat against a tense body.
  — Tail is motionless but jerks when aroused.
  — When stalking, tail will be down.
  — When playing, tail will be up, arched, or in an inverted U-shape.
  — Will either be silent or elicit teeth chattering or lip smacking when excited.

A useful book for understanding cat communication is *The Cat Whisperer* (Bessant, 2001). Some simple illustrations of five cat postures are provided in Appendix D of this book that may help to distinguish between different expressions.

Horse Behavior

The primary means of horse communication are tail switches (swishing), head position, ear position, and facial expressions—such as widening or narrowing of the eyes, and nose and lip movements (Delta Society, 2002; Weeks and Beck, 1996). Common horse vocalizations include soft puffing or snorting, but strong snorts, neighs, and screams are given when horses are distressed or aggressive (Delta Society, 2002). When a horse is relaxed it usually carries its head low with a slow swinging motion, the horse's muscles are soft or loose, and the gait is smooth and fluid (Delta Society, 2002). Visual communications used by the horse to indicate agitation include the following: nose wrinkles upon the upper caudal edge of the nostril, which indicates disgust, agitation, or aggression; ears flatten back, which indicates aggression, defense, or a ritualized posture for irritation; head tossing, which indicates irritation or frustration; and tail swishing, which indicates tension, frustration, or agitation (Weeks and Beck, 1996, p. 24).

Following are some guidelines to interpret different behaviors of horses (Delta Society, 2002, pp. 1–2):

- Relaxed Horse Posture:

  — Head is level or lower than the top of the shoulder.
  — Makes eye contact.
  — Tail is swishing or hanging loose.
  — Lips hang loosely.
  — Nostrils are relaxed.
  — Weight is evenly distributed but may rest all hind weight on one leg and cock the relaxed leg.

- Aggressive Horse Posture:

  — Head is held high and the neck is tense.
  — Eyes are wide and may show whites.
  — Ears are pricked stiffly forward or pinned back.
  — May bare teeth or wrinkle the nose.
  — Lips may be tense and stiff with the chin flattened.
  — Nostrils are flared.
  — May snort or whistle.
  — Tail is held out or thrashing.
  — Weight is on the front legs with hindquarters tucked and tense, and may include stomping.

- Fearful or Submissive Horse Posture:

  — Eyes are rolling.
  — Head is up and pulled back.
  — Nostrils are flared.
  — Lips are pulled back.
  — Tail is tucked.
  — Hindquarters are hunched.
  — Weight is on the hindquarters.

- Displacement or Calming Horse Signals:

  — Tossing the head.
  — Shaking the mane.
  — Pawing the ground.
  — Grazing.
  — Yawning.
  — Turning away.

Horses can be easily startled by objects because they have binocular vision in front and monocular vision on either side, which can make things in their environment change shape and become frightening:

> Horses are a prey species with a highly developed flight response. Horses routinely flee a situation and turn to analyze it later.
>
> (Delta Society, 2002, p. 1)

Paul McGreevy, author of *Equine Behavior* (2012), provides useful descriptions of horse communication. For instance, he describes that a horse typically flicks or points its ears in the direction to which it is paying attention. If both ears are forward then attention is being paid, for the most part, to what is in front of the horse. If one ear is forward and the other ear is directed to the side or back, then this may reflect that attention is divided with some attention being paid to what is in the front and some to what is at the side or back of the horse. When both ears are pointing back, this may indicate the horse is paying attention, for the most part, to the rider or what is behind the horse. Ears laid or pinned back can indicate the horse is angry or distressed about something anywhere in the horse's perceptual field. Ears laid back can also mean the horse is ready to bite or kick (McGreevy, 2012).

Over a 2-year period, Brandt (2004) observed women and horses working together in various horse barn settings and conducted 25 in-depth interviews with women regarding their communication with their equine companions. Based on the information gathered through these observations and interviews, the researcher presented the argument "that humans and horses co-create a language system by way of the body to facilitate the creation of meaning" (p. 299).

> For both species, the body is a tool through which they can communicate a wide range of emotions and desires. Both horses and humans can learn a complicated system of body language different from the elements of spoken language, thus enabling each to express a subjective presence to the other and work together in a goal-oriented fashion.
>
> (Brandt, 2004, p. 304)

Humans can learn about how horses communicate by observing their behavior with other horses. Horses are highly sensitive to body language expressions by other horses and also by humans. Horses have highly sensitive bodies because their bodies are their primary vehicle for communication. Likewise, humans experienced at working with horses,

> develop a similar heightened awareness about their body language . . . and are careful to think about the messages they are conveying, or intend to convey, to the horse by way of their bodies.
>
> (Brandt, 2004, p. 306)

Birke (2007) wrote of a current rise of what is popularly called "natural horsemanship," describing it as "a definitive change within the horse industry" (p. 217). The way of natural horsemanship is not to force a horse to participate in activities through outdated tactics of fear and dominance but rather to gain a horse's cooperation to participate in activities by learning to better understand and communicate with a horse.

> This drive toward what advocates generally call "natural horsemanship" is a significant shift in the horse-world, both in Europe and in North America. . . . The emphasis is on kindness, with particular emphasis on communicating with and learning to understand from the horse's point of view—the natural behavior of horses.
>
> (Birke, 2007, p. 218)

A great many horse-owners and handlers turn to the way of natural horsemanship in the belief that its methods offer something that will give them a closer, more trusting relationship with their horses (Birke, 2007; Roberts, 2008).

Horses are capable communicators of their feelings and intentions. Similar to humans, chimpanzees, and dogs, horses can signal their intentions via referential communication. In their investigation of a horse's ability to communicate referentially, Malavasi and Huber (2016) determined that horses communicated with a human observer about the location of a food bucket that was out of reach. The horses appeared to use both indicative (pointing) and nonindicative (nods and shakes) head gestures in the test conditions. The investigators concluded that horses used referential gestures to manipulate the attention of a human recipient in order to obtain an unreachable resource.

Incorporating knowledge on horse communication will assist a therapist and client to work with a horse in harmony, in ways that are respectful, positive, and congruent with the natural way of the horse. Understanding how to communicate with a horse encourages people to be authentic, real, and honest with themselves and the horse. This facilitates a nurturing mutual relationship between human and horse. A brief video that illustrates horse calming signals is *Calming Signals of Vosje* by Rachel Peters (August 12, 2014; 2 minutes 45 seconds; showing licking; empty chewing; head turning; sniffing; ears sharply forward; quick and varied ear movement [ears sharply forward, ears sharply back, ears divided]; eye blinking; turning away; and showing neck and look back): https://vimeo.com/103271203.

Animals and Emotions

It has generally been accepted by scientists that animals experience the primary emotion of fear as an instinctual survival mechanism. However, whether animals experience complex secondary emotions like love, sadness, or grief has been much debated in scientific circles. In an attempt to better understand dogs, Sanders (1993) systematically observed his interactions with his own dog and interactions by other dog owners with their dog, and interviewed dog owners about their understanding of their dogs. In regard to the dog as minded actor Sanders described:

> The owners with whom I spoke had little doubt of their dogs' cognitive abilities, and all could recount examples of what they defined as minded behavior. Dogs' thought processes were generally seen as fairly basic ... and to a certain extent, thoughtful intelligence was seen as varying from animal individual to individual and from breed to breed.
>
> (Sanders, 1993, p. 212)

In regard to the dog as individual Sanders described:

> Although many caretakers did see certain personality characteristics as breed related, they regularly spoke of their own dog as unique individuals. ... Owners were adept at describing their dogs' unique personal tastes ... likes and dislikes in food, activities, playthings and people.
>
> (Sanders, 1993, pp. 215–216)

In regard to the dog as emotional and reciprocating, Sanders described:

> [O]wners typically understood their dogs as having subjective experiences in which some form of reasoning was linked with emotion. The most common theme that emerged ... was that dogs are eminently emotional beings. Dogs were, for example, described as experiencing loneliness, joy, sadness, embarrassment, and anger.
>
> (Sanders, 1993, p. 216)

In conclusion:

> The dog owners studied by Sanders regularly described interactions with their dogs which clearly and reasonably demonstrated to them the ability of animals to be minded, insightful, and empathetic. Their dogs typically were characterized as creatively employing learned gestural signs in symbolic ways; they organized their behavior so as to communicate new ideas in novel situations.
>
> (Sanders and Arluke, 1993, p. 380)

Scientific technology that allows for the examination of brain chemistry and brain imaging is providing supportive evidence for the experience of complex secondary emotions in animals. Researchers discovered that animals have similar neurochemical responses as humans when seeming to express affection, facial stress, or the loss of a companion (Daley

Olmert, 2009; Panksepp, 2005; Tangley, 2000; Uvnäs-Moberg, 2010). This objective evidence compounded with subjective observations of animal behavior strongly suggests that animals do in fact experience complex secondary emotions. In addition, some behaviorists suggest that domesticated animals, such as pet cats and dogs, have evolved to a social level of actively expressing a large variety of secondary emotions to their owners, for instance, a dog exhibiting a play bow to express a desire to frolic or cuddling on the couch to express affection, or a cat curling up in a lap and purring and rubbing a cheek against your hand as an expression of affection (Schultz, 2000).

Animals and Social Interaction and Expression

Though AAT is not limited to canines and equines, it is established that dogs and horses are keenly aware of both subtle and obvious social cues that communicate intention and interaction, and their repertoire of vocal, facial, and bodily expressions makes them especially capable social communicators (Gosling, Kwan, and John, 2003; Hill, 2006; Hoffman, 1999; Roberts, 2008).

> Horses have highly developed herd relationships and excellent communication skills. Most communication is in the form of subtle body language.
>
> (Delta Society, 2002, p. 1)

There is increasing recognition that many animal species adapt vocal signals to social situations, as evidenced by the article titled "Acoustic Interaction in Animal Groups" (Schwartz and Freeberg, 2008), published in a special issue of the American Psychological Association's *Journal of Comparative Psychology*. Research on animal vocalizations in a within-species social context has included the study of insects, fish, amphibians, birds, and mammals (including dolphins), just to name a few. In their discussion of some of this research, Schwartz and Freeberg (2008) concluded the following:

> The vocal behavior of individuals obviously impacts the social behavior of other individuals in a group of animals. It is also becoming clear that the social behavior occurring within groups—indeed, the social structure of the group—can impact the vocal behavior of individuals in the group.
>
> (p. 234)

Various animal studies indicate that influences from a sufficient number of individuals in a group can affect the structural complexity of individuals' social vocalizations in the group. Indeed, animal studies demonstrate the common phenomenon of within-species vocal convergence in a social context; this is where vocal signals of individuals within a group tend to become acoustically more similar to one another over time. Thus, with enough individual influence, the social vocalizations and social structure of a group can change, and over time the influence of the group can result in changes in the social vocalizations of an individual (Schwartz and Freeberg, 2008).

It has therefore been shown that animals are natural social communicators and that their social communications can influence and be influenced by others of their own kind within a group social context. How does this knowledge about the social communication abilities of animals help us understand and appreciate the influential possibilities of human–animal interaction? When different species interact, and especially when they learn to communicate with one another, such as humans with dogs or humans with horses, can one expect that there may be potential for these interactions to influence the social behavior of the two different species? These are questions some have tried to address and others are still trying to address through research on human–animal interaction, AAA, and AAT.

Based on what we think we know so far about animal behavior, it seems that understanding and expressing what we think a therapy animal is communicating in a social interaction can further facilitate the human–animal relationship and enhance the clinical efficacy of human–animal social interactions. Understanding what animals are communicating can also assist with recognizing when a therapy animal is stressed and requires attention or rest and when the therapy animal is distressed or uncomfortable with a person or situation. As mentioned earlier in the chapter, when a therapy animal, such as a dog, is stressed, it presents with calming signals, such as averting the head and eyes, lip licking, blinking, and yawning. For various reasons it is important to understand how an individual therapy animal communicates. An informative film by Rugaas (2005), *Calming Signals*, demonstrates how to interpret signals from your dog.

Horse–Human Interaction

A demonstration of how a horse may respond to certain human attitudes and behaviors was performed by Chamove, Crawley-Hartrick, and Stafford (2002). They were specifically interested in assessing the effects of human confidence levels on horse behavior. A total of 40 veterinary students participated in the study with a horse. Assessment of human confidence levels was achieved before and during interaction with the horse. Prior to participant–horse interaction, participants were asked to complete a three-part questionnaire. The first part included relative items from the Personal Evaluation Inventory (PEI), used to measure self-confidence in working with horses; relative items from the PEI to assess recreational and work experience with large animals; and selected items from the Attitudes Towards Animals: Species Rating Scale. Participants were then videotaped while they led a horse around a predetermined course, and the video recordings were viewed for assessment of human and horse behavior. The following human behaviors were measured from the video recordings: looking at the horse; hand position on the lead rope in proximity to where it connected to the horse's halter; and lead tension. Horse behaviors that were measured from the video recordings were: head position, ear movements, ear position, and horse's resistance (i.e., any pause of movement exhibited by the horse while being led or any movement away from the person leading the horse). Multivariate analysis was performed on the data. The results showed that:

> a positive attitude towards the horses related to infrequent ear movement in that horse (accounting for 46% of the variance); positive attitude, together with low lead tension, related to a horse's forward ear position (47%); loose lead tension related to both a horse's low resistance (66%) and low head position (11%).
> (Chamove, Crawley-Hartrick, and Stafford, 2002, p. 323)

The results demonstrated that the horse exhibited less ear movement and had a forward ear position more frequently when led by people with a positive attitude toward horses. Low lead tension was strongly associated with a horse's low resistance, less ear movement, and a low head position. The researchers used only one horse for all trials and thus suggested that further studies are needed to generalize the results. The researchers concluded that the mare could detect the experience and confidence of the person leading her and that, relative to these, the mare was relaxed, calm, interested, and more compliant (Chamove, Crawley-Hartrick, and Stafford, 2002).

Additional studies describe the effect of human–horse interaction. Weeks and Beck (1996) found a significant increase in specific agitation behaviors in horses ridden by beginner riders, in comparison with intermediate and advanced riders (presumably more confident and more positive toward the horses). Hama, Yogo, and Matsuyama (1996) found that horse heart rate was less reactive and human heart rate was slower when horses were touched by people who were both confident with horses and held a positive attitude toward animals (compared with groups who had a negative attitude toward animals or who had a positive attitude toward animals but little or no contact with horses).

We have known for some time that a horse's heart rate changes with different types of interactions with humans; for instance, the heart rate of horses goes up markedly from baseline (for a transient period) when they notice a human entering or exiting their area, but the heart rate of horses goes down significantly from baseline and stays lower when the same person is petting them (Lynch et al., 1974). The question remains: just how perceptive and sensitive are horses? As one way to address this question, the Institute of HeartMath teamed up with Dr. Ellen Gehrke of San Diego to measure heart rate responses in horses and humans interacting (HeartMath, 2006). In their pilot study involving four horses, the researchers wanted to find out if horses' inner state was reflected in their heart rhythm patterns and to determine if there were any indications that the horses were responding to a change in human emotional states. A 24-hour ambulatory heart rate (ECG) recorder was placed on Dr. Gehrke and the four horses to measure their heart rate during a series of different conditions and interactions. There were periods when the horses were alone (e.g., eating) and periods when they were individually with Dr. Gehrke (e.g., being groomed and being ridden; or Dr. Gehrke sitting quietly in the same area). The researchers were specifically studying heart rate variability (HRV). The researchers found that HRV patterns did reflect a change in a horse's inner state but recommended further research to confirm this in a more scientifically rigorous manner. The researchers also found clear indications that the horses responded differently to Dr. Gehrke's changing states. The most interesting example of heart rate pattern synchronicity between the horses and Dr. Gehrke occurred during a "Heart Lock-In" period generated within Dr. Gehrke while she was sitting quietly in the same area with each individual horse. Heart Lock-In is when there is heart rate and breathing coherence within the same individual, occurring when a person is internally generating positive feelings and intentionally sending thoughts and feelings of care, love, or appreciation to someone with the outcome intended to be beneficial (HeartMath, n.d.). During the Heart Lock-In periods:

> Three of the four horses spontaneously walked over to Ellen and nudged or licked her after she started the Lock-In. One of the horses, Shiloh, even placed his nose in Ellen's lap and stayed beside her for the majority of the Heart Lock-In period. More importantly, these three horses' HRV patterns became more ordered.
>
> (HeartMath, 2006, p. 4)

The researchers were especially pleased with the results because they believed they possibly had recorded the first example of horse heart rate coherence. An example of how the horses' heart rate variability patterns shifted based on different types of interactions is demonstrated with the horse Rusty. Rusty's heart rate variability shifted and became much more coherent after Dr. Gehrke petted him and hugged him compared with when she was riding him. From this exploratory study, it seems that the heart rate patterns of horses change according to their state, and their heart rate patterns can shift to reflect the type of interaction occurring with a person. Furthermore, it seems a person can positively influence the heart rate pattern of a horse by behaving in nurturing ways (petting and hugging the animal) or by simply intentionally sending nurturing thoughts to the horse (HeartMath, 2006). If heart coherence in horses occurring during social interactions with humans means the same thing for the horses that it does for the humans, could it be that while a human is generating positive feelings and intentionally sending care, love, or appreciation to the horse that a horse can simultaneously experience similar positive feelings and intentionally send back to the human the same kind of care, love, or appreciation? It would be very useful to discover if this is possible and measureable, and thus it is certainly deserving of further research inquiry.

Given that horses provide observable different reactions to humans who have more or less confidence or more or less positive attitudes toward them, we can, to a degree, discern the states and traits of a human relative to these characteristics by observing a horse's reaction to the person. It is likely that the horse is picking up on external and internal cues given off by the human with whom the horse is interacting. Recognizing horse reactions to a person can be very useful for a therapist performing equine-assisted therapy. Further, by pointing out the horse's reactions to the client, a therapist may facilitate enhanced awareness for the client and potentially a shift in human attitude and behavior. The way a horse can mirror the external and internal state of a client can serve as a powerful therapeutic tool for personal awareness and change.

While some may debate whether a dog, horse, or cat actually experiences emotions like love, happiness, sadness, and grief, I prefer to land on the side of the argument which assumes that animals do experience more complex emotions and to more meaningful levels than we currently can understand. If the suggestion by research is correct that animals are potentially capable of experiencing complex emotions, then the potential benefits and risks to AAT may be enhanced. Risks may be enhanced in that a therapy animal may actually take on some of the emotions of a human client with whom it works, such as the client's depression or anxiety, or that, after termination of counseling, an animal may miss a client it has interacted with on a regular basis. Benefits may be enhanced in that as we learn better to accurately interpret animal expressions, we may better understand how a therapy animal's interactions with and reactions to a human client can provide valuable information about and for that client.

Animal Personalities

Research has determined that animals have a distinct personality that is unique to each animal (i.e., not species- or breed-specific), and is in fact manifested in much the same way as human personality. In a direct comparison between dogs and humans, it was determined that judgments of specific and uniform criteria measuring personality were found to be consistently and accurately applied for dogs and for humans, leading the researchers to conclude with confidence that personality differences do exist and can be measured in animals other than humans (Gosling, Kwan, and John, 2003). A total of 78 dogs and their owners were recruited from a dog park to participate in the research. A four-factor model was used to examine dogs' personalities: (1) neuroticism, represented by dogs' emotional reactivity; (2) extraversion, represented by dogs' energy; (3) openness to new experience, represented by dogs' intelligence; and (4) agreeableness, represented by dogs' affection. This four-factor model was based on the well-accepted five-factor model used to measure personality for humans, with the factor of conscientiousness omitted for dogs. The standardized assessment for the five-factor model, the Big Five Inventory (BFI) (John and Srivastava, 1999), was used to measure the personality of dogs' owners, and the slight modification of this same instrument was used to measure dogs' personalities by both dogs' owners and objective observers. The research determined that dogs' personality traits observed while they were interacting were not based on mere looks or appearance, because distinct personality traits were not found when a separate group judged the same dogs only by examining still photos of the dogs. Furthermore, the dogs' personality traits were measured consistently across time by different observers (Gosling, Kwan, and John, 2003). This evidence supports the premise that each dog has some unique personality characteristics that can distinguish it from dogs of the same breed.

Research has shown that the personality of horses can differ according to their working role (Morris, Gale, and Howe, 2002). A total of 210 owners completed the short version of the NEO Personality Inventory/Five Factor Inventory as it described their horse (items were modified from first person to third person). This instrument was designed to measure five factors of human personality: (1) neuroticism; (2) extraversion; (3) openness to experience; (4) agreeableness; and (5) conscientiousness (Costa and McCrae, 1992). When the researchers performed their analysis on the completed NEOs, there were two factors delineated for extraversion, one consistent with the original instrument, NEO extraversion, and one additional factor specific to this study that was labeled factor 2: social extraversion, which measured specifically the tendency to be sociable (Morris, Gale, and Howe, 2002).

The horses were subdivided according to their main working roles and functions (dressage, teaching, ceremonial, show jumping, and eventing). There were no significant differences found on personality factors by breed (Thoroughbred and Thoroughbred cross, Irish draft and Irish draft cross, Arab and Arab cross, warm bloods and cobs, and other breeds). Instead, analysis showed the following differences in personality factors based on working roles of the horses. Regarding the factor NEO extraversion, horses used for teaching were significantly less extroverted than show jumpers, and ceremonial horses were significantly less extroverted than show jumpers. Regarding factor 2: social extraversion (sociable), ceremonial horses were less sociable than all other groups, and this difference was significant for dressage, show jumpers, and event horses. Regarding the factor openness to experience, show jumpers were significantly more open to experience than horses used in teaching and ceremonials. Eventing horses were also significantly more open to experience than horses used in teaching. There were also some differences found based on the level of sophistication at which horses were used (novice, club, area, intermediate, and international). Regarding NEO extraversion, horses became progressively less extroverted the higher the level of use, but the only significant difference was between the novice horses and international horses. Regarding factor 2: social extraversion (sociable), the same pattern was found as for NEO extraversion. Regarding conscientiousness, the opposite pattern was found with horses becoming progressively more conscientious the higher the level of use, but the only significant difference was between novice horses and international horses. The researchers concluded that the study provided some evidence for differentiation in horses' personality structures based on their working role and the level of sophistication of the working role (Morris, Gale, and Howe, 2002).

The research findings, that an animal can have some distinguishing personality characteristics that are not breed-specific and are somewhat unique to that animal (as described for dogs) or to its working role (as described for horses), are very relevant to AAT applications. A therapist who is very aware of his or her pet's unique personality characteristics and how these are presented in the therapy setting can make more meaningful interpretations of human client–therapy pet interactions. This could result in additional valuable information for facilitating client recovery. Also, a therapist can make more accurate predictions of anticipated animal and human behavior in a therapy session based on an understanding of the personality traits presented by a therapy animal that is interacting with a human client. Increased ability to interpret and predict animal and human behavior in a therapy session enhances the benefits and reduces the risks of the AAT process.

PREVENTING INJURY AND INFECTION DURING AAT

Minimizing the risk of injury to the therapy animal and to the clients the animal works with is imperative. For this reason, all therapy dogs should be kept on a leash, and small animals should be provided a small crate or basket in which to be carried. Only the trained handler should ever control the therapy pet and supervise the animal's interaction with clients. The therapy pet should never be left alone with a client or with a staff member with whom the pet is unfamiliar. If there is a need to leave the pet, it should be properly crate-trained so it can be safely secured in a crate and is comfortable being left alone for short periods.

A colleague of mine who was a director of a counseling clinic told me of an incident involving an intern who brought a therapy dog to her clinic to perform AAT. The intern had attended a 1-day training workshop, and she and her dog were nationally registered for volunteer work in AAA. However, this is not sufficient training to perform professional AAT. The intern performed a series of serious mistakes. First, the intern brought the dog to the counseling clinic without the knowledge or permission of the clinic director or any supervisor. Second, the intern did not screen or inform clients in advance before bringing the dog, nor did she properly evaluate which clients would be appropriate for AAT. Given these errors, the clinic director informed the intern that she could not work with the dog that day when seeing her clients. The student had not brought any type of dog crate with her and did not want to cancel with her clients; plus, there was no time to take the dog home and get back in time to see her first scheduled client that day. Thus, the clinic director agreed to let the intern place the dog in the director's office with the door closed so the intern could counsel her clients down the hall in a therapy room. So the situation presented was a young, playful, and inexperienced therapy dog, placed alone in an unfamiliar environment, away from the owner, under no proper supervision, and not properly confined in a dog crate. This is a condition that can likely lead to some kind of trouble. The dog did what many other dogs might do in a similar situation: it looked for something to do to entertain itself. It spotted a squirrel outside the window of the director's office and began jumping at it, an exercise that resulted in destroying an entire wall of expensive window blinds before the dog and squirrel game was discovered. The irresponsible actions of the intern resulted in the dog being banned from the clinic. Given a similar situation, the best action would have been to simply cancel the intern's clients for the day or for the time it would take to send the intern home so the dog could be left in a safe and familiar environment, given that the intern had not brought a crate for the dog. This type of incident creates the potential for the dog to injure itself and to give a bad reputation to AAT. It is imperative that animal-assisted therapists act responsibly to ensure the safety of a therapy animal, the safety of clients, the safety of facility staff and furnishings, and to demonstrate the best side that AAT has to offer.

Properly trained and socialized therapy pets are highly unlikely to cause injury to a client. However, it is possible for accidents to happen. For instance, what if a client did not see the dog's leash between you and the animal, and the client tripped and fell to the ground? It is important to have a well-thought-out plan of action in place just in case injury to a client does occur during AAT. Pet Partners (2014) has a clear policy for handling injury to a client for its registered Pet Partners. The animal should be safely secured as soon as possible so you can manage the situation. Do not tie the animal to furniture. This invokes nightmarish images of a chair chasing a frightened dog down a hallway that can only escalate the situation by implying the animal is out of control. The animal should, preferably, be secured safely in a crate in an office. If the person you are visiting is injured, get help for them as quickly as possible. Get an appropriate staff person to administer or call for medical aid if necessary. Only properly trained facility staff or medical personnel should administer medical treatment of any kind, including the application of a simple bandage on a scratch. If the incident occurred in an agency or facility, the pet's handler should report the incident to the appropriate facility supervisor or administrator, and all proper paperwork should be completed. The handler should also report the incident to any sponsoring AAT organization to which he or she belongs, such as Pet Partners. There should be no more therapy work involving the animal for the rest of the day. Animals are very sensitive to stress, and the situation calls for giving the animal the rest of the day to relax.

To keep the animal safe from injury, the handler must scan the environment for objects that might harm it, such as stray food, sharp objects, or contaminated objects on the floor. The handler must be careful that the animal does not run into any furniture or knock over objects in the room. On one visit with Rusty, Snowflake, and Dolly to the juvenile detention center where I volunteered with assistance from two of my graduate students, it was the winter holiday season and the adolescents had made cardboard fireplaces and strung yarn in the shape of Christmas trees in the individual section units of the facility. Seeing the changes to the areas that the pets had frequently visited, I supervised the adolescent residents while they slowly walked the therapy animals around so the animals could see the new obstacles in the room. Even given such precautions, during a ball fetch exercise that day Rusty got briefly tangled in the yarn Christmas tree, and Snowflake jumped on top of a flimsy cardboard fireplace mantel, which brought the whole structure tumbling down. No person or animal came near to being injured that day, and it would have been difficult for that to happen given my assessment of the lack of danger presented by the objects. However, the incident demonstrates the importance of being aware of the working environment and keeping it safe.

Sometimes danger to the therapy animal can be invisible. Rusty frequently accompanied me to my office at the university where I work. On one occasion, we had been there about 10 minutes when I noticed his usually light pink and brown freckled stomach was a fiery cherry red and extremely warm to the touch. I immediately rushed him to my veterinarian, who diagnosed and treated him for an unidentified allergic reaction. Rusty recovered quickly, and I took him to the university office again the next day. Again, shortly after our arrival his stomach turned fiery red. This second time the veterinarian suggested that it was likely something at the office that was causing Rusty's reaction. I called the administrative staff and reported the vet's suggestion. Being animal lovers and Rusty fans, the staff began to examine what Rusty might have been reacting to in the office suite. The discussion revealed that all of the staff had been suffering with respiratory problems for several days that they had thought was just a bad cold being passed around. It was further discovered that the head administrative assistant had gone to the hospital for emergency treatment of a severe asthma attack. Convinced something was terribly wrong with the office environment, the staff contacted the environmental management office on campus, reporting Rusty's reactions and their own illnesses. The environmental office was hesitant to take the case seriously, but the staff insisted that based on the dog's reactions something was seriously amiss. Environmental management investigated and discovered that a new member of the custodial staff had recently cleaned the carpet in the office suite but had inadvertently used the pure concentrated form of a cleaner instead of diluting it as instructed on the ingredient container. In its concentrated form, the cleaner was dangerously toxic. After the office suite was treated to neutralize the toxins, the administrative staff's respiratory ailments cleared up, and Rusty had no reactions while at the office. Rusty was credited with being a bit of a hero for this incident.

Unfortunately, a second, similar incident occurred several months later during a therapy visit to a juvenile detention center. This detention center was divided into sections with about five to ten juveniles in each section. Each of the juveniles in the section had a private room that opened into a shared, larger meeting area. My therapy team (trained graduate students, my three therapy animals and I) conducted weekly group animal therapy visits to three sections dedicated to the long-term residential post-adjudication program—two sections of boys and one section of girls. During one visit with Rusty and Snowflake, a trained assistant and I noticed after about 10 minutes of arriving in one section that Snowflake's ears were turning a dark, cherry red. We watched him and Rusty closely. Then the cat's nose and paws became dark red, and he began to have difficulty breathing. Rusty's stomach turned red. A rushed visit to the vet followed with treatment for Snowflake and Rusty for an allergic reaction. I reported the incident to the facility staff and clarified it was only in the last section we visited that day. The therapeutic programs coordinator reported back to me that the investigation of that section revealed residents and staff had been suffering from some type of respiratory problems thought to have been a cold or something else being passed around. It was felt that the allergic reaction by the therapy animals in combination with the respiratory problems of residents and staff suggested a possible environmental problem. An investigation by environmental management staff ensued that narrowed the possible causes to either mildew caused from a recent plumbing problem in that section or to a misuse of concentrated cleaning materials. The section was thoroughly cleaned to neutralize the problem. However, on a subsequent visit to that section, both the cat and dog had a strong allergic reaction, and the visit was quickly ended. These allergic reactions subsided on their own several minutes after leaving the facility. Finally, after several cleanings, it was safe again to visit with Rusty and Snowflake in that section. Many types of chemical agents, including a variety of common cleaning materials, are toxic to animals. It is very important that a counselor working with a therapy pet be aware of possible toxic agents that must be avoided for the safety of the therapy animal.

Zoonoses are diseases that can be exchanged between people and other animals (Delta Society, 2000). The risk of a therapy pet infecting someone that it works with can be minimized by the owner keeping the pet up to date on routine vaccinations and free from parasites (e.g., fleas, ticks, and worms). Also, the pet should never work if it is ill or has an open wound. At the work site, a designated location should be established for the pet to relieve itself, and all feces should be removed immediately following defecation and disposed of properly. Clients should wash their hands before and after visiting with a therapy pet as germs can be spread from person to person via the animal's fur (Pet Partners, 2014). If no sink is available for hand washing, then antibacterial hand wipes or gel can be used, but these may not be as effective as hand washing for killing germs.

PREPARING FOR AAT WORK TIME

When working with a therapy animal, the therapist must make sure the animal is clean and well groomed. Dogs and cats should also have their nails trimmed and filed smooth before a therapy visit. A therapy animal kit should be carried at all times or maintained at the location of the therapy facility. The kit should include waste bags for disposing of dog excrement and paper towels and a stain and odor remover in case an accident happens indoors. The cleaner should be safe for animals, should kill bacteria, and should not discolor carpet or flooring. The local pet store is a good source for this. The pet should drink only bottled water or water brought from home and served in a dish you have brought. Toys, chews, and treats should be included in the kit so if a client wants to offer the pet a treat it is one that is healthy for the animal. A small, very soft bristle grooming brush can be included for clients to safely brush the pet. A spare leash and collar are necessary in case the current one wears out. The leash and collar for therapy visits should not be made of metal but rather of leather, cloth, or nylon. The leash should not be more than 6 feet in length. No choke collars or pinch collars can be used during therapy. Buckled neck collars, chest harnesses, or head halters are permissible. Also, have available a pet first-aid kit for handling small emergencies if the pet becomes ill or gets injured. Your local veterinarian can recommend some good contents for this first-aid kit, but this usually includes some bandages, antiseptic, and something to stop bleeding as well as something to counteract a severe allergic reaction. It is also useful to include in the therapy kit a lint brush for participants to remove animal hair from their clothing after the visit as well as antibacterial hand wipes or gel for participants to clean their hands with, if soap and a sink are not handy, before and after visiting the therapy animal.

ETHICAL CONSIDERATIONS FOR AAT

Competent and ethical AAT counseling practice requires compliance with: (1) ethical codes and standards of practice established by animal welfare and AAT organizations; (2) ethical codes and standards of mental health organizations; (3) local, state, and federal guidelines governing the welfare and protection of humans and animals and the recognition of the professional practice of AAT and qualified therapy animals; and (4) standards and guidelines that consider sensitivity to cultural, racial, ethnic, and other individual differences, especially differences in attitudes toward animals. Organizations that provide training and credentialing for AAT provide a foundation for professional ethical standards. Professional animal-assisted applications, such as AAT, have been described as a more formal process than nonprofessional animal-assisted applications, such as AAA (Pet Partners, 2014).

AAT is overseen by a human service provider as part of a professional practice and must be goal directed and documented. The animal may be handled by the professional or by a volunteer under the direction of the professional. Pet Partners' (2014) "Code of Ethics for AAA and AAT" covers issues of competency, fair treatment, responsibility, and compliance. In addition, Pet Partners outlines types of unsatisfactory professional conduct including breach of client confidentiality, any type of abuse or harassment of clients or animals, and misrepresentation of practice credentials, or qualifications for counselors or animals. Pet Partners (2014) outlined clear policies and procedures for practice. The Pet Partners standards cover the following areas: facility assessment; risk management and compliance with existing laws and regulations; provider organizations including recommendations for personnel involvement along with policies and procedures; service delivery including clients' rights; selection, health, and management of animals; and research. The equine-assisted therapy organizations Professional Association for Therapeutic Horsemanship, International (PATH, Intl., n.d.c) and Equine Assisted Growth and Learning Association (EAGALA, n.d.c) both have their own code of ethics covering issues of competency and professional conduct. Also, EAGALA's certification program outlines standards for practice for equine-assisted mental health professionals that include a requirement for university- and college-level mental health training and professional practice credentials.

Mental health professionals who practice AAT should follow the ethical codes and standards of practice for their profession. These include, but are not limited to: the American Counseling Association's *Code of Ethics* (ACA, 2014); the American Psychological Association's *Ethical Principles of Psychologists and Code of Conduct* (APA, 2010); and the *Code of Ethics of the National Association of Social Workers* (NASW, 2008). Currently these ethical codes and standards do not directly address AAT, which denotes a need for attention to this matter, and consideration should be given to addressing AAT in each of these documents in the near future. The Association for Multicultural Counseling and Development's *Multicultural and Social Justice Counseling Competencies* (AMCD, 2015) is another important document that does not address work with animals in counseling but probably should since there is diversity in attitudes about animals. Given that differences in individual and cultural attitudes toward animals exist, counselors should apply AAT in a manner that is culturally sensitive by considering cultural, racial, ethnic, and other individual differences before and during application of AAT with a particular client and in a particular environment.

It is important to be aware of laws pertaining to animal welfare, treatment, and rights, including recognized status for public access. A valuable resource to stay updated on such laws, both in the United States and in other countries, is the Animal Legal and Historical Center (ALHC, n.d.); through its website current laws related to animals can be checked and tracked. In the United States, many states have legislative provisions for the definition, function, and protection of official service or disability assistance animals, but rarely can one find any legislation to define and protect the work of a therapy animal. It is important to clarify that an animal working as a therapy animal is not serving the same function as an animal working as a service animal or a disability assistance animal. Service or disability assistance animals (which are most often dogs) live with and assist the animal's owner who has an emotional or physical disability for which the animal is trained to respond (for example, epilepsy seizure detection dogs, vision or hearing assistance dogs, wheelchair assistance dogs, and emotional assistance dogs), as well as dogs that assist with the owner's clinical condition (for instance, anxiety or panic attacks, or autism). In contrast, a therapy animal is a domesticated pet, most frequently owned by the therapist, and works under the direction of the therapist to provide AAT services for clients—for instance, a therapy dog that is present in a therapy session and made available for the client to pet or hold. The most common therapy animals are dogs, and the second most common are horses. Other animals that often work as therapy animals include cats, rabbits, birds, gerbils, hamsters, llamas, donkeys, and farm animals (Lipin, 2009). An award-winning documentary film, *Kids and Animals* (2006), demonstrates the efficacy of AAT with farm animals, such as a cow and pig, and with aquarium animals, such as a dolphin and sea turtle.

The practice of AAT is growing throughout the world. Given that the therapy involves animals that are highly dependent on humans for protection and care, some ethical concerns arise regarding the potential exploitation of these creatures:

> Questions have arisen over the past few years about the ethics of using animals in some or all therapy programs. While some animal protection groups encourage programs involving animal visitations or animal-assisted therapy, others view this use of animals as yet another form of exploitation. . . . However, people who participate in animal assistance programs are more often than not aware of animal welfare and animal rights, and many either support animal protection activities or consider themselves to be sensitive to those issues.
>
> (Iannuzzi and Rowan, 1991, p. 154)

Dangers for Residential Animals in Elderly Care Facilities

In an attempt to clarify issues regarding potential exploitation or abuse of animals in AAA and AAT, a survey was conducted by two researchers with an assortment of individuals involved in programs across the United States (Iannuzzi and Rowan, 1991). Although most programs had a relatively benign impact on the animals, the surveyors uncovered some troubling cases. For instance, at one elderly residential care facility, animals suffered from excessive feeding and too little exercise, with some animals dying prematurely as a result of congestive heart failure. Some dogs were left to roam outside another facility and were killed by cars. At another facility, one dog froze to death when left outside on a winter's day. An animal at another facility strangled to death when left tied on a leash unattended (Iannuzzi and Rowan, 1991).

Dangers for Residential Animals in Prison Programs

For animals at residential programs, fatigue of the therapy animal was found to be a concern when the animal was not allowed enough time to rest (Iannuzzi and Rowan, 1991). At prisons, animals ran the risk of abuse, and some incidents involved even the guards abusing therapy dogs when they were in the kennel. Some incidents of birds being killed and eaten in a prison facility were also reported. Providing adequate supervision of therapy animals for their protection was found to be of great concern in a long-term residential facility (Iannuzzi and Rowan, 1991).

Dangers for Animals in Visitation Programs

Visitation programs are the most widespread type of AAT program. Visitations were found to be stressful for the visiting animals, and the ability to cope and manage the stress varied greatly from animal to animal (Iannuzzi and Rowan, 1991). A lack of ability to control the atmosphere and availability of water was found to be problematic in visitation programs. The combination of heat and dehydration was stressful and in some cases led to exhaustion of the animal (Iannuzzi and Rowan, 1991).

Dangers for Dolphin Programs

Survey researchers uncovered several concerns regarding dolphin swim programs (Iannuzzi and Rowan, 1991). Dolphin swim programs have been used as possible assistance for autistic children. Dolphins are very social animals, and isolation from other wild dolphins can be extremely stressful as can confinement in a pool without unlimited access to their natural habitat. Dolphins fed by humans have lost the ability to hunt and feed for themselves. Dolphins have very sensitive hearing, and loud environments may create stress for them. Captive dolphins, especially those exposed to many human beings, show enlarged adrenal glands. Thus, it is clear that dolphin swim programs are a potential danger to dolphins (Iannuzzi and Rowan, 1991).

Brensing et al. (2005) observed wild captive dolphins in two swim-with-the-dolphins programs. The swimmers were adults, children, and children with mental and physical disabilities. The researchers observed 83 unstructured sessions with five dolphins at Dolphins Plus in the United States and 37 sessions with 13 dolphins at Dolphin Reef in Israel. Both facilities are fenced sea pens with ocean water. Researchers observed notable differences in the behavior of the dolphins in the two programs. The dolphins at Dolphins Plus showed some signs of stress such as avoidance, speed increase, higher metabolism, and intensification of a subgroup. These signs were most evident when the dolphins were with adult swimmers. In contrast, the dolphins at Dolphin Reef seemed to be attracted to adult swimmers. In the Dolphin Reef program the size of the swimming enclosure was more than 20 times larger than the pen at Dolphins Plus. In addition, the Dolphin Reef enclosure was divided into three parts (not materially), with an entry area, an area where dolphins and humans could interact, and a huge refuge area for the dolphins to be away from the humans. The provision of this refuge area has been shown to reduce aggressive, submissive, and abrupt behaviors of the dolphins during swim-with-the-dolphins programs. Another difference in the enclosure area of the two programs was that the dolphins at Dolphin Reef could leave the enclosure to return to the open sea, offering an additional refuge area. A further difference between the two study sites was the size of the groups of swimmers. In the Dolphin Reef program, groups were comparably smaller (average of 3.2 swimmers compared with an average of 5 in Dolphins Plus) and were always guided by a staff member who was well known to the dolphins.

The researchers concluded that the dolphins at Dolphins Plus showed notable levels of agitation and stress not observed in the dolphins at Dolphin Reef due to the previously noted differences in the enclosure and number of swimmers (Brensing et al., 2005). From this study we can conclude that programs that involve human–wild dolphin interaction should provide opportunity for dolphins to choose to be away from humans by providing a very large refuge area, should be exposed only to small numbers of humans during interaction opportunities, and should be allowed to come from and go to the open sea freely and in a manner that is safe for dolphins. This seems to be the most humane way to provide a swim-with-the-dolphins program.

GUIDELINES FOR ANIMAL PROTECTION IN AAT

Based on the previously reported cases, it is clear that ethical concerns for the use of therapy animals are warranted. A therapist who uses a therapy animal should follow basic guidelines for animal protection and welfare. It is best that only domesticated animals and not wild animals be incorporated into therapy programs, with exceptions being wildlife rehabilitation and care programs that are under the supervision of a licensed wildlife rehabilitator or wildlife care expert. The therapy animal should always be adequately supervised during therapy work, for the animal's safety, and provided sufficient rest, and proper care and nutrition. In addition, the handler of the therapy animal should be properly trained and educated in animal welfare and risk management.

Hatch (2007) interviewed volunteers of AAA programs regarding concerns for the animals' welfare. From these interviews some important considerations were presented. In keeping the welfare of animals in mind, there is reason to be cautious about people who are visited. Handlers should avoid people who can and do express their dislike for animals, and animals may be in harm's way if they are exposed to people who cannot voice their dislike or fear. Certain populations may be inappropriate for animal visitation, especially those with aggressive tendencies. Further, risk is posed to animals in AAA or AAT inadvertently by handlers without proper training or who have a lack of sensitivity to an animal's needs:

> For example, if an animal who fears wheelchairs and walkers is pulled toward them (instead of learning to be comfortable with them) the handler could create anxiety in the animal and thereby reinforce the fear. Another example, seen several times in this study, is the handlers' failure to provide the dogs water due to concerns about the dog urinating in the facility. While not intentionally malicious, the handlers' are in effect dehydrating the dogs and creating an unhealthy experience for them. The handlers' lack of knowledge about calming signals and other stress reactions could result in their failure to read, or their misreading of, the behavioral cues the animals display. In AAA [or AAT], the potential for handler mistreatment, mishandling, and ignorance exists, regardless of how well intentioned the human may be. Without proper knowledge about animal behavior, handlers may not know when to take an animal from a situation. Without proper knowledge, handlers may reinforce fear or stress reactions [in animals].
>
> (Hatch, 2007, p. 45)

Stress can suppress reproductive functioning, impair immune functions, and have other ill effects on animals (Hatch, 2007).

In the practice of AAT, it is of paramount importance that we carefully consider the safety and welfare of the animal, as well as the type of experience that the animal will have in its role as a therapy animal. If AAT is not a positive experience for a therapy animal, then we should not require the animal to participate. In considering the facilitator's responsibility for the therapy animal, the international organization Pet Partners requires that handlers abide by the following policies in the performance of AAA/AAT: "I will be responsible for my animal at all times, considering its needs and humane care first" and, "I will always stay with my animal and remain in control of the situation" (Pet Partners, 2014, p. 45).

Preziosi (1997) presented a facilitator code of ethics for pet assisted therapy. Following is a summary of the major points that apply to the welfare of the therapy animal:

- A therapy animal's welfare must be the priority of the AAT facilitator.
- A therapy animal must never be forced to leave the home to go to work.
- In the therapy environment a therapy animal must never be forced to perform an action that the animal does not initiate willfully.
- A facilitator should know a therapy animal well enough to recognize when it is and is not comfortable and should not place the animal in a situation where the animal is not comfortable.
- The therapy animal must be allowed to adjust to travel and to the therapy environment gradually before engaging in therapy work.
- The activities for animals during therapy should involve the types that are safe and enjoyable for the animal.
- The therapy animal must be given a place and time to rest.
- The facilitator must never leave the animal alone or out of sight during a therapy session.
- A facilitator must ensure the environment is safe for the therapy animal.
- The facilitator must ensure that no one offers food to the therapy animal without the facilitator's expressed permission and supervision.
- A client who has a disease that can be transmitted to the therapy animal should not be allowed contact with the animal.
- The facilitator must provide for the vaccination and other healthcare needs of the therapy animal.
- An "ethical" facilitator or therapist "does not 'use' a therapy animal," meaning that there must always be a demonstration of respect for the animal and its natural traits and temperament.

With these 13 points, Preziosi (1997) provided a foundation for an ethical approach to AAT that considers the welfare of the therapy animal to be a priority.

MORAL IMPLICATIONS OF AAT

The bioethicist Peter Singer of Princeton University helped to launch what became known as the animal rights movement with the 1975 publication of his book titled *Animal Liberation*. He argued that the ability to suffer is a great cross-species leveler, and we should not inflict pain on or cause fear in an animal that we would not want to experience ourselves:

> If a being suffers there can be no moral justification for refusing to take that suffering into consideration. No matter what the nature of the being, the principle of equality requires that its suffering be counted equally with the like suffering—in so far as rough comparisons can be made—of any other being. If a being is not capable of suffering, or of experiencing enjoyment or happiness, there is nothing to be taken into account. So the limit of sentience (using the term as a convenient if not strictly accurate shorthand for the capacity to suffer and/or experience enjoyment) is the

only defensible boundary of concern for the interests of others. To mark this bound-ary by some other characteristic like intelligence or rationality would be to mark it in an arbitrary manner.

(Singer, 1975, p. 9)

There has never been universal agreement about Singer's premise, but new scientific stud-ies are revealing that animals are much more consciously aware than we had previously given them credit for (Kluger, 2010). Apes are capable of communication with humans through sign language and by arranging symbol icons to form complex sentences. Crows excel at tool use and have a complex social structure. Dogs demonstrate personality char-acteristics that are unique to that animal and not breed-specific. Elephants have demon-strated grief and bereavement for deceased family members. In fact, many animal species have similar neurochemical responses to humans when these animals seem to be express-ing complex emotions such as affection, stress, or grief over loss (Kluger, 2010). Since humans are consciously aware of how we treat animals, we have a moral obligation to avoid treating them in ways that cause suffering, and we should do this regardless of whether we view ourselves as intellectually or rationally superior to animals. Thus, with this in mind, practitioners of AAT and AAA should try to ensure that the animal's participation in AAT or AAA is something the animal wants to do and is something that does not distress or harm the animal.

Zamir (2006) examined the moral basis of AAT and concluded that, while certain types of AAT are morally unobjectionable, some modes of AAT should be abolished. Zamir described six primary reasons for animal liberationists to hold the position that using animals to treat humans is potentially immoral:

- Since animals need to be kept by a therapist to perform therapy they may suffer from "limitations of freedom."
- Turning an animal into a companion animal is a life-determining action; that is, it involves making a decision for the animal on how it will live its life.
- Getting animals to assist humans requires prolonged periods of training for the animal.
- Animals that serve or assist humans are socially disconnected from their own kind.
- An animal may become injured in the process of providing therapy.
- Animals should not be considered objects for use by humans, such as petting, touch-ing, riding, and interacting in other ways.

Zamir is not in agreement with animal liberationists that all AAT is immoral. For animal species that are traditionally domesticated and live with humans as pets (e.g., dogs or horses), these reasons do not necessarily cause harm to the animal and they allow humans and ani-mals to live in harmony and the animals to thrive. Responsible pet ownership would provide for the needs of the animal and protect the animal as a beloved pet:

Forms of AAT that rely on horses and dogs are continuous with the welfare of these animals. Without a relationship with humans, an overwhelming number of these beings would not exist. Their lives with human beings exact a price for them. But given responsible human owners, such lives are qualitatively comfortable and safe, and they need not frustrate the social needs of these creatures. A world in which practices like AAT exist is an overall better world for these beings than one that does not include them, and this provides a broad, moral vindication of forms of AAT that rely on these beings.

(Zamir, 2006, p. 195)

However, for other species of animals that are not traditionally domesticated, Zamir (2006) concludes that AAT is not appropriate for their welfare:

> On the other hand, rodents, birds, monkeys, reptiles, and dolphins gain little by coercing them into AAT. Such practices are therefore exploitative. Since the human interests that are involved can be easily met without exploiting these beings, the moral conclusion is that such forms of AAT should be abolished.
>
> (p. 195)

We may conclude from works regarding ethical considerations and moral implications that AAT or AAA should be performed only if the experience that the therapy animal will have as part of the AAT or AAA will be safe and enjoyable for the animal, and that this is more readily assured if we limit participation in AAT or AAA to animal species that are more easily socialized to human interaction. In striving to provide for the needs of humans through the modalities of AAT or AAA, we should carefully consider the welfare of the animals and maintain high moral ground when considering interacting with these beings who cannot speak for themselves. AAT, with the benefits it has to offer both humans and animals, provides opportunity for moral evolution regarding humans' attitude and behavior toward animals as well as greater appreciation for the social gifts of animals. Animals who desire to cooperate with humans in sharing their comforting gifts of love and companionship have much to teach us about living in harmony—as opposed to abashed exploitation—only if we are willing to learn. Consistent with respect for animals, AAT researchers and practitioners today should, and many do, avoid the attitude and terminology of *use of animals* or *using animals* in science and practice and instead adopt more respectful and appreciative attitudes and terminology, such as *working with animals* and *interacting with animals*.

In his 1969 book entitled *Pet-Oriented Child Psychotherapy*, Levinson's words of concern regarding humans' attitude and behavior toward animals still have relevancy today and emphasize a need for more harmonious companionship between humans and animals:

> Alienation is widespread in our society. Man finds that he is a stranger to himself. He surfeits in his largess and cries out in his anxiety. He apparently lost the key to self-understanding. Man's anxiety is partly due to his withdrawal from the healing forces of nature and its foremost representatives, the animal kingdom. No longer able to identify with nature and its representatives, man finds himself in a psychological no-man's land. He may be able to regain some of his emotional harmony by reestablishing his bond with the animate and inanimate world. Through identification, this process proceeds in three stages; first with inanimate nature, then with the animate nonhuman world, and finally with human beings.
>
> (p. xiii)

For the historical section in Chapter 1 of this book, I corresponded with Olivia Corson for permission to use lengthy excerpts from the 1975 work of her parents, Samuel Corson (1909–1998) and Elizabeth O'Leary Corson (1920–2004). In her reply, Olivia Corson shared reflections on the transformation she observed to occur in her parents' work once they discovered the benefits of pet-facilitated therapy. Prior to their discovery of pet-facilitated therapy, the Corsons had been engaged in Pavlovian-type experimentation on animals that could be cruel at times. With her permission, I have reproduced the correspondence with Olivia Corson here. Her words have both educational and spiritual value and reflect humanity's moral obligation to respect and protect animals and nature.

November 11, 2010

Dear Cynthia,

Thank you for your great work! Yes I give you permission to use the quotes and have signed below. I am thrilled you are including my parents' work in your textbook on animal-assisted therapy. And I am so glad and touched that such a wonderful field now exists, and that my parents were pioneers in establishing this field. My mother, Elizabeth O'Leary Corson, died 6 years ago in my home, at the age of 84. I miss her still. A flood of memory opened for me as I read the quotes. I wanted to share a little of it with you. I named that Fox Terrier Arwyn—from Tolkien's trilogy—when I was in junior high school. Before that, I talked my dad into letting me bring several of his research dogs home. We had Beagle and Fox Terrier puppies tearing about the house at times, and somehow I also convinced them to let me bring some of the grown dogs home to live, at least for a while. The research dogs at his work, and the Pavlovian work itself, actually broke my heart and taught me/gave me so much insight into the depths of need and brokenness between the human and the more-than-human world, particularly between human beings and the rest of the creature world. Arwyn and the other Fox Terriers, Beagles, and Border Collies came from John Paul Scott's research labs in Bowling Green, Ohio, where they were bred for Scott's and other scientists' experiments. I don't know where Buster, the very sweet, patient and sad Labrador mix came from. Nor where Whiskey, the lively Shepherd/Husky mix came from. All of them were beings I witnessed and walked, touched, groomed, talked with—and as a child longed to liberate. I visited Scott's labs with my father, saw the dogs and the conditions in which they were raised (not good), and witnessed the ways the scientists treated them, talked about them, etc. I clearly remember sitting through a difficult (for me) dinner with these grown-ups—John Paul Scott, his quiet, attentive wife, my father, and me. Both these men had grown up in tough times and were born into that disastrous, and for far too long dominating, cultural/spiritual belief system that humans (particularly urbanized men of wealth) were more intelligent and vastly superior to other life-forms; that creation was made FOR humans to use and consume as they pleased—especially those with violent power to back them up.

I loved my parents. And I was traumatized by aspects of their early work—by the Pavlovian experiments on dogs, and by being taken to other researchers' labs where I witnessed suffering that was being inflicted on helpless animals. I remember being in Florida as a young child in the early '60s where a researcher had a living dolphin trapped in a box where she or he was silently and clearly screaming to me. I think it was John Lilly's lab. When I was 18, in 1971, I was taken along to a primate lab in Soviet Russia that has haunted me my whole life. I was helpless at the time to stop these cruel injustices, and unable to express directly how this felt to me, let alone how it so obviously felt to the animals involved. I also witnessed and began to understand that there was a massive burying and twisting of emotions with all the people involved in this work as well. Thankfully, some of these researchers evolved. I have met several people who once worked with Lilly on his captive dolphin projects and later became marine mammal advocates and educators—dedicated to protecting and revering ocean life.

Eventually I realized that I too had gotten to contribute to the wonderful evolution of my parents' work—totally away from Pavlovian experiments, which, while they were definitely early mind–body research, were cruel by nature. My parents held their dogs in respect. My mother loved them despite that being unheard of in vivisection work and difficult for her to hold. She played the key role in this great transformation of their work. She had a palpable, positive rapport with humans and animals, especially those in mental and spiritual distress. Kind to her core, and highly empathic, she played the main role in actually allowing, encouraging, and working with the powerful energy and communication flow between human and nonhuman animals (which indeed exists between all beings and elements). Dad was amazing at articulating the work in a way that could communicate with mainstream science and policymakers. He was a fabulous extrovert, world traveler, linguist (who spoke six languages fluently), passionate dancer and singer—utterly fearless when it came to communicating across differences; talking, writing, publishing, energizing situations, pushing things along and getting them done! He loved and admired nature and took himself outdoors daily—often calling the rest of us to come and behold a baby snapping turtle, the first intoxicating lilac blooms, a family of ducks . . . or branches covered in ice and lit by the winter sun. . . . He died in my arms, in my sister's home in 1998. I am grateful for my beloved parents' pioneering work in establishing the vibrant and important field of pet-facilitated therapy/animal-assisted therapy. I value their contributions to the essential repatterning of our old, destructive, and false belief system, in which humans are somehow contrived to be separate from, and better than, all other forms of life. In fact, we are physically and spiritually bereft and doomed if we do not reinhabit our bodies, lives, and earth with simplicity and gratitude and with direct communing, reverence, and respect for other life-forms—to whom we are utterly beholden. May we quickly and surely reweave our habits, our policies, institutions, priorities and our hearts to include ourselves within the complex, sacred web of Earth life.

I have worked for decades founding a healing art form, Body Tales, which weaves together intuitive movement and personal and cultural story. Many of my movement theater pieces are about the extraordinary numinous powers of the nonhuman animals—their lives, gifts, intelligences, needs, and plight in this era of catastrophic loss of biodiversity. I have created and performed so many pieces about my childhood, my small and mighty family, and the all-encompassing, more-than-human realm especially the creature world. My parents gave me such strong grounds for my life and for my work. I miss them both hugely and am very grateful for who they were, what their work and lives evolved into, and [how they] gave back to the world—including, so generously, to me.

Sincerely,
Olivia Corson
Oakland, California
www.bodytales.com

RECOMMENDED ADDITION TO ETHICAL STANDARDS FOR COUNSELORS

If we consider ourselves partners with our companion animals who work with us in a therapeutic environment, then we must advocate for the safety and welfare of therapy animals in much the same way as we advocate for humans. Being a social advocate for those we work with and those we serve is a professional obligation for counselors (ACA, 2014). Perhaps the following excerpt from the *ACA Code of Ethics* (ACA, 2014) should be adapted as a model to apply to the welfare and status of therapy animals with which a counselor works:

Counselors are expected to advocate to promote change at the individual, group, institutional, and societal levels that improve the quality of life for individuals and groups and remove potential barriers to the provision or access of appropriate services being offered.

(ACA, 2014, Section C, Professional Responsibility, p. 8)

I propose that ACA adopt something similar to the previous statement as advocacy for therapy animals and the practice of AAT. The statement could read something like this:

Counselors are expected to advocate to promote change at the individual, group, institutional, and societal levels that improve the welfare and quality of life for therapy animals and remove potential barriers to the provision or access of appropriate services being offered that include a therapy animal.

A statement such as this would support a partnership of animals and handlers in the provision of appropriate AAT services, but at the same time would clarify a stand against inappropriate exploitation of animals for therapy work or for other human preferences that are not healthy for a therapy animal.

Another area that needs to be addressed in the ethical standards of professional counseling organizations includes that of competency to practice AAT. However, one could assume that this is covered by a global competency statement regarding all practices and modalities of counseling. The current ACA ethical standards state the following about competence:

Counselors practice in specialty areas new to them only after appropriate education, training, and supervised experience. While developing skills in new specialty areas, counselors take steps to ensure the competence of their work and to protect others from possible harm.

(ACA, 2014, Section C.2.b, New Specialty Areas of Practice, p. 8)

Regarding competence, it must be understood by the practitioner of AAT that AAT is much more than simply taking your pet to work and inviting clients to interact with your pet. To practice AAT one should obtain training in AAT practices. AAT involves certain risks to people and animals that must be understood and thus avoided as much as possible. A most important issue of competency is knowing when and when not to practice AAT. Some clients are not appropriate candidates for this type of counseling, and some animals are also not appropriate to work as therapy animals. Individual and cultural differences in attitudes toward animals may impact if or how AAT is incorporated with a client. Also, human–animal interaction presents additional psychodynamics that should be recognized and addressed by a counselor to enhance clients' therapeutic gains. Regarding documentation when therapy animals are involved, the animal and the AAT practice should be described in the professional's disclosure statement and in the client's informed consent for services, in client treatment plans, and in therapy session notes. Additionally, the impact of the AAT practiced should be noted in the therapy session notes and in the final treatment summary (termination summary). Assuming the responsibility of competency to practice AAT contributes to the safety and advocacy for all AAT participants; this includes people and animals.

7

Animal-Assisted Interventions and Counseling Theories

A counselor who does not adequately comprehend the multiple ways AAT can increase and enhance therapeutic opportunities will not be able to take full advantage of the therapeutic potential of this modality. Furthermore, a failure to understand the value of AAT in a counseling setting can actually jeopardize acceptance of its practice. For instance, at the beginning of one of my AAT-C training courses, a graduate student, having had some experience at counseling that did not involve AAT, expressed her concern that the presence of a therapy animal in the therapy room would be a negative distraction for a client that would interfere with therapeutic progress, a concern she was repeating from a former professor who had no knowledge or experience in AAT. I began my lecture on applications of AAT in mental health and explained how AAT-C actually had the opposite effect of the student's expressed concern. Instead of interfering with a client's progress, human–animal interactions enhance a client's therapeutic experience in such ways that significant progress occurs.

For example, AAT has been shown to be effective at motivating clients to attend sessions and promoting a safe and nurturing environment. Holcomb and Meacham (1989) reported that the nondirective presence of a therapy dog increased motivation of psychiatric patients to attend rehabilitation sessions. Lange et al. (2007) reported that the nondirective presence of a therapy dog in a counseling group of adolescents increased motivation to attend sessions, had a calming effect on clients, and increased clients' sense of safety. According to Reichert (1994, 1998), the nondirective presence of a therapy dog in a sexual abuse recovery group of female children was reported to increase a sense of safety and calm in participants. The clients would often pet and hold the dog while talking about their distress and often found it easier to talk directly to the dog, with the counselor listening. VanFleet (2008) described how canines added to the emotional safety of a therapeutic environment in a play therapy setting due to the dogs' seemingly accepting and nonjudgmental nature with people. Fick (1993) reported that the opportunity to interact socially with a therapy dog increased positive social behaviors in a group of nursing home patients. Richeson (2003) demonstrated how the nondirective presence of a therapy dog decreased agitation and increased positive social behaviors in older patients with dementia. Heindl (1996) described how having a therapy dog available for play and petting was effective in decreasing behavior problems and increasing positive social behaviors in children at a community-based children's day treatment program. Friedmann et al. (1983) reported that people tend to exhibit lower blood pressure and to verbally express feelings of relaxation in the presence of a dog. Thus,

DOI: 10.4324/9781003260448-7

including a therapy animal in a counseling session is far from a hindrance to client progress, as some may unknowingly fear; rather, AAT serves to assist clients' progress by enhancing their therapeutic experience.

Another important consideration is how the presence of a therapy animal may positively influence the formation of a therapeutic alliance between client and therapist. Schneider and Pilchak Harley (2006) investigated how the presence of a dog influenced the evaluation of psychotherapists. The study used an experimental design in which participants viewed a video recording of one of two therapists who were either with or without a dog. There were 85 participants who were college students (51 females and 34 males). The participants were assigned to view either a male or a female psychotherapist in one of two conditions: either alone or accompanied by a dog. The same male and female psychotherapist was used for the dog and no-dog conditions. The dogs, a Golden Retriever and a black Collie/Labrador cross, belonged to the psychotherapists. The verbal content of the presentations by the psychotherapists was kept consistent in both the dog and no-dog conditions. Each participant completed the Counselor Rating Form—Short Version, a 12-item adjective instrument designed to measure the perception of the therapist as trustworthy, expert, credible, attractive, powerful, and an overall "good guy." Participants also completed the Disclosure to Therapist Inventory—III, a 101-item inventory that covers a range of topics normally discussed in therapy. Two other instruments completed by participants were the Pet Attitude Scale, developed to measure favorableness of attitudes toward pets, and a background questionnaire, to obtain demographic information and past companion animal ownership. It was discovered that people responded more positively to psychotherapists when accompanied by a dog; specifically, they were more satisfied and more willing to disclose personal information. These effects were not influenced by the participants' attitudes toward pets and only minimally influenced by participants' prior history with pets. The researchers demonstrated that the presence of a companion animal, in this case a dog, enhances perceptions of therapists and the willingness to disclose to therapists (Schneider and Pilchak Harley, 2006). From these findings, we can suppose that working with a therapy animal can further the facilitative properties of therapy.

At the conclusion of my lecture explaining how AAT-C is beneficial while citing supportive research, the same student was in awe of the magnitude of potential therapeutic benefits. Even at the beginning of learning about AAT-C, the student's attitude switched from reservation to anticipatory excitement. It is apparent that a lack of familiarity with AAT-C may cause some to misjudge it. Thus, it is the responsibility of those of us who practice AAT-C and perform research to explain the therapeutic value of AAT-C and how it works. After all, the key to accessing the potential benefits of AAT is understanding how to facilitate this type of treatment with therapeutic intention. Thus, I have dedicated this chapter to describing how AAT is performed in the counseling environment and for what purposes. I will begin by describing my conception of the basic psychodynamics of AAT-C.

PSYCHODYNAMICS OF AAT WITHIN COUNSELING

The phrase that possibly best explains the value of AAT is *increased and enhanced therapeutic opportunity*. The word "therapeutic" derives from the Greek *therapeutikos* and relates to "the treatment of disease or disorders by remedial agents or methods," and the term "opportunity" refers to "a good chance for advancement or progress" (Merriam-Webster.com, n.d.). Thus, placed together, therapeutic opportunity means a good chance for advancement or progress of treatment by remedial agents or methods. AAT is a method whereby the use of human–animal interactions advances or progresses the recovery of a human client. The therapeutic method of AAT-C is human–animal interaction. The primary therapeutic agent of AAT-C is a human therapist who facilitates interactions between a therapy animal (a secondary therapeutic agent) and a human client. The value of incorporating an additional therapeutic agent, a therapy animal, and an additional therapeutic method, human–animal interaction, adds to the potential progress that can be made in therapy. Notice how the word *additional* is used here. AAT does not replace or substitute for counseling, nor does a therapy animal replace or substitute for a human therapist. AAT is a method incorporated into counseling, giving us AAT-C, for additional therapeutic gain. A concept key to understanding additional opportunities for therapeutic gain offered by AAT-C is that of psychodynamics. The word "psychodynamics" is "the aggregate of motivational forces, both conscious and unconscious, that determine human behavior and attitudes" (Dictionary.com, n.d.); an *aggregate* is a collection or combination of particulars or parts (Dictionary.com, n.d.). Vital particulars of psychodynamic process include the relationship experiences of those involved, experiences facilitated by a therapist and processed with a client.

In AAT-C counselors perform similar types of individual and group process that they are trained to perform in non-AAT sessions, but when human–animal interactions are incorporated as they are in AAT there are more particulars made available to the counselor and client to experience, which increases and enhances opportunities to impact human attitudes and behaviors. Given that an interpersonal relationship is an emotional connection or association between two social beings, in a non-AAT counseling session where one therapist and one client are present there are two interpersonal relationship experiences occurring: a client's experience of a therapist and a therapist's experience of a client. Many of my students first guess that there is one relationship, forgetting that a client's experience of a therapist is not exactly the same as a therapist's experience of a client. While a therapist and a client share the relationship experience, each has his or her own perspective of that experience. So how many interpersonal relationships are being experienced in a session including one therapist, one client, and one therapy animal? There are six, with the addition of the client's experience of the therapy animal, the therapy animal's experience of the client, the therapist's experience of the therapy animal, and the therapy animal's experience of the therapist (Figure 7.1). Each of the six interaction dyads provides opportunities for meaningful experience for the parties involved, including valuable observation of interactions by each party. Interactions

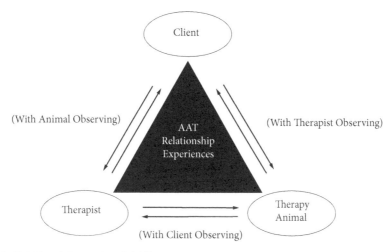

Figure 7.1 Relational dynamics of AAT.

might happen consecutively or concurrently; for example, a client and therapist might both be interacting with a therapy animal at the same time.

A client's observation of interactions involving a therapist with a therapy animal can be meaningful to a client in a number of ways including affecting the formation of a client's beliefs about a therapist, such as one who is kind and caring. Such beliefs are founded on how a therapist treats an animal along with the animal's attitude toward a therapist. Further, therapist–therapy animal interactions model for a client nurturing relational dynamics with appropriate boundaries. A therapist's observation of client–therapy animal interactions may be useful to the therapist in a number of ways, such as in providing a therapist with significantly more opportunities to assess a client's inner state as well as relational capacity and to impact client self-awareness by reflecting impressions of the client's and animal's responses to one another. A therapy animal's observation of therapist–client interactions can be meaningful to the animal in any number of ways, such as providing the animal with information regarding when and how to engage with a client based on the client's presentation or on the therapist's and client's responses to one another.

What does it mean for a client to experience a therapy animal? Many possibilities exist, but one example is the soothing touch and affection an animal can provide when a client pets the animal while discussing distressing concerns. Researchers have discovered that positive touch causes skin sensors to stimulate release of the hormone oxytocin in the brain, which has multiple positive effects, including calming, uplifting mood, and social bonding; this works in a similar way for both humans and animals because the oxytocin molecule along with its release and effects is the same in all mammals (Handlin et al., 2011; Uvnäs-Moberg, 2010; Uvnäs-Moberg, Arn, and Magnusson, 2005). Animals can experience contact with humans and animals as nurturing in much the same way; this mechanism underlies an animal's desire to seek and provide affection that is so beneficial to a client. The stress response of humans and animals is also similar. When humans and animals perceive there is a reason to be distressed, then stress-related hormones such as aldosterone, cortisol, and adrenalin are released into the body that result in fight, flight, or freeze responses (Panksepp, 1998). These responses will be maintained until the human or animal no longer perceives there is a need to be distressed. Thus, animals can experience distress from negative social interaction in much the same way as humans, and when the animal's behavior reflects this in response to a client the event can promote self-insight for a client. What does it mean for a therapy animal to experience a client? Well, one instance would be an episode I observed where a therapy horse refused to lift its hoof for grooming until an adolescent shifted her attitude toward the horse from bullying to calming and reassuring because the horse did not feel safe enough with the adolescent's initial attitude and thus was unwilling to cooperate. After the adolescent calmed herself and spent time reassuring the horse with a soothing touch and voice then the horse became cooperative. In summary, with six interpersonal relationship experiences and accompanying observations occurring in an AAT-C session where one therapist, one client, and one animal are participants there exist significant additional opportunities for therapeutic processing and therapeutic gains compared with a session where an animal is not involved. Therapeutic opportunities increase even more when the number of human or animal participants slightly increases, as in animal-assisted couples counseling, family therapy, or small group therapy.

The Therapy Animal's Role as a Transitional Being and Therapeutic Agent

One role of a counselor involves recognizing and processing therapeutic relational dynamics with a client to assist a client to become more self-aware in relation to others, and a therapist can also assist a client to generalize this information to other persons and situations in a client's life outside of therapy. In this respect, a therapist serves as a transitional object for a client by way of client–therapist interactions, and this mechanism assists a client to transition to greater levels of insight, awareness, and healing. An object or being becomes a transitional object to a client when a client takes a subjective experience, such as a relational experience, and projects it onto a real object or being in a manner that derives personal meaning for the client. A transitional object can be another human such as the therapist or other clients present in a session, a toy or other inanimate therapy tool, or a therapy animal. Including a therapy animal as a participant in a counseling session creates unique therapeutic opportunities as a result of the animal's value as a transitional object capable of impacting client awareness, insight, development, and healing:

> Animals make good transitional beings because they move and show intentional behavior, behaving more like a person than a stuffed toy who just lies there unless moved by the child. Unlike stuffed toys who provide soft touch, animals are capable of giving active affection and seeking out the child. But most importantly they can never contradict the attributes projected onto them with words.
>
> (Katcher, 2000b, p. 468)

I am of the opinion that therapy animals have great transitional potential. Perhaps therapy animals make the best of all transitional objects because they are affectionate and responsive, unlike a toy, and genuinely accepting and nonjudgmental in a manner unlike most humans. As transitional objects, therapy animals combine the best therapeutic attributes of both toys and humans while avoiding the obvious limitations that toys and humans may present. It is important to understand the concept of a therapy animal's tendency to be genuinely accepting and nonjudgmental in a manner unlike that of most humans. Humans tend to judge and respond to other humans based both on their own relationship with that person and on what they know about that person's behavior in situations outside of the immediate relationship. In contrast, an animal does not comprehend information about a person's behavior outside of its own experience with and observation of that person; thus, an animal can be genuinely accepting and nonjudgmental of a person regarding those aspects about which the animal does not know. Basically, clients get a fresh start with a therapy animal with opportunities to learn about the consequences of their immediate attitude and behaviors that are reflected by an animal's response to these. The relative simplicity of human–animal relationship dynamics makes engaging with a therapy animal more inviting and less emotionally threatening for a client. An animal will judge and respond to a client based on what it comprehends about the client, and an animal will place conditions on a relationship with a client based on those judgments. However, unlike human tendencies, an animal's responses to a person are mostly limited to its own experience of that person. Also, unlike human tendencies, an animal will always be very immediate and honest in its reactions, which makes the consequences of one's attitude and behavior readily apparent.

With the use of human–animal interactions, therapeutic opportunities are made available to a therapist and client when there is comprehension of the sorts of conditions an animal will place on a relationship with a person. This requires an appreciation for the natural tendencies of animals. A therapy animal that has been properly trained and socialized has learned that it can, for the most part, feel comfortable and safe around humans. Yet a therapy animal has survival instincts and will not disregard cues from its environment that help it to thrive and survive. A therapy animal will signal with positive behaviors that it perceives someone as safe and potentially rewarding; such as, a dog wagging its tail in a relaxed manner and moving toward a person for petting. A therapy animal will also signal with cautionary behaviors that it perceives someone is in distress or is unsafe to be near; such as, a dog moving toward someone who is in distress to offer nurturance, or moving away from someone who might be threatening. A therapy animal may ignore stimuli that it perceives to have no reward and is capable of choosing one object over another based on its perception of which stimulus offers the greatest reward. If a therapy animal perceives a human's presentation as uncomfortable, it may choose to not approach a human, to not cooperate with a human, or to demonstrate signs of distress around a human. For example, if a client is speaking in an angry tone of voice, a therapy dog may hesitate to approach the client. Or if a client runs directly toward a therapy horse, the horse is likely to run away from the client. If one client holds a dog treat and another client does not, the therapy dog is most likely going to choose to interact with the client holding the dog treat.

Animals can also retain memories of past events based on the perceived thrive or survive value of the event. For instance, in a small group session where clients spend a few minutes first playing fetch with a therapy dog, the dog may prefer to bring a ball to one client for play instead of another because the dog remembers that one of those persons frequently teased the dog by only pretending to throw the ball instead of actually throwing the ball for the dog each time so it could retrieve it. An ability to learn and recall the reward value of specific environmental stimuli or, as in the previous case, the actions of specific people is what allows animals to thrive and survive.

So the thrive and survive instincts of therapy animals can place conditions on a relationship with a client. However, the conditions placed by a therapy animal on its relationship with a client are usually confined to that relational experience, in that an animal does not typically judge a person outside the parameters of its interactions or observations with that person, unless of course that person reminds the animal of someone else or the animal has generalized previous experiences with other people onto the current person with whom it is interacting. A therapy animal does not know that a particular client has a history of failed relationships prior to coming into the therapy animal's world, or is in a detention center as a result of acts of vandalism, or feels abandoned by a parent after a divorce, or is a victim of child sexual abuse or whatever precipitating event or events brought the client to therapy. The animal knows and cares about the client only in relationship to it and its environment. If a therapy animal consistently experiences a client behaving in a manner the animal understands to be comfortable, rewarding, and nonthreatening, then it is likely to behave in positive ways toward the client. A client who consistently offers no reward value might be ignored by a therapy animal. When a therapy animal experiences a client behaving in a manner that makes the animal uncomfortable, then it will act distressed around or avoid the client. Though a therapy animal has a memory for negative events it experiences, relationships with a therapy animal can still be formed or repaired if a client commits to consistently providing the therapy animal with sufficient evidence that it is worthwhile to interact with the client, that is, many positively rewarding experiences in the absence of negative experiences.

An animal's limited capacity to judge a client beyond its experience with or observation of a client is what allows a client and therapy animal relationship to form much more quickly than a client and human therapist relationship. Clients may be hindered in the relationship-building process with a human therapist because they typically understand that humans tend to negatively judge or be critical of other humans based on things they have done or experienced in their past and may fear that a human therapist will do likewise. Clients can be very anxious about how a human therapist's judgment of them may negatively impact them, so clients may be slower to form a trusting relationship with a human than with a therapy animal. Forming a relationship with a therapy animal is much simpler than forming a relationship with a human. While the expectations of the therapy animal must be met in order for a client to form a positive relationship with the animal—expectations of safety, comfort, and reward—these expectations are much easier for a client to comply with than the complexity of expectations that humans have for other humans. The client–therapy animal relationship is more easily formed and maintained when compared with the more complex client–human therapist relationship. The fact that it is fairly easy for clients to understand that therapy animals do not intentionally respond to clients in ways that may minimize, embarrass, humiliate, or otherwise threaten them emotionally, means clients are likely to be more authentic in their relationship with a therapy animal. Experiences of success while being authentic with a therapy animal contribute to clients' understanding of how this is beneficial and facilitates them being more authentic with the human therapist as well. A therapist can use the dynamics of the client–therapy animal relationship to assist clients in generalizing relational experiences to other events, such as contributing to the formation of a strong therapeutic alliance between the client and the human therapist, interacting more positively with other humans, and facing other life challenges.

Given that clients may more closely associate with and relate to a therapy animal than a human therapist, at least in the earlier stages of the therapeutic process, this connection between client and therapy animal may facilitate conditions that foster client recovery. Clients' connection with the therapy animal may contribute to a warmer and safer atmosphere for the clients. They may experience the therapy animal as a support mechanism during sessions, feeling comforted by the animal's presence or from touching or holding the animal. Clients may experience quicker and deeper trust for the human therapist seeing how the therapy animal and human therapist interact. The therapy animal can be an additional mechanism to convey the human therapist's empathy for clients, especially when the human therapist reflects the interactions between clients and the therapy animal. It is of primary importance that human therapists establish rapport and convey empathy for clients to form a therapeutic relationship. This therapeutic relationship is necessary for client recovery to occur. A therapy animal can enhance the establishment and continuation of a therapeutic relationship between clients and the human therapist. The incorporation of a therapy animal into a counseling session should not serve as an excuse for failing to foster a close, caring relationship between a human therapist and clients. The relationship between the therapy animal and clients is not meant to be a substitute for the relationship between clients and the human therapist. In fact, it is meant to do the opposite—to facilitate the relationship between clients and the human therapist. Witnessing the nurturing relationship between the counselor and the therapy animal, the client's fondness for the animal extends to the counselor.

The greatest assets a therapy animal brings to a counseling session that make it such a powerful therapeutic agent for change for human clients are: (1) its ability and desire to give and receive emotional and physical nurturance with humans; and, (2) its ability to perceive and desire to signal emotional experiences of humans, especially those emotional experiences of humans that are not outwardly observable. It is incredibly useful the way a therapy animal can "sniff out" and signal nonvisible emotional distress in humans, making the invisible available for consideration and processing in the session.

The more capable a counselor is at recognizing therapeutic opportunities and facilitating processing of psychodynamics of human–animal interactions, the more therapeutic benefit can be had from including an animal in a counseling session. Counselors should apply the observation and processing skills they use in non-AAT sessions to AAT-C sessions by additionally acknowledging the impact that human–animal interactions have on clients, therapy animals, the counselor, and the therapeutic environment. To further understanding of how human–animal interaction can be effectively utilized to benefit clients, I will now describe a theory I developed, and first presented in the spring and summer of 2015, that is designed to guide the practice of animal-assisted counseling and psychotherapy; I call it human–animal relational theory (HART) (Chandler, 2015b, 2015c, 2017, 2018).

HUMAN–ANIMAL RELATIONAL THEORY (HART)

We know from scientific research, such as was presented in Chapter 1, that all mammals, both humans and animals, share similar psychophysiological systems: a social response system and a stress response system. These two systems can be activated at different times during human–animal interaction. During AAT, therapy animals may provide service in the role of nurturer via activation of their social response system, which is involved in positive relational activity, for example approaching or making positive physical contact with a client or therapist. This type of engagement may, in turn, activate the social response system of the client or therapist. And this gives rise in the client or therapist hormones associated with a sense of wellbeing, these hormones being oxytocin, dopamine, and endorphins. Likewise, the client or therapist may serve this same role of nurturer for the therapy animal. Therapy animals may also provide service in the role of emotional distress detector via activation of their stress response system, which is involved in signaling their perception of a stressor presented by a person, another animal, or in the environment. Activation of the stress response system means there is an increase in production of hormones such as cortisol, adrenalin, or aldosterone. A therapy animal will communicate via body language or vocalizations their perception of a stressor, including their perception that a person is stressed or anxious, and so forth. These alerting signals from the animal assist the client and therapist in determining that something needs to be attended and explored, thus encouraging introspection followed by emotional and behavioral change by a client or therapist so that the animal may feel safer and more comfortable. The roles a therapy animal may serve as nurturer, via activation of the social response system, and as emotional distress detector, via activation of the stress response system, are fundamental to understanding the impact of human–animal interaction and its potential therapeutic benefits. A therapy animal's service in the roles of nurturer and emotional distress detector during a counseling session are fundamental to ideas presented in human–animal relational theory (HART).

HART is a set of constructs I designed to explain the value of therapeutic process and resulting therapeutic impact of human–animal interaction. The practice of HART is referred to as human–animal relational therapy. Here I shall describe theoretical constructs and practice concepts of HART. I begin with the idea that, when a therapy animal is present during a therapy session the people and animals involved in the session are relating to one another, and we can observe that a series of human–animal relational moments (RMs) occurs. These can be between the animal and client, or between the animal and therapist, or between all three at the same time (see Figure 7.1). HART assigns greater value to the more significant human–animal relational moments (SHARMs) that occur during human–animal interaction, along with effective processing of those moments by a client and a therapist. The processing of a SHARM is what I call human–animal relational processing (HARP). The more effective the processing is of a SHARM by a therapist and/or a client, the greater the therapeutic impact is likely to be obtained. Effective HARP can be accomplished individually and silently by a therapist or a client. This internal processing is what I refer to as I-HARP. Effective HARP can also occur with a therapist and a client processing out loud and together. This external processing is what I refer to as E-HARP. Both I-HARP and E-HARP may occur regarding a human–animal interaction. I encourage a counselor to facilitate E-HARP when deemed appropriate to aid a client's comprehension of how a human–animal interaction that occurred may reveal something of value to the client. The degree of human–animal relational therapeutic impact (HARTI) is dependent upon the recognition of a SHARM by a therapist or client, along with the effectiveness of the processing of that SHARM, individually and/or together. Sometimes the client, and not the therapist, is the first to recognize a SHARM during human–animal interaction. But most of the time, especially in the early phases of therapy, the therapist is first to recognize a SHARM, due to the therapist's experience and knowledge. Processing is the action of going forward to enact change or make progress. The action of going forward in a counseling session can involve increased insight, enhanced awareness, furthered understanding, and emotional and behavioral changes. When a SHARM occurs and a person consciously processes that moment, individually and/or together with someone else, the consideration is in regard to what the human–animal interaction may reveal for or about the person with whom the animal is relating. Any new insight or awareness facilitated by this revelation is moving the client forward.

I chose the terms "relating" and "relational" as descriptors in HART because I believe they best represent the social dynamic that occurs in therapeutic human–animal interaction. Relating involves bringing into or establishing association, connection, or relation with some other being, while relational is a feeling of being close or connected to another being. SHARMs represent impactful events between a person and animal, an animal with which that person feels a connection or desires to feel a connection. Feelings of connection and desires for connection can result in either nurturing or challenging moments of interaction. Someone who wants a dog to bring a ball back after the person throws the ball may feel rejected if the dog takes the ball to someone else. Someone grooming a horse that refuses to lift its hoof for cleaning may feel frustrated by the horse's lack of cooperation. Someone who has a cat snuggling in the lap may feel comforted. Both nurturing and challenging relational moments can assist conscious and unconscious motivational forces of the client, originating from past or present experiences, to be presented in the here and now, thus providing opportunity for therapist and client to process these constructively. Each of the examples just described reflects actual cases. When the adolescent felt rejection because my dog Rusty did not bring the ball back to him, this provided opportunity to process his feelings in the moment with me as his therapist and for him to gain insight on these same feelings that were present in relationship with his family members. The adolescent who felt frustrated by the horse's lack of cooperation immediately recognized the situation was similar to the one she presents to her mother and declared, "Now I know what I put my mother through!" From her internal processing of this experience with the horse, the adolescent gained significant new insight and became motivated to change her problematic behavior at home; within one week she and her mother both reported she was much more cooperative and pleasant. The adolescent who felt comforted by my cat Snowflake in her lap processed with me, her therapist, how it was the most relaxed she had been in a long time and elaborated on her anxiety, providing opportunity for her to gain important insight.

I believe human–animal interaction can be more impactful, and thus more therapeutic, if a social connection or even a desire for social connection with the animal is present. When AAT is applied in counseling, it is possible that the people and animal involved with one another can form a sympathetic association, that is, caring about each other's emotional welfare. This is why it is important the therapeutic environment allows for social relatedness to occur between client and therapy animal. The animal should not just be considered an object for interaction, as this limits the potential benefit that may be gained. A therapist must appreciate the animal as a social being and social stimulus, honoring the contribution the animal may make to the psychodynamics of therapy.

The values in my simple, descriptive HART formula for studying and practicing human–animal interaction, SHARM + HARP = HARTI, are subjective values. First, there must be recognition that a SHARM has occurred. Many human–animal relational moments are likely to be presented during a session, thus a therapist or a client must discern which human–animal relational moments hold significance for potential benefit. Once a SHARM has been recognized it must be processed to be effective. As mentioned, this processing can be done internally by either the therapist or the client, and/or it can be done externally with therapist–client interactive dialogue. How effectively a SHARM is processed determines the therapeutic impact that can be had from that human–animal relational moment; this is the HARTI. While the values of the formula are subjective, one could suppose the more significant the moment (SHARM) is in combination with the more effective the processing (HARP), then the greater the impact of these two values combined is likely to be—thus, the greater the HARTI. The HART formula may be used in a qualitative manner to determine efficacy of AAT-C intervention.

When a SHARM is processed externally, that is, using interactive dialogue between therapist and client, the observed or potential therapeutic impact may become very apparent to both client and therapist. When a SHARM is processed internally, that is, via a private dialogue within either the therapist or client, the therapeutic impact may not be apparent in the moment to both the therapist and the client, but may be very useful in benefiting the client, nonetheless. Consider the following examples. A therapy dog moves from a resting position during a counseling session to an alert position near the client signaling that something about the client needs attention. A counselor may facilitate an external dialogue with a client about the observation of the dog's behavior in wondering aloud what it could mean. During this external process the client might reveal he/she became anxious about something just prior to the dog's shift in position, when the dog directed attention toward the client. Through continued interactive processing of the observed SHARM, the potential impact may become very apparent to both client and therapist. In contrast, internal processing is not shared in the moment but can still be beneficial. For example, a therapist may observe a therapy horse shy away from a particular client and internally process or privately speculate that this might reflect the client has a distressed emotional state. However, a therapist may choose to withhold this information from the client in the moment, while keeping it in mind during succeeding human–animal interactions. The reason a therapist might withhold the awareness from the client in the moment would be unique to the assessed needs of the client. Perhaps a therapist is waiting to see if sometime during the session the client notices for himself/herself how the horse is behaving toward him/her as a determinant of the client's emotion-recognition ability. Another instance of how internal processing alone may benefit a client would be when a client experiences a friendly greeting from a therapy dog and internally processes that it feels good that the dog likes him/her, thus the client feels likeable or worthy.

When facilitating human–animal interaction we must also consider the client's capacity or readiness for insight as a variable in determining therapeutic impact. Additionally, therapeutic impact may be difficult to measure due to its nature. Therapeutic impact may be immediate or delayed and it may be obvious or less obvious. Therapeutic impact may not be stationary, but rather increase (progression) or decrease (regression) across time. Or, the impact of therapy may present only in unique circumstances. Of course the client's capacity or readiness for insight as well as the many variations of therapeutic impact are the same issues confronted whether or not therapy involves human–animal interaction.

I am the first to admit that human–animal interaction can still be therapeutic even if a therapist and client never recognize or process SHARMs. We know from past researchers that just a few minutes' visit with a therapy dog can have a great deal of positive impact on human participants, such as, calming, uplifting mood, increasing positive social connection and so forth; this being accomplished through the natural physiological changes that occur from positive human–animal interaction. What HART provides is an approach for increasing the potential benefits that human–animal interaction provides. After years of practicing AAT-C and providing supervision for my graduate students who practice AAT-C, it became much clearer as to the significant contribution the therapy animal made to the relational dynamics of the counseling session. I developed HART in an attempt to convey how much more therapeutic impact can be gained during an AAT-C session by consciously attending to and processing the social–relational dynamics contributed by a therapy animal. By understanding that human–animal interaction involves the occurrence of a complex series of human–animal relational moments, one can then examine these relational moments, identify those of greater significance or relevance to the client's state or wellbeing, and discern meaningfulness for the client of those relational moments. This involves describing and processing observed human–animal relational dynamics and how they reflect something significant for the client. The constructs of HART—SHARM, HARP, and HARTI—were designed in an effort to help researchers, practitioners, and beneficiaries of human–animal interaction appreciate the tremendous amount of therapeutic opportunity presented when animals participate in therapy. HART recognizes the value of a therapy animal as a social–relational being whose participation may significantly impact the relational dynamics of therapy, giving rise to potentially greater therapeutic gain.

The descriptive formula SHARM + HARP = HARTI may be enacted several times during a therapy session, depending upon how many SHARMs are recognized and processed. However, a therapist must not choose quantity over quality. One must remember, it is not the number of SHARMs that are recognized during a session that determines therapeutic impact (HARTI). Rather, it is how effectively the processing (HARP) is performed related to a SHARM that determines therapeutic impact. The HARP of a SHARM gives personal meaning and relevance to the event. Without effective HARP, the meaning and relevance of a SHARM may be missed or quickly forgotten. The more effective HARP is regarding a SHARM, then the more HARTI is gained for the session. I have enacted the formula only once during a session and found it to be a very powerful session based on the amount of insight provided for the client. In this case, the recognition of just one SHARM alone resulted in a full session of HARP, and the therapeutic impact (HARTI) or gain for the client was transforming. However, the formula can be applied more than once during a session if therapeutic opportunity is presented.

The art of processing is a standard skill that is required learning in counselor training programs. The level of this skill increases with practice, in that the more experienced counselor is often a more effective processor with a client. To be an effective processor, a counselor must keep in mind the presenting concern or concerns of a client relevant to how the client engages as a social being. With this in consideration, counselors attempt to help a client identify conscious and unconscious motivational forces, that is, the psychodynamics that are presented in a therapy session, so these may be reflected to the client in a manner that increases client self-awareness, self-insight, and self-understanding. In-depth client–therapist discussion that follows can lead to additional client insights. The more opportunities presented to identify and process client psychodynamics, the more potential therapeutic gain. Incorporation of human–animal interaction in counseling gives rise to additional social–relational dynamic forces for a therapist and client to identify and process. This is what I mean when I say integrating a therapy animal into a counseling session presents additional therapeutic opportunities. In Figure 7.1, I present how during a therapy session, relational moments with a therapy animal can occur within all dynamic pairings (separately or at the same time, meaning integrated): between client and animal (with therapist observing), between therapist and animal (with client observing), and between therapist and client (with animal observing). During a therapy session, observations are made on how a therapy animal, therapist, and client are relating to one another at any given moment and the potential impact of this relating upon all possible relational dynamic pairings. As mentioned earlier, the significance of a relational moment can be identified by a client or a therapist.

A therapist facilitates human–animal interaction and resulting relational moments by bringing a therapy animal into a session. Spontaneous relational moments occur (e.g., dog walking up to client), as well as those that may be more directed by the therapist (e.g., game of fetch between client and dog). A therapist may guide or direct the client or therapy animal in interactions to achieve certain goals, while at the same time keeping in mind the need to allow the client and animal to interact naturally. While the therapist is facilitator of AAT-C, the modality works best if we honor, value, and respect the natural state of the animal and work within those parameters: yet set limits on animal and human behaviors for preservation of the safety and welfare of therapy animals and humans engaged in the therapy. The state, attitude, needs, desires, ability, or disability of humans and animals must be taken into consideration during AAT-C. Many human-directed activities are not too inconsistent with the natural behaviors of animals. It is not too unnatural or too inhibiting, in many cases, to ask a therapy dog to respond to simple commands such as *sit*, *down*, *stay*, and *come* and to walk politely on a leash. In fact, there are a variety of activities a therapy animal, such as a dog, can engage in that are consistent with the natural ability of the animal. Thus, much opportunity with a variety of social activity is available with which to work, i.e., petting, fetch, seek and find, walk on a leash, etc. Similarly with other species of animals many human-directed activities are not too inconsistent with the animal's innate makeup and thus, do not interfere much with the opportunity for the animal to interact naturally with a client. However, it is important to remember the fewer restrictions placed on an animal's natural social–relational behavior during therapy, within safe and comfortable limits for humans and animals, the freer the animals and humans are to relate to one another naturally, and thus greater relational opportunity can be presented for possible therapeutic gain. Human-directed activities are effective in AAT-C, but be mindful of how directed activities may either facilitate or interfere with relational opportunity between client and therapy animal. For example, a therapy dog that strictly adheres to *sit*, *stay* commands in a therapy room may not feel free to signal emotional distress it perceives in a client, a signal it normally would give by, for example, walking over to the client and licking the client's hand. The key is to not restrict or overly direct a therapy animal's behavior in such a way that the animal may not provide us with extremely valuable signals about a client that we might otherwise miss.

Facilitating engagement between a therapy animal and a client can be accomplished with or without utilizing additional objects such as treats, toys, or agility challenges. However, treats, toys, or agility challenges can be used to gain the animal's attention and direct the animal's interaction. These objects are very helpful when a therapist wishes to have the client engage in command giving or play behavior with a therapy animal as part of the therapy session. However, when these objects are brought into the therapy session these objects will direct the animal's focus, attention, and behavior, and to some extent predetermine the amount and type of the animal's social engagement. What may be lost in these directed activities, since the animal is otherwise occupied, is the degree to which the animal may sense, reflect, or attend to the internal state of the client or the internal state of the therapist. It is likely that more information about internal personal dynamics may be discerned and signaled by the animal when the animal's attention or behavior is less preoccupied or directed. I rarely bring food treats into my AAT-C sessions. I do not want the dog to be preoccupied with the food treat. I want my dog to interact with me and my clients for social reward, not for food reward. Without the presence of food to distract, my dog's interactions with myself and my client serve as a valuable mirror reflecting our state of being. The only time I bring food treats into a therapy session is when I determine it would be valuable for a client to experience the reward of a dog complying with obedience or trick commands, which can build confidence and a sense of self-efficacy in a client. In this case the dog is motivated to comply with client commands for want of a food treat, yet the directed human–animal interaction still has great benefit for the client.

In committing an error, a therapist may under-utilize or over-utilize human–animal interaction. In over-utilizing, the therapist over-directs human–animal interaction in a manner that does not allow for a significant relational dynamic to occur between the therapy animal and the client. In under-utilizing, the therapist fails to recognize when a significant relational dynamic is actually occurring or has occurred and the therapist misses an opportunity to point out and process that relational moment with a client. Both over- and under-utilization are two sides of the same coin. Both over- and under-utilization can limit therapeutic opportunities in human–animal interaction. They are both symptoms of a therapist undervaluing the potential contribution of the therapy animal as a relational being capable of significantly contributing to therapeutic dynamics.

When a therapy animal is present in a session it attends to the social dynamics of all beings present, including other animals and all humans. During a therapy session, the animal is not only discerning the client's emotions and behaviors but also those of the therapist. If a therapist is frustrated with a client, the therapy animal may sense and signal the therapist's frustration in some manner, such as attending to the therapist in a nurturing way or trying to break the tension by redirecting attention. This became apparent to one of my graduate students and myself as we watched a video recording of her counseling performance with a client and observed the behavior of her dog during the session. The graduate student counselor was confused about why her dog behaved the way it did and asked my opinion as to why the dog ignored the client and focused engagement with her instead. While we watched the video recording of the session I inquired as to the emotional experience of the graduate student counselor at these moments of working with her client and experiencing the curious behavior of her dog. The graduate student conveyed her frustration with the client's resistance and how her frustration with the client grew across the session. In hindsight, we could see on the video recording how the dog's behavior exactly paralleled the rising frustration in the graduate student counselor. At first the dog kept going over to the counselor's lap and sniffing her face. When this did not yield a satisfactory result for the dog, it started trotting back and forth between the therapist and the door. With still no satisfactory result, the dog resorted to bringing her toy to the therapist and shoving it in the therapist's face until she got the therapist to start laughing at the dog's silly behavior. With the tension release, the atmosphere felt better for the dog and the dog settled down at the therapist's feet and took a nap. The therapist confirmed she recognized and released her frustration with her client at that moment during the session and relaxed for the remainder of the session. The therapist confirmed that her dog behaved in a similar fashion at home when the therapist experienced frustration or stress, but she had not recognized it in the session with her client. Now the therapist is more aware of her own presentation with her client, thanks to the signals from her dog working as a therapy animal.

If a therapist is feeling insecure or anxious about her/his own performance during a session, a therapy animal may attend to the therapist in an attempt to calm or reassure the therapist. It may not want to leave the therapist's side, or it may want to lick the therapist's hand or face. This was observed on multiple occasions of reviewing video recording of counseling sessions with my graduate student counselors, with confirmation of their internal experience that likely triggered the dog's behavior toward them. The point I am making here is that a therapy animal may signal relational dynamics in all beings present, often choosing to signal the experience that seems most intense or uncomfortable in either the counselor or the client. This makes the animal's communication all the more valuable as it assists both the therapist and the client to be more aware of their emotional and behavioral presentation in a session. It also assist therapists to better recognize and regulate their emotional state so that the animal is not distracted by the emotional state of the counselor, and the animal may instead feel freer to attend to the client and communicate how the animal experiences the client's emotional and behavioral presentation.

A key in correctly interpreting an animal's communication is to place the animal's behavior in context within a session. For instance, a therapist or client must attempt to discern if a dog is bringing a client a toy to play with because the dog is merely bored and wants to play, or is the dog trying to lighten the distressed mood of the client. Most of the time we can only guess at what the animal is conveying, but the more familiar you are with the animal you are working with, the more often you will accurately comprehend the animal's behavior in a session. In observing my animals work, I have learned they have certain patterns they present in relation to others that are consistent with certain moods presented by clients, and these patterns are repeated with different persons with which the animal works. So, the more I work in partnership with a particular animal, the better I get at discerning what the animal is signaling in relation to me or the client with whom I am counseling. The easiest way to discern what the animal may be signaling is to simply ask the client what he or she believes the animal is communicating in relation to what the client is feeling or thinking at that moment and, regardless of whether the client's speculation about the animal is accurate or not, something of value is usually revealed about the client.

A therapy animal can discern a complex set of social dynamics occurring in an environment and choose to attend to one or more of these social dynamics based on perceived need to bring the atmosphere, and the beings present in the atmosphere, back to a more comfortable state. This means that performing a live public demonstration of AAT is a very difficult thing to accomplish. This is because the animal will not just attend to the client's emotional and behavioral presentation during the demonstration, but will also attend to the therapist, and be simultaneously distracted by everyone in the room who is watching the demonstration. When an animal experiences sensory overload like this, it may just resort to exploratory behavior or calming signals (i.e., sniffing all around the room), or it may try friendly engagement with several persons present. When demonstrating the therapeutic value of human–animal interaction, I prefer to show video recording of role play demonstrations or, with permission of clients, film clips of real AAT therapy sessions. It is impossible to ask an animal to be selective in its focus and attention, thus live demonstrations of AAT-C for public consumption rarely approximate the value of human–animal interaction that occurs in a more private therapy session where fewer beings and distractions are present to draw the animal's attention.

Human–animal relational dynamics can be quite complex and difficult to identify. If a therapy animal senses that a significant emotional experience occurs in the client and/or therapist, the therapy animal will likely signal the need for this to be attended to or resolved. Furthermore, if this dynamic does not get attended to or resolved in a timely manner (within seconds or sometimes minutes), a therapy animal may make repeated attempts with similar or varied behaviors until the psychodynamic is attended to or resolved. For example, if a client experiences an intensity in emotion, such as greater emotional pain when reflecting upon a memory or fear, a therapy animal is likely to sense the intensity of the client's experience. The animal may sense this as an olfactory (smell), gustatory (taste), visual (see), auditory (hear), or kinesthetic (feel) perception. Animals, such as dogs and horses, have very well-developed olfactory systems, much more developed than humans', and this well-developed olfactory system possibly permits these animals to smell emotions through the endocrine secretions perceptible by the animal in the breath, sweat, and urine of humans.

Their enhanced olfactory ability suggests why animals can perceive emotions occurring in humans quicker and more efficiently than human observers. Likewise, an animal may taste endocrine secretions by licking the air or the skin of a person.

Once an animal perceives emotional intensity, then the animal may choose to alert by demonstrating a signal, such as a shift in body posture, body language, or with some type of vocalization. The animal may move toward or away from the client, the animal may look toward or away from the client, the animal may demonstrate another type of social signal, calming signal, or displacement signal, and so forth. For example, during one session my Cocker Spaniel Jesse was lying quietly on the couch snuggled next to my client who was gently petting her. My client had been sharing with me her exhaustion from school and work and her need for self-care, along with her struggle to actually provide herself with that self-care. I asked my client to introspect deeply about why she was not able to prioritize giving herself self-care. The client became very quiet and began to introspect. After just a few seconds Jesse sat up quickly and turned her face toward my client. She then did four quick "calming signals" in a row (that is, behaviors that exhibit the experience of stress or distress)—a look away and look back, an eye blink, lip licking, and a yawn—all of these taking place within a few seconds of each other. She finished by gazing at the client while continuing to sit next to my client. Unfortunately, in the moment I missed these initial, very overt calming signals from Jesse that she was sensing strong emotional reactions and I did not recognize them until later when reviewing the video recording of the session. However, fortunately for me and the client, when her initial signals went unnoticed in the session Jesse continued to give alerting signals that reflected her perception of distress in the room. As the client sat silently in continued contemplation, teetering on the precipice of resistance versus insight, Jesse leaned heavily against the client's side, rolled over on to her back staying pressed against the client's thigh, and then engaged in active wriggling with her little paws flopping in the air, as if to say "come on, get into it, you will feel better, let's talk about it, it will be okay." When Jesse did this snuggling roll over against the client's side, the client smiled at Jesse and made a deep sigh. I commented on the client's recognition that Jesse was signaling her concern and expressing encouragement for the client. The client nodded and courageously began to explore intense personal concerns while gently rubbing Jesse's belly and chest. Jesse then settled in quietly enjoying her belly rub. My client reflected upon how difficult it was for her to give herself time and space for self-care as a result of her fear of performance failure. She felt she had to push herself hard or she would not achieve her goals. This was complicated by the fact that she was experiencing an emotionally unsafe work environment at the time. She came to the realization that the more unsafe she feels, the harder she pushes herself. So, therapy dog Jesse had accurately signaled the client's emotional distress. Jesse had mirrored the client's experience of distress by demonstrating alerting signals and persisted with variations in signaling until the client and I acknowledged Jesse's behavior as signaling that some distress in the client needed attention. I am thankful that Jesse persisted in expressing alerting signals until we noticed she was signaling us. Jesse's signals reflected the level of distress the client was experiencing during her hesitation (resistance) to introspect and express, and simultaneously Jesse's signals encouraged the client to decrease her resistance and engage in therapeutic processing. Furthermore, when a client initiates a catharsis the animal often senses the emotional pressure in the client is subsiding and with this sensation the animal usually settles down in a more relaxed posture, which is what Jesse did after the client lowered her resistance and began fully expressing herself while rubbing Jesse's belly.

The reality that I did not see those initial four alerting signals given by Jesse with the client (the look away and look back, eye blink, lip licking, and yawn) until later while reviewing a video recording of the session is a demonstration of how difficult it can be sometimes to recognize what a therapy animal may be communicating in the moment with a client. The point here being that in realizing its fuller potential, AAT is an advanced and complex form of therapy that provides a therapist and client with numerous and varied cues for processing. Even if cues signaled by the animal are initially missed by a therapist and client, the animal will likely provide additional signals until proper attention is paid by the therapist and client to whatever is causing the animal to feel a need to generate certain social or alerting signals. Even if an animal's behavior is misinterpreted by the client or therapist, it can still be therapeutic in the way clients imagine what the animal may be feeling or thinking, in that clients project their inner experience onto the behavior of the animal.

To increase potential in recognizing social or alerting signals from a therapy animal you should become familiar with common behavioral signals known to be generated by the species of animal with which you work with in therapy. For instance, a look away, eye blink, yawn, and lip licking by a dog are well-known "calming signals" reflecting the experience or perception of the animal of stress and/or distress. Having this knowledge allowed us to recognize that Jesse was giving these common calming signals in relation to perceiving a client's distress. Additionally, you should be familiar with and pay attention to personality and behavioral traits unique to your animal that help you recognize signals from it about what it may be experiencing from any humans present in a therapy session, as well as signals that may represent the animal itself has a need that wants attending.

Significant Human–Animal Relational Moments (SHARMs)

We have established that integration of human–animal interaction into therapy provides additional opportunities for therapeutic impact from SHARMs that may occur. It is important to recognize, describe, and process these moments to enhance therapeutic impact. In my work as a counselor and supervisor I began to identify and classify SHARMs that can tend to occur in animal-assisted counseling sessions as well as animal-assisted supervision sessions. I present some of my observations here. I do not consider this an exhaustive list of possible SHARM categories, but by presenting these as examples in the context of when they occurred I may provide you with a better understanding of how to identify and process a SHARM and assess the potential therapeutic impact of performing this exercise. The categories I have identified for SHARMs that occurred in either my own or my student counselor's sessions are: Greeting, Acknowledgment, Speculation, Interpretation, Comfort, Assurance, and Checking In. Remember, different animals have different personalities and may be communicating different things with their behavior. For instance, a particular behavior by one dog may mean something different when enacted by a different dog. It is important to become familiar with your own animal's behavior. In addition, it is not always necessary to accurately comprehend what an animal may be communicating because therapeutic benefit may occur when clients project their own meaning onto the animal's behavior. All of the following vignettes are true stories provided by a therapist who was working with a therapy dog. The client participants in each of the following vignettes verified at some point during the session the significant relational moment with the animal and the resulting therapeutic impact from processing the moment with the therapist.

Greeting

For a Greeting SHARM, a therapist facilitates a greeting between client and therapy animal each time the client comes to a session where the animal is present. The therapist comments on the animal's body language in response to the greeting and the possible meaning or value of this body language. This aids in conveying acceptance and warmth to a client.

Additionally, a client may get a feeling of "I'm likeable" because the animal, which is authentic in its interactions, wants to engage with the client. The greeting interaction may also assist in the forming and strengthening of the relationship between the client and the therapist. See Figures 7.2 and 7.3 for an example of a Greeting SHARM.

Example vignette (provided by myself as therapist working with my dog Jesse, a buff and white Cocker Spaniel):

> The therapist and her therapy dog, Jesse, meet the client in the waiting area. The therapist signals Jesse to say "hello" to the client. Jesse wags her tail and enthusiastically moves to the client, who then smiles and reaches down to pet Jesse. Jesse responds to the petting with a faster tail wag, body wiggle, and a broad smile. The therapist comments on how happy Jesse is to see the client. The therapist, therapy dog, and client then walk back to the therapy room together. As the client takes a seat, Jesse walks over to the client and continues to interact with a tail wag and broad smile. The client mirrors the dog's behavior with a broad smile of her own while petting Jesse. The client comments on how soft Jesse's fur is and how good it feels to touch her. The counselor reflects on how Jesse enjoys the client petting her and feels comfortable with the client. Jesse then jumps on the couch and lays down next to the client. The counselor inquires as to how it feels to have Jesse relax next to her. The client replies that it is very comforting and relaxes her body posture while petting Jesse. The therapist suggests that Jesse can serve as a support for the client while she shares what is on her mind today. The client begins discussing her presenting concerns, occasionally glancing toward the dog who has settled next to her on the couch. The client continues to pet and glance at Jesse as she presents and works through her concerns.

In the example above, the SHARM was the greeting facilitated by the therapist between the client and animal in the waiting area through to the point where the dog settled next to the client on the couch in the therapy room at the start of the session. The therapist described the SHARM and briefly processed what the SHARM could mean for the client (HARP), to "provide support." The processing was intended to enhance the therapeutic impact (HARTI) of the therapy animal's engagement with the client, that is, to encourage the client to share her presenting concerns. In this case, the HARP was quite brief, yet the HARTI was still important and maintained its importance throughout the remainder of the session. The amount of HARP that accompanies a SHARM is not relevant to the type of SHARM, rather it is relevant to the need presented by the client. Thus, HARP can be brief or can be more in depth, depending upon the need of the client and the resulting HARTI.

Acknowledgment

For an Acknowledgment SHARM, a therapist acknowledges the animal is communicating something of value to the client, the therapist, or about the animal itself. The animal is communicating something of value that needs to be attended to about a person present in a session or about the animal itself, for example, by the animal's demonstration of a stress signal, calming signal, or an alerting signal. This is one of the most valuable assets of a therapy animal; to signal when it detects an intense emotional experience of a client, even one that is not apparent from the client's outward appearance. It is most likely that the animal can see, smell, hear, or feel the client's emotional experience. Since human therapists lack the ability to detect emotions masked by a client's outward appearance, when a therapy animal is present, issues can be addressed in the moment that might not otherwise be attended. Common stress signals, calming signals, or alerting signals in dogs include lip licking, eye blinking, looking away, yawning, quick and vigorous shake of the body, moving toward or away from the source of distress, quick bark or other vocalization, and so forth. Other species have some stress and alerting signals similar to dogs and also some that are different from dogs. What a therapy animal is communicating is highly valuable and when this communication is acknowledged and explored by counselor and client it may significantly benefit the client. An animal's contribution should be acknowledged with the animal also, by petting and thanking the animal, thereby reinforcing its tendency to serve this positive role. An untrained therapist working with a therapy animal might find the animal's stress signaling and alert signaling behavior annoying or distracting and might either ignore or correct the animal. This error not only devalues the animal's contribution but also discourages the animal from providing these important signals in the future. See Figure 7.4 for one example of an Acknowledgment SHARM.

Example vignette (provided by therapist Tiffany Otting working with her dog Wally, a black Schnauzer–Poodle mix or Schnoodle):

> Therapy dog Wally is pacing back and forth between the client and therapist. Then he sits down by the therapist, looks at the client and barks once. From experience the therapist knows this is how Wally signals there is unexpressed anxiety. The therapist thanks Wally for letting the client and therapist know that something needs attending. The therapist explains the reason for Wally's behavior and asks the client what she thinks: "Wally is letting us know that something needs attending, meaning there is a thought or feeling in a person that may reflect discomfort, anxiety, or something else. Do you know what that might be?" The client then begins to express feelings that were previously suppressed. Wally relaxes on the floor and falls asleep while the client expresses the previously unshared feelings or thoughts that the client believes reflect what the animal was sensing.

In the example above, the SHARM was the dog pacing back and forth and vocalizing the bark. The therapist acknowledged Wally for his contribution to the session and described the SHARM to the client, which involved Wally making the therapist and client aware that something needed attention. The therapist then began to process the SHARM with the client by asking the client what it was that needed attention (HARP). The client agreed that there was indeed something she was holding back, and then began to share the previously suppressed feelings and concerns. By sharing these concerns, the client was able to experience some relief and work on her issues; this was the resulting HARTI.

Speculation

For a Speculation SHARM, a therapist may wonder aloud what the animal is thinking or feeling in an effort to make a point that may provide insight or awareness to the client. Alternatively, the therapist may ask the client to speculate about the animal's thoughts or feelings to provide a medium through which the client may project the client's internal experience. The speculation does not have to be accurate to be of value. See Figure 7.5 for one example of a Speculation SHARM.

Example vignette (provided by myself as therapist working with my dog Jesse):

> Therapy dog Jesse is fast asleep on the floor between the therapist and the client. The therapist and the client notice that Jesse seems to be dreaming. The dog is making small running motions with her feet, vocalizing muffled whimpers, and barking softly while she sleeps. The therapist wonders aloud as to whether Jesse may be having a good

dream or a bad dream and what Jesse may be feeling. "Jesse seems to be dreaming. I wonder if she is running toward something or away from something. I wonder if she is happy, or I wonder if she is scared." The client then shares her thoughts, projecting the client's own desires or fears into the speculation about the dog's behavior. The therapist and client continued to process, eventually exploring how the experience of the dog might resemble the client's own life experience.

In the example above, the SHARM was Jesse dreaming, making small running motions with her feet, vocalizing muffled whimpers, and barking softly while she slept. The therapist pointed out the dog's behavior to the client and speculated about what it meant. In responding to the therapist's inquiry, the client projected her own inner experience onto the dreaming behavior of the dog (HARP). As the therapist and client continued to process, they explored how the experience of the dog resembled the client's own life experience; the resulting awareness and insight gained by the client was the HARTI.

Interpretation

For an Interpretation SHARM, a therapist offers an interpretation of the animal's behavior, or asks a client to interpret an animal's behavior to imply what the animal is experiencing or may be communicating. In this instance we are looking to offer an accurate interpretation of what the animal is likely experiencing or communicating. See Figure 7.6 for one example of an Interpretation SHARM.

Example vignette (provided by myself as therapist working with my dog Jesse):

At the beginning of the session, therapy dog Jesse jumps up next to the client who is sitting on the couch and greets her by moving her nose up near the client's face. The client pets Jesse on the head and Jesse lays down on the couch next to the client. After a few moments, Jesse jumps down off the couch and walks a few steps across the room and jumps into the lap of the therapist. The therapist strokes Jesse a few times and then Jesse jumps off her lap and goes back over onto the couch and lays next to the client who gently pets her. In a few moments, Jesse jumps off the couch and goes back over to the therapist's lap. After observing the back-and-forth behavior of Jesse, the therapist conveys to the client that Jesse is experiencing a dilemma: "Jesse is conflicted, she wants to be near you, but at the same time she wants to be near me. This seems to be a dilemma for her. I wonder if we can help her with a solution." The client and therapist then explore Jesse's desire to be next to both the therapist and client. Together they resolve that since the couch is very big that the therapist would sit on one end, the client would sit on the other end, and Jesse would be able to be in the middle if she desired. The therapist moves to the couch and Jesse spontaneously jumps between the client and therapist, lays down, and stretches her body out lengthwise so that she is making physical contact with both people at the same time. The therapist asks the client to explore what thoughts and feelings are invoked in the client by Jesse's conflict and ultimate resolution and relate this to the client's own life. The client expresses a dilemma she is experiencing and explores her conflicted feelings.

In the example above, the SHARM was Jesse's conflicted feelings and resulting behavior. The therapist pointed out the dog's behavior to the client and interpreted the perceived meaning. The therapist and client processed this and worked together toward a solution of having Jesse lay down between the client and therapist (HARP). As they continued to process, the therapist asks the client to explore a similar situation in the client's own life regarding conflict and necessary resolution. The client's sharing and exploration of her conflicted feelings about a dilemma in her own life was the HARTI.

Comfort

For a Comfort SHARM, a therapist reflects on the animal spontaneously engaging in comforting physical touch with the client, such as snuggling, laying in the lap, or trying to lick the face or hands. With this SHARM we can convey the animal's perception of a client's need for comforting, and/or we can convey the animal's desire to be comforted by a client with whom the animal feels safe. See Figure 7.7 for one example of a Comfort SHARM.

Example vignette (provided by myself as therapist working with my dog Jesse):

> Therapy dog Jesse moves to the client and tries to lick the client's face. She then curls her body around, leans in, and snuggles her back against the client's side. Jesse then glances back toward the client. The therapist comments on Jesse's caring behavior and suggests to the client that the animal senses the client is needing comforting or nurturing: "Jesse is caring for you; she senses you need to be comforted right now." The client then expresses her feelings of discomfort, vulnerability, and emotional pain. With the client's revelations the therapist is able to assist the client through conveyance of empathy and support.

In the example above, the SHARM was Jesse's nurturing behavior toward the client. The therapist pointed out the dog's behavior to the client and explained that Jesse sensed the client needed comforting (HARP). In response to the therapist's comments the client shared significant distressful feelings she was having. With the client's presentation of distressful feelings, the therapist was then able to utilize clinical knowledge and skills to assist the client (HARTI).

Assurance

With the Assurance SHARM, a client experiences assurance or self-assurance as a result of the animal's behavior around the client or from a client observing some behavior of the animal. This SHARM involves primary issues of (1) worth, (2) self-efficacy, or (3) safety. A therapy animal who chooses to engage with a client contributes to feelings of worth for that client. So, a horse that willingly follows a person around with no rope attached assures a client they are worthy or have value to the horse; the client feels "I'm worthy because the horse wants to follow me." The assurance for the client stems from the horse's trust and feeling safe with a client. Another example is a dog that complies with commands given by a client to perform a trick or command. This conveys the animal is willing to work with a client, and success with the task boosts a client's confidence and sense of self-efficacy, leaving a client feeling "I'm capable." Also, a client who feels vulnerable may avoid or resist participation in therapy, but then may choose to participate when in close contact with or accompanied by a therapy animal whose presence increases the client's sense of safety; the animal's presence or behavior encourages a client to feel "I'm safe." For two examples of an assurance SHARM see Figures 7.8 and 7.9.

Example vignette 1 (provided by myself as therapist working with my dog Jesse):

> During the session, therapy dog Jesse, who has been sleeping next to the therapist on one end of a long L-shaped couch, spontaneously gets up and walks to the other end of the couch where the client is sitting, jumps up on the back of the couch, and lays down

nestling her body against the back of the client's neck and head. The therapist reflects, "Jesse feels very comfortable with you. She senses you are a safe person she can trust right now." The client smiles, gently reaches back to pet Jesse and then shares with the counselor how she feels about herself in regard to a certain situation where she feels unsafe with a person in her life. While speaking, the client occasionally reaches back behind her head to stroke Jesse's soft fur.

In the example above, the SHARM occurred when Jesse moved over to the client and lay down on the back of the couch with her body nestled against the back of the client's neck and head. The HARP involved the therapist explaining that Jesse felt safe and comfortable with the client, along with the client reaching back to pet Jesse before and during her sharing how she feels about herself in regard to a painful experience. The resulting HARTI was how the client seemed encouraged to express herself as a result of Jesse's close contact. As she continued to reach back to touch Jesse, the client was both providing and receiving assurance of comfort and safety. This added emotional support for the client to explore a situation where she felt vulnerable.

Example vignette 2 (provided by myself as therapist working with my dog Dolly, a red and white Cocker Spaniel):

When I was co-counseling adolescents from the county juvenile detention center utilizing equine-assisted counseling, my dog Dolly would often accompany me to the therapy ranch. The juveniles already knew and trusted Dolly from her many visits with me to the detention center for either recreation or counseling with the adolescents. This trusting relationship with Dolly greatly benefited many adolescents when participating in equine-assisted counseling. For example, some of the adolescents would be afraid of the horses and hesitate to interact with them in the corral upon first contact. Yet when the adolescents saw Dolly's comfort level with the horses, the adolescents commented on this and became assured of their own safety and would then stand exactly next to Dolly and risk reaching out to pet the horses.

Checking In

For the Checking In SHARM, a therapist points out the animal is checking in to make sure the client is okay or the therapist is okay. Alternatively, the therapist or client can check in with the animal to see if the animal is okay in order to model care or facilitate sharing. A dog checking in is demonstrated by the animal moving toward a client and sniffing or licking the client's face or hand. Licking often provides additional olfactory information for some animals if that species has an additional olfactory pathway in the mouth (like dogs and cats); so, licking can increase the animal's ability to discern emotion through smell. Horses will also sniff and lick, either the air or a person or object, to gather information. Horses can increase their sense of smell by curling their upper lip to capture and hold odor molecules in the upper regions of their long nasal cavity; so this flehmen response by a horse may signal that a horse is checking in, that is, gathering information about a client's emotional state. See Figures 7.10 and 7.11 for examples of a Checking In SHARM.

Example vignette (provided by therapist Mickey White working with his dog Bolt, a blonde Labrador–Golden Retriever mix):

Therapy dog Bolt greets the client at the beginning of the session and eventually lays down on the floor and closes his eyes. Then at one point in the session when the client is feeling emotional Bolt gets up on his own initiative, walks over to the client, and nuzzles the client's hand with his nose. Bolt continues to nudge the client's hand until the client pets him. The therapist explains that Bolt is checking in to see if the client is okay with this expression of concern: "Bolt is checking in with you to see what is going on with you right now, to see if you are okay." The client then expresses to a deeper level how he is at that moment, what he is feeling and thinking, and how he is managing his state.

In the example above, the SHARM occurred when Bolt walked over to the client and nuzzled the client's hand until the client petted him. The HARP involved the therapist explaining that Bolt was checking in to see if the client was okay. The client then expressed to a deeper level how he was at that moment, what he was feeling and thinking, and how he was managing. The resulting HARTI was increased awareness for the therapist and client about the client's feelings and thoughts and how he was coping. A Checking In SHARM can be a potent conveyor of empathy, and offers powerful encouragement for client expression.

The Checking In behavior most commonly exhibited by my dog Jesse is to get close to a person's face and smell their breath. She may even try to lick the air near a person's face to get a better sense of the smell of the emotions of the person. Jesse commonly does this Check-In behavior at two times with a client. She performs this behavior when greeting a person to initially surmise how they are doing, making this also a part of her SHARM of Greeting, and she performs this Check In during a session when she perceives a client is

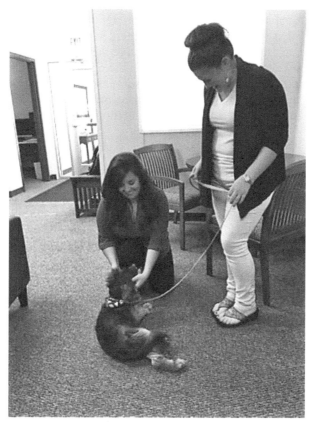

Figure 7.2 An example of a Greeting SHARM. A therapist facilitates a greeting between a client and a therapy animal. Greeting the animal sets a positive therapeutic mood for the session.

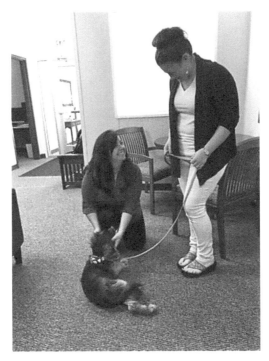

Figure 7.3 A Greeting SHARM also enhances the connection between the client and the therapist.

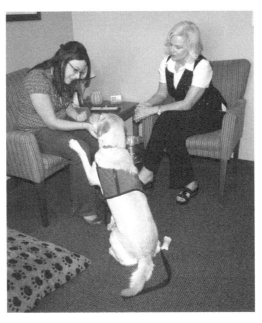

Figure 7.4 An example of an Acknowledgement SHARM. A therapist and client acknowledge the therapy dog is conveying something important during a counseling session when the dog stands, walks over, and places a paw on the client's knee. Therapy dog Dakota and Dr. Pam Flint (right) working with a client at the Student Counseling Center at the University of North Texas.

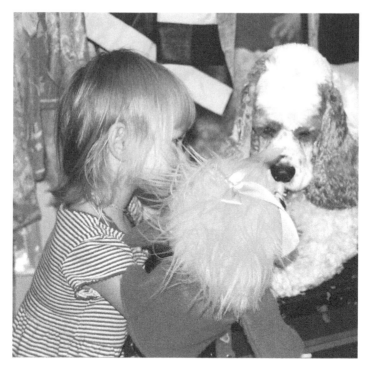

Figure 7.5 An example of a Speculation SHARM. During an animal-assisted play counseling session, the child client speculates about what the therapy dog Rusty might be thinking or doing. Speculation does not have to be accurate as it is a projection from the inner state of the client.

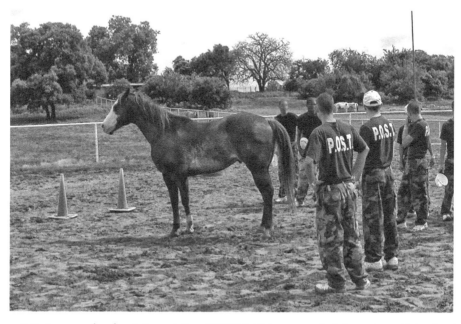

Figure 7.6 An example of an Interpretation SHARM. This group of adolescents participating in an equine-assisted counseling session attempt to accurately interpret a horse's body language and other behavior so as to better understand and communicate with the horse so the horse will move between two orange cones without being touched or offered a bribe.

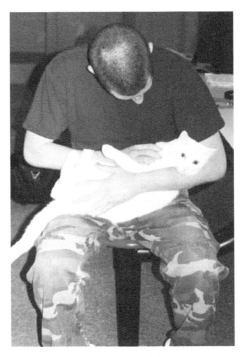

Figure 7.7 An example of a Comfort SHARM. This adolescent in a juvenile detention center finds comfort from holding and petting my therapy cat Snowflake.

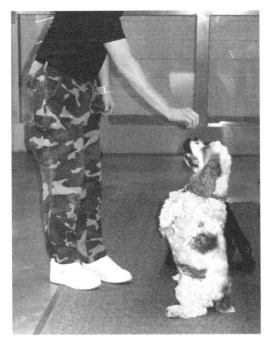

Figure 7.8 An example of an Assurance SHARM. This adolescent in a juvenile detention center potentially gains some assurance of self-efficacy by successfully performing a trick with my therapy dog Rusty.

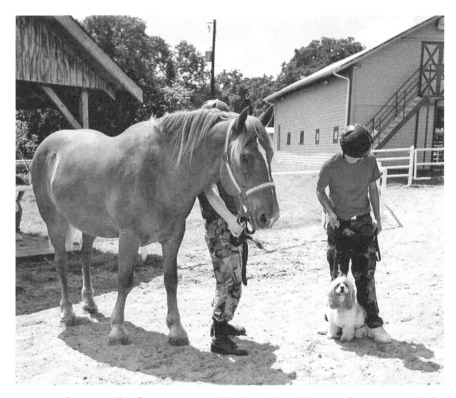

Figure 7.9 Another example of an Assurance SHARM. This adolescent from a juvenile detention center was at first hesitant to participate in equine-assisted counseling, but he found assurance of safety when accompanied by my therapy dog Dolly, whom he already knew very well, because Dolly demonstrated she was comfortable being around the horses.

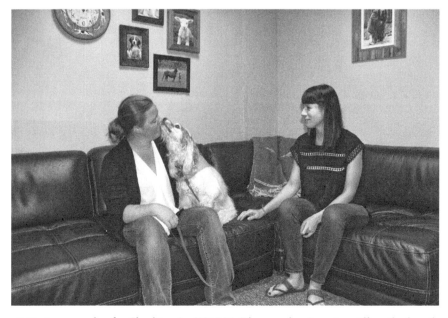

Figure 7.10 An example of a Checking In SHARM. Therapy dog Jesse is sniffing the breath of the client to detect emotions of the client.

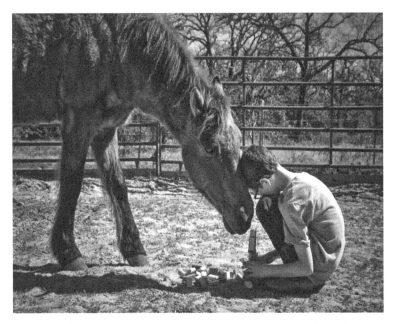

Figure 7.11 An example of a Checking In SHARM. A horse checking in with a client during an equine-assisted play therapy session.

(*Source:* photo courtesy of Hallie Sheade.)

experiencing some significant emotion, such as a need for support, making this behavior part of her SHARM of Checking In. Jesse also licks a hand in a show of providing comfort, making this also a part of her SHARM of Comfort. A therapy animal's behavior may be exhibited for different, but often related, circumstances such as in the example just provided where Jesse licks near a person's face or on the hands, both as an instance of checking in and as a show of comfort.

The Utility of HART

There may be times when more than one SHARM is presented during an episode of human–animal interaction. Any SHARM may initiate internal and/or external processing by a client and/or therapist regarding the meaning or value of that SHARM. I developed HART as a means for assisting counselors and psychotherapists to better understand and recognize the contribution a therapy animal makes to the social–relational dynamics of a therapy session. Attending to social–relational dynamics is a primary medium for helping clients to grow, develop, and heal in counseling and psychotherapy. Thus, the additional social–relational dynamics provided by a therapy animal can be of great assistance.

Though I designed HART for application in the fields of counseling and psychotherapy, the basic constructs and formula, SHARM + HARP = HARTI may be of use to therapists and clients working together in other fields, such as occupational therapy, speech therapy, and physical therapy. The amount and type of HARP would likely be different given that a different type of HARTI is hoped for; a HARTI specific to the needs of a client in treatment for either occupational skill development, speech development, or physical recovery, and so forth. The value of HART is more pronounced when working with therapy animals that have interest in social engagement with humans. The more social engagement that occurs, the greater the likelihood of SHARMs.

AAT TECHNIQUES AND INTENTIONS

To make the most of AAT applications in counseling it is highly beneficial for a counselor to understand when, how, and why to facilitate the animal interventions. Let us examine some techniques and intentions for AAT designed to facilitate therapeutic progress. A number of different types of animal-assisted therapeutic interventions are described in the literature. In its most basic form, a therapeutic intervention can be divided into two parts: the technique used by a therapist; and the intention for using the technique. The intention is the purpose or reason for using the technique, or otherwise stated as what a therapist hopes to accomplish by facilitating a particular type of AAT-C technique. O'Callaghan (**2008**) conducted a comprehensive review of literature related to AAT applications in mental health and identified 18 techniques and 10 intentions or purposes for using AAT techniques. The 18 AAT techniques are:

1. Therapist reflects or comments on client's relationship with therapy animal.
2. Therapist encourages client to interact with therapy animal by touching or petting therapy animal.
3. Therapist encourages client to play with therapy animal during session.
4. Therapist encourages client to tell therapy animal about client's distress or concerns.
5. Therapist and client engage with therapy animal outside of a traditional therapeutic environment, i.e., taking therapy animal for a walk.
6. Therapist interacts with therapy animal by having animal perform tricks or follow commands.
7. Therapist encourages client to perform tricks with therapy animal.
8. Therapist encourages client to perform commands with therapy animal.
9. Therapist comments or reflects on spontaneous client–animal interactions.
10. Information about therapy animal's family history (e.g., lineage, breed, species) is shared with client.
11. Any other history related to therapy animal is shared with client.
12. Animal stories and metaphors with animal themes are shared with client by therapist.
13. Therapist encourages the client to make up stories involving the therapy animal.
14. Therapist uses the client–therapy animal relationship, such as, "If this dog were your best friend, what would he know about you that no one else would know?" and/or "Tell Rusty (therapy dog) how you feel, and I will just listen."
15. Therapist encourages client to recreate/re-enact experience where therapy animal plays a specific role.
16. Therapy animal is present without any directive interventions.
17. Therapist creates specific structured activities for a client with a therapy animal.
18. Therapy animal engages with client in spontaneous moments that facilitate therapeutic discussion.

The 10 AAT intentions are:

A. Building rapport in the therapeutic relationship.
B. Facilitating insight.
C. Enhancing client's social skills.
D. Enhancing client's relationship skills.
E. Enhancing client's self-confidence.
F. Modeling a specific behavior.
G. Encouraging sharing of feelings.
H. Behavioral reward for client.
I. Enhancing trust within the therapeutic environment.
J. Facilitating feelings of being safe in the therapeutic environment.

Using the 18 techniques and 10 intentions identified from the literature review by O'Callaghan (2008), a survey was developed and then distributed to mental health therapists who practiced AAT to determine how many of the therapists used these techniques and with what intentions (O'Callaghan and Chandler, 2011). To summarize the survey results, of those mental health therapists ($N = 31$) who reported using a technique either "often" or "always," most respondents reported using AAT techniques 1 (90.3 percent), 2 (77.4 percent), 9 (87.1 percent), 16 (74.2 percent), and 18 (83.8 percent); a majority reported using techniques 10 (61.3 percent), 11 (58.1 percent), and 12 (54.9 percent); some reported using techniques 3 (48.4 percent), 5 (42 percent), 6 (41.9 percent), 7 (32.3 percent), 8 (48.4 percent), 14 (35.5 percent), and 17 (45.2 percent); and only a few reported using techniques 4 (22.6 percent), 13 (12.9 percent), and 15 (16.1 percent) (O'Callaghan and Chandler, 2011). The survey also asked survey participants to endorse for what intention they had used the techniques. The number of therapists surveyed who reported using a particular technique for a particular intention is summarized in Table 7.1 using the following format: high number of therapists (70 percent and over), medium number of therapists (40 percent to less than 70 percent), low number of therapists (10 percent to less than 40 percent), or very low number of therapists or none (less than 10 percent). It is clear from the results reported in Table 7.1 that AAT techniques were applied for a variety of intentions, but some intentions

Table 7.1 Number of Surveyed Mental Health Therapists Who Reported Using a Specific AAT Technique for a Specific Intention

Techniques[a]	Intentions[b]										
	A	*B*	*C*	*D*	*E*	*F*	*G*	*H*	*I*	*J*	*K*[c]
1	H	M	M	H	H	M	M	L	M	M	V
2	H	L	M	M	M	M	L	L	M	M	V
3	M	L	M	M	M	L	L	L	L	M	V
4	L	L	V	L	L	V	M	V	M	M	V
5	L	L	L	L	L	L	L	L	L	L	V
6	M	L	V	L	V	L	V	L	L	L	V
7	L	L	L	L	M	L	V	L	L	L	V
8	L	L	M	L	H	M	L	L	L	L	L
9	M	M	M	M	M	L	L	V	L	L	V
10	H	L	L	L	L	L	L	V	M	L	L
11	H	M	L	L	L	V	L	V	M	L	L
12	M	M	L	L	L	L	L	V	L	L	V
13	L	L	L	L	L	V	L	V	L	L	V
14	L	M	L	L	L	V	M	V	L	V	V
15	V	L	L	L	V	V	L	V	L	V	V
16	M	L	L	L	L	V	L	V	M	M	V
17	L	M	M	M	M	M	L	V	L	L	V

Source: Adapted from O'Callaghan and Chandler, 2011.

Note: H = high; M = medium; L = low; and V = very low or none. Technique 18 is not listed here since it inquired about spontaneous moments. $N = 31$.

[a] See techniques listed in the text of this chapter.
[b] See intentions listed in the text of this chapter.
[c] Other intention as identified by the surveyed respondents.

were clearly more common than others; for instance, one of the most commonly used intentions for techniques 1, 2, 10, and 11 was that of building rapport in the therapeutic relationship (O'Callaghan and Chandler, 2011).

The study by O'Callaghan and Chandler (2011) is useful in a number of ways. The information provided describes a variety of AAT techniques and provides an indication of how frequently these techniques were used. Further, techniques are matched with intended reasons for using them. This type of information is helpful in furthering an understanding of AAT-C and provides a valuable tool for training practitioners of AAT-C. Additionally, the information may serve as a guide in treatment planning. For instance, a counselor who works with a therapy animal and has a client who is deficient in self-confidence can examine the information provided in Table 7.1 to get ideas on which techniques have been used for this intention and by what number of therapists from the surveyed sample of mental health therapists. For example, by looking down column E, the intention for enhancing client's self-confidence, one can see that a majority of the therapists surveyed by O'Callaghan and Chandler (2011) used the following techniques to assist with this intention: 1 (used by a high number for this intention, in this case by 74.2 percent of surveyed therapists); 8 (used by a high number, in this case by 71 percent); 7 (used by a medium number for this intention, in this case by 51.6 percent of surveyed therapists); and 9 (used by a medium number, in this case by 51.6 percent). Also, three more techniques were used for this intention (intention E) by a medium number of the surveyed therapists: 2 (used by 48.4 percent); 3 (used by 45.2 percent); and 17 (used by 48.4 percent). For exact percentage of use for all technique–intention pairs, see the results reported in O'Callaghan and Chandler (2011).

Using information provided from the literature review by O'Callaghan (2008), researchers proposed ways in which AAT could be applied within the parameters of a variety of counseling guiding theories, including; person-centered, cognitive-behavioral, behavioral, Adlerian, existential, choice, psychoanalytic, gestalt, and solution-focused (Chandler et al., 2010; see Tables 7.2 and 7.3). This presentation of AAT applications within counseling theories is not meant to imply that an AAT technique or intention is limited to practice within a particular theoretical orientation; rather, it is meant to demonstrate the versatility of AAT applications. In fact, many of the techniques and intentions discussed have useful application with several theories.

In the following sections, information is provided on how AAT techniques and intentions facilitate the therapeutic relationship, along with discussion on how AAT techniques and intentions are compatible with practice from various counseling theoretical orientations. Numbers and letters in parentheses that have been placed adjacent to techniques and intentions in the text refer to the lists from O'Callaghan (2008) and Chandler et al. (2010) presented earlier in this chapter. Also, the next sections give brief summaries of real cases used to exemplify AAT applications consistent with various counseling theories. In many of these cases, I was the counselor working with one of my therapy dogs. I often use techniques from a variety of theoretical approaches to meet the unique needs of clients and to accommodate the particular circumstances presented. It is important to note that the animal's safety and welfare along with the client's safety and welfare were always considered a priority by the counselor during each AAT session.

AAT AND THE THERAPEUTIC RELATIONSHIP

Consistent with many theoretical orientations is initial emphasis on building a therapeutic relationship with a client. This therapeutic alliance between counselor and client is thought by many to be necessary to promote client therapeutic progress. A number of AAT intentions may facilitate the counseling relationship—for example, building rapport (A), enhancing

Table 7.2 Matching AAT Techniques with Counseling Guiding Theories

Counseling Theories	AAT Techniques[a]																	
	1	2	3	4	5	6	7	8	9	10	11	12	13	14	15	16	17	18
Person-centered	×								×							×		×
Cognitive-behavioral	×		×			×	×	×	×					×	×		×	
Behavioral	×	×	×		×	×	×	×	×								×	
Adlerian	×	×	×	×	×	×	×	×	×	×	×			×	×	×	×	×
Psychoanalytic	×	×							×			×	×					×
Gestalt				×									×				×	×
Existential	×											×						
Choice	×	×	×				×	×	×					×	×	×	×	×
Solution-focused	×						×	×	×						×		×	×

Source: Adapted and modified from Chandler et al., 2010.

Note: [a] See techniques listed in the text of this chapter.

Table 7.3 Matching AAT Intentions with Counseling Guiding Theories

Counseling Theories	AAT Intentions[a]									
	A	B	C	D	E	F	G	H	I	J
Person-centered	×	×			×		×		×	×
Cognitive-behavioral	×	×	×	×	×	×	×		×	
Behavioral			×	×		×		×		
Adlerian	×	×	×	×			×		×	×
Psychoanalytic		×					×			
Gestalt		×					×			
Existential		×	×	×	×		×			
Choice	×	×	×	×	×		×		×	×
Solution-focused	×		×	×	×	×			×	×

Source: Adapted and modified from Chandler, et al., 2010.

Note: [a] See intentions listed in the text of this chapter.

trust (I), and facilitating feelings of safety (J) (Chandler et al., 2010). This can be accomplished by using any number of AAT techniques, such as reflecting on the client's relationship with the therapy animal (1), encouraging the client to interact with the therapy animal (2), and sharing information about the therapy animal with the client (10, 11) (Chandler et al., 2010).

Regardless of a counselor's primary theoretical orientation, a therapist-facilitated SHARM of Greeting can assist in establishing rapport in the first session as well as creating a warm atmosphere at the beginning of all sessions. Putting the client at ease with this SHARM may help a client to share important concerns earlier in a session and to a greater depth. A spontaneous SHARM of Checking In initiated by the therapy animal conveys warmth, caring, and empathy. This can add to the therapeutic support experienced by a client in a session.

The effects of SHARMs of Greeting and SHARMs of Checking In contribute to the establishment and strengthening of the therapeutic alliance. AAT can be very useful in establishing a vital relationship link between the counselor and the client.

AAT AND PERSON-CENTERED COUNSELING

The nondirective approach of person-centered counseling is ideal for the use of spontaneous human–animal interactions. A person-centered counselor can make use of additional relational dynamics provided from human–animal interactions by reflecting on the therapist's observation of the potential meaning and result of these interactions. Following is a brief synopsis of person-centered counseling and a presentation of how certain AAT techniques and intentions are compatible with a person-centered approach. Some basics of person-centered counseling are as follows (Tudor and Worrall, 2006):

- Primary goal: To move clients toward self-acceptance.
- Nondirective approach.
- Primary use of reflection and clarification of client's verbal and nonverbal communications.

INTERVENTIONS AND THEORIES • 177

- Primary aim: To enhance client insight.
- Therapist's presentation: unconditional positive regard (congruent, authentic, genuine, caring, accepting, warm, and empathic).
- Therapist's attitude and presentation style assist client to feel safe and nondefensive and to trust oneself more, thereby freeing client from past and facilitating greater self-acceptance as client moves through therapy.

Some AAT techniques that are consistent with a person-centered approach to counseling include (Chandler et al., 2010): reflecting on the client's relationship with the therapy animal (1), reflecting on spontaneous client–therapy animal interactions (9), having a therapy animal be present without any directive interventions (16), and therapeutic discussion of spontaneous interactions between the client and therapy animal (18). Some AAT intentions that are consistent with a person-centered approach to counseling include (Chandler et al., 2010): building rapport in the therapeutic relationship (A) and enhancing trust within the therapeutic environment (I), which enhances clients' sense of safety (J) and thereby encourages them to share their feelings (G), which may facilitate client insight (B) and, in turn, foster client self-acceptance or self-confidence (E).

Following is a summary of a case scenario of an animal-assisted person-centered counseling intervention involving me as the counselor and my dog Rusty as the therapy animal (also described in Chandler et al., 2010).

Person-centered AAT Intervention

Therapeutic Event: A female adolescent being newly processed into a juvenile detention center is being interviewed by a probation officer and is acting uncooperative and uncommunicative. By happenstance, the therapist is walking by accompanied by her dog Rusty. The probation officer and therapist notice the harsh expression of the adolescent soften significantly when she sees the therapy dog, a Cocker Spaniel, near the interview room. The probation officer invites the counselor with her therapy dog into the room. After the counselor asks the adolescent if she would like to pet the therapy dog, the adolescent gets down on the floor, and the dog spontaneously crawls into her lap and leans its head against her chest. The adolescent then begins to cry as she holds the dog. Sensing the tears, therapy dog Rusty nuzzles his head up high onto her shoulder and presses against the neck of the adolescent. With this act of care the teen girl begins to sob heavily. The counselor makes soft, intermittent reflections on the client–therapy dog interaction and on the client's presentation; i.e., "Rusty cares about you." "Rusty knows you are having a bad day." "Rusty knows you are going to be okay." The client responds with a head nod. After a few moments the teen has a calm demeanor and expresses gratitude for the time allowed with the therapy dog. After this several-minute intervention by the counselor and therapy dog, the counselor and dog depart. The therapist was informed days later that the interaction had a lasting effect on the adolescent who was calm, polite, and cooperative with the probation officer after the therapy team's departure.

Therapeutic Opportunity: An animal-assisted therapeutic opportunity was initiated when the probation officer and the counselor noticed a spontaneous positive shift in the adolescent's expression when she saw the dog near the interview room.

SHARM: The adolescent gets down on the floor, and the dog spontaneously crawls into her lap and leans its head against her chest and shoulder. The adolescent then begins to cry heavily as she holds the dog. This is an example of a SHARM of Comfort.

HARP: The counselor makes intermittent reflections on the client–therapy dog interaction and on the client's presentation. The client responds with a calmed demeanor and expresses gratitude for the time allowed with the therapy dog.

AAT Technique: The counselor gently and warmly reflected on the client's feelings for several minutes while the client held and petted the therapy dog during a client–therapy animal interaction.

AAT Intention: To increase the client's sense of safety, comfort, and trust in the environment.

HARTI: The probation officer later reported her appreciation for how this spontaneous intervention with a counselor and her therapy dog lowered the adolescent's defenses so that she became much more communicative and cooperative in the remainder of the intake interview with the probation officer.

AAT AND COGNITIVE-BEHAVIORAL COUNSELING

A counselor can use human–animal interactions to achieve many goals of cognitive-behavioral counseling. Following is a brief synopsis of cognitive-behavioral counseling and a discussion about how certain AAT techniques and intentions are compatible with a cognitive-behavioral approach. Some basics of cognitive-behavioral counseling are as follows (McMullin, 1986):

- Primary goal: To identify and challenge irrational beliefs of clients which contribute to maladaptive feelings and behaviors.
- Directive approach.
- Methods: Identify and challenge irrational thoughts, shame-attacking exercises, change communication style, model and role play new behaviors, and cognitive homework to generalize lessons outside of therapy.
- Therapist is viewed as a teacher and practice partner for clients to challenge self-defeating beliefs, thoughts, and behaviors, and to learn and integrate new ways of believing, feeling, and behaving.
- Some cognitive-behavioral therapists, such as Aaron Beck, recognize the importance of rapport and trust in the client–therapist relationship, where others like Albert Ellis do not believe this is necessary.

Many animal-assisted techniques and intentions are well suited for a cognitive-behavioral counseling approach (Chandler et al., 2010). The counselor can use the client–therapy animal relationship to assist a client in expressing feelings or identifying beliefs (14). Clients could be guided to practice certain social skills with a therapy animal (15). The counselor can model appropriate social behaviors with a therapy animal (6). The counselor can ask a client to practice new and more functional behaviors with a therapy animal when engaging the animal to perform tricks or commands (7, 8). Similarly, the therapy animal can be involved in structured activities (17) to assist a client in learning and practicing new skills. Practicing new, positive behaviors with an animal first may be much more fun and much less threatening than trying them out on other humans. The use of appropriate humor by a counselor is an aspect of cognitive-behavioral counseling and can be assisted through encouragement of playing with an animal during a session (3). A counselor's feedback on all client–therapy animal interactions (1, 9) can assist a client in identifying functional and dysfunctional behaviors and reinforce client adaptation of more prosocial behaviors. Each of the following AAT intentions is consistent with the goals of cognitive-behavioral counseling: building rapport (A) and enhancing trust (I) in the therapeutic relationship; encouraging sharing of feelings (G); gaining insight (B) about the consequences of feelings, thoughts, and actions; developing social and relationship skills (C, D); modeling specific behaviors (F); and enhancing client's self-confidence (E) with successful interactions.

Following is a summary of a case scenario of an animal-assisted cognitive-behavioral counseling intervention involving me as the counselor and my dog Rusty as the therapy animal (also described in Chandler et al., 2010).

Cognitive-behavioral AAT Intervention

Therapeutic Event: An adolescent male in a juvenile detention facility chose to tease a therapy dog instead of playing with it. In this scenario, the dog brought a toy ball to the adolescent and dropped it in his hand and started to turn in expectation of chasing a thrown ball. Instead of throwing the ball, the adolescent reached out and grabbed the dog by its collar and waved the ball in front of its nose. The dog signaled the boy to change his behavior by tugging against the boy's hold on the dog's neck collar. The counselor reflected on the dog's desire for the adolescent to change his behavior, and then instructed the adolescent to let go of the dog and throw the ball. When retrieving the ball, the dog acted suspicious toward the adolescent and dropped the ball over a full arm's length from the boy and stayed this distance away, not allowing the boy to pet or touch him anymore. The adolescent complained of the dog's behavior to the counselor, who in turn spent time assisting the adolescent in understanding how he had damaged the trust in his relationship with the dog as a result of his over-controlling and teasing behaviors. Regretting that the dog did not want to come near him anymore, the client committed to changing his attitude and behavior toward the dog. After a few more sessions during which the counselor facilitated positive interactions between the client and therapy dog, whereby the adolescent consistently acted with respect and caring toward the dog, the therapy dog began to spontaneously initiate, on its own, approaching the adolescent and letting him pet and hold it, and the dog would once again drop the ball in the client's hand during a game of fetch. The counselor's processing of the experience with the adolescent assisted him with self-discovery—to become aware of and challenge his irrational thoughts and self-defeating beliefs that he needed to be a bully to feel in control and be successful. The counselor assisted the adolescent in generalizing what he had learned from his interactions with the dog to his interactions with other people. The adolescent was able to rapidly learn from this experience and successfully modified his former bullying and teasing behaviors toward other people and became much more respectful and caring in his interactions with both people and the therapy dog.

Therapeutic Opportunity: An adolescent experienced the negative impact of his bullying and teasing behaviors on his relationship with a therapy dog and was motivated to modify his behaviors to be more prosocial in order to repair the relationship with the therapy dog.

SHARM: When the dog would no longer come near the boy and the boy expressed his frustration at this, the therapist explained to the client that the dog demonstrated he no longer trusted him because he had teased the dog. This is an example of a SHARM of Interpretation.

HARP: The therapist processed with the adolescent how he had damaged his relationship with the dog and explained what he would have to change in order to repair the relationship. Additionally, the therapist helped the adolescent generalize his lesson with the dog to other relationships in his life.

AAT Technique: Therapist-facilitated interactions of a client playing with a therapy dog.

AAT Intention: To facilitate client insight to enable challenge of a client's irrational thoughts and self-defeating beliefs.

HARTI: The therapist with her therapy dog assisted the adolescent client to become aware of and challenge his irrational thoughts and self-defeating beliefs, resulting in the client successfully modifying his behaviors.

AAT AND BEHAVIORAL COUNSELING

Behavioral counseling and AAT are very compatible, especially since AAT provides multiple opportunities for modeling new behaviors for clients. Some basics of behavioral counseling are as follows (Wilson, Gottfredson, and Najaka, 2001):

- Goal-focused therapy to improve client's quality of life by altering behavior that restricts client's social, work, and other activities.
- Directive approach with continual assessment of progress toward goals.
- Therapist role is to teach new skills by: providing instructions, modeling new behaviors, designing opportunities for behavioral rehearsal, and providing feedback on client performance.
- Homework assignments help to generalize lessons outside of therapy.

Many animal-assisted techniques and intentions are well suited for behavioral counseling (Chandler et al., 2010). Opportunities to interact with a therapy animal via petting (2), playing (3), or performing tricks or commands (7, 8) can serve as motivating forces for clients to participate in the counseling process; client willingness and motivation to change are essential in behavioral counseling. Petting, playing, or performing with the animal are fun and rewarding, and use of interactions with a therapy animal can serve as a behavioral reward for a client (H) to increase target behavior. A counselor can create specific, structured activities with the therapy animal (17) that allow the client to experience or practice new behaviors. The counselor's feedback on client performance of newly learned behavior is essential for client growth and development and can be facilitated by commenting on client–therapy animal interactions (1, 9). Further, a counselor may model social behaviors (F) by demonstrating appropriate touch of the animal, using positive verbal and nonverbal communication with the animal, and having a therapy animal perform tricks or commands (6). Additional generalization of what a client learns can be assisted by the counselor and client engaging with a therapy animal outside of the traditional therapeutic environment (5), such as taking the animal for a walk. AAT intentions regarding enhancing clients' social (C) and relationship (D) skills are also consistent with the goals of behavioral counseling.

Following is a summary of a case scenario of an animal-assisted behavioral counseling intervention involving me as the counselor and my dog Rusty as the therapy animal (also described in Chandler et al., 2010).

Behavioral AAT Intervention

Therapeutic Event: One day in a juvenile detention center where I volunteered my counseling services, several male clients in a small group session were complaining about losing a number of merit points in the days prior to the session because they had failed to comply with rules that required some self-discipline and impulse control (e.g., no teasing or bullying peers, and no talking out of turn). The clients claimed the rules were unfair because they could not help themselves. Thus, I demonstrated to the group the capacity of a therapy dog for self-discipline and impulse control—two behavior areas that the adolescents struggled with in many areas of their life. One demonstration was where the therapy dog was consistently able to wait until instructed to retrieve a food treat or dog toy placed just a few inches from him. The animal's desire for the treat or toy was very apparent to the adolescents, which further demonstrated to them the dog's ability to resist temptations upon request. Clients were further impressed by the therapy dog's ability to wait with a food treat lying on the bridge of his nose until the dog heard the command to flip the treat up in the air and catch it in his mouth. I processed with the group how if a dog could demonstrate such control, then so could the clients because they had far more intellectual capacity than a dog. For weeks following these demonstrations, group members spontaneously reflected in and between counseling sessions on how the therapy dog's abilities revealed for them their own potential for self-discipline and impulse control and discussed situations where they were able to maintain these by remembering the therapy dog's performance.

Therapeutic Opportunity: Clients' focus and attention are gained, and client insights are facilitated by way of an entertaining interaction between a therapist and her therapy dog.

SHARM: Adolescents' observations of a dog demonstrating self-discipline and impulse control during the performance of a demanding trick gave them greater self-assurance that they too could demonstrate self-discipline and impulse control under demanding circumstances. This is an example of a SHARM of Assurance (of the self-efficacy type).

HARP: The therapist processed with the adolescents their observations and impressions of the dog in a manner that assisted the adolescents to gain greater assurance of their potential for self-discipline and impulse control.

AAT Technique: Therapist-facilitated commands and tricks with a therapy dog.

AAT Intention: Therapist facilitation of a therapy animal modeling specific self-discipline and impulse-control behaviors.

HARTI: Clients became aware of their own capacity for self-discipline and impulse control by observing these behaviors in a therapy dog.

AAT AND ADLERIAN COUNSELING

The Adlerian approach to counseling emphasizes understanding a client's style of striving for significance in relation to others. A client's perceived frustrations or failures within a social system can result in discouragement that may move a client away from social connectedness. It is the role of the Adlerian counselor to assist clients in understanding and adapting their private logic that contributes to or interferes with social successes. Social interactions with a therapy animal are ideal for revealing a client's private logic. Some basics of Adlerian counseling are as follows (Carlson, Watts, and Maniacci, 2005; Dreikurs, 1950; Kottman, 2003):

- Primary focus: Humans are motivated by social relatedness—an innate striving for social significance (superiority) that is motivated by clients' inferiority feelings within family and community. This striving can be functional (healthy) or dysfunctional (unhealthy).

- Therapist role is to establish an egalitarian relationship that assists clients to examine private logic behind lifestyle choices and to adapt or change logic to achieve greater satisfaction in major life tasks: work/school, love, and friendship.
- The basis for the client's private logic that drives unhealthy striving can be determined by examining a client's perception of events from early childhood (where origin of motivation lies) and throughout life.

A number of animal-assisted techniques and intentions are well suited for Adlerian counseling (Chandler et al., 2010). To establish an egalitarian therapeutic alliance, a counselor can use AAT to facilitate rapport (A), trust (I), and feelings of safety (J) for a client. Adlerian counselors may use opportunities for social interaction among client, counselor, and therapy animal to facilitate insight (B), to enhance the client's social and relationship skills (C, D), and to encourage sharing of feelings (G). The Adlerian emphasis on social connectedness is consistent with nearly all AAT techniques. For example, all techniques involving interaction with a therapy animal are social in nature (1–9, 14–18). The Adlerian technique of gathering information on a client's family history can be facilitated by the counselor first sharing information about the therapy animal's family history (lineage, breed, or species) (10) as well as other personal history related to the therapy animal (11).

Following is a summary of a case scenario of an animal-assisted Adlerian counseling intervention involving me as the counselor and my dog Rusty as the therapy animal (also described in Chandler et al., 2010).

Adlerian AAT Intervention

Therapeutic Event: An adolescent in a juvenile detention center, who had a voice tone and accent very different from those of the counselor, became very frustrated that the counselor's therapy dog would not perform a complex trick for him that the dog had just performed for the counselor. The dog was friendly and socially engaging with the client and was performing various behaviors when the client spoke, just not the specific trick the client was asking the dog to perform. After only a few attempts, the client quickly became discouraged, gave up trying and disappointedly claimed that he just was not capable of getting the dog to do the trick and felt the dog did not want to do the trick for him anyway. The counselor pointed out how hard the dog was trying to please the client and asked the client to consider any other possible reasons the dog did not perform the trick other than the client was not capable or the dog did not want to do the trick for him. The client could not come up with any other explanations. So the therapist explained to the client that dogs do not understand the meaning of words but rather associate specific sounds with rewarded behaviors. So, instead of the client being incapable of performing the trick with the dog he might just need to try a little longer so the dog could become familiar with his voice and associate the sound of his particular command with that trick. The client re-engaged with the dog and tried commanding the dog to perform the trick. After repeated attempts that involved patient guidance by the client, the dog did become more familiar with the client's voice tone and accent. Not very long after, the client had multiple successes performing many tricks with the dog, reinforcing the idea that the client was indeed capable. The counselor processed with the adolescent why he was so quick to initially decide that he was not capable or that the dog did not want to perform for him. This counselor-facilitated processing assisted the client to gain new insight that challenged the self-defeating private logic of the adolescent; for instance, by first asking him to consider what else it could be that was interfering with the client's success with the dog, and then providing an interpretation of the dog's behavior for the client. To help generalize the client's insights, the counselor discussed with the client other areas of the client's life where similar dysfunctional logic might be interfering with healthy striving for significance.

Therapeutic Opportunity: The client's private logic for unhealthy striving was revealed when the client prematurely gave up on trying to direct a therapy dog to perform a trick because he mistakenly presumed that he, the client, was not capable.

SHARM: In this case there were two most significant human–animal relational moments: (1) the therapist attending to the adolescent initially giving up, and then (2) the therapist attending to the adolescent leading the dog through the trick successfully. With the first event the therapist initially tried to facilitate a SHARM of Speculation to assist the client in considering alternative explanations for the dog's behavior. The therapist wanted the client to be an active part of the discovery process. However, the client could not come up with any alternative explanations. Thus, the counselor then utilized a SHARM of Interpretation to assist the client with an accurate understanding of the dog's behavior that challenged the adolescent's presumptuous and defeating private logic. After the second event, the client's persistent attempts and ultimate success with the dog, the therapist facilitated a SHARM of Assurance to assist the client to be encouraged by his efforts and generalize this lesson to other areas of his life.

HARP: Processing of the first SHARM encouraged the adolescent to consider alternative possibilities about his capability in order to challenge his mistaken and discouraging belief about himself. Processing of the second and third SHARMs encouraged the adolescent to consider a healthier perception of self.

AAT Technique: A therapist facilitated a client performing tricks with a therapy animal to create opportunities for success or failure that might reveal a client's healthy or unhealthy striving for significance that the therapist could process with the client.

AAT Intention: To facilitate the client's insight by challenging his private logic that led to discouragement and retreat from social interaction. Also, to encourage the client's healthy striving for significance with experiential opportunities for success in a social interaction.

HARTI: The counselor was able to help the client understand how the client's dysfunctional private logic led the client to perceive the initial outcome with the dog as a personal failure and a misperception of self-worth. With new insight, the adolescent was encouraged to re-engage with the dog long enough to experience significant success and gain self-confidence from the interactions.

AAT AND PSYCHOANALYTIC COUNSELING

According to psychoanalytic theory, people are mostly unaware of why they feel or act the way they do. Through animal-assisted psychoanalytic counseling, clients can gain conscious awareness of the unconscious patterns of their thinking, and this enables them to work through their trauma and relieve internal pressure. Some basics of psychoanalytic counseling are as follows (Hall, 1954; Singer, 1973):

- Unconscious biological and instinctual drives result in irrational motivations. People are mostly unaware of why they feel or act the way they do.

- Dysfunction occurs because something has threatened to throw off the balance of power in the client's psyche.
- Freudian theory: Anxiety comes in two forms, either neurotic anxiety (pressure from id) or moral anxiety (pressure from superego).
- Jungian theory: Anxiety occurs when a client's life experience is difficult to accommodate into an existing structure of the psyche (archetype).
- Therapist role is to assist a client to become consciously aware of unconscious patterns that impair functioning.
- Transference and countertransference are major tools.

AAT is very compatible with psychoanalytic theory, given that psychoanalytic counselors' primary roles are to use the dynamics of the therapeutic relationship to facilitate client insight (B) and encourage client sharing of feelings (G) (Chandler et al., 2010). Counselors may do this by reflecting on the client's relationship with the therapy animal (1), reflecting on spontaneous client–animal interactions (9), and reflecting on how the animal engages with the client in spontaneous moments (18) (Chandler et al., 2010). The counselor can ask a client to make up stories about the therapy animal (13), allowing opportunity for the client to reveal unconscious thoughts and feelings by projecting them into the story. Animal stories and metaphors with animal themes may be shared with a client by a counselor (12) to access unconscious processes that are well defended by the client.

Following is a summary of a case scenario of a psychoanalytic counseling intervention described to me by a counselor who works with therapy horses (D. Goodwin-Bond, personal communication, April 2004; also described in Chandler et al., 2010).

Psychoanalytic AAT Intervention

Therapeutic Event: An adolescent male client was paired with a similar-aged male to work with a sorrel and white paint horse in a therapy session. His partner interacted comfortably with the horse, but each time the client approached the horse to engage with it, the horse behaved as though it was distressed—pulling back its ears, stomping the ground, and shying away from the client. This was very frustrating for the client, especially in contrast to his partner, with whom the horse seemed to be very comfortable. A counselor inquired with the client about his perception of what he thought was going on with the horse, whereby the client replied that he thought the horse did not like him. The counselor asked the client why he thought the horse did not like him, and the adolescent said he did not know. The counselor encouraged the client to think about this and let the counselor know if he figured anything out. For the remainder of the session the client's partner performed most of the interactions with the horse while the client watched from nearby. The following week the client rushed up to the counselor and excitedly exclaimed that he had figured out why the horse did not like him. When the counselor encouraged the adolescent to share his insight the client said, "Because I do not like myself." The counselor processed this in depth with the client individually and in a small group session where the client received support and encouragement. The client expressed his appreciation to the counselor and his peers and said he was going to work on liking himself better. Interestingly, immediately after the group process that day, the client and his partner began interacting with the same therapy horse from the previous week and the horse was now very receptive to both adolescents. The client shared he was convinced the horse liked him better now because he liked himself better.

Therapeutic Opportunity: A challenging dynamic occurred in an interaction between a client and a therapy horse.

SHARM: A client became frustrated with a horse that acted uncomfortably with the client's presentation. The therapist asked the client to consider reasons why the horse might be acting that way toward him. The client exclaimed that he felt it was because the horse did not like him. The therapist asked the client to consider reasons why he thought the horse did not like him. Both inquiries by the therapist are utilizations of a SHARM of Speculation.

HARP: Two HARPs occurred that allowed the client to gain self-insight and greater self-acceptance. The first was brief and involved the counselor asking the client to consider why he thought the horse did not like him. The client took a week to consider the question, and followed up the next session with the insight that the horse did not like him because he did not like himself. This set the stage for further therapist-facilitated processing involving the client and the client's peers in the counseling group.

AAT Technique: Counselor-facilitated client interactions with a therapy horse.

AAT Intention: To provide opportunities for the occurrence of therapeutic relationship dynamics, such as transference.

HARTI: The client transferred his inner anxiety onto his interactions with the therapy horse. The horse perceived the client's anxiety and responded by signaling discomfort. Counselor-facilitated processing with the client promoted client insight that assisted the client to work through some of his personal anxiety and achieve greater self-acceptance.

AAT AND GESTALT COUNSELING

Gestalt theory promotes the idea that clients may reach an impasse or stuck point that interferes with life satisfaction or functioning. In the gestalt counseling process, it is necessary for clients to fully explore an impasse, to accept life circumstances, and to become fully present and aware in the here and now. Gestalt counseling assists clients to develop awareness regarding patterns that are incongruent with feelings and experiences; in essence, clients become free to see things more completely by gaining more complete images of the here and now. Since gestalt counseling often involves a number of exercises and experiments that create opportunities for clients to move toward self-determined goals, AAT is a useful tool for facilitating awareness and self-discovery in clients. Some basics of gestalt counseling are as follows (Perls, Hefferline, and Goodman, 1980):

- Primary goal: To assist clients to clear away all that may be distracting them from being fully present and aware in the here and now.
- Unexpressed feelings result in unfinished business that may cause a client to get stuck (an impasse), and this may interfere with functioning or life satisfaction.
- Therapist role is to encourage client to attend to their sensory awareness, body sensations and body language, and verbal language patterns in the present moment as a signal for the existence of what needs attention.
- Gestalt exercises can facilitate awareness and focus.

The gestalt counseling approach can benefit from a number of AAT interventions to facilitate sensory awareness and self-discovery in clients (Chandler et al., 2010). Clients having difficulty attaching words to internal states may be assisted to process their bodily sensations and feelings when petting and interacting with a therapy animal (2, 18, G). Counselor-facilitated activities for a client with a therapy animal (17) may assist a client to become more aware of verbal and body language patterns that may assist client insight (B) regarding life areas where the client has become stuck. Further, clients who have difficulty expressing personal challenges and unfinished business may find it easier to first share their distress or concerns with the therapy animal in the presence of the counselor (4). Finally, counselors may assist clients to access internal conflicts by requesting that they make up stories involving the therapy animal (13) (Chandler et al., 2010).

Following is a summary of a case scenario of a gestalt counseling intervention facilitated by counselors working with a therapy horse (also described in Trotter et al., 2008).

Gestalt AAT Intervention

Therapeutic Event: A group of fourth-grade girls with a history of emotional and behavior problems were participating in equine-assisted counseling. For one small group counseling session they were asked to get a horse to walk over a low jump placed in an arena. The only rules given for the activity were as follows. While engaging with the horse there can be no physical touching of the horse, no halters or lead ropes used, no bribing the horse with food, and no verbal communication with each other. The group members were allowed to verbally communicate with one another to form a plan before the task began and during time-outs called by the therapists. Time-outs were called infrequently so as not to interrupt the participants' efforts and were used to allow the participants to briefly rest and process what was and was not working. There is no one right solution to this activity. It can be solved in any number of ways, but it is up to the participants to work together to come up with a solution. Arriving at a solution requires participants to acknowledge the needs of the therapy animal in gaining the animal's cooperation, as well as acknowledging the need for group members' cooperation to achieve a goal involving the therapy animal. To achieve group cooperation, individuals in the group have to examine their success or failure at being a productive member of the group. This activity was designed to symbolically recreate life situations with which participants may be struggling. The rules of the activity inhibited group members from using devices they commonly employed in relationships—physical manipulation (no touching the horse), bribery (no food offerings for the horse), and verbal coercion (no talking to one another during interactions with the horse). The rules were designed to challenge participants to move away from old dysfunctional patterns and help them discover new solutions and healthier ways of doing things.

Completion times for this activity can vary depending on the interpersonal dynamics of the group. I have observed some groups that completed this exercise relatively quickly, in about 45 minutes or so, but it took this group of fourth-grade girls three sessions (6 hours over 3 weeks) to be successful with this task. They would make a plan, but no one would follow the plan. Interactive communications deteriorated to blaming and finger pointing, which made this an emotionally uncomfortable experience. They knew that they had to be successful at this task before they could move on to another one, and they all were anxious to progress. Finally, the tendency to rely on old dysfunctional verbal and body language patterns was interrupted when one girl said, "You guys. We have to get this done to move on. We're going to have to work together. Let's just try saying please to each other. We'll see if that works!" They started addressing each other with "please," resulting in a more respectful tone that changed the temperament of the group. With better communication the participants presented with a calmer and more respectful attitude toward each other and toward the horse. The girls constructed a plan that quickly led to success. Using other jumps in the arena, the group constructed an elaborate labyrinth that guided the horse to step over the target jump pole as the group walked slowly behind encouraging the horse's forward movement. The counselors processed with the clients the thoughts and feelings they had during and upon completion of the exercise. Clients expressed enhanced awareness of their personal patterns that impeded their relational functioning and additionally discussed specific life areas and relationships where this new awareness could be applied.

There exists any number of possible solutions for this particular equine-assisted counseling activity. The amount of time and effort it takes group members to succeed in this task is directly related to how their internal state manifests through their communications and interactions with others to either impede or facilitate the task and how their current level of self-awareness or unawareness allows them to generate solutions. Patterns of communication and interaction during this exercise, including ideas that clients design and rules they choose to impose on self and others, can reflect ways in which clients have become stuck or stagnant in their life. For instance, participants often erroneously assume that they cannot move the jump or other objects in the arena as part of a solution. At the conclusion of the task a counselor shares observations and encourages clients to share their experiences with the intent of helping clients to become much more self-aware both in this task and in other areas of life.

Therapeutic Opportunity: Clients were asked to complete as a group an activity involving clients' interactions with a therapy horse, and the challenge revealed personal and interpersonal dysfunctions.

SHARM: During a challenging group exercise involving interactions with a therapy horse, several SHARMs were presented as clients struggled in their attempts to achieve a goal. The challenge of the exercise allowed opportunity for dysfunctional client communication and social interaction patterns to be presented and eventually acknowledged. A culminating SHARM was when the group achieved success with the horse after modifying their own attitude and behaviors. This is an example of a SHARM of Acknowledgment. Acknowledging the animal's behavior in relation to the clients' presentation resulted in clients' acceptance that something needed attention within each individual self and the group as a whole.

HARP: Therapist-facilitated processing at the conclusion of the event assisted clients' self-awareness regarding several social dynamics that resulted in intrapersonal and/or interpersonal failure or success. Processing included asking the participants to generalize beyond the exercise with the horse to other relationships and challenges in their life.

AAT Technique: The counselor facilitated a challenging structured and goal-oriented small group activity for clients involving interactions with a therapy horse.

AAT Intention: To facilitate client insight and awareness of dysfunctional verbal and body language patterns, to encourage clients' sharing of feelings, to enhance clients' social skills, and to enhance clients' relationship skills.

HARTI: Clients became more self-aware of dysfunctional patterns of communication and interaction that hindered completion of an equine-assisted therapeutic activity. After many frustrated attempts and processing of those attempts, clients finally adjusted their patterns of interaction and communication with one another and with the horse to be more respectful and functional and thereby succeeded with the task. Additionally, clients were assisted by way of therapeutic processing to apply new insights in other life areas.

AAT AND EXISTENTIAL COUNSELING

From an existential perspective, feelings of anxiety, guilt, dread, despair, and unsettled-ness are responses to the reality of human living. However, individuals try to avoid these uncomfortable experiences by pretending they do not exist via a process referred to as inauthentic living. A primary goal of existential counseling is to assist clients to recognize the ways in which they are not living fully authentic lives and to make choices that will lead to becoming what they are capable of being. Human–animal interactions in AAT create additional opportunities for clients to become aware of the impact of uncomfortable experiences that they are trying to deny. Some basics of existential counseling are as follows (Cooper, 2003):

- Assist clients to recognize ways in which they are not living fully authentic lives and to make choices that will lead to becoming what they are capable of becoming.
- Therapist role is to assist clients to attend to the whole life experience, including the painful, so that they may free themselves from anything that interferes with personal freedom and complete authentic living.
- Frustration, emptiness, depression, and neurosis arise from being lost in one's pursuit of meaning in life.
- No specific techniques. Often borrows techniques from other approaches.

AAT is compatible with the basic tenets of an existential approach to counseling (Chandler et al., 2010). The existential goals of enhancing self-awareness and searching for meaning are consistent with the AAT intention of facilitating insight (B). Clients' movement toward greater personal freedom and responsibility is achieved by letting go of hindrances resulting from feelings of guilt and anxiety: this can be facilitated by the AAT intention of encouraging sharing of feelings (G). Achieving greater personal freedom and responsibility contributes to the AAT intention of enhanced client self-confidence (E). The existential proposition of striving for identity and relationship with others is consistent with the AAT intentions of enhancing clients' social and relationship skills (C, D). By allowing spontaneous interactions to occur between client and therapy animal (18) and commenting on the nature of these interactions (1), counselors may assist clients to become aware of fears or feelings that impair authentic living (Chandler et al., 2010). Animal stories and metaphors with animal themes may be shared with a client by a counselor (12) as examples of authentic or inauthentic living.

Following is a summary of a case scenario of an existential AAT intervention where I was the counselor and my dog Rusty was the therapy dog (also described in Chandler et al., 2010).

Existential AAT Intervention

Before describing the scenario for existential counseling I would like to clarify that the session was not presented to the client or observers as an existential session; it was just a general demonstration of an AAT session (non-theory specific). Also, the counselor did not have a reputation as an existential counselor. The reason this is important is so that you can appreciate the natural potency of the AAT session described.

Therapeutic Event: One day I was doing a brief demonstration of AAT for a colleague's doctoral counseling practicum course. A student in the class volunteered to be the client for the demonstration, and she, my therapy dog Rusty, and I (the counselor) sat on the floor as there were no comfortable chairs or couches for the therapy dog to get up onto to be next to the client in the classroom. With the whole class looking on, the counselor invited the client to interact with the therapy dog by petting as she talked about whatever she wanted to talk about. The counselor directed the therapy dog to lie down next to the client. The client sat there making quick, long strokes down the fur on its back while she talked about fairly superficial things regarding her day and her week. The counselor made appropriate reflections regarding what the client was sharing. After just a couple of minutes, the therapy dog got up, walked in a tight circle, nuzzled the client's hand, and lay back down next to her in the same spot as before. The client then resumed talking about superficial things while making quick, long strokes down the therapy dog's back. After about two more minutes had passed the therapy dog repeated this behavior; it got up, walked in a tight circle, and lay back down next to her.

The counselor then reflected on the therapy dog's behavior and asked the client what she thought about it. The client responded, "I think Rusty is unsettled." The counselor asked her why she thought so. The client said, "Because I am unsettled." The counselor encouraged her to elaborate on her feelings of being "unsettled," and then noticed a significant change in the client's presentation. She shifted her eyes slightly to the side, took a deep breath, and sighed. She slowly, perhaps subconsciously, moved her hand up to the therapy dog's neck and began gently massaging it. The client then began to speak about how she was very stressed by a family situation that was frustrating her and creating a lot of inner turmoil for her. The counselor encouraged her to continue sharing. The more she talked about her distressing concerns, the more she altered her voice and body tone to suggest she was becoming more introspective—that is, she spoke and moved more slowly. The therapy dog responded to the client's internal and external shift by laying its head down and closing its eyes while continuing to lie next to the client as she massaged its neck. As time passed the client explored her concerns more deeply. As she did so the counselor noticed her hand had moved to gently stroking and rubbing the therapy dog's long Cocker Spaniel ears. The client seemed to be petting without thinking much about it. She was focused on herself while conveying her personal concerns. The client was very intent and focused on telling her story while gently rubbing the therapy dog's ears as it lay quietly snuggled next to her and drifted off to sleep.

At the conclusion of this approximately 30-minute demonstration, the counselor asked the client if she would like to share with the group how she experienced the session. She said she was nervous about being in front of the class and at the same time very anxious about issues in her life. She had been putting off things and trying not to deal with them or even to think about them. She felt that the therapy dog could sense her anxiety and so was unsettled around her. She further conveyed that when she did acknowledge to herself that she needed to face and talk about her concerns she began to sense some internal relief and that is when the therapy dog settled down. She felt she and the therapy dog were very in tune with one another; the therapy dog being at first a source of providing self-awareness for her and then later a source of affirmation and soothing comfort for her. She felt that by observing the therapy dog's unsettled behavior she was confronted with having to face her issues instead of running away from them because she too felt very unsettled. Her unsettled feeling was mirrored by the therapy dog's unsettled behavior. She further explained that at the point that she began to acknowledge her issues and express her feelings, the therapy dog settled down, and that affirmed for her that she was releasing some anxiety by expressing herself. She felt that the therapy dog then served as a source of soothing comfort for her as she rubbed its soft, warm ears and observed its relaxed, slowed, easy breathing as she shared her uncomfortable personal issues. She went on to say that if this had been a more private counseling session she would have put her arms around the therapy dog and cried for a bit.

Even so, she said she felt better after spending just a few minutes engaged in AAT as part of the class demonstration. Thus, in just one short classroom exhibition, the therapy dog assisted in demonstrating how a therapy animal can assist a human counselor to provide greater self-awareness for a client, to encourage client expression, and to contribute to a client's experience of some relief.

Therapeutic Opportunity: By observing the unsettled behavior of a therapy dog, the client became more self-aware of her own unsettled feeling.

SHARM: Two SHARMs were presented here. The first was the therapist and client's observation of the dog's unsettled behavior and the client recognizing that it was because the dog sensed the client herself was feeling unsettled. This is an example of a SHARM of Acknowledgment. Acknowledging the animal's behavior in relation to the client's presentation resulted in the client's acceptance that something needed attention within herself. The second SHARM was the client observing the dog had eventually settled down and she recognized that as affirmation that she herself was at that moment feeling calmer. This is an example of a SHARM of Assurance. The client was assured it was best to attend to, rather than neglect, the concern in her life that was causing her distress.

HARP: When the therapist acknowledged the dog's behavior and asked the client why she thought the dog was behaving in that manner with the client, the client responded that the dog was sensing and reflecting the client's own inner experience of being unsettled. This opened the door for the client to address what she previously had been avoiding in her life. Additional processing occurred when the client described how comforted and soothed she felt from petting and hugging the therapy dog, which, in contrast, was very different from the experience of anxiety she felt by avoiding addressing her stressful life situation. This, too, enhanced her awareness of the need to address the concern causing her distress.

AAT Technique: Inviting a client to pet a dog during a counseling session and asking the client to share her thoughts and feelings about the dog's behavior.

AAT Intention: To promote client self-awareness and insight.

HART: Enhanced client's self-awareness of the detriment in avoiding uncomfortable issues and the resulting relief experienced when the client began to explore those issues.

AAT AND CHOICE COUNSELING (REALITY THERAPY)

According to choice theory (reality therapy), all behavior is chosen and purposeful, and individuals work to satisfy needs through total behavior: acting, thinking, feeling, and physiology. Reality counseling emphasizes client choice and responsibility for choosing behaviors that meet clients' needs. Human–animal interactions offer multiple opportunities for clients to experience the consequences of their choices and to make and practice new choices that achieve more desirable results. Some basics of reality counseling and choice theory are as follows (Glasser, 1999):

- Basic premise: All behavior is purposeful and chosen.
- Total behavior is made up of four components: acting, thinking, feeling, and physiology.
- Emphasizes choice and responsibility.

- Therapist role is to challenge and teach clients to self-evaluate through a positive relationship, which instills hope in a client that change is possible.
- Therapy focus: Focuses on the present, contending that whatever mistakes were made in the past are no longer important and that we can satisfy our needs only in the present.

Several AAT techniques and intentions may facilitate progress from a reality perspective (Chandler et al., 2010). Human–animal interactions can assist with the formation and maintenance of the all-important therapeutic alliance between the counselor and the client (A). Clients' motivation to attend and participate in counseling may be assisted by their desire to spend time with the therapy animal for reasons that range from having fun in human–animal interactions (2, 3, 7, 8) to appreciating the animal's role in easing self-evaluation and change, such as facilitating insight (B), encouraging sharing of feelings (G), enhancing trust within the therapeutic environment (I), and facilitating feelings of being safe in the therapeutic environment (J). Interactions with the therapy animal may challenge clients in ways very similar to challenges in their life with people; however, these challenges can appear to be less threatening with animals than they are with people (C, D, 1, 9). Counselor-facilitated examinations of the consequences of actions, thoughts, feelings, and behaviors in human–animal interactions (14, 15, 16, 17, 18) can assist clients to learn lessons that can be applied with greater confidence (E) to relationships with people (Chandler et al., 2010).

Following is a summary of an equine-assisted reality counseling intervention I have observed and participated in on several occasions (also described in Chandler et al., 2010; Trotter et al., 2008). The following activity is appropriate for most groups that are at least school age and older, though for safety reasons small children may need to be more closely accompanied by an adult therapy team member.

Choice/Reality AAT Intervention

Therapeutic Event: In this therapeutic activity each pair of clients is provided a halter and a lead rope and instructed to go out into a pasture where a small group of horses are roaming freely. Ongoing observation by horse experts and counselors of the interactions assure the safety and comfort of all human and horse participants. The clients are simply instructed to put a halter on a horse and lead the horse back to the stable. No specific instructions are given on how to halter a horse or how to succeed in this task, but prior to the task clients are advised about safety issues around horses and reminded to recall an earlier lesson on the thrive-and-survive instincts of horses. Clients who have loud, manipulative, threatening, or otherwise dysfunctional approach behaviors will have difficulty with the task and will need to learn to make adjustments in their interaction style in order to succeed. To accomplish the task, clients' mannerisms must reflect sensitivity to the horse's self-preservation need and responses, and the clients must successfully alter their own attitude, posture, walking tempo, and approach style in a fashion that instills feelings of trust and safety in the horse.

During this task, a counselor's role includes watching out for the safety of participants, encouraging participants, and, if asked to do so, providing only slightly suggestive clues that may assist a client in achieving the task. However, it is not the counselor's role to rescue the client from the challenges of the exercise or to give step-by-step instructions. The primary goal of the exercise is not to teach a client how to halter and lead a horse but to give rise to the types of dysfunctional thoughts, feelings, and behaviors that a client struggles with in life and to create opportunities for the client to learn and practice new, more functional attitudes and behaviors. This activity also provides opportunities for lessons in creative thinking, in that as long as clients complete the instructions given, simply "put a halter on a horse and lead the horse back to the stable," then the clients are successful, no matter if the halter was put on the horse's head the correct way or not. One pair of clients working together realized the halter they had been given was too small for the horse they had successfully approached, so they creatively looped the lead rope around the horse's neck, laid the halter on the horses back, and led the horse to the stable; the halter was on the horse, albeit on the horse's back instead of the horse's head. At the end of the task, the counselor processed the experience with the clients, and they discussed lessons learned and how these lessons could be generalized to other areas of the clients' lives. Clients explored new awareness regarding performance anxiety, frustration tolerance, impatience, self-efficacy issues, and lack of self-confidence.

Therapeutic Opportunity: Clients' desire to succeed in the task motivated enduring participation because they wanted to spend time with a horse. This same desire enhanced clients' receptivity to altering attitudes and behaviors that were interfering with success.

SHARM: While a series of relational moments occurred during the clients' approach of the horses and interactions with the horses, each client experienced one or more SHARMs relevant to their unique experience with the horse challenge. Most of the SHARMs were of the nature of Interpretation and/or Acknowledgment. Clients who were most successful gained insight from interpreting their horse's behavior toward them, acknowledging their need for attitude adjustment and behavior change, and choosing to make necessary adjustments for successful engagement with the horse.

HARP: The therapist processed with the clients the various emotions regarding struggle, success, failure, and so forth that were experienced from the human–horse interaction challenge. During processing clients discussed moments of most profound frustration from failure and/or feelings of great elation from success and how these moments were personally relevant and meaningful. Clients were asked to generalize this experience to other life areas where performance challenges may be presented.

AAT Technique: The counselor facilitated a goal-oriented client–therapy horse interaction.

AAT Intention: To facilitate client insight about the consequences of dysfunctional and functional interaction styles, and to enhance clients' social and relationship skills.

HARTI: The equine activity was effective at demonstrating the consequences of dysfunctional attitudes and social behaviors, and at assisting clients to adapt more positive attitudes and social behaviors better suited to meet their needs.

AAT AND SOLUTION-FOCUSED COUNSELING

Solution-focused counseling views humans as competent with a therapeutic focus on what is possible. A main goal of solution-focused therapy involves helping clients to shift from talking about problems to focusing on finding solutions. AAT offers many opportunities for clients to experience success that may be generalized to other life areas. Some basics of solution-focused counseling are as follows (Macdonald, 2007):

- Primary focus: Humans are competent, and thus therapy focuses on what is possible (i.e., no in-depth exploration of problem is necessary).

- Primary goal: To assist clients to shift from talking about problems to finding solutions.
- When clients are able to arrive at a satisfactory solution to enhance their lives, the counseling is terminated.
- Quality of trust in the therapeutic relationship is a determining factor in the outcome. Trust is essential so clients will return for further sessions and follow through on homework assignments.

A solution-focused counseling approach is quite compatible with AAT (Chandler et al., 2010). Given that trust in the therapeutic relationship is a determining factor in the outcome of solution-focused counseling, AAT techniques and intentions that foster a therapeutic relationship can be very valuable, including building rapport in the therapeutic relationship (A), enhancing trust within the therapeutic environment (I), and facilitating feelings of being safe in the therapeutic environment (J). With solution-focused counseling there is an emphasis on here-and-now situations rather than on the past, and client–therapy animal interactions can be helpful with clients' focus, attention, concentration, and skill building (1, 7, 8, 9, 18). Additionally, solution-focused counseling emphasizes finding solutions to problems, and interactions with therapy animals provide opportunities to learn and practice new social and relationship skills (15, 17, C, D, F) that can result in enhanced client self-confidence (E) (Chandler et al., 2010).

Following is a summary of an equine-assisted counseling group in which I was assisting. I observed how a solution-focused approach generated much-needed self-confidence in an adolescent who was a resident at a juvenile detention facility (also described in Chandler et al., 2010).

Solution-focused AAT Intervention

Therapeutic Event: A 16-year-old male was viewed by the counselors and staff at a detention facility as intelligent, articulate, and creative, but he had low self-worth that was impeding his achievement. He was doing the minimum effort necessary to get by and get out of the facility. The counselors and staff felt he was capable of so much more than the effort he was demonstrating, but the adolescent was not very responsive to counselors' or other staff's efforts to get him to break free of his stagnating attitude. The adolescent's case manager decided the adolescent could benefit from spending time in a different environment, one with different types of challenges that could help the client realize his potential by experiencing successes in skill building and forming more functional relationships. With the client's permission, he was enrolled in an equine-assisted counseling program at a nearby therapy ranch. He was transported for weekly visits to the therapy ranch, along with some of his peers, to attend group counseling sessions once a week for 8 weeks. The therapy sessions were 3 hours long, and sometimes just a bit longer. The client had never been around any horse before this opportunity with equine-assisted counseling. From his first arrival at the ranch the client showed great interest in the horses and very much enjoyed being around them. He worked very hard at forming positive relationships with the horses. He was very attentive to the counselor's instructions during equine-assisted activities and often sought out additional advice and guidance to build on his relationship skills with the horses. Motivated by a desire to learn how to form a positive relationship with the horses, the client quickly emerged from his protective shell and formed and practiced positive relationships with the counselors. The horses readily responded to the client's enhanced interaction style. Appreciating the client's positive attitude and comforting demeanor, the horses gravitated toward him and readily cooperated with his requests. This meant the client accomplished equine-assisted counseling activities with much ease and comfort, which was greatly admired by his peers. His peers reinforced the benefits of the client's growth and development from their frequent requests for his help and guidance during tasks and from their encouraging remarks about his abilities that were shared during group process with the counselors of the equine program. With much opportunity to succeed and positive encouragement from the counselors, the horses, and his peers, the client began to believe in himself; and in a just a few weeks he developed into a competent, caring leader of his peer group. This translated into enhanced achievement in the juvenile detention program, and the client graduated much ahead of the pace he had been moving prior to his participation in equine-assisted counseling. The benefits experienced from the equine-assisted counseling sessions had a lasting effect on the adolescent. After returning to his neighborhood school, he chose to fulfill a class community service assignment by volunteering at the therapy ranch as an assistant to the caretaker of the horses, from which he received very positive evaluations.

Therapeutic Opportunity: An adolescent, who was stagnated in his development by a lack of desire to strive, was motivated to adapt a more prosocial attitude and to develop more functional social behaviors out of a desire to form and maintain positive relationships with therapy horses.

SHARM: Several SHARMs occurred for the client during the course of therapy when he engaged in interaction with the horses. The most significant of these were reflected in the horses' desire to be with and interact with the client, along with the client's frequent successes in engaging with the horses in various activities—for example, efficiently approaching and haltering a horse that was loose in an open pasture, effectively leading a horse around an arena without a lead rope (the horse voluntarily follows close behind the client), and grooming a horse while it remained calm and highly cooperative. Additional valuable SHARMs were presented when his peers recognized and valued his social gifts with horses and recruited his assistance with their own horses. Therapists recognized how the client was assured by his social engagement with the horses, which desired and valued his presence and social interaction. Therapists also recognized the client's transformation to a more sociable, engaging, and helpful individual by patiently and effectively assisting his peers. Therapists provided opportunity for and facilitated SHARMs of Assurance to assist the client to enhance his self-worth, as well as to appreciate his worth as a social being.

HARP: Therapists were cognizant of processing SHARMs relevant to the client's presenting concerns and treatment goals. Such processing gave SHARMs greater meaning for the client and positively impacted his self-concept and ways of relating with other people. With processing, these gains generalized outside of the therapy environment in interactions with family and peers.

AAT Technique: Therapist-facilitated client–therapy horse interactions.

AAT Intention: To motivate a client to learn and practice more functional social and relationship skills and to provide opportunities for the client to experience the benefit of successes achieved from using these skills.

HARTI: The client was able to change a stagnating self-centered attitude and accompanying behaviors to be more prosocial and compassionate. This was accomplished after experiencing benefits from practicing a more functional attitude and behaviors with the horses and counselors with which he worked, and with peers in his equine-assisted counseling group.

POTENTIAL IMPACT OF AAT ON OUTCOME FACTORS OF COUNSELING

Conclusions made from the result of meta-analytical research were that psychotherapy outcome variance is attributable to the following factors in discernible proportions (Asay and Lambert, 1999; Lambert and Ogles, 2004):

- 40 percent: Client and extratherapeutic factors (e.g., client's ego strength, amount of social support).
- 30 percent: Therapeutic relationship (the client's experience of respect, empathy, warmth, acceptance, collaboration, validation, and encouragement of risk taking from the counselor).
- 15 percent: Expectancy of outcome and hope of a client.
- 15 percent: Techniques and models of individual approaches by therapists.

According to this research, the bulk of client improvement is attributable to factors that are not limited to a specific therapeutic approach but rather to factors that are common to all different types of counseling and psychotherapy: client and extratherapeutic factors, therapeutic relationship, and expectancy of outcome and hope of client. A smaller proportion of client improvement can be attributed to the factor of how effectively a therapist performs techniques and models of a specific approach.

An argument can be made for the potential of AAT-C to positively impact all of the aforementioned factors of therapy, both common and specific. In prior sections of this chapter, descriptions and examples were provided to demonstrate how AAT-C techniques can be facilitated within a variety of specific theoretical models and approaches. In addition, a presentation of the psychodynamics of AAT-C earlier in this chapter described how AAT-C can positively impact the therapeutic relationship. Further, we discussed earlier in this chapter the increased and enhanced therapeutic opportunities and resulting client experiences made available from AAT-C to affect, for example, client awareness, insight, learning, and growth, which suggest that AAT-C can significantly impact clients' expectations and hope for a positive therapeutic outcome. It is also interesting to consider how extratherapeutic factors may interact with AAT-C to affect therapeutic outcome in that clients who enjoy the company of animals may be highly motivated to attend and participate in AAT-C, where they may not be so motivated without an animal.

A SUMMARY OF THE BENEFITS, ROLE, AND FUNCTION OF AAT WITHIN COUNSELING

AAT-C is not meant to be a standalone profession. Rather, AAT-C is an adjunct modality that is meant to enhance the efficacy of existing professional practice, such as counseling (Chandler, 2009). In the use of AAT-C,

> [the] therapist must identify clients who are motivated by contact with animals as well as identify animals appropriate for the clinical applications. The therapist's creativity is an essential component for incorporating the approved animal into treatment sessions in such a way that the client achieves specific clinical goals.
>
> (Gammonley et al., 2007, p. 1)

Many benefits have been demonstrated through research that exemplifies how AAT may be incorporated into the counseling process as well as the potential therapeutic impact of

AAT-C. The most notable benefits of AAT-C include: (1) increasing client motivation to attend and participate in therapy sessions; (2) enhancing clients' sense of emotional safety and calm during sessions; (3) increasing client focus and attention during sessions; (4) receiving nurturance; and (5) facilitating growth and healing for clients through client–therapy animal interactions. The role and function of AAT-C that contribute to its beneficial properties include: (1) increasing environmental stimuli during a counseling session; (2) increasing interpersonal dynamics during a counseling session; and (3) the animal's service as a transitional being and therapeutic change agent. Support for the premises of the benefits, role, and function of AAT-C is provided throughout this book.

When performing AAT-C, therapists should be cognizant of the potential impact of a therapy animal on a client's experience, whereby a significant increase in sensory stimuli occurs, such as new and different smells, sights, sounds, texture, and movement. While additional sensory stimulation from interaction with a therapy animal has been shown to enhance the therapeutic experience and contribute to therapeutic gains by increasing clients' motivation to participate and clients' focus and attention to task, therapists must be cautious of how added stimuli may, potentially, negatively impact specific clients in a particular way. There are three notable reactions clients may have to a therapy animal: attraction, fear, or indifference. The most common reaction is attraction. Most people find that interacting with or touching a therapy animal is a nurturing, soothing, and enjoyable experience; thus, clients who are comfortable with animals will most likely have a very positive reaction to the presence of a therapy animal. However, some people may be afraid of animals, and so therapists should proceed cautiously and respect personal space when accompanying a therapy animal and remain astutely aware of people nearby and their reaction to the therapy animal. Where appropriate, therapists should diffuse anxiety by explaining about the therapy animal and making invitation for someone to approach the animal or ask permission before approaching someone while accompanied by a therapy animal. Refusals to approach or interact with a therapy animal by a client should always be honored and responded to with polite understanding. Some individuals have a neutral or indifferent reaction to a therapy animal, and, though they may not fear the animal, they may prefer not to interact with or work with a therapy animal; this too should be met with polite understanding.

When a therapy animal is participating in the counseling process, there are multiple additional inter-relational dynamics available through which a counselor can facilitate client awareness, insight, and change. In the counseling process the therapy animal often serves as a transitional being to the client who takes subjective experience and projects it onto a real object, such as in this case a therapy animal—demonstrated by interactions with, or thoughts expressed about, the animal. Understanding and using the unique relationship dynamics that AAT-C affords greatly enhance its potential impact.

Effective integration of AAT into the counseling process by a therapist involves: (1) assessing clients' needs that may be met through AAT intervention; (2) developing counseling treatment goals and plans that integrate AAT; (3) having knowledge and skill in the application of AAT interventions; (4) assessing the efficacy of AAT interventions in moving a client toward treatment goals; and (5) staying current with, describing, and critically evaluating qualitative and quantitative counseling-related research on effective AAT applications. Establishing treatment goals and plans that integrate AAT into counseling is done in much the same way as one would establish non-AAT interventions. Decisions regarding if, when, and how a therapy animal should be incorporated into counseling depend on: (1) the client's desire for AAT along with the appropriateness of the client for AAT; (2) the counselor's capacity to integrate AAT interventions consistent with a client's treatment goals; and (3) the therapy animal's ability and desire to socially engage and/or perform activities that assist in moving a client toward treatment goals. When completing counseling treatment session summary forms, counselors should describe AAT-C interventions that occurred including any perceptible impact of such interventions. The effects of AAT-C interventions should be assessed, both during and at the conclusion of the course of treatment for a client.

The potency of AAT-C lies in the many ways it can positively impact factors that are attributable to client improvement. This is why AAT-C is considered such a valuable modality by many and why the popularity of AAT will continue to rise in the future. When I conduct training for people just starting to learn about AAT-C, a common question is, "Why is it useful to have an animal in a counseling session?" Another common question is, "What do you do with an animal in a counseling session?" This chapter was designed to address these questions as well as others about integrating AAT into the counseling process. As practitioners and researchers of AAT-C, we must understand the when (therapeutic opportunity), why (intention), and how (technique) of performing AAT-C and share our knowledge with others so they too may reap the benefits of animal-assisted practice.

COUNSELING SUPERVISION AND AAT

There are two applications of supervision related to the practice of counseling where a therapy animal may be involved. One application is the supervision of AAT-C, that is, to supervise counselors in training for their practice of AAT. In supervision of AAT-C, a therapy animal does not have to be present during the supervision session, but an animal does need to be present during the counseling session or sessions practiced by the supervisee. The second application is animal-assisted supervision of counseling (AAS-C). That is, to have an animal assist a supervisor in the provision of supervision regardless of whether the supervisee practices animal-assisted counseling. In AAS-C, a therapy animal is present in the supervision session, but a therapy animal does not have to be present in any of the counseling sessions practiced by the supervisee.

Supervision of AAT-C

Supervision of AAT-C does not require the presence of a therapy animal during the supervision meeting. Supervision of AAT-C means the supervisor is assisting one or more supervisees in their practice of AAT during their counseling sessions; that is, counseling sessions where a therapy animal will be present. A supervisor assisting supervisees in their practice of AAT-C should have knowledge, skill, and, preferably, experience in the practice of AAT-C because it is an advanced and complex counseling application. Not only does the counselor need to attend to the presentation of the client, but the counselor must also attend to the presentation of the therapy animal. The supervisor must assist the counselor-in-training to recognize and appropriately act on all useful psychodynamics in a counseling session presented by all social beings, including animals, and to do this in ways that benefit the client. Supervision of AAT-C requires that a supervisor highly values the contribution an animal makes to a therapy session because the animal's presence and social engagement with the counselor and client are often significantly impacting past and present, conscious and unconscious, relational and motivational forces of the client. The greater knowledge, skill, and experience a supervisor has in practicing AAT-C, the more effective a supervisor will be for supervisees. Information presented in this book, especially in this chapter, is very useful for guiding supervision of AAT-C.

Animal-Assisted Supervision of Counseling

AAS-C is the incorporation by a supervisor of a qualified therapy animal into the counseling supervision process. In the practice of AAS-C, it is not necessary that the supervisor's supervisees practice AAT-C. In AAS-C, a therapy animal is present during the supervision meeting and the animal's presence and social engagement with the supervisor and supervisees during the supervision meeting assist in the process of supervision. Given that the psychodynamics involved in counseling clients is somewhat similar to the psychodynamics that occur in a supervision relationship, AAS-C functions in a manner very like AAT-C, but with a different goal in mind. Instead of facilitating personal awareness and insight in clients for their personal growth, development, and healing, AAS-C assists supervisees with their personal and professional awareness and insight to facilitate their growth, development, and performance as counselors-in-training. Following is an example of how AAS-C, that is the inclusion of a therapy animal in a supervision session, can be beneficial to supervisees.

I directed the supervisor training of the doctoral student in this story, Tiffany Otting, and together we reviewed video recordings of her supervision sessions to obtain my feedback. Tiffany was supervising, with the assistance of her dog Wally, two master's-level graduate student counselors-in-training. Neither of these supervisees were practitioners of AAT-C, but they were in a graduate-level counseling techniques course that required they practice counseling with clients. During one supervision session, Wally was sleeping on the couch next to his owner/handler Tiffany, the supervisor. Two supervisees were present during this triadic session; one was sitting on the couch a few feet from Wally and Tiffany, while the other supervisee was sitting on the floor near an audio-visual cart. The supervisee near the audio-visual cart began introducing a videoclip of a counseling session she performed that she was intending to show during the supervision session for feedback from Tiffany and the other supervisee. The supervisee was about 2 minutes into her prelude to showing the video when Wally suddenly woke up, sat up quickly, jumped off the couch, walked over to the supervisee sitting on the floor who was speaking, where he smelled her breath, wagged his tail, sat down next to the supervisee, and then looked over to the supervisor, Tiffany. The supervisee petted Wally who then briefly walked away only to come right back to the student again to show similar concern. Tiffany verbally acknowledged Wally's behavior to the two supervisees in the room and to Wally himself by reaching out to pet and reassure Wally. The supervisor asked the supervisee if she wanted to continue her plan to show the videoclip or process what Wally was picking up regarding her internal emotional experience. The supervisee chose to discuss her internal emotional experience. She revealed that immediately before Wally woke up and came over to her she began experiencing a great deal of anxiety over a memory in her past that resembled feelings she had regarding the client in the videoclip she was just about to show. Prior to Wally's engagement she had not demonstrated any outward signs of this anxiety, nor had she verbalized anything about her experience of anxiety; nonetheless Wally had signaled that he had discerned her anxiety. The supervisee went on to describe her extreme anxiety about an upcoming parent consultation with an emotionally unstable parent. She felt distress because this parent reminded her of an experience she had with an emotionally unstable parent when she was a teacher in the past. Two years prior, a troubled parent of one of her students had committed suicide and she was carrying a large amount of residual anxiety with her today from that past experience. She was holding that in the back of her mind during the introduction of her videoclip and had not thought it relevant to bring up in the moment because it originated from two years ago before she started her counselor training, but Wally's signaling his perception of her current emotional distress suggested immediate relevancy. The valuable supervisor–supervisee processing that came from that SHARM assisted the supervisee to gain significant insight that alleviated her anxiety and enhanced her upcoming counseling and consultation performance. Once the supervisee began to process the SHARM, Wally sensed that the necessary catharsis was taking place and settled down back to sleep next to the supervisor.

At the end of the semester both supervisees included in their evaluative comments of their supervision with Tiffany how much they enjoyed having Tiffany's dog Wally in supervision sessions. Each described how they experienced support and comfort from his presence and their interactions with him. Indeed, one of the supervisees declared how wonderful it was that Wally "did not let us get away with anything," meaning that is was difficult to avoid addressing that which needed to be addressed due to Wally's keen perceptual skills. This is just one example of how AAS-C can be very beneficial. Any type of SHARM can be appropriate for sessions with clients or with supervisees.

I have found that the presence of my therapy dog during my supervision sessions with my supervisees is very facilitative of the supervision process, with relevance to both supervisees that do and that do not practice AAT-C. AAS-C is beneficial in a number of ways. First, a supervisor accompanied by a therapy animal may seem less threatening to a supervisee and, thus, the formation of a positive supervisor–supervisee relationship may be hastened and strengthened. Supervisee observations of supervisor and therapy animal interactions may confirm for the supervisee that the supervisor is kind, compassionate, nurturing, and trustworthy. Second, interaction with a therapy animal during supervision meetings may calm and soothe anxiety a supervisee may experience regarding performance and evaluation. And third, a therapy animal may alert a supervisor and supervisee to concerns that the supervisee may have that are not readily apparent without the alerting response of the therapy animal, and, thus, deeper and more meaningful supervisee growth and development can be accomplished in supervision.

It is important to respect the right of any supervisee to choose not to have a therapy animal present in a supervision session; especially because the supervisee may have an allergy or phobia related to the therapy animal. I have rarely had a supervisee request that a therapy animal not be present in supervision. However, this reminds me of an interesting dynamic that occurred in supervision sessions of doctoral student supervisor-in-training Tiffany Otting, with a particular pair of supervisees she was training. She was working in triadic supervision with two supervisees enrolled in a master's-level counseling techniques course where they practiced counseling clients. Initially, both supervisees expressed enthusiasm about wanting Tiffany's dog Wally present during supervision meetings. At the first supervision meeting, Wally became very busy with attending to one of the supervisee's needs while that supervisee described her professional development goals for supervision. I have described before how Wally is very good at alerting when unobservable and unattended anxiety is present in a room. Wally moved over next to the supervisee and signaled anxiety in her by staring at her, wagging his tail, initiating a soft bark, and then looking back at Tiffany. It was as if Wally was declaring, "Hey Tiffany, this person is upset. Can we help her feel better?" Tiffany explained the likely meaning of Wally's behavior to the supervisees and invited the designated supervisee to elaborate on what she might be feeling. Yet the supervisee denied she was feeling any anxiety or other discomfort. Tiffany invited Wally to lay back down next to her on the couch, which he did: but moments later Wally moved back over to the supervisee, stared at her, wagged his tail, barked once, and looked back at Tiffany. Whereupon Tiffany again invited the supervisee to share anything that Wally might be signaling. The supervisee repeated her denial that she was feeling any anxiety or other form of discomfort. Tiffany reassured Wally and invited him to lie down at her feet. Moments later, Wally went over for a third time to the same supervisee who was still speaking, stared at her, wagged his tail, barked once, and looked over at Tiffany. The supervisee once again assured Tiffany and the other supervisee that she was feeling okay and she tried to reassure Wally by petting him. Then the supervision session time was up for the day. The next day, the supervisee who was pointed out by Wally three times the previous day sought Tiffany out and told her she preferred not to have Wally present in supervision meetings anymore. In a caring and respectful tone, Tiffany said she would certainly oblige the supervisee, apologized for any discomfort Wally may have caused for the supervisee, and said the supervisee need not explain why she did not want Wally present. However, the supervisee immediately volunteered the reason. She said that Wally was fine and did not cause her to be uncomfortable at all; it was just that she had not been honest in yesterday's supervision meeting. She explained that Wally had been correct when he signaled that she was experiencing anxiety. She did in fact have a lot of anxiety about performance and being evaluated but could not bring herself to be authentic about that anxiety in the immediate moment. She was afraid acknowledging her anxiety would make her look incapable. She was not used to talking about her inner anxiety, of which she had a great deal. She was also afraid she was making Wally uncomfortable and was concerned she would take too much time away from the other supervisee if she processed her anxiety out loud. So in her explanation as to why she did not want Wally in supervision anymore, the supervisee revealed to her supervisor a number of very valuable things—personal issues of the supervisee that could potentially inhibit her growth and development. Tiffany addressed the supervisee's concerns and assured her that performance anxiety was normal and typical for counselors-in-training, that it would be beneficial for her professional development to process out loud her internal experiences in supervision, and that she as the supervisor would make sure that Wally and the other supervisee were cared for and had their needs met. She encouraged the supervisee by saying she would never be pressured to share her internal emotional experiences but would always be invited to do so. The supervisee chose to continue supervision meetings with Wally present and became much more comfortable with sharing. She in fact credited Wally's presence and interaction in supervision sessions as a major stimulus for much of her personal and professional growth that semester.

CONCLUSION

As with animal-assisted counseling, animal-assisted supervision is a valuable tool for facilitating growth and development. The keen sensory perception of animals and their willingness to signal their perceptions is a tremendous aid in counseling and counseling supervision. Animals need no training to signal their perception of emotions in humans because it is part of their natural biology to elicit these signals through behaviors and vocalizations. Some animals will do this more overtly than others; and animals who are encouraged and rewarded for signaling their perceptions will be more likely to continue this behavior. I have experienced canines and equines as some of the more prolific vocal and behavioral communicators when signaling and attending to the emotions they perceive in other animals and in humans. This is one of the reasons why dogs and horses are the two most frequently utilized species in animal-assisted counseling and supervision.

I created HART and its many constructs to aid practitioners, supervisors, researchers, and educators to implement, guide, study, and teach AAT-C more effectively. As with any new constructs, it is important they be validated through investigation. The first investigation of the credibility of my constructs of HART was performed by Tiffany Otting (2016) for her doctoral dissertation. Otting (2016) investigated ways in which constructs of HART manifested in AAT-C practice. The four constructs of HART to be investigated by Otting were RMs, SHARMs, HARPs, and HARTI. The major findings in Otting's study were: (1) Chandler's (2015b, 2015c) constructs of RMs, SHARMs, HARPs, and HARTI were consistent with counselor and client participants' experiences of AAT-C (discerned from postintervention interviews with counselors and clients); (2) client-initiated HARPs produced more meaningful HARTI for clients than counselor-initiated HARPs; (3) the research team (who coded video recordings of the counselor–client AAT sessions) produced rich descriptions of SHARMs, HARPs, and HARTI; (4) counselor and client participants identified interactive experiences of AAT-C; and (5) there was identification of types of client resistance in the context of HART (Otting, 2016). Based on the results of Otting's study, my constructs of HART have been found to be credible within the context of AAT counseling practice (Otting, 2016; Otting & Chandler, 2023).

To achieve some of the greatest benefits that animal-assisted counseling or supervision has to offer, a practitioner must: (1) be able to recognize and to some extent interpret an animal's vocal and behavioral communications; (2) appreciate the potential value of an animal's vocal and behavioral communications; and (3) assure, acknowledge, and reward an animal for its vocal and behavioral communications by responding to the animal with a nurturing touch and soothing verbal response. Someone who is not appropriately trained in AAT is prone to fail in these three principles. Without the knowledge to recognize and to some extent interpret animal vocalizations and behaviors, a practitioner will fail to comprehend valuable information being presented. A lack of appreciation for the potential value of animals' vocal and behavioral communications will cause much therapeutic opportunity to be missed. Finally, failure to assure, acknowledge, and reward an animal for its willingness to signal and respond to what it has perceived may discourage a therapy animal from sharing these valuable gifts.

8

Animal-Assisted Counseling Practices

AAT is a therapeutic modality with goals that are consistent with all of the basic counseling theoretical orientations. It is considered an adjunct to therapy in that it encourages and facilitates client motivation and participation, enhances the client–therapist relationship, stimulates client focus and attention to task, and reinforces positive client change. AAT can be integrated with any style of counseling practice, be it directive or nondirective. It offers a variety of techniques that are flexible enough to be applied in individual, group, or family therapy formats. One important therapeutic aspect of a pet practitioner can be its presence in the therapy room. The pet can contribute significantly to an atmosphere of cozy comfort and lessen the negative impact for the client of being in an unfamiliar environment. A pet practitioner is a therapeutic agent of warm and cuddly feelings. In AAT, I have observed clients pet and snuggle with an animal in a therapy room and report that the animal makes them feel safer and more secure. With AAT, the client seems to engage with the therapist faster because the client observes a positive relationship between the therapy animal and the therapist. Clients also report that petting the animal is soothing and comforting. I have observed clients become more expressive in therapy and introspect more as they search for personal insights when a therapy animal is present to interact with as compared with when an animal is not present. The presence of a therapy animal may soothe clients' pain to allow them to explore their issues and concerns longer and more deeply. For those who may argue that an animal in a therapy session may impair the therapeutic process because clients need to feel the full extent of their pain to recover from it, I reply that I do not perceive that the therapy pet interferes with the therapeutic process but instead temporarily soothes clients' pain or directs attention away from their pain enough to allow them to examine issues more closely. Even with the number of benefits the presence of a therapy animal can offer, it is important to note that it is not just the mere presence of the therapy animal in the room that contributes to client change. The therapist's processing of interactions between the client and the therapy animal, as well as between the client and the therapist, are vital components to the success of therapy that incorporates the use of a therapy animal. The effects of AAT are not magical, mystical, or mysterious. Effective AAT requires facilitation by a knowledgeable and skilled therapist: only then can AAT be an integral and powerful contribution to therapeutic progress.

DOI: 10.4324/9781003260448-8

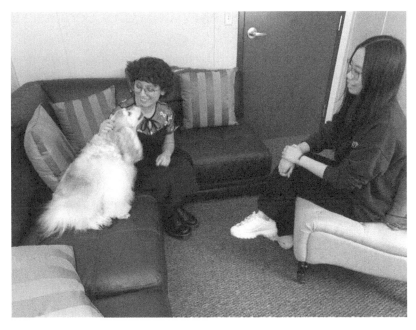

Figure 8.1 A client in a counseling session receives nurturing attention from therapy dog Jesse.

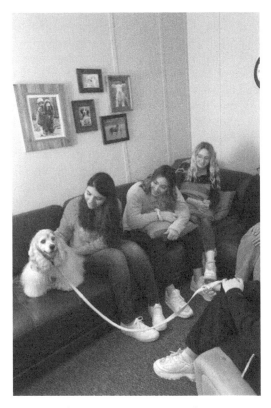

Figure 8.2 Therapy dog Jesse contributes to a positive atmosphere in a group counseling session.

WORKING AS A TEAM WITH A THERAPY ANIMAL IN A COUNSELING ENVIRONMENT

A counselor who wishes to work as a team with a therapy animal must be able to: (1) demonstrate competency in facilitating opportunity for human–animal interaction between a therapy animal and a client, and be effective at processing such human–animal interaction for therapeutic impact; (2) create or evaluate a facility or counseling environment for appropriateness of AAT; (3) educate and inform facility and program staff regarding the intent and activities of therapy animals; (4) develop policies and procedures or follow existing program policies and procedures regarding the practice of AAT; and (5) evaluate client appropriateness for participation in AAT.

During client–therapy animal interactions, the handler should be proactive in limit-setting for behavior to protect both the animal and the client. The handler should be assertive in telling people, "No, my therapy animal cannot do that," or "No, do not do that with the therapy animal." Also, for the safety of people and therapy animals, therapy animals must be well behaved; for example, a therapy dog must not jump up on or place paws on people without being instructed to do so. Therapy animals must respond to appropriate commands when necessary; for instance, therapy dogs should most especially respond consistently to basic obedience commands such as *sit, (lie) down, (get) off, wait, stay, come,* and *leave it* (leave an object alone, such as food on the ground), and be able to walk politely on a leash. Also, a facility must be conducive for the application of AAT. The grounds should accommodate a place for the animal to relieve itself and to stretch its legs or exercise. The facility must provide a safe and accessible location for AAT interventions. Where applicable, the facility must provide for a safe and secure location for the therapy animal to rest. Guidelines for the evaluation of a facility's appropriateness for AAT are provided by Pet Partners (2014), and the Professional Association for Therapeutic Horsemanship, International (PATH, Intl., n.d.b). Prior to the implementation of an AAT program, approval should be obtained for the practice of AAT at the site, and all relevant facility and program personnel should be consulted. This includes supervisors, directors, and staff of clinical programs and facilities, including those from custodial and other facility or human services (Pet Partners, 2014). Policies and procedures for AAT practice should specify important things "to do" and "not to do" relevant to AAT practice in a particular facility or program, and also should provide safety guidelines for health and risk management. Sample policies and procedures for AAT practice can be found in the Appendices of this book: Appendix E is for a counselor education and training program, and Appendix F is for a clinical agency or private practice. Consulting with other established AAT counseling practices and programs is also a good source of information for the development of policies and procedures.

Not all clients are appropriate candidates for AAT. Recommended client screening guidelines were discussed in Chapter 6 and are also presented in Appendix B. Some of the most important issues to consider regarding evaluation of client appropriateness for AAT are: (1) clients who have a fear or phobia of the animal as they are probably not appropriate candidates for AAT with an animal species consistent with the fear or phobia; (2) clients who are aggressive or who have poor reality orientation as they are unlikely candidates for AAT due to the danger posed to the therapy animal; and (3) clients with animal allergies, and if the allergy is severe (poses a health risk and cannot be controlled with medication) then the client is not an appropriate candidate for AAT with the species to which they are allergic.

ANIMALS AS SURROGATES FOR THERAPEUTIC TOUCH

For the most part, it is prohibitive for a human therapist to touch a client as a result of real or perceived danger of client exploitation. Yet there are occasions during a therapy session when a client could greatly benefit from the nurturance that appropriate, genuine, and caring physical contact can offer. This is another instance where an affectionate therapy animal can be very beneficial. A therapy animal may work well as a surrogate for therapeutic touch. Clients can hug, pet, and appropriately touch a therapy animal when the need or desire may arise without fear of landing in a compromising position. The advantage of hugging or petting a live animal over that of hugging a toy is that the animal responds in kind with affectionate behaviors that reinforce the therapeutic benefits of the touch. Remember that I presented research in Chapter 1 on how positive touch of the skin releases the hormone oxytocin in the body of the animal and human involved in the touch, and that this hormone has many psychosocial and physiological benefits—enhancing social connection, calming, and lowering anxiety—all of which increase a sense of safety.

When I took a therapy pet with me to the juvenile detention facility for animal-assisted visitation or counseling, the adolescents initiated touch with the therapy pet as soon as we entered their area. Furthermore, the juveniles continued to reach out and pet, touch, and hug the therapy animal during the duration of the counseling session or the visitation time. It is obvious that touching or petting an animal in nurturing ways is enjoyable for most humans. When a client is in special need of nurturance, therapeutic touch with an animal can provide comfort for the client.

On some days at the juvenile facility when a juvenile was emotionally distraught, staff members sought me out with one of my therapy animals for a few moments of nurturing companionship to help console the adolescent. For example, one day a really young juvenile was admitted to the detention facility; he was 10 years old, but his size and expression made him seem even younger. He was pretty scared to be in the facility on his first day. A program counselor sought me out and brought the young man to meet Rusty and visit him for a few minutes to help soothe the child's nerves. As is common with this intervention, the child managed a small smile, brighter eyes, softer face, and slower breathing as he knelt down and petted Rusty on the head and scratched behind his ears. Seeing and petting a friendly dog in an otherwise scary place may help a client to feel a bit safer.

On another day, the juveniles who were more advanced in the rehabilitation program had just returned from a field trip to a local Holocaust museum—a museum for the preservation of evidence of the horrific assault on Jewish and other declared "undesirable" people by the oppressive German Nazi regime of the 1930s and 1940s. One of the senior adolescents was especially distraught over the experience. Rusty and I had stopped by his section to drop off another adolescent we had been counseling. Rusty immediately sensed the overwhelming sadness in the senior juvenile and walked over to the young man while slowly wagging his tail. He was a large, husky 17-year-old fellow who typically presented a strong, quiet presence, but on this day he was crying. Rusty gingerly put his head on the knee of this fellow and stared up at him with his big brown eyes. The kid reached down and scratched Rusty's ear with one hand while he held his head with his other hand and continued to cry. I stood by quietly. After a few brief moments, the young man began drying his tears and looked down at Rusty who was still looking up at him while his ears were being scratched. The kid simply said, "Thanks, Rusty," and then looked over at me a few feet away and said thanks to me. We left while the young man continued to dry his tears. A therapy animal can extend a silent kindness to help soothe a saddened soul.

ANIMAL-ASSISTED RAPPORT BUILDING

Rapport is defined as "a close or sympathetic relationship; agreement; harmony" (Agnes, 2002, p. 1188) and as "relation; connection, especially harmonious or sympathetic relation" (Dictionary.com, n.d.). The quality of the therapeutic relationship is thought of as a key to a successful therapy experience for the client. Thus, building and maintaining rapport with a client by a counselor is vital for effective counseling. Following are some real case scenarios shared with me by various counselors of how animal-assisted rapport building facilitated a therapeutic process.

The Intuitive House Cat

Flower was a black-and-white house cat that stayed in an old renovated southern-style mansion used as an office suite by a handful of counselors in Denton, Texas. One of the counselors, Dr. Anetta Ramsey, specialized in helping clients with eating disorders. Soon after a client entered Dr. Ramsey's office, Flower could often be heard meowing at the door. She always showed up at the beginning of sessions. The counselor asked the clients if they would like Flower to join them, and the answer was almost always yes. According to Dr. Ramsey, Flower had a keen sense of which clients to visit; she invited herself to only those sessions of clients who liked cats or were not allergic to them. How the cat seemed to know this no one could figure out, but it constantly amazed the clients and counselor alike. On those days when Flower was a little tardy in attending the session, some clients requested that Flower attend, and the session was slightly delayed until Flower was found. The counselor reported that her clients found comfort in holding the cat during therapy. The clients said that holding Flower helped them to feel safe and helped them to better get in touch with their feelings.

The Irresistible Pup

Several years ago, play therapist Nancy Innis was working with a young girl who was a selective mute. The child had chosen not to speak to anyone in her life, including her parents. After several sessions of seemingly no progress, the play therapist was running out of ideas. On a whim the counselor decided to bring her Boston Terrier to the session to see if the girl would show any interest. The child immediately responded verbally to the dog and very soon thereafter responded verbally to the therapist. The child began to show steady progress in therapy with the dog present and eventually overcame her choice to be mute. Nancy was convinced that the child and dog interactions led to greater rapport between the child and the human therapist, allowing for progress to occur. Convinced of the therapeutic benefits of AAT, Innis practiced AAT for many years as a school counselor in north Texas with her Boston Terrier therapy dog.

The Fuzzy Bunny

A counselor relayed this story to me at a workshop I was leading. She was working with a young child who had severe depression. The child was unresponsive to the techniques the counselor had usually found to be very effective with a client of this age. However, she had never before worked with a child with this deep level of depression. The counselor had a light brown dwarf bunny named Fuzzy that she had rescued and adopted as a pet; Fuzzy had been abandoned by its former owner who had received the rabbit as a gift the previous Easter. The counselor decided she would see if Fuzzy could break the girl's strong resistance to therapy. Fuzzy began going to work with the counselor to visit with this child. In the first session with the bunny, the child responded for the first time with a slightly brighter mood as she held and petted the rabbit. With a brighter mood, the child then responded much better to the counselor. Fuzzy became a regular part of therapy sessions, and the child made steady progress in therapy. Sessions ended a few weeks later after the child's dark mood had lifted and she presented as happy and interactive in therapy sessions with the rabbit and therapist, and she was now also happy and interactive at home and school. As a result of the success with this child, the counselor began receiving numerous referrals from parents with similarly depressed children. The therapist claimed that Fuzzy was an integral part of the progress made in therapy by each of these children.

The Purposeful Poodle

Denette Mann, a private practitioner in Dallas, Texas, was working with a 5-year-old boy who was engaged in group play therapy with two other boys his own age. The other two boys were engaged in an activity that had this one boy feeling left out. He felt rejected and chose to hide under a table across the room. Rosie, a lap-sized white therapy Poodle, had been resting on her bed in the play therapy room observing the boys play. She followed the dejected boy with her eyes as he disappeared under the table. Rosie got up and leisurely strolled over to the table to see what the boy under the table was doing. She stopped just at the edge of the table, sat down, looked at the boy, and wagged her tail. A few long seconds passed before a small hand reached out from under the table to lightly pet Rosie's head. Rosie responded with an accelerated tail wag. After a few more seconds, an elbow became visible as the boy petted Rosie a little more vigorously. The shoulder was soon sticking out followed by both arms, which engulfed Rosie with a hug. The boy then spent a moment giving Rosie a good petting. Rosie was up on all four paws wagging her tail and enjoying the rubdown immensely. The young boy confidently made his way back over to the other boys, followed close behind by Rosie, and asserted himself nicely in the play. The three boys played well together for the remainder of the session with Rosie looking on.

The Friendly, Furry Face

My dog Rusty and I had been volunteering our services for individual and group AAT-C and group AAA at a juvenile detention facility for about 6 months when we were called on to spend some one-on-one time with a young man aged 15 years whom we will call Larry. Larry had a reading difficulty and a speech problem resulting from low self-esteem and poor self-concept. In conversation with adults, he would not make eye contact, and he mumbled in a very low and oftentimes inaudible voice. Larry had been observed in detention as having great difficulty relating well with peers and authority. He had been very resistant to counseling and was easily prodded by his peers into fights. He came from a very abusive home and had a quick temper and hypersensitive nature. He did have a positive interest in animals and missed his own dog while he was in confinement. Sensing an opportunity, the therapeutic programs coordinator referred Larry to me for AAT.

Rusty and I saw Larry once a week for 1 hour. During that time, he played with and petted Rusty for about 10 minutes, practiced reading a book aloud for 20 minutes, was counseled for 20 minutes, and played with and petted Rusty for 10 more minutes. While Larry practiced his reading and participated in counseling, Rusty slept with his head resting on Larry's leg while Larry petted him. Larry often verbalized how Rusty helped him be less anxious while practicing his reading and talking about painful things in counseling. Larry said he felt more comfortable with me as a counselor because he could see what a positive relationship I had with Rusty. He said he trusted dogs more than people and he could see that Rusty loved and trusted me, so he decided to risk trusting me too. With Rusty present, Larry began to share things with me as his counselor that he had not shared with anyone else. His experiences of abuse at home were multiple and included a horrific event of being physically held by one adult male relative and forced to watch as another male relative raped his younger sister. After a few sessions of therapy, Larry started saying goodbye to

Rusty with an "I love you, Rusty" whispered in the dog's ear. Larry responded very well to this type of AAT intervention. After only 6 weeks, his reading skills had greatly improved, and when conversing with others he could make good eye contact and speak in clear and audible tones. His temper was much better and he was getting into significantly fewer physical altercations. Larry credited Rusty with his motivation to attend and work hard in weekly therapy sessions. It is important to note that while Larry had great difficulty trusting and liking people, he found it much easier to trust an animal, especially a dog. It was easier and more comforting for him to spend therapeutic time with Rusty and me than time with a therapist not accompanied by a dog.

Rusty was a very affectionate Cocker Spaniel with a very friendly, furry face. His spotted red-on-white coloring gave him a nonthreatening appearance. When you added a scarf around his neck, those red freckles on his face gave him a canine "Howdy Doody" appearance (Howdy Doody was a red-headed, freckle-faced cowboy puppet from a popular American children's television show in the 1950s). Rusty's friendly and outgoing personality, affectionate nature, and really cute appearance attracted a lot of people to him for petting, which he just loved.

One day Rusty and I were walking Larry back to his room at the juvenile detention center when we passed an interview room with the top half of the wall made of glass. Inside were two female probation officers trying to communicate with a belligerent-looking teenaged girl, whom we will call Stacy. As we passed the room, one of the officers saw us and came out to greet us. She introduced herself to me as Larry's probation officer and said she had heard many good things about Rusty the therapy dog and wanted to meet him. I asked Larry to introduce Rusty to his officer, and he did so with beaming pride, a big smile, and in clear and coherent speech. While we were conversing, the other probation officer had been called out of the interview room to take a phone call, leaving the teenaged female alone in the room with the door open. A few moments passed as Larry, his probation officer, and I were conversing when the three of us looked down at Rusty to see that he had stretched the limits of his leash to move to the open doorway where he had made eye contact with Stacy who was sitting alone in the small interview room. Stacy's face had changed since I had first seen her through the glass only a few moments before. Initially the muscles in her face were tight, her forehead deeply furrowed, her lips frowned, and her eyes angry. Yet now her face was different as she looked back at Rusty: her eyes were soft and had a longing look, her frown had slipped into a slight smile, and her forehead was more relaxed and smooth. She looked very much like she wanted to pet Rusty, who was actively wagging his tail in an expression of wanting to greet her.

The probation officer and I made eye contact in recognition that something very special was taking place between Stacy and Rusty. The officer asked Stacy if she would like to pet Rusty, and without hesitation she gave a nod and moved from the small room down to the floor in the doorway. Rusty accelerated the speed of his tail wag, which caused his whole body to wag with it, and crawled into her lap and snuggled up against her chest. Stacy put her arms around Rusty and began to cry. As the heavy teardrops hit Rusty's curly coat, he pushed his head up to her shoulder and nuzzled his nose against her neck as if to say, "It's okay; I am here for you." With Rusty snuggled against her body, Stacy began to sob heavily. Rusty continued to snuggle with Stacy as her tears of anger and fear poured out of her. Larry and his probation officer stood quietly for these few precious moments while Rusty provided therapeutic affection to Stacy. I had slowly knelt down beside Rusty and Stacy when Stacy started to cry and I waited patiently. When Stacy's tears began to slow, I made a few simple intermittent reflections: "Rusty cares about you," "Rusty knows you are having a hard time right now," and "Rusty knows you are going to be okay." Stacy's tears subsided and she dried her tears on her shirtsleeve. She thanked Rusty and he hopped from her lap. Then she and the probation officer resumed their interview while Rusty and I escorted Larry back to his room.

After Rusty and I were back in the car ready to leave for home, I allowed myself to release my feelings, and as my eyes teared up I told Rusty what a very, very good dog he was. My heart was full of joy and compassion, and once again it was affirmed to me that my choice to work with Rusty as a partner in therapy was indeed a very good one. I received a phone call a few days later from the therapeutic programs coordinator, who told me that the two probation officers were saying glowing things about AAT. They said that after just a few moments of empathy exchange with Rusty, Stacy had become cooperative with the officers. The belligerent and resistant attitude she had only moments before her visit with Rusty had disappeared after her visit with Rusty. Sometimes, it takes a friendly, furry animal face to help people who are frightened of other people to feel safer.

ANIMAL-ASSISTED PSYCHOSOCIAL GOALS AND TECHNIQUES

AAT goals and techniques can be applied in all four domains of human growth and development: (1) physical; (2) speech and communication; (3) cognitive; and (4) psychosocial. A number of psychosocial goals can be achieved using a variety of AAT techniques (Gammonley et al., 2007, pp. 43–47; 2003, p. 38), including:

- Common animal-assisted psychosocial treatment goals:

  — Improve social skills.
  — Brighten affect and mood.
  — Provide pleasure and affection.
  — Improve memory and recall.
  — Address grief and loss.
  — Improve self-esteem and self-worth.
  — Improve reality orientation.
  — Improve cooperation.
  — Improve problem-solving ability.
  — Improve concentration and attention.
  — Decrease manipulative behaviors.
  — Improve ability to express feelings.
  — Reduce general anxiety.
  — Reduce abusive behavior.
  — Improve ability to trust.
  — Learn about appropriate touch.

- Common animal-assisted counseling techniques:

  — Give and receive affection with an animal (pet or hold the animal).
  — Learn gentle ways to handle an animal.
  — Learn to communicate with an animal.
  — Learn about how animals learn.
  — Observe and discuss animals' responses to human behavior (immediate consequences).
  — Generalize animal behavior to human circumstances.
  — Brush the animal.
  — Learn about proper care, feeding, and grooming of an animal.
  — Engage in play with the animal.
  — Talk to the animal.
  — Talk about the animal.
  — Learn and repeat information about the animal and other animals.

- — Share animal stories.
- — Ask the animal to do tricks or commands it knows.
- — Teach the animal a new trick or command.
- — Follow a sequence of instructions with an animal.
- — Take the animal for a supervised walk.
- — Introduce the animal to others.
- — Recall information about the animal.
- — Recall information about client's own pets, past and present.
- — Discuss how an animal might feel in certain situations.
- — Learn about animal behavior.
- — Predict or forecast animal behavior.
- — Develop a cooperative plan to accomplish something with the animal.

These animal-assisted techniques can be incorporated into counseling sessions to help meet a variety of psychosocial treatment goals. For example, to work toward the goal of improving a client's social skills, the client can practice interacting with a therapy dog by sharing nurturing touch, playing together, and teaching the pet commands or tricks. The client can describe or demonstrate the accomplishments to someone else or teach another person these same skills. Self-esteem can be enhanced by the successful accomplishment of a difficult task with a therapy animal, such as cleaning a horse's hooves or teaching a dog tricks or agility commands. Compassion and gentleness can be taught and reinforced in a client who must learn to enter a pasture with a posture and attitude that instills a sense of trust in a horse the client must approach and successfully halter. A client's sense of self-worth can be enhanced by a therapy animal that desires to interact or play with a client. Clients who work together in animal-facilitated team activities, such as dog obedience or horsemanship, must practice good communication and cooperation to achieve efficacy with the animal activity. Reducing general anxiety in a client can be accomplished through petting and hugging a therapy cat. Improved reality orientation can be achieved through brushing a pet or asking a pet to do a trick or command. Concentration can be improved in a client learning and repeating animal information. Motivation to attend and participate in counseling is potentially enhanced by a client's desire to interact with a therapy animal. The positive benefits to be gained from therapy can be more immediate when a therapy pet is involved, especially to a client who may have initial resistance to therapy that can likely be reduced by a desire to be with the therapy pet.

A therapist who wants to reinforce the importance of proper communication in getting oneself understood might invite a client to ask a pet to do a trick. The pet's response to the client can be entertaining for the client but also affirm or refine the client's skill at communication. I frequently used this approach with the juveniles with whom I worked at the detention center. I am left-handed and have trained my dogs to respond to verbal commands in conjunction with left-hand signals. Most of the juveniles are right-handed. So when they gave a right-hand signal to Rusty and he did not respond, I worked with the juveniles to teach how specific and clear communication must be in order to get themselves heard and understood. When the juveniles used a different word with my dogs from what I had used in training them and the dogs did not respond, we discussed how one must be willing to match communication language and style to the recipient for greater success at being heard, so that the message one intends is the message that is received. If you asked Dolly or Rusty to *lay,* a word with which they were not familiar, they would stare blankly at you. On the other hand, if you asked the dogs to *down*, they would plop down to the ground and lie there until released. I processed this exercise with the juveniles to relate the lesson to real-life experiences involving different communication approaches people can use to convey messages in a way that might serve a better purpose for them. Sometimes this involves not only being clear in one's communication but also discovering the best way to actually be heard depending on to whom one is speaking.

My dogs are most familiar with my vocal tone, speed, and accent. Some of the juveniles spoke very differently from me, such as at a faster or slower speed, more or less clearly, more or less loudly, or with a different accent. Thus, sometimes the dogs did not respond to the verbal requests of the juveniles as well or as quickly as they do for me. I sometimes watched juveniles struggle to get Rusty to do a trick. Rusty tried to understand the juveniles and sometimes even attempted a few different things he knew in hopes of hitting on the right one. The juveniles at times got frustrated easily and gave up. This happens very quickly in this population, after only about two or three tries. This makes for a great opportunity to teach and reinforce patience and frustration tolerance. I encouraged the juveniles to stay with the dog and keep practicing. I shared a few suggestions to help. The juveniles were motivated to keep trying because it was obvious that they really wanted to experience the sense of self-efficacy that comes with successfully completing the command or trick with the dog. After several more tries, success was achieved, and we processed what the juveniles did to finally achieve that success. They were smiling with a sense of accomplishment and relayed their understanding about the event with great interest and pride. I would often see these same juveniles carefully instructing another juvenile who was struggling as they first did. The second juveniles were motivated to be receptive to the instruction from their peers, as opposed to being closed-minded and mouthing off to reject assistance, because they were motivated to complete the exercise with the dog. Thus, a previous attitude of coercion, manipulation, or "one-upmanship" that is common with this population was replaced with a sense of mutual cooperation being built between the juveniles due to their desire to interact positively with the dog and to experience accomplishment with the dog.

AAT can contribute to a decrease in a variety of antisocial behaviors. Adolescents and teenagers in the juvenile detention post-adjudication program in which I was involved were not allowed to participate in animal-assisted social activity if they misbehaved too much. Misbehaving juveniles "go off program" for a while, meaning they are not currently earning points toward release from the facility. To "get back on program," the adolescents need to demonstrate proper behavior for a designated time period, and then they can once again participate in recreational types of activity such as animal-assisted social visits. I had reported to me, and had observed myself on numerous occasions, juveniles making conscious decisions to correct behavior or to remind a peer to correct behavior so they could continue to spend time with the animals. Social workers, counselors, and probation officers at the facility all reported to me how sad juveniles were when they found out their behavior was going to prevent them from participating in upcoming AAT or AAA and that the juveniles worked hard to correct the situation so they could once again interact with the therapy dogs, cats, or horses involved with the juvenile rehabilitation program. AAT is a powerful motivational force for engaging and maintaining engagement of at-risk youth in behavioral rehabilitative therapy.

The concept of animal-assisted behavioral rehabilitation is so effective that sometimes simple information about animals can reinforce good behavior maintenance or encourage behavior correction. One day, I brought to the detention facility an article for each adolescent on the history of the various dog breeds classified as Pit Bull. The kids had been asking for an article on this topic for some time and were excited for me to get around to this variety of dog breeds when bringing educational articles about animals each week. When it was time for me to bring information about Pit Bull dogs, one particular juvenile was not allowed to have the article because he was "off program," and standard procedure prohibited him from receiving it. His disappointment was profound. Sensing an opportunity for reinforcing rehabilitation, I shared the juvenile's disappointment about not getting the article with the adolescent's caseworker at the facility. So the caseworker made a deal with the juvenile: he would keep the article for the adolescent and give it to him as soon as he got back on program. The adolescent verbalized he would start immediately with his behavior correction. He worked really hard and was back on program within a day, and he was as happy as he could be about the article he got to have and read. On my next weekly visit, he told me all he had learned about the dogs from the article in great detail. He had not realized that so many of these types of dogs were gentle pets that served as therapy dogs. He was quite proud of himself for learning all of the information and verbalized that he was maintaining his good behavior because he missed playing with the pets when I visited, and he wanted to keep getting the information articles about different dogs. He then made a request for a dog breed he wanted me to bring information on when I could, an Australian Shepherd. I made a special effort to bring that information the next week to reinforce the good progress the juvenile was making in the program.

Many of the adolescents in detention came from homes that had a Pit Bull-type dog as a pet, or tragically a family member had chosen to fight these dogs. Sometimes the youths were just intrigued by a stereotypical reputation that Pit Bull dogs have as being the toughest, meanest dogs. I shared information about this breed with the juveniles in detention to reeducate them about the cruelty of dog fighting and also to highlight these dogs' positive characteristics that should be nurtured. In fact, several dog breeds are often referred to as "bully breeds." Primarily, these include the American Pit Bull Terrier (also called a Pit Bull), American Staffordshire Terrier, Bull Terrier, Staffordshire Bull Terrier, miniature Bull Terrier, and American Bulldog (Christie, 2002). The dog breeds typically classified as "bully dogs" vary in personality characteristics, some more friendly than others, and some more affectionate than others. However, most of these dogs, when appropriately trained, properly socialized around people and animals, and raised by a loving family, make affectionate and well-behaved companions (Coile, 1998). In fact, the 1999 winner of the prestigious Delta Society (now Pet Partners) national special service award "Beyond Limits" was the animal therapy team of owner Linda Bates and her American Pit Bull Terrier named Rowdy, who enriched the lives of the people they visited in a California psychiatric hospital (NAPBTA, 2000). Some cities, counties, and states consider bans of certain breeds appropriate, such as Pit Bulls; this has been referred to as canine racism by the late Franklin Loew, dean of both the Tufts and Cornell Veterinary Schools (Rollin, 2009, p. 6). In an article in the *Journal of Animal Law*, Rollin (2009) challenged the ethics of breed-specific legislation and pointed out that in an objective temperament testing, Pit Bulls fared just as well as many other breeds:

> An objective measure of temperament is the breed testing done by the American Temperament Testing Society, a non-profit group that evaluates the temperament of dogs by a uniform test. In the 2006 tests, 84.1% of American Pit Bull Terriers passed the test, 83.9% of American Staffordshires, and 85.2% of Staffordshire Terriers. In contrast, only 71.4% of Chihuahuas passed, 79.2% of Collies and 75.5% of Pomeranians passed. This, of course, must be taken with a grain of salt, as the numbers of each breed varied widely. But it helps belie the view that all pit bulls are vicious.
>
> In fact, any dog can be made vicious by owners, depending on treatment. Beating the animal, tying them on a short leash, not socializing and many other ways of managing the animal can make a dog mean or bitter. Breed reputations are garnered largely by public hysteria fueled by the media.
>
> (Rollin, 2009, pp. 13–14)

Several dogs associated with the "bully breeds" have achieved positive notoriety in the United States. Sharing stories of positive accomplishments by a breed of dog with a really bad reputation helps to overcome this and place into perspective how any dog from any breed can achieve good and sometimes wonderful feats, despite any reputation the breed might have. This metaphor may instill hope in juveniles who wish to overcome a bad reputation they have developed for themselves. Following is a list of some well-accomplished "bully dogs" that I share with my juvenile clients (Deneen, 2002; Orey, 2002; Thornton, 2002):

- The well-known commercial image of a dog sitting next to an RCA gramophone in 1900 and later a television, was that of a dog named Nipper, a mutt that was part Bull Terrier with a trace of Fox Terrier.
- For several years in the early 2000s, a well-known department store named Target featured in its advertisements and on gift certificates a white Bull Terrier with a red bull's-eye.
- A well-known beer company named Budweiser debuted during the 1987 Super Bowl a television commercial on its Bud Light product starring a Bull Terrier they called Spuds Mackenzie. The commercial ran until 1989, and during the period the commercial ran, the popularity of the breed largely increased.
- A dog that starred in the popular 1930s "Our Gang" comedies was Pete, an American Staffordshire Terrier.
- A Bull Terrier appeared in the 1996 Disney movie *Babe*.
- A Bull Terrier appeared in the 1963 original version of the movie *The Incredible Journey*, and an American Bulldog starred in the 1993 remake of the film.
- Prominent people who have owned Bull Terriers include the famous World War II general George S. Patton, famous actress Dolores del Rio, famous author John Steinbeck, and former U.S. president Woodrow Wilson.
- Famous actors Humphrey Bogart and Lauren Bacall owned a Pit Bull-type dog named Harvey.
- The famous author and teacher Helen Keller (who was both blind and deaf since early childhood) owned an American Pit Bull Terrier.
- An American Staffordshire Terrier mix named Popsicle, left for dead after a pit-fighting past, achieved fame in 1998 as a narcotics detection dog due to the dog's tremendous nose and resilient spirit.
- A Bull Terrier named Lady Amanda was inducted into the Purina Animal Hall of Fame in 1987 for saving her sleeping female owner by leaping at and pinning an intruder against a wall until the police arrived.
- A Pit Bull named Weela was recognized as a Ken-L Ration Dog Hero in 1993 for her bravery in saving 30 people, 29 dogs, 13 horses, and a cat during heavy floods in Southern California.
- An American Pit Bull Terrier mix named Buddy was a stray puppy found on the carport and adopted by a family he later saved from a devastating house fire in their Florida home in 2000.
- An American Staffordshire Terrier named Norton saved his owner's life when he went for help after she collapsed from a deadly allergic reaction in 1997. He was later inducted into the Purina Animal Heroes Hall of Fame in 1999.
- An American Staffordshire Terrier named Cheyenne was an abandoned, abused, and mange-covered 4-month-old puppy in California and was going to be put to death simply as a consequence of her breed as a Pit Bull. The dog was rescued by her current owner, who had a life-threatening illness. The dog was instrumental in the owner's recovery, providing emotional support and physical assistance, such as licking

the owner's forehead when she was feverish and retrieving household items needed by the disabled owner. Cheyenne's nurturing abilities encouraged her owner to share the dog's gifts of healing with others. Cheyenne worked as a therapy dog in a hospital. With her owner, she visited patients in recovery along with a second "bully dog" adopted into the family, an American Pit Bull Terrier named Dakota.

Hearing or reading about accomplished dogs can inspire an individual to achieve: "If a dog can be a contribution to society, why can't I?"

There is no doubt that, as a group, "bully dogs" have been unfairly stereotyped as bad dogs. Any dog that is trained to be aggressive or is not trained to be a good citizen and therefore is undisciplined and unruly is potentially a dangerous dog. Even a badly behaving Chihuahua can inflict a painful bite. However, a small, badly behaving dog does relatively little damage, whereas a strong and powerful badly behaving dog can maim and kill. Initially, it is not the dog's fault if it is a danger to society; rather, it is the owner's fault. All dogs should receive proper socialization, nurturance, and training to be good companions and well-behaved citizens in a community. On a rare occasion, a dog may be born with something neurologically wrong with it, and successful social training is not possible. Normally, though, dogs are genetically wired to be intelligent and social creatures that desire companionship and respond well to socialization and obedience training (Alderton, 2000a). Helping adolescents to realize the damage that can be done by bigoted stereotyping of animals is a helpful tool for teaching fairness in judgment and proper management of the responsibility that comes with pet ownership.

During AAT sessions clients frequently tell stories about their own pet or a former pet. In order to emphasize how facilitative a therapy pet can be for stimulating conversation about a client's pet, I would like to point out that in my experience with my therapy pets, about 90 percent of the people who engage with me while I am accompanied by a pet, whether a stranger on the street or a client I am working with in therapy, initiate a discussion, without any query from me, about their own pet or a pet of a family member or friend. If it is a former pet, opportunity to discuss grief and loss issues is presented. If it is a current pet and the client is confined in a facility that separates the owner from the pet such as a hospital, nursing home, or detention facility, opportunity is presented for the client to process how much he or she misses the pet. If it is a current pet waiting at home, the discussion usually centers on the special feelings a client has for the pet and the personal needs the pet fills in the client's life. Each of these is a significant relationship issue that can stimulate client exploration and sharing of very deep emotions. The significance of a client–pet relationship or a client's loss of a pet is too often overlooked by a therapist. Much can be discovered about a client by exploring client–pet relationships. Opportunity to heal bereavement from pet loss can contribute to greater wellbeing for a client. Also, discussion about client–pet relationships or feelings a client has for a living or deceased pet easily leads into exploration about relationships with people.

A number of additional activities can be useful in AAT (Delta Society, 1997):

- Gain knowledge about animals.
- Learn humane animal care.
- Develop motor and physical skill through human–animal interactions.
- Learn animal training.
- Practice appropriate discipline and correction.
- Incorporate an attitude of kindness and compassion.
- Learn about nurturance.
- Practice loyalty and responsibility.
- Experience human–animal bonding.

- Learn responsible pet ownership.
- Learn AAT and AAA training and activities.

As mentioned earlier, I brought information about animals to share with the juveniles in detention, and this became a very popular activity among these adolescents. They very much looked forward to receiving handouts or copies of articles that described information about dog and cat breeds or that told interesting and true animal stories. If I forgot to bring an article or could not because the photocopy machine was broken, the juveniles' disappointment was apparent. A good source for dog stories was the American Kennel Club's *AKC Gazette* magazine. *Dog Fancy* and *Cat Fancy* magazines are also full of good animal stories. My veterinarian saved his old issues and gave them to me for my counseling work. Dog and cat breed information was obtained from Alderton's *Cats* (2000b) or *Dogs* (2000a) or from Coile's *Encyclopedia of Dog Breeds* (1998). A source for stories on AAT is Pet Partner's *Interactions Magazine*. Also, at the local pet store, I found entire magazine volumes dedicated to one specific dog breed that contained a history of the breed and some fascinating true stories about dogs of that breed achieving some type of fame, notoriety, or act of heroism. It is possible that accomplished dogs portrayed in true stories serve as surrogate positive role models for clients.

It is important that articles shared with clients be appropriate for the population. For instance, for juveniles in a detention center, all animal-related material was screened for curse words. Even the word "bitch," which typically refers to a female dog, was not allowed in materials handed to the juveniles as a precaution against misuse of the word by the juveniles in the facility. No addresses or contact information or advertisements were allowed in the materials to be shared with juveniles in the facility. All reading material was age-appropriate and served a positive educational or therapeutic purpose. Also, no staples or paper clips were used to hold multiple pages together as these could be used as instruments of harm toward self or others. Having the pages three-hole punched before distributing them made it easy for the juveniles to store the information in their notebooks of collected educational material provided by the facility.

ANIMAL-FACILITATED LIFE-STAGE DEVELOPMENT

Therapeutic work involving a therapy animal may facilitate an individual's progression through primary stages of psychosocial development:

> Within the first series of life stages, the primary goals that need to be achieved pertain to a child's needs to feel loved and to develop a sense of industry and competence. In a practical sense, the animal's presence in therapy . . . may assist a child in learning to trust. Furthermore, the animal may help the clinician demonstrate to the child that he is worth loving. Unfortunately, for some children, their reservoirs of life successes are limited and they feel incompetent. This sense of incompetence may be acted out aggressively toward others or internally against oneself. A therapist may utilize an animal to help a child see value in life.
>
> (Fine, 2000b, p. 190)

It is important to consider that the various core conditions required for a person to adequately assimilate one or more stages of development might be aided by social interaction with a therapist working in conjunction with a therapy pet. Following is a developmental model for psychosocial development proposed by prominent psychologist Erik Erikson in 1968 (found in Kolander, Ballard, and Chandler, 2005, p. 30). Let us examine Erikson's model in conjunction with suggested AAT interventions to facilitate life-skill development.

For purposes of discussion we will hypothetically assume that for some reason in a child's or person's life there might have been some impairment in the development of a particular stage or stages of normal psychosocial development or there was a desire to expand upon a current normal level of development.

Erikson's Stages of Psychosocial Development

If the life task is mastered, a positive quality is incorporated into the personality. If the task during each stage is not mastered, the ego is damaged because a negative quality is incorporated (found in Kolander, Ballard, and Chandler, 2005, p. 30):

1. Trust vs. distrust (0–1 year of age): Learning to trust caregivers to meet one's needs; or, developing distrust if needs are not met.
2. Autonomy vs. shame and doubt (1–2 years of age): Gaining control over eliminative functions and learning to feed oneself; learning to play alone and explore the world and develop some degree of independence; or, if too restricted by caregivers, developing a sense of shame and doubt about one's abilities.
3. Initiative vs. guilt (3–5 years of age): As intellectual and motor skills develop, exploring the environment, experiencing many new things, and assuming more responsibility for initiating and carrying out plans; or, if caregivers do not accept the child's own initiative, instilling a feeling of guilt over labeled misbehavior.
4. Industry vs. inferiority (6–11 years of age): Learning to meet the demands of life, such as home and school, and developing a strong sense of self-worth through accomplishment and interaction with others; or, without the proper support and encouragement, beginning to feel inferior in relation to others.
5. Identity vs. role confusion (12–19 years of age): Developing a strong sense of self; or, becoming confused about one's identity and roles in life.
6. Intimacy vs. isolation (20s and 30s for males only; and 12–19 years of age for females. Intimacy develops in conjunction with identity in females but intimacy development follows identity development in males): Developing close relationships with others; or, becoming isolated from meaningful relationships with others.
7. Generativity vs. stagnation (40s and 50s): Assuming responsible, adult roles in the community and teaching and caring for the next generation; or, becoming impoverished, self-centered, or stagnant.
8. Integrity vs. despair (60 years and over): Evaluating one's life and accepting oneself for who one is; or, despairing because one cannot determine the meaning of one's life.

The first stage of psychosocial development proposed by Erikson, that of trust versus distrust, requires the experience of a relationship with a caregiver or care provider in which a child can trust that the provider will not harm the child and will in fact ensure the safety and welfare of the child. This would typically be the child's parents. However, the child may not have had nurturing parents or may have had an abusive experience with an adult or older child, or perhaps a divorce or death involving a parent has caused distress for the child; any of these types of events could potentially impair development of attachment, trust, or safety for a child. This early developmental impairment may cause psychosocial difficulty for the client at any time or throughout the client's life. A counselor may be able to help a client to repair early childhood impairment through a therapeutic process. The therapist is trained in basic relational skills that assist to convey empathy to the client and to facilitate a trusting relationship. Even so, an impaired client may have difficulty trusting the therapist's presentation given that some individual in the client's life was neglectful or betrayed trust. Thus, any additional information that may reinforce the client's ability to observe and experience trust with the therapist can be most beneficial. When a client observes the trust conveyed between a therapist and the therapist's pet this provides the client with strong evidence that the therapist might be trustworthy. Furthermore, a therapist can teach a client what an appropriate nurturing and loving interaction looks like by demonstrating that type of interaction with the therapy pet. Additionally, the client experiences the genuine affection offered by a therapy pet to the client, showing the client that he or she is in fact lovable. Finally, a client can take initial risks in expressing trust, love, and affection in the safe environment of the therapy room by interacting with the therapy pet, giving and receiving nurturance and affection, and developing a trusting relationship with the pet; and transferring that trust to the pet's handler, the therapist.

The second of Erikson's stages, autonomy versus shame and doubt, describes the developmental process whereby the child either develops the necessary confidence and courage to explore the world or instead is inhibited by self-imposed shame regarding one's perceived inadequacies and doubt about one's abilities. Progression toward proper development in this stage or rehabilitation regarding impairment of this stage may be facilitated with AAT. Interactions with a therapy pet can offer a client opportunity to demonstrate competency; for example, the client may teach a therapy pet a trick or train the animal in basic commands.

The third stage of Erikson's model for psychosocial development, initiative versus guilt, implies that children either receive support and encouragement for the behaviors they initiate on their own or feel guilty because their initiative is labeled as misbehavior and they become discouraged. A child can easily become discouraged without proper support and encouragement regarding their choices about behavior. This discouragement can play a dominant role in determining the client's healthy versus poor behavior choices throughout life. A discouraged person may lack a sense of meaning or worth and feel her or his life has no important purpose. Opportunity to initiate productive behaviors with rewarding effects can be offered through the care of animals. Choosing to participate in the daily care of an animal through feeding, grooming, training, and cleaning its bedding offers positive evidence for clients that they can make good choices and participate in productive and rewarding behaviors. AAT that incorporates care and compassion for animals can facilitate a sense of purposefulness for a client. Grooming a horse for its comfort and health, caring for farm animals, training an unruly dog from the shelter to increase the dog's chances for adoption, are examples of therapeutic avenues for instilling or reinforcing a sense of meaning and usefulness for a client.

The fourth stage in Erikson's model for psychosocial development is industry versus inferiority. In this stage, clients must develop a sense that they are worthwhile people who can successfully interact with others and accomplish things of importance. An example of animal-assisted facilitation or rehabilitation of the life tasks in this stage is assisting clients to teach a therapy animal some advanced skills that can result in rewards for them and the animal. This might include obedience training or agility training for a dog, or riding skills with a horse. Some of the horses and dogs trained by the client can have been rescued by the humane society or other rescue groups and need training for adoption. Thus, the client's sense of self-worth is further reinforced by accomplishing a task for self and by doing something valuable for someone else; the animal and the animal's future adopted family.

The fifth stage of psychosocial development proposed by Erikson is identity versus role confusion. A client must develop a sense of self in this stage; failure to do so can result in confusion and a lack of direction in life. Providing a client with opportunities to participate in AAIs can lead to greater life direction. For instance, vocational skills can be developed regarding dog or horse exercising, training, and grooming, plus veterinary technical skills can be acquired as well as knowledge and experience in animal boarding and kenneling. In addition, assisting clients to team with a pet, obtain training, and pass evaluation so they can visit patients in a nursing home or hospital can demonstrate for them the benefits of integrating the role of community service provider into their identity development. This may eventually lead to a profession directly or indirectly related to human services or other types of benevolence.

The sixth stage in Erikson's model of psychosocial development is intimacy versus isolation. A therapist might encourage a client who is lonely or isolated to get and care for a pet. The pet can provide good companionship for the client. In addition, walking a pet out in the community stimulates social interaction for a client with others who may want to engage with the client's pet, talk about the client's pet, or discuss their own pet with the client. This introduction may lead to the establishment of acquaintances or friendships that offer opportunity for additional social interactions. The person with their pet can become a volunteer and provide AAA service by visiting with their pet at schools, nursing homes, and hospitals. They can join a local group of animal handlers who do this on a regular basis. Even if individuals do not want to volunteer with their own pet, or if their pet does not have the proper temperament for becoming a therapy animal, they can volunteer to assist others who provide AAT; for instance, to volunteer to be a side-walker for a client who is participating in equine-assisted therapy. A side-walker walks along the ground, keeping pace at the side of the mounted rider to help assure that a young rider or a rider with a physical disability can maintain balance on the horse. All of these types of animal activities can provide additional social contact opportunities for an individual. Opportunity for interaction with a therapy animal can be a motivating force for a socially challenged client to take personal risks and engage in therapeutic activities for developing interpersonal and relationship skills.

Generativity versus stagnation is the seventh of Erikson's stages for psychosocial development. An individual can find personal and financial fulfillment through the practice of animal-related professional activities, hobbies, or community service. Perhaps if you are reading this book, you are considering incorporating animals into your professional practice. Many clients are attracted to the idea of working with a therapist who partners with a therapy animal; thus, AAT may increase your client base. Furthermore, some therapeutic goals might be more easily accomplished with a client with the assistance of a therapy animal, thus enhancing the efficacy of your practice with particular clients. In addition, you may be sought out for contract work by other agencies such as schools, hospitals, prisons, or detention centers for training faculty or staff in AAT techniques or in providing AAT. Thus, working with animals can foster the professional development and satisfaction of an individual, including you.

The final stage of psychosocial development described by Erikson is integrity versus despair. AAT is a common practice with elderly clients. Therapy animal visitations can increase the social interaction and brighten the mood of an elderly client. In addition, the therapist's animal may encourage the client to discuss pets they have had in their life, thus initiating a life review process for the elderly client. This life review can reinforce for clients the many interesting experiences and productive accomplishments they have had throughout their life and can reassure them that their life has been a meaningful one. Elderly clients may be somewhat isolated or may no longer have anyone to care for. Suggesting that they get a pet to care for, such as in their own home or maybe a resident therapy dog or cat in a senior care facility, can give them chances to experience being important and meaningful to another living being.

This brief presentation of how AAT can facilitate normal psychosocial development or rehabilitate impaired psychosocial development for clients is meant to demonstrate just a few ways in which a therapist incorporating animal-related interventions into a counseling practice may assist a client at any stage of life. Many different types of AAI or AAA might be incorporated into a therapeutic practice to assist a variety of clients with a variety of concerns.

TYPICAL ANIMAL-ASSISTED COUNSELING SESSION

As mentioned previously in this chapter, AAT is an adjunct tool that may be used by a therapist during an individual or group counseling session. A nondirective therapist may simply introduce the therapy pet to the client and explain that petting or playing with the pet during the session is a standing invitation during any point of the client's session. A more directive therapist may build in a few minutes at the beginning or end of the counseling session, or both, specifically as a time dedicated for the client to interact with the therapy pet, but also invite the client to interact with the pet during the session by petting or holding it. Also, a directive therapist may actually structure interventions for the client aided by interaction with the pet, all done with the permission of the client. This might include any number of activities or interventions, for example: helping the client to feel more comfortable in the therapeutic environment by facilitating a response to the client's request for the therapy dog to perform certain tricks; relieving tension by having the therapy dog catch a ball tossed by a client; and guiding a therapy dog to snuggle with a client who is sad, or placing a cat in a client's lap to soothe the client's anxiety.

It is quite acceptable for a therapist to pet a therapy animal that seeks nurturing affection from the therapist during a therapy session. This nurturing interaction provides useful information to the client about the positive and trusting relationship between the therapist and the pet and may help the client to feel more comfortable with the therapist after observing such kind and gentle behavior. Ideally, showing nurturing affection toward a therapy animal may strengthen the therapeutic alliance with a client who perceives the therapist as kind and trustworthy. Also, the client may be encouraged to interact with the pet simply by observing the therapist's and pet's nurturing interaction.

I once read an absurd belief written by someone claiming to be an animal-assisted psychotherapist. I paraphrase here her statement that she never petted her dog if it walked up to her for affection during a therapy session because she wanted to teach the dog it was only going to get petted if she initiated the interaction. I completely reject this idea of ignoring or rejecting a therapy animal who is seeking nurturance or affection during a therapy session. This action places harsh conditions on what should be a natural, loving relationship. It is not only sad and mean for the animal, it is terrible modeling of relationship for the client. It also basically tells the client that if you can reject your animal in a moment of need then you can also reject me, the client. The rejection or ignoring of an animal seeking nurturance or affection can only damage the opinion a client has of a therapist. It also discourages the animal from social engagement during a therapy session, thus depriving all human participants of the greatest gift a therapy animal has to offer: its ability to give and receive nurturance.

In a group therapy setting, the same approaches, nondirective or directive, can be incorporated into a session depending on the therapeutic style of the therapist, the nature of the group, and the goals for that particular group therapy. Again, the therapist may direct specific, structured interventions between the pet and the clients or simply have the therapy pet in the therapy room or therapy area for when the clients might choose to interact with the pet. A unique aspect of AAT group therapy is how group members' interactions with the pet might reflect the formation of cohesion and role development among group members. Some group members may ignore the pet altogether, whereas other group members may focus a great deal on the therapy pet. There may even be some competition among group members vying for the pet's attention. The addition of a therapy pet in a group therapy session requires the group leader to be aware of the potential dynamics presented as a result of the pet's presence and a need to assimilate this information to better understand the group. The group leader may sometimes reflect this information back to the group, when appropriate, to assist the group members' awareness of self and others.

A university colleague of mine was teaching a graduate class studying group counseling. As a class activity they visited an equine facility to learn more about group equine-assisted counseling. A counselor from the facility invited the class to participate in a couple of actual equine-assisted interventions. The first activity was to pair up and approach one of the horses loose in an arena and halter it. The second activity was, together as one group, to get a specific horse to move between two orange cones on the ground that were about 10 feet apart without touching or bribing the horse or talking out loud to one another in the group. After each exercise, the counselor processed the experience with the group class. Several individual and group dynamics were shared by participants that exemplified enhanced awareness of self and others. For instance, one student shared that she was aware of some performance anxiety because the other classmates knew she had some previous experience with horses, and they were looking to her for information and leadership. She was very nervous about messing up because she wanted to get it "right." The therapist asked her how this need for perfection played out in other aspects of her life. Self-insight was gained as the student integrated a new perspective regarding the pressure she puts on herself, caused by not allowing room in her life for any mistakes.

Having introduced the topic of a "typical" AAT session, I would like to point out that there really is no typical session. The manifestation of animal-assisted individual or group therapy depends very much on; (1) the therapist's preferred style of therapy, (2) the clients' needs and wants, and (3) the therapy animal's desire and abilities. There is no "cookbook" for performing AAT. The therapy animal is basically an assistant to the human therapist. Though therapy animals are referred to as pet practitioners and co-therapists, they are under the direction and guidance of the human therapist and assist in facilitating counseling sessions. The human therapist has to decide if, when, and how a therapy animal may fit into a counseling session or sessions to facilitate clients' recovery, taking into consideration the welfare of both clients and therapy animals. AAT intervention strategies are provided as ideas for a therapist who might choose to incorporate AAT into counseling practice at certain times with certain clients.

INTRODUCING THE PET PRACTITIONER

A counselor who involves pets in the therapeutic process must disclose this information to clients in advance of their attendance at an AAT session. Thus, if clients do not wish to have a therapy animal present in the session, the counselor has ample time and opportunity to make arrangements for the therapy pet to be secured in the pet's crate or bed in a corner of the counselor's therapy room, or in another room altogether, or left home that day. The therapy pet should always be secured in a safe and comfortable place when not engaged in a therapy session. For clients who do wish to work with the therapy pet, the first introduction to the pet should be made outside of the therapy room if possible, such as in a waiting area, with plenty of personal space between the client and the animal. After introductions with the pet, the therapist then may invite the client and the pet to meet and greet one another. The therapist has the responsibility to make sure the therapy dog understands not to jump up on clients in their enthusiasm of meeting them. Experienced and well-trained therapy dogs will meet and greet with all four paws on the floor. It is okay if the therapy dog rolls over on its back for a tummy rub because this is acceptable behavior. After everyone has had a chance to meet for the first time and seems to be okay with the relationship, then the therapy team can proceed into the therapy space for a counseling session.

ANIMAL-ASSISTED BASIC RELATIONAL TECHNIQUES

Every effective counselor uses four basic listening responses in a helping relationship to convey empathy and facilitate a therapeutic relationship: reflection, paraphrase, clarification, and summarization. *Reflection* is the counselor responding to the feelings expressed by the client. A counselor will reflect these feelings to the client by rephrasing the affective part of a client's message. The intended purpose of reflection is to assist the client to be more expressive and more aware of feelings, to acknowledge and manage feelings, and to accurately discriminate between feelings (Cormier and Nurius, 2003). *Paraphrase* is the counselor responding to the content expressed by the client. A counselor will accurately rephrase the content of the client's message in the counselor's own words. The intended purpose of paraphrase is to assist the client to focus on the content of the client's message and to highlight content when attention to client feelings is not appropriate (Cormier and Nurius, 2003). *Clarification* is the counselor requesting more information from the client. Clarification frequently takes the form of a counselor asking the client a question. The most effective therapeutic questions are open-ended questions that allow for comprehensive answers by the client and usually begin with "how," "what," "when," "where," or "why." The intended purpose for clarification is to encourage more client elaboration, to check the accuracy of what the therapist heard the client say, and to clear up vague or confusing messages (Cormier and Nurius, 2003). *Summarization* involves the therapist joining together two or more paraphrases or reflections that sum up the client's messages partway through the session or at the end of a session. The intended purpose of summarization is to tie together multiple elements of client messages, to identify common themes or patterns presented by clients, to interrupt excessive rambling by a client, and to review client progress (Cormier and Nurius, 2003).

In an AAT session, it can be very therapeutic to reflect, paraphrase, clarify, and summarize the behaviors and expressions of the therapy pet, the client, and the interactions between them. The therapist must be astutely in tune with the therapy pet to be able to observe and oftentimes acknowledge even the most subtle reactions of the pet for therapeutic purposes. Most dogs demonstrate keen perceptions in their relations with others. The therapy pet's interactions with and reactions to the client can provide a therapist with additional information about what is going on with the client. Also important are the client's interactions with and reactions to the pet; these can provide extremely useful information about the client's emotional state, attitude, and relational style and ability.

To draw a clearer picture of what some animal-assisted relational responses may look like, I have provided a few examples from my own experience:

- Reflections:
  - "When you got very quiet, Rusty walked over and placed his head on your knee and looked up at you and your eyes filled with tears."
  - "A moment ago you seemed a little anxious, and your voice was fast and high-pitched. Now as you sit there stroking Rusty's fur, you seem quieter and more introspective."

- Paraphrases:

  - "When you began to focus inward I saw you look over at Dolly sleeping on the floor; you took a deep breath, and then you shared how painful losing your mother was for you as a child."
  - "Each time, as you begin to talk about your father and seeking his approval, you start scratching Rusty's ears a little more vigorously."

- Clarifications:

  - "There are certain times during the session that Dolly walks over to you, looks up at you, and wags her tail; this seems to make you smile. What are you experiencing?"
  - "Rusty was a bit wiggly when you first arrived, and you seemed a bit anxious. But now as you sit there rubbing his ears you seem calmer and he seems calmer as you both have slowed down your breathing; you both seem more relaxed as he rests next to you. How do you experience yourself differently now compared with when the session first began?"
  - "When you talk about your mother you cuddle with Rusty; when you talk about your father you pick up the ball and roll it back and forth with Rusty. How is your relationship with your mother different from your relationship with your father?"

- Summarizations:

  - "You have spoken a great deal today about how important it is for you to regain your father's confidence in you—that you are not sure he realizes how hard you have been working on your issues and how much you have changed. You have reached out to pet Rusty a lot in the session, mostly during the times you talked about your father. This is a deeply emotional issue for you."
  - "You have shared today how you have been putting off dealing with some family issues in your life, and it is getting to the point you feel you can no longer avoid these issues. But you are unsure as to how to begin to address them. You said you did not realize how much you had been negatively affected emotionally by avoiding the issues until you noticed in yourself during the session how much comfort you got from sitting close to Rusty and petting him. You realized you have really been stressing out and not wanting to acknowledge it."

The intent of these examples is to demonstrate how occasionally including useful information during a session about the client—therapy animal interactions can provide additional information that may benefit the client. These animal-assisted relational statements are not meant to take the focus off the client but rather to further the client's self-understanding and reinforce the client's introspective process. These animal-assisted relational statements are also designed to communicate to the client that you are very aware of what is going on with the client in a session, and the inclusive empathy conveyance may increase the client's confidence in your therapeutic ability. You may recall what it was like for you when you took your first basic counseling techniques course and you not only had to learn how to properly reflect, paraphrase, clarify, and summarize but also had to sense when it was most appropriate to do so for the maximum therapeutic benefit. It is equally true for animal-assisted reflection, paraphrase, clarification, and summarization; timing is very important. Incorporate animal-assisted relational techniques when they can specifically enhance the therapeutic process for the client. Animal-assisted relational techniques should be used strategically during a session to retain their potential benefit. You may recall, I described in Chapter 7 a theoretical practice model, referred to as HART, which can assist a therapist in identifying a significant human–animal relational moment (SHARM) and facilitating processing of that moment to achieve therapeutic impact.

ACCESSING FEELINGS THROUGH THE USE OF AAT

Sometimes it is difficult for a client to get in touch with or to express feelings. Having an animal present can often help a client with this. Techniques to facilitate emotional expression can be very subtle or very direct. One direct technique is to ask the client a question from a therapy animal's perspective. For instance I might say, "Dogs have a keen sense of perception and oftentimes know people better than other people do. So, if this dog could talk, what would he say about you or how you are feeling?" Or: "If this dog were your best friend, what would he know about you that nobody else would know?"

One subtle technique for accessing clients' feelings is to have them briefly focus on the animal and try to empathize with it. For instance, when a client is scratching Rusty's ear and Rusty is relaxed, eyes closed or drooping, with slowed breathing, I will ask the client to observe and describe Rusty's emotional state and guess how Rusty might be feeling right then. We will discuss what has to happen for Rusty to feel safe, relaxed, and content and what would interfere with that state. Likewise, I proceed to have clients relate the same types of condition in their lives where they feel safe and relaxed and when they do not. So the client–animal interaction serves as a lead to initiate expression of feelings that the client may be struggling to recognize or to share.

I learned from experience that Rusty was sensitive to the internal state of the client, and if the client was anxious, nervous, or angry, Rusty became a little unsettled and wiggled a lot or got up, walked around, and lay down several times. This made for a great opportunity to suggest that the client focus inward and become more aware of what feelings were inside of the client and what impact these feelings had, even though the client may have tried to hide the feelings from self or others. When a client was sad, Rusty seemed to know this and gravitated toward the client and put his head in the client's lap or against the client's knee in a snuggle-like pose. This elicited tears from clients on many occasions.

I observed an interesting and fairly consistent phenomenon between Rusty and the clients with whom he worked. At the beginning of the session, the client mostly stroked Rusty's back. As the client got deeper into personal issues, the client's hand moved up to rubbing Rusty's neck and shoulders. When the client was talking about the most intense personal issues or was in touch with emotional pain, the client gently rubbed Rusty's ears, starting at the tips and then moving to rub the base of the ear where it connected to the head. Rusty progressively relaxed both posture and demeanor through this touching process, moving from friendly and calm to relaxed, and then to deeply relaxed. This relaxing touch progression happened without any direction from me. I do not know why it happened, but I can speculate. Back stroking or patting a dog may be a more superficial acquaintance interaction by a client that began the process of connecting with Rusty while a client considered how to approach discussing an issue of concern; both the client and Rusty demonstrated alertness during this rapid active petting. Rubbing Rusty's neck and shoulders reflected a progression of connecting with the animal while a client described the issue of concern; it was also a more soothing activity that helped both the client and Rusty to become calm. Finally, rubbing Rusty's ears reflected a much stronger connection with the dog and initiated a deep relaxation response in Rusty that was further soothing and comforting for the client and made it somewhat easier for the client to go deeper into the issue of concern and share painful memories, introspect, and gain personal insights. Many behavior specialists recommend rubbing a dog's ears to relax a dog, especially at the base where the ear meets the head. I find it interesting that clients intuitively interacted with Rusty via touch in a progressively comforting manner that soothed and relaxed the dog and then likewise soothed and comforted the client. There seemed to be a natural pacing and matching process of human and animal emotional and behavioral energy levels that did not require conscious awareness to occur. Therapeutic reflection of observations when this did occur was very facilitative of insight and growth for a client.

Deb Goodwin-Bond, a very talented and insightful equine-assisted counselor, who worked at an equine facility in north Texas, often pointed out to a client how a nervous horse was responding to the nervous energy generated from a client, or a horse that was acting stubbornly was likely responding to a client's attempts to bully the horse. She taught her clients the importance of looking within themselves to become aware of any negative emotional energy they were projecting and to modify that energy to project a more positive energy, resulting in the presentation of a more positive and friendly posture. This counseling technique assisted clients to learn to be more aware of negative internal emotional states, to recognize the importance of resolving issues that give rise to such states, and to modify a destructive or counterproductive internal negative emotional state to a more positive and constructive emotional state.

A friend of mine, and a private practitioner in north Texas, Dr. Sara Harper, relayed a story to me about how her blond Labrador Retriever therapy dog, Brie, really got one family's attention regarding the family's dysfunctional communication. As I remember the story, the therapy session began when family members were greeted merrily by the friendly therapy dog, and all was cordial. Then the family members raised their voices and started accusing and blaming behavior patterns. The dog eventually tired of it and went to the corner of the room and lay down on her bed. The family's mutual word barrage continued and escalated loudly. Just then Brie got off her bed, walked to the center of the therapy room, and regurgitated. Everyone stopped talking instantaneously. Before the therapist could share the apology posed on the tip of her tongue, the family members became concerned for the dog and began to direct kind and nurturing words and pats toward Brie. All family members spontaneously began to discuss how they felt they had made the dog sick with their angry words in the therapy room. Recognizing this as a metaphor for how they were treating one another, the family focused the remainder of the session on how they were hurting each other with their words and behavior and how they needed to behave better. The session became very productive, and the therapist had great success with this family as the lessons learned in the therapy session generalized to the home. The family members were always nurturing of Brie in continuing therapy sessions and were careful to keep their communications healthy for fear of upsetting Brie. In speaking with me about this story, Dr. Harper conveyed that she was not sure if Brie vomited because she coincidentally had an upset stomach or if the family's extremely dysfunctional interaction had actually made her ill. Brie had not become ill before in sessions and had not since, but she also had not experienced such poor behavior from clients as she had from this particular family. A therapy dog vomiting in a therapy session is not supposed to be a therapeutic intervention and should be avoided for the welfare of all, but sometimes accidents do happen. It is difficult to tell why Brie vomited since she could not tell us, but the incident served to help one family become more aware and motivated family members to work and grow together. Though she never became ill in another session, therapy dog Brie remained a good barometer of anger for clients as she would gracefully exit the therapy session when voices were raised, an action that made it difficult for clients to deny dysfunctional behavior.

Dr. Harper's AAT work was featured in the *Dallas Morning News* (McKenzie, 2003). In addition to Brie, she also worked with two Tonkinese cats, Katherine and Elliot. Along with animal-assisted individual and family counseling, Dr. Harper often combined biofeedback-assisted relaxation therapy with pet therapy to help patients recover from a variety of conditions. Adult as well as child clients were calmed when they petted one of the therapy cats who were more than willing to sit and purr in their laps while they learned and practiced the therapy skills taught by Dr. Harper. Also, children who might not otherwise want to come for therapy instead looked forward to playing ball with the dog Brie, who was very adept at pushing a tennis ball back and forth during the child's therapy session.

DePrekel and Welsch (2000b) designed a structured activity that can be used in an individual or group format to assist with the recognition and expression of affect. It consists of providing clients with a simple line drawing of a dog or horse on a sheet of paper and asking them to color the various body parts based on the following schema. Colors represent the following feelings: blue = sad; red = angry; orange = happy; green = confused; yellow = scared; and purple = curious. The body parts represent the following topics: tail = friends; head = family; ears = school or work; feet = myself; body = love; and neck = left blank to be filled in by client. The resulting discussion about the client's end product can initiate the sharing of important issues and the feelings surrounding them.

I prefer a slightly different format for using animal illustrations for accessing client feelings. I ask clients to choose their own colors and label what feelings each represents within them. Likewise, I ask them to label the animal's body parts to represent significant areas in their lives. See the illustrations of a dog, a cat, a horse, a rabbit, and a parrot along with accompanying exercise instructions provided in Appendix D for your convenient use.

Another helpful exercise to access feelings is to provide clients with a picture of a dog or a cat posed in different expressive positions, for example, an angry dog barking with hackles up or a fearful dog with its tail tucked and ears back. After exploring together what the animal in the picture might be feeling, the therapist can guide the client in a discussion about how the client may feel. Also, the client and therapist can discuss how animals typically show how they feel. In contrast, sometimes humans express how they feel, and sometimes they hide their feelings. The therapist may inquire when and under what circumstances clients hide feelings and when they show feelings genuinely. See the illustrations of a dog and cat in expressive poses along with accompanying exercise instructions provided in Appendix D for your convenient use.

Sometimes it is easier to stimulate a conversation for clients to talk about themselves when they have something to compare with how they see themselves. The therapist can provide a photograph or picture of certain dog breeds with accompanying descriptions of common characteristics for that breed. Clients can pick out one or more dogs to represent shared characteristics of how they see themselves and the dog as similar. Coile (1998) thoroughly describes over 150 breeds in her text; Table 8.1 gives a sample list of just a few contrasting dog breed characteristics that can be useful.

For example, if I were to compare myself to one of the dog breeds characterized in Table 8.1, I would have to say that I am most like a Great Dane. You can also have a client describe a breed or characteristics of different breeds that they would aspire to be more like to assess the self-acceptance level of the client. For example, I am pretty happy being a Great Dane, but I would prefer to have the personality of a Cocker Spaniel and the protection ability of a German Shepherd. I guess in my ideal world, this would make me something like a Spaniel–Shepherd. You can also have the client pick out which family members share certain characteristics with certain dog breeds or a combination of dog breeds. This stimulates a discussion around family dynamics and potential family misunderstandings and conflicts. A therapist can also use this exercise in a team-building workshop to help participants describe their perceptions of self and of the colleagues they work with in an effort to build a greater understanding of how one is perceived and how this impacts working relationships. It is also a good exercise to inquire as to what type of dog characteristics clients see themselves as having in different situations, such as home versus work, or with friends versus with family or a spouse. It would be interesting to discover that the client is more like one dog at home and a different dog at work and so forth. This exercise explores the potential dichotomies within the client's life. The exercise should be introduced with the idea that no dog breed is a bad dog breed; every dog breed's unique characteristics make it special.

Some other structured activities I have developed and use to assist clients with accessing feelings are described in the following vignettes: "Doggone Different" and "Animal Tales."

Table 8.1 Dog Breed Characteristics

Dog Breed	*Characteristics*
American Cocker Spaniel	Considered a medium-sized dog. Average weight 24–28 pounds. Average height 13.5–15.5 inches. Watchdog ability high but protection ability very low. Medium energy level. Extremely friendly and playful. Easy to train. Very high affection level. Grooming requirements very high. Cheerful, amiable, sweet, sensitive, willing to please, and responsive to its family's wishes. Also inquisitive and loves outings in the country, but is equally at home in the city and happily walks on a leash for its exercise. (pp. 30–31)
American Staffordshire Terrier (Pit Bull-type dog)	Considered a large dog. Average weight 57–67 pounds. Average height 17–19 inches. Watchdog ability and protection ability very high. Medium energy level. Not very friendly. Low training ability. Medium affection level. Low grooming requirements. Sweet, trustworthy, docile, and playful with its family. Friendly toward strangers as long as its owner is present. Generally good with children. Aggressive toward other dogs—especially those that challenge. Stubborn, tenacious, and fearless. Loves its owner's fond attention. (pp. 146–147)
Bloodhound	Considered a very large dog. Average weight 90–110 pounds. Average height 23–27 inches. Watchdog ability high but protection ability low. Medium energy level. Friendliness high. Ease of training very low. Affection level very high. Playfulness very low. Grooming requirements very low. Gentle and placid, calm manners, and extremely trustworthy around children. Tough, stubborn, and independent. A great tracker used for hunting and search and rescue. (pp. 64–65)
Border Collie	Considered a medium-sized dog. Average weight 30–45 pounds. Average height 18–23 inches. Watchdog ability high and protection ability medium. Energy level very high. Friendliness medium. Training ability very high. Affection level medium. Playfulness high. Grooming requirements medium. A bundle of energy. One of the most intelligent and obedient breeds. Needs lots and lots of exercise. A dependable and loyal companion. (pp. 288–289)
Bulldog	Considered a medium-sized dog. Average weight 40–50 pounds. Average height 12–15 inches. Watchdog ability very low and protection ability low. Energy level very low. Friendliness high (but not toward other dogs). Training ability low. Affection level very high. Playfulness high. Grooming requirements low. Jovial, comical, docile, and mellow. Willing to please although does have a stubborn streak. (pp. 246–247)
Chihuahua	Considered a very small dog. Average weight 6 pounds or less. Average height 6–9 inches. Watchdog ability very high but protection ability very low. Very high energy level. Not very friendly or playful. Not easy to train. Not very affectionate. Low grooming requirements. A saucy dog with intense devotion to a single person. May try to be protective but is not very effective. Often temperamental and may bark a lot. (pp. 204–205)

Table 8.1 (continued)

Dog Breed	Characteristics
Dachshund	Considered a small dog. Average weight 16–22 pounds. Average height 8–9 inches. Watchdog ability extremely high but protection ability extremely low. High energy level. Friendly and playful. Hard to train. Affection level medium. Grooming requirements low. Bold, curious, and likes adventure. Likes to track and sniff things out. Independent but likes to join in on family activities. Reserved with strangers and may bark a lot. (pp. 68–69)
German Shepherd	Considered a large dog. Average weight 75–95 pounds. Average height 22–26 inches. Watchdog and protection ability extremely high. Medium energy level. Somewhat friendly (but aggressive toward other dogs). Easy to train. Very playful. Affection level medium. Grooming requirements low. Very intelligent with great ability as a working dog. Very devoted and faithful to its owner but suspicious toward strangers. May try to be domineering. (pp. 298–299)
Golden Retriever	Considered a large dog. Average weight 55–75 pounds. Average height 21.5–24 inches. Watchdog ability medium and protection ability low. Energy level medium. Extremely friendly, playful, and affectionate. Very easy to train. Medium grooming requirements. Friendly, devoted, and obedient. Needs lots of exercise and active nature outings. Overly exuberant, boisterous, and enthusiastic about everything. Eager to please and enjoys learning new things. (pp. 16–17)
Great Dane	Considered a very large dog. Average weight 100–120 pounds. Average height 28–32 inches. Watchdog ability high and protection ability medium. Low energy level. High friendliness and very playful. Easy to train. High affection level. Low grooming requirements. Gentle, loving, easygoing, and sensitive. Generally good with children and friendly toward other dogs. A powerful dog (and can be hard to handle if not properly trained), but it is very responsive to training. A pleasant and well-mannered family dog. (pp. 116–117)
Poodle (miniature)	Considered a small dog. Average weight 12–18 pounds. Average height 10–15 inches. Watchdog ability is very high but protection ability is very low. Energy level, friendliness, and affection levels are high. Playfulness is very high. Easy to train. Grooming requirements are very high. A lively and playful dog that is eager to please. Responsive, smart, and obedient. (pp. 264–265)
Yorkshire Terrier	Considered a small dog. Average weight 7 pounds or less. Average height 8–9 inches. Watchdog ability is very high but protection ability is very low. Energy level medium. Somewhat friendly toward strangers but not too friendly with other pets. Training ability is low. Playfulness is high. Affection level medium. Grooming requirements high. Seems oblivious to its small size. Eager for adventure and trouble. Very busy and quite inquisitive. Bold and stubborn and can be aggressive to strange dogs and small animals. (pp. 236–237)

Source: Coile, 1998.

I have used these exercises often with a variety of participants, and the exercises are very well received. In fact, the group that participates often asks to repeat the exercise a few weeks later in the group because they found it so beneficial the first time.

ACTIVITY 1: DOGGONE DIFFERENT

PURPOSE

Clarify personal change, growth, or personal goals.

POPULATION

Clients or students (most often a group activity). I have most frequently performed this activity with adolescent therapy groups in the juvenile detention center and with graduate students taking my AAT course.

AGE SPECIFICATION RECOMMENDATION

Adults or adolescents.

MATERIALS NEEDED TO APPLY THE ACTIVITY

Numerous and varied pictures of different dogs at different places performing different activities. It is best if the dogs have varied expressions that could represent a vast array of emotions. I use a stack of 365 pictures from a calendar of dogs. No people are in the photographs, just dogs. Each calendar picture is approximately 5 inches square. Some are in color, and some are in black and white. Numerous breeds and ages of dogs are represented. A few examples of variety include: a dog covered with diamonds and jewelry wearing sunglasses and sitting in the front of a convertible parked outside a casino in Las Vegas; a dog covered with soap suds in a bathtub; a dog flying high to catch a Frisbee; and a dog walking down a dark and deserted alley in the rain. These types of images can invoke a variety of feelings in a client.

DESCRIPTION OF THE ACTIVITY

1. Give a small stack of photographs to participants and encourage them to share their stacks with one another as they go through and pick out two dog photographs per participant based on the instructions given in part 2.
2. The two dog photographs each participant picks are to represent either a change that has taken place or can take place in the participant's life. Depending on the particular group you are working with, the two photographs can represent one of the following:

   — A change from past to present—the person they were and the person they are now (examples: before being brought to the detention center and currently; before the stressor or trauma and now; before deciding to come to graduate school and now in graduate school; or 5 years ago and today).

— A personal goal—the two photographs can represent who they are now and who they aspire to be in the near future (for example, how they hope to be different or what they hope to accomplish).

3. Participants share with the group their choice of dog photographs and what they represent for the participant.

SPECIAL CONSIDERATIONS

You need to have a small group of participants and you will have to encourage participants to pick their animal pictures quickly to have sufficient time for the exercise. I use dog photographs because I perform AAT with a dog that is usually present during this activity. However, this activity can be performed outside of any reference to AAT. The symbolic use of animals makes it easier for participants to get in touch with and share their feelings. This activity can be performed with photographs of any species of animal.

ACTIVITY 2: ANIMAL TALES

PURPOSE

Clarify personal feelings and values. The inner workings of a person can be reflected in a story the person tells about an animal.

POPULATION

Clients or students (best done as a group activity of no more than seven to ten people). I have most frequently performed this activity with adolescent therapy groups in the juvenile detention center and with graduate students taking my AAT course. (For teaching and demonstration purposes: in larger groups, the remaining participants can watch.)

AGE SPECIFICATION RECOMMENDATION

Adults or adolescents.

MATERIALS NEEDED TO APPLY THE ACTIVITY

About twelve 8-inch by 10-inch photographs of dogs and a few cats (or you can use photographs of horses if you wish). Each is pasted on cardboard and laminated. The color photographs are varied pictures of different dogs and cats at different places performing different activities. I use pictures cut from an old calendar my veterinarian gave me. Examples of the photos are: a blonde Labrador Retriever fetching a stick from the ocean; a Husky standing atop a snowy hill; an Australian Shepherd wearing a bandana sitting in front of a wagon wheel that is leaning against a barn; a brown dog coming from a grassy field climbing through a wooden rail fence; two orange kittens peeking out over the edge of a small wooden bucket; and a multicolored cat playing on a wooden porch.

DESCRIPTION OF THE ACTIVITY

1. Without being too specific, ask the small group to choose one photograph to use today in a group discussion activity. After the group chooses one, set the other photographs aside as they will no longer be used.
2. While holding the selected photograph up to the group, give the following instructions. "The group is going to tell one story about this picture. Each member of the group will contribute to the story" (with the exception of you the group leader). Go on to say, "When you add your part of the story, try to speak for no more than 2 or 3 minutes; less is okay. You can say whatever you want, but you have to take up the story where the previous person left off. We will not go in any order. Please raise your hand or speak up when you want it to be your turn. Be respectful of the person talking, and do not try to influence that person's part of the story while they are telling it. The last person to speak will end the story. Who will volunteer to begin the story?"
3. After each person has contributed to the story, say the following. "Take a moment to reflect and ask yourself, what is going on for you that influenced you to say what you said as your part of the story?"
4. Encourage participants to share what they think or feel has happened or may be happening in their lives that is related to why they contributed the content they did to the story.

SPECIAL CONSIDERATIONS

It is a good idea to keep the number of participants in the group small. The symbolic use of dogs and cats (or, if you prefer, horses) makes it easier for participants to get in touch with and share their feelings. This activity can be performed within the context of AAT or in a non-AAT context and with photographs of any species of animal.

ANIMAL-ASSISTED FAMILY HISTORY GATHERING

Many clients own a pet and consider their pet a close family member that they spend a lot of time with and from which they receive emotional support. Research by Chandler et al. (2015) found that pet owners reported eight domains where pets impacted their personal wellbeing. With a therapy animal present in a session, it seems natural for a therapist to inquire as to whether clients have a pet. This type of discussion can easily segue into a discussion about their support system and how well they are using personal resources.

AAT can be useful for gathering family histories or facilitating clients' creation of a family tree. The family tree exercise in counseling involves clients listing all significant persons in their lives, most predominantly relatives, and describing various remembrances they have had about them, positive and negative influences (direct or indirect) these persons have had upon the clients, and any significant mental health issues or other pertinent history of these persons. The exercise is useful for helping clients understand the social influences that have impacted their own growth and development. One type of common family tree exercise used in counseling is clients' construction of a genogram:

> The genogram is a pictorial representation of the client's family tree. It quickly shows a family's history by depicting current and past relationships. . . . The genogram is therapeutic when a client's main concerns are family problems because the client gains insight into the issue by describing them to the helper as the genogram is constructed.
>
> (Young, 2005, p. 210)

Young (2005) describes basic reasons to consider using the genogram, including the client and therapist gaining a greater understanding of the following:

- Cultural and ethnic influences.
- Strengths and weaknesses in relationships.
- Intermarriage and generational influences.
- Family disturbances including addictions, divorce, and mental illness.
- Sex and gender role expectations.
- Economic and emotional support and resources.
- Repeated patterns in clients' relationships.
- Effects of birth order and sibling rivalry.
- Family values and behaviors including dysfunctional patterns.
- Problem relationships.
- Family traumas, such as suicides, deaths, and abuse.

When the therapy animal has a pedigree with some type of registry, such as the American Kennel Club for dogs, sharing the animal's family ancestry is a fun way to introduce the clients' family tree exercise. When the animal's family ancestry is unknown, then the counselor can use a history of the breed of the animal. For a history of individual dog breeds, *Encyclopedia of Dog Breeds* (Coile, 1998) is a good resource, and for a history of individual cat breeds I recommend *Cats* (Fogle, 2000). Even if the therapy animal's particular breed history is unknown, an exploration of the history of the animal's evolutionary rise can serve as a substitute.

Alderton (2000a) describes a brief history of the species of the domestic dog. It is believed that all dogs, wolves, jackals, and foxes are members of the Canidae family and can be traced back some 30 million years. Today there are 13 genera and 37 recognized species spread all over the world. It is thought that all modern domestic dogs are descended from the grey wolf. Wolves and domestic dogs share the same social, territorial, hunting, and guarding instincts. The socialization of the domestic dog is thought to have begun over 12,000 years ago, probably in the Northern Hemisphere when wolves were in greater number and spread over a wider territory than they are today. There are now more than 300 different breeds of domestic dog.

Cheetahs, panthers, ocelots, wild cats, and cats are all part of the Felidae family. There are a number of wild cats spread over the world, but it is thought that all domestic cats are descended from the African wild cat (Alderton, 2000b). The domestic cat has had a varied history:

> During the 9,000 years or so since the domestication of the cat began in the Middle East, these remarkable creatures have provided a mixed reception. Although worshiped

in ancient Egypt, and treasured in the Far East, they suffered undeserved persecution in Europe during the early Christian era because of their associations with the old pagan religions. However, the role of cats in destroying the rats that carried the Black Death across Europe regained them some status.

(Alderton, 2000b, p. 6)

AAI AND CLINICAL DIAGNOSES

There is no comprehensive scientific resource that delineates how specific AAIs can be applied to clients with a particular clinical diagnosis. However, in their workbook, DePrekel and Welsch (2000a) described over 14 clinical disorders for which they believe AAT can be effective. The workbook also includes information on specific AAT goals, interventions, precautions, and contraindications. The diagnoses they address are based on the *Diagnostic and Statistical Manual for Mental Disorders*, 4th edition, published by the American Psychiatric Association, and include general anxiety disorder, attention deficit/hyperactivity disorder, bipolar disorder, borderline personality disorder, conduct disorder, eating disorders, major depressive disorder, narcissistic personality disorder, obsessive-compulsive disorder, oppositional defiant disorder, post-traumatic stress disorder, reactive attachment disorder of infancy or early childhood, separation anxiety disorder, and substance- related disorders. Verifying the accuracy of the information in the DePrekel and Welsch text would make an interesting research project. Many of the interventions are recommended for more than one of the diagnoses. A common contraindication for participation is a history of animal abuse. A few examples of the recommended diagnosis-based interventions by DePrekel and Welsch (2000a) are:

- Generalized anxiety disorder:

  — Undertake slow-breathing exercise with an animal.
  — Walk an animal to the tempo of relaxing music.

- Attention deficit/hyperactivity disorder:

  — Identify parts of an animal.
  — Participate in dog exercising and agility activities.

- Bipolar disorder:

  — Compare own behavior with the turtle and the finch.
  — Compose a journal about how learning from animals helps to understand self.

- Borderline personality disorder:

  — Substitute self-destructive behaviors with productive animal care behaviors.
  — Work one-on-one with an animal to form an attachment.

- Conduct disorder:

  — Study herd behavior of horses.
  — Engage in proper play or other interaction with animals.

- Major depressive disorder:

  — Groom an animal and discuss need for daily self-care.
  — Learn riding and horsemanship skills to build competence.

- Oppositional defiant disorder:

  — Train in basic dog obedience.
  — Play with and exercise an animal.

- Post-traumatic stress disorder:

  — Hold or pet an animal while talking about own trauma.
  — Observe and discuss flight or fright responses in animals.

ANIMAL-ASSISTED METAPHOR AND STORY-TELLING

AAIs such as animal images, stories, and metaphors used as symbols paralleling clients' experiences can be very beneficial for facilitating client insight and growth. Metaphor has been defined as "a thing regarded as representative or symbolic of something else" (Jewell and Abate, 2001, p. 1074), and as "a figure of speech containing an implied comparison, in which a word or phrase ordinarily and primarily used for one thing is applied to another" (Guralnik, 1980, p. 893). Stories and metaphors can work like distraction methods getting around client defenses and resistance. The client relates to the image or metaphor but finds it less threatening to consider because it is presented about someone or something else.

Milton Erickson used imagery, stories, and metaphor to speak with the client's "unconscious mind" (Bandler and Grinder, 1975; Zeig and Munion, 1999). When Erickson refers to speaking with "the unconscious part of the mind," he is referring to the mute or nondominant hemisphere of the brain. The left side of the brain, considered the dominant hemisphere for functioning in most humans, synthesizes language whereas the nondominant right side of the brain synthesizes space. The left hemisphere perceives detail, and the right hemisphere perceives form. The left hemisphere codes linguistic descriptions and the right hemisphere codes sensory input in terms of images. Thus, if one wants to surpass the defenses established by the logic and language of the dominant left hemisphere, this is best done through the use of imagery or symbolic metaphor processed by the nondominant, right hemisphere.

The success of the use of animal-related metaphor and story-telling in therapy is based on the idea that even though the imagery and metaphor briefly shift the focus to the animal, clients will still tend to process the animal's experience or animal's story through their perspective, which is formed around their life experience. It is my belief that this side-door technique inviting clients to imagine what the animal's experience is like helps to tap more deeply into suppressed and even repressed client feelings and experiences. Animal-assisted metaphorical intervention sidesteps clients' barricaded self-awareness and gains access where it is typically limited when using more directive inquiry. Animal-assisted metaphors must be brief and used somewhat sparingly so clients do not tire of them. These techniques are most powerful when the client and the therapy animal have established a positive relationship because then the client will relate more strongly with stories and metaphors relating to animals. Following is an example of a therapeutic metaphorical animal story I developed and used effectively in therapy to encourage adolescents in a detention center to be open to learning and practicing positive communication.

A Failure to Communicate: A Story about the Value of Positive Communication

Let me tell you a story about a friend and his dog, an 8-month-old German Shepherd. My friend would get very frustrated when his dog did not understand him. When they went walking the owner would get tangled up in the leash, or he would go on one side of a telephone pole and the dog would go on the other side. Sometimes he would almost trip on the leash and fall down. The dog pulled on the leash most of the time and would drag him down the street. Back at the house, when he would give the dog a treat he would get his fingers nipped by the dog's haste to get the treat because the dog had poor manners. When my friend wanted to add something to the dog's food bowl while he was eating, the dog growled at him and he was afraid he would bite him. He resisted the idea of obedience training for the dog because he did not think it was the right thing to do to a dog. He would say it was unnatural and thus not fair to the dog. Finally, out of desperation, he decided to go see what obedience training was all about. The obedience trainer started by explaining:

> Owners and their dogs need to develop a form of communication between one another. Without the ability to communicate, there can be no mutual understanding or cooperation. If you and your dog had a shared language, you would get along much better and like each other's company a great deal more. In addition, you and your dog could go more places together. You are frustrated because your dog does not behave the way you want him to. But dogs do not naturally know the English language. They have to be taught. In fact they can learn some simple words in any language. I have a friend in Seoul, Korea, whose dog is actually bilingual, responding to commands in Korean and English. So people with their dogs need to go to school for several weeks to learn a shared language, called obedience training. It is positively rewarding for the dog and the trainer; whenever your dog understands you, give him lots of praise and reward him with petting, a food treat, or a toy treat. Learning can be fun for both you and your dog. In addition, watch your dog's body language. He has no words to express his feelings, but he can say a lot: with his tail up and tense he tells you he is alert to something, or his tail tucked between his legs demonstrates he is afraid or cautious, or his tail can be relaxed and wagging, sharing that he is calm and friendly. He can say a lot with his ears that will be perked up when he is alert, drawn back when he is afraid or cautious, or relaxed when he is calm and friendly. So not only does your dog need to learn your English-language obedience commands, but you need to learn his "dog speak" so he can communicate with you. It is a shared venture of learning and training to benefit your relationship and what you can get from it.

Well my friend fell in love with the obedience training, and not only do he and his dog now have a shared language of understanding and cooperation, but they also enjoy going just about everywhere together. My friend is so proud of his dog and his relationship with his best furry friend. Sometimes you just have to figure out how to communicate to have a better relationship with someone. And if you cannot figure it out by yourself, going to school or getting counseling are good places to get the information and guidance you need to be successful.

There are several symbols, images, and messages presented in this metaphorical story. It is likely that clients will self-select those symbols, images, and messages that are most meaningful for them. Several phrases in this animal metaphor story that clients might notice are "would get very frustrated," "did not understand," "get tangled up," "trip and fall down," or "drag him down." These phrases symbolize how things are not going very well in clients' lives. The next few phrases could symbolically represent their life fears: "would get his fingers nipped," "growled at him," and "afraid he would bite him." Phrases that might symbolically address clients' potential resistance to change are: "he did not think it was the right thing to do," "it was unnatural," and "not fair." The following phrases could stimulate clients' openness to gain insight or initiate change: "need to develop a form of communication," "mutual understanding and cooperation," "shared language," "get along much better," "like each other's company," and "go more places." The next set of phrases is designed to construct the change goals and process into perceptively achievable steps so clients feel less overwhelmed: "have to be taught," "simple words," "go to school," "positively rewarding," "praise and reward," "learning can be fun," "shared adventure of learning," and "benefit your relationship." Finally, the last set of phrases is designed to reflect the positive outcome likely to occur from clients achieving the change goals: "shared language," "understand each other," "going everywhere together," and "proud of his dog." It is possible that the dog in the story is a symbolic representation of one aspect of clients' self or represents some other significant person in their life.

Following is another example of a metaphorical story I developed and have used effectively in counseling with clients to encourage them to be open to change in their life.

Shedding the Old to Make Room for the New: A Story to Encourage Openness for Change

My Cocker Spaniel, Rusty, has a lot of hair. His coat is very thick and wavy. But his coat changes when it needs to, with the changing of the seasons. For instance, in the winter his coat becomes thicker to keep him warm when the weather is cold, and in the summer his coat becomes thinner to help keep him cooler in the heat. He changes his coat when the need arises. His thinner summer coat has to be shed before his thicker winter coat can grow in, and vice versa. His coat changes naturally, but sometimes the change works much better for him when he gets help. If he gets brushed and combed regularly, then his coat stays smooth and soft. If grooming is neglected, then his hair can become so tangled that combing it takes a great amount of effort that can sometimes be uncomfortable for the dog. Sometimes to get a smooth coat again a piece of tangled fur has to be trimmed out. The trimmed piece of fur leaves space for a healthier coat to grow in its place. Thus, regular attention to grooming, especially during the more drastic seasonal changes, makes his coat healthier and more functional. But no matter what, sometimes tangles happen. And when they do, we deal with them in the best way we can so his coat becomes soft and smooth once more.

This animal metaphor story is also designed with key symbolic phrases to facilitate client insight and initiate the change process. The phrases "has a lot of fur" and "very thick and wavy" might represent the complexities of clients' issues. The next phrases may serve as encouragement for clients' desire and ability to change along with reinforcing the idea of seeking help with the process: "He changes . . . when the need arises," "has to be shed," "can grow," "change naturally," "combed out," "trimmed a little bit," and "works much better for him when he gets help." The following phrases may represent clients' fears: "neglected," "so tangled," and "very painful." Finally, these last phrases may represent expected outcomes for change and thus motivate clients: "space for a healthier coat to grow," "healthier and more functional," "deal with them in the best way," and "becomes soft and smooth."

Creating a Metaphorical Story

It is easy to create an animal-assisted metaphorical story. Think of the basic elements you want to convey to your client, and think about animal behavior or situations that would reflect those elements, and string them into a story for your client. Be careful to include metaphors that are appropriate for your client's unique needs, for example, the part in the "shedding" metaphor about trimming out a tangle may not be appropriate for a client that self-mutilates but may send a message for someone else to change a negative behavior or to distance oneself from negative influences. Metaphors do not require interpretation by the therapist. In fact, they work best when the interpretation is left solely to the client so greater personalization can occur. Sometimes clients ask me what the story means. I simply tell them, "It is just a story that may have meaning for you. Think about it over time if you like, and if you want we can discuss what it means for you." When using the animal metaphor story, some clients respond immediately with personal insights; but sometimes clients seem to dismiss the story only to come back in a later session with some meaningful insights the story stimulated for them.

Use of metaphor and therapeutic story-telling is the use of symbolic representation to bypass a person's resistance to healing, growth, and change. Many symbols used in a story are designed to have meaning and purpose specific to the client's concerns. The symbolically framed words are meant to facilitate in-depth client understanding and motivation for change in a manner that is less threatening than direct and nonsymbolic conversation. Therapeutic stories are intriguing and have an element of truth so they are accepted by the client; for instance, consider the power of just this brief statement I compiled that can assist someone who has experienced a trauma or loss and is stuck in sadness or grief: "There was a terrible storm during the fall harvest that stripped the great tree bare of its colorful foliage. The tree shivered, cold and alone without its golden fleece of leaves, but felt reassured that there will be a place for newer, stronger, more vibrant leaves when the inevitable next season of change draws near." The person hearing the metaphor uses his or her imagination to consider how a tree might feel cold and alone. Exercising the imagination in the presence of a therapeutic message leaves the client more open to hear or receive the message on either a conscious or even subconscious level. In comparison, the message that is attempting to be sent through the following nonsymbolic, intellectually framed statement, "You need to consider when it is time to move forward with your life," is much easier for a client to resist than the therapeutic message implied through the symbolism of the earlier statement, that is, that the suffering tree will gradually, inevitably recover and bloom again in spring.

Symbolically framed words can be more powerful than nonsymbolic, intellectually framed words because symbols affect a person directly at the emotional level, instead of the intellectual level. Affecting someone at the emotional level bypasses many of a person's argumentative, irrational defenses. So when using symbolically framed words, therapeutic messages can have a more effective impact. With symbolically framed words a counselor can plant important ideas for the client to consider. It is much easier for a client to be defensive and argumentative against intellectually framed words. With symbolically framed words in a story, therapeutic messages get through to a person to a deeper level than the intellectually framed words because the first step in interpreting symbols by a client is to explore the feelings and values invoked by the symbols. Therapeutic story-telling is a form of expressive art therapy. Expressive art therapy is designed to bypass intellectual resistance to allow for meaningful emotional recovery for a client. When I create a therapeutic story, one that takes from 3 to 5 minutes to share, I symbolically incorporate into the story the following important elements that are designed to have meaning and purpose for the client and the client's particular concerns:

- Phrases describing how things are not going very well in the life of the story's main character, in order to convey understanding to a client.
- Phrases addressing fears and pain and other emotions a character in the story may have, in order to convey empathy to a client.
- Phrases that address potential obstacles or resistance to change or action, to prepare a client for potential setbacks or guard against self-sabotage.
- Phrases to suggest what might lead to change or action, to facilitate insight for a client.

- Phrases to construct change or action to achieve a goal or achievable steps toward a goal, to motivate and encourage a client.
- Phrases to reflect the likely positive outcome, to instill hope in a client.

Use of therapeutic metaphor and story-telling can be pre-planned or spontaneous. As one gets more practiced in the technique it becomes easier to create a story in the moment that will benefit the client.

TELEHEALTH AND AAT

Telehealth is a mode of delivering services over the Internet using an electronic device with good audio and visual quality. Telehealth has the benefit of making counseling intervention possible when a client cannot come to a session in person. Most state government laws in the United States prohibit a counselor from providing therapeutic treatment for a client who is not present, at the time of the session, in the same state where the counselor is licensed to practice. Also, the Internet and web services the counselor utilizes to provide a telehealth session must be compliant with all federal and state government regulations for security and the protection of confidentiality and privacy of the client and the client's records.

Telehealth is not a favored medium for the delivery of AAT services. Primarily because most of what makes AAT so efficacious is the in-person interaction between the client and the therapy animal. The primary roles of nurturer and emotional distress detector in which a therapy animal may serve are not available if the client and therapy animal are not together in the same space. At most, during a telehealth counseling session a client may experience some semblance of vicarious benefit from watching a therapy animal on their screen during a session. Watching a therapy animal on a screen may evoke feelings of warmth or enjoyment for a client. And the client may experience a more positive connection with a therapist who has a therapy animal visible on a screen.

A study performed with university students examining the effects of virtual canine comfort on undergraduate wellbeing (Binfet et al., 2022). The researchers utilized a randomized-controlled trial design.

> Participants (n = 467) were recruited from undergraduate psychology classes at a mid-size Western Canadian university and were randomly assigned to either synchronous (i.e., live Zoom) or asynchronous (i.e., pre-recorded YouTube videos) sessions with or without a dog present. An abbreviated, small group dose intervention of five minutes was used and handlers across conditions followed a script that mirrored as closely as possible the dialogue shared during a typical live, in-person visit (i.e., shared information about their dog, asked participants to reflect on their wellbeing, etc.) . . . . Regarding the impact of platform delivery, participants reported greater campus connectedness following their participation in the synchronous (live) conditions. . . . As hypothesized, undergraduate students in this study did report feeling less stressed at the end of the intervention when a dog was present.
>
> (Binfet et al., 2022, p. 809)

For the most part, I do not recommend AAT services be delivered via telehealth if possible as it is less effective than AAT in-person. But sometimes telehealth becomes necessary. For instance, when the COVID-19 pandemic caused a shutdown of services in the spring of 2020, for safety reasons counseling practitioners had to shift to delivering interventions to clients via telehealth. Thousands of people were dying from the epidemic and there was no vaccine developed for many months. Most people were isolated in their homes. Many developed some degree of anxiety and or depression from the isolation and fear of being infected by the dangerous virus.

Scheck, Williamson, and Dell (2022) reported positive results when an in-person AAT program had to switch to a virtual format when the COVID-19 pandemic struck. The in-person AAT program had been offered since 2014 at an in-patient psychiatric center with therapy dog and handler teams. They transitioned to a virtual format with the onset of the COVID-19 pandemic in March 2020. Their exploratory research examined whether and how a virtual offering of AAT could provide positive benefits to forensic psychiatric patients. Overall, their findings reveal an understanding of the virtual sessions from patient, handler, and clinician perspectives, including:

> (a) differences between connection in virtual versus in-person facilitation, (b) the role of technology, (c) the unique role of the handler, and benefits for patients, including (d) emotional support, (e) positive effects on mental health, and (f) feelings of hope, normalcy, and deinstitutionalization despite the COVID-19 pandemic. Using an online platform allowed patients who had had preexisting interactions with the therapy dog teams to form or continue their connection/bond and benefit from AAT during the COVID-19 pandemic, a time when in-person contact was not possible. Therefore, this research provides support for the use of web-based video conferencing in facilitating AAT sessions with incarcerated psychiatric patients.
>
> (Scheck, Williamson, & Dell, 2022, p. 1)

Virtual AAT sessions with the therapy dog teams were described by patients as beneficial to their mental health, resulting in less stress, anxiety, and depression, and helped them better express their emotions (Scheck, Williamson, & Dell, 2022, p. 5).

The graduate students in training that I was supervising in north Texas at the time of the COVID-19 pandemic tried to adapt from providing AAT in person to providing AAT via telehealth. The counselors had the therapy animal (dog or horse) visible on the counselor's screen during the session. The counselor provided a few reflections about the animal, and clients remarked about the animal or the animal's behavior. In the instance of equine-assisted counseling, a third person was often involved where the horse expert was in the presence of the horse in the arena at the ranch and kept the horse visible on the screen while the counselor and the client each had their own screen, which made this simultaneous counseling on three different screens at three different locations.

One of my counseling interns relayed an instance to me when equine-assisted telehealth counseling was shown to be very therapeutic. The counselor was counseling from the computer at her home office and joining via the computer at her own home was an adolescent client. During this session, the horse expert was in the horse arena at the therapy ranch keeping her electronic tablet camera pointed at the therapy horse. The horse would frequently come over to the horse expert to spontaneously interact and socialize with her. As the counselor and client were engaging, sometimes either the counselor or the client would make a remark about the horse and its behavior. The client had been working with this horse in counseling prior to the epidemic shutdown and spoke about missing the horse and her frustration of not being able to be in the horse's presence. As the client was commiserating at length about being tired of the isolation and having to wear a mask when going outside and absolutely hating having to use antibacterial gel, in that exact moment the horse walked over to a barrel in the arena and grabbed in its mouth the top of a plastic bottle of antibacterial gel that was sitting on the barrel, waved the gel high in the air a few times and then threw the bottle from its mouth high into the air with it landing about 10 feet away on the ground. The counselor, client, and horse expert all simultaneously erupted in laughter and made humorous comments about how the horse must also be fed up with the epidemic. The client had received validation, empathy, and stress release from the horse's behavior. The horse had not been trained to perform this behavior, nor had the horse been cued by the expert in any way. It was a marvelous therapeutic coincidence.

While some clients continued AAT via telehealth during the COVID-19 epidemic with the interns I supervised, most clients said it wasn't as beneficial without being able to touch, pet, and otherwise interact with the animals. Some clients even took a vacation from counseling until they could get back to experiencing AAT in person. Telehealth can be a viable medium for counseling services, but, in my opinion, telehealth is not as effective as AAT delivered in person.

Utilizing Pet–Owner Interactions during Telehealth

While the delivery of AAT via the Internet is challenging, therapists who are trained in AAT can utilize their skills to incorporate pet–owner interactions into counseling sessions in effective ways. Tiffany Otting, one of my former students, has a private practice in Georgetown, Texas where she incorporates AAT. She graciously provided me with instances to share with you where she effectively incorporated spontaneous pet–owner interactions into a telehealth counseling session for therapeutic impact. Having been trained in my HART model (see Chapter 7), Tiffany utilized my constructs from HART in describing three cases. She did not use the real name of her clients.

TIFFANY OTTING'S TELEHEALTH SESSION WITH KASON AND HIS FISH

Kason was a long-term client who participated in several years of outpatient counseling. Kason's presenting concerns were social anxiety, difficulty communicating needs to caregivers, and depressive symptoms. We began working together onsite at our practice with Stella, our therapy dog, when he was 13. Kason also developed therapeutic relationships with other animals including our rabbits, Whiskers and Spot, our beta fish, Rainbow, and another therapy dog, Pearl. During the course of treatment Kason identified and came out as transgender, was evaluated and diagnosed with attention-deficit hyperactivity disorder (ADHD), and later diagnosed with autism spectrum disorder (ASD). When treatment concluded, Kason was 16, scored in a healthy range of functioning on the YOQ-SR assessment, and reported feeling healthy enough to move to a maintenance relationship with me. When Kason was 18, he returned to services with me for support via telehealth after moving to a new city with his family. One of Kason's struggles was attending to his own hygiene and activities of daily living (ADLs). During this time, Kason and I began telehealth for the first time. Kason introduced me to his gecko, cat, dog, and his aquarium full of various fish—marine biology had always been a special interest. Kason shared the names of his fish and care procedures for his fish: cleaning the aquarium, watching for fin rot, and the feeding and activity patterns of the fish. Kason demonstrated that he could hold fish food at the surface of the water and the fish would come to take it from his hand.

APPLICATION OF HART WITH KASON

SHARM: Kason initiated contact with his fish and integrated me into their relational dynamic by using the forward-facing camera on his phone during our session. The fish swam around the aquarium, flipping their fins in front of the camera. I was able to see the markings on their bodies and the beauty of their fin span in the water.

HARP: I reflected the effort Kason must have invested in creating such a pristine and interesting environment of the aquarium as well as knowing how to recognize the needs of the fish. I also reflected that the fish appeared to see him as a safe human as evidenced by their taking food directly from his hand. I identified this strength of Kason to recognize the needs of the fish and reflected his gentle compassion toward their needs. I then invited him to explore how he could recognize the needs of his own body. Kason began to share the underlying problems that kept him from maintaining his ADLs. He described teeth brushing as the feeling of tiny needles in his mouth. He described increased gender dysphoria when taking a shower, and feelings of overwhelm and dizziness when closing his eyes to wash his hair. We discussed the process of sensory overload and identified solutions to help him manage his felt sense of his body when completing self-care tasks. We identified that the discomfort of the tasks contributed to his avoidance of the tasks.

HARTI: Kason was able to have compassion for his own struggle when framed through the lens of sensory issues related to ASD. He expressed relief that avoiding self-care tasks was not a moral failing, rather, a human response toward an unpleasant experience. Kason experimented with strategies to help him maintain a sense of regulation such as listening to music through headphones when brushing teeth, experimenting with showering in a bathing suit, and using a shower chair when washing his hair. Moreover, he independently began studying polyvagal theory to help himself regulate his body during other times of sensory overload. We ended that episode of counseling after 6 months because Kason had processed the underlying problems that were keeping him from self-care tasks, and he had developed strategies to cope with the related discomfort.

TIFFANY OTTING'S TELEHEALTH SESSION WITH STAN AND MIMI THE CAT

Stan was a 16-year-old who identified as nonbinary (their/they/them) and was referred to me for AAT by their mother when they were 16 years old. Their presenting concerns were chronic sensory integration, identity development, and social problems related to level 1 autism spectrum disorder (ASD). Stan's previous counselor could only accommodate bi-weekly sessions and recommended the need for a higher dose of therapeutic intervention. Stan began in-person weekly counseling and worked with Pearl, our therapy dog. Occasionally, Stan's mother requested an online session for Stan to accommodate mom's work schedule. The example below occurred in one of those online days and was session 25 in the treatment sequence. Stan struggled with looking at themselves on camera. They experienced gender dysphoria as well as sensory overload when seeing themselves reflected on the screen.

Stan decided to turn off the camera about two-thirds of the way through our session. So, I set a limit with Stan for keeping the camera on because having the video on during telehealth is needed to maintain activity-based engagement through the virtual platform. Though this client was 16 years old, their primary form of communication remained in the realm of activity. They were still on the learning curve of expressing themselves with words. I acknowledged that Stan felt uncomfortable looking at themselves on the video, and that this was a video session, so "the camera was for staying on." I began to offer the option of having the camera facing away from Stan so that I could see the activities in which they were engaging; i.e., playing with plushies on their bed and playing with Mimi, the cat. Stan interjected before I finished the targeted alternatives and asked, "Can I just focus the camera on Mimi?" I replied that they could choose where they would like to focus the camera during our time, as long as it remained on.

APPLICATION OF HART WITH STAN

SHARM: Mimi was grooming herself for most of the 5 minutes she had been on camera. Stan exclaimed, "Mimi, can you stop cleaning yourself for a minute and just acknowledge us?!" Mimi continued grooming while Stan petted areas of her fur that were not being cleaned.
   HARP:

Stan: She doesn't care. She just cares about being clean.

Tiff: Mimi seems focused on getting clean.

Stan: Maybe she's just a germophobic cat? No, wait. She ate some of her own puke once. She's not a germophobe. That can't be it.

Tiff: Hmm. I wonder if you relate to this feeling. Mimi is deep, deep into a task. It doesn't matter what you do or say, she seems unable to transition out of that task. She is solely focused on finishing what she has in mind.

Stan: Gasp! Mimi is Autistic?! [laughing]

Tiff: [Laughing with] Sounds like you recognize that feeling!

Stan: You hear that, Mimi, we've both got the 'tism! You got it from me.

Tiff: I wonder if you are able to show her some compassion? Are you able to give her some empathy and allow her the space she needs right now?

Stan: Yeah! That thought just crossed my mind!

HARTI: Stan recognized that they were behaving toward Mimi in a way that other people behave toward them. For example, demanding that they be present in ways that make sense to others, but may be uncomfortable for Stan (i.e., eye contact, physical touch, physical closeness). Stan realized that similar to themselves, cats' behaviors are often misunderstood. Stan became curious about whether or not cats really could be autistic. For the last few minutes of the session, Stan researched this topic online. They confirmed that autism is not diagnosed in cats, *and* that persistent licking could be a sign of stress. They realized that their behavior toward Mimi may have contributed to Mimi's distress. They modeled compassion, empathy, and repair with Mimi. Through this SHARM, Stan was able to practice relational universality with Mimi (shared experience of self-soothing and hyper-focus), have curiosity about Mimi rather than making assumptions about Mimi's behavior, and demonstrate empathy toward and repair with Mimi. These are all skills that Stan was working on in their relationships with people!

TIFFANY OTTING'S TELEHEALTH SESSION WITH PAULA AND PARKER THE PUP

Paula was a long-time adult client and mental health professional who referred herself to me to work on concerns related to life transitions and professional development. With Paula, I worked with Wally, our therapy dog, in a nondirective manner until we transitioned to telehealth during the COVID-19 epidemic. Paula reported finding telehealth to be equally effective, and more convenient to her schedule. Paula has two dogs who occasionally make their presences known during our sessions. Through the years I observed relational moments, which I perceived as SHARMs, such as her dogs nuzzling her leg, wanting to sit in her lap, or barking to alert her about important sounds. Historically, when I attempted to process those relational moments, Paula dismissed them as distractions or "just dogs being dogs." From my research addressing the credibility of HART (Otting & Chandler, 2023), I remembered that dismissing SHARMS can be a sign of resistance in clients. Put another way, I had reflected a dynamic, or dynamics, that she was not ready to explore. The events below occurred in the fifth year of our therapeutic relationship, and the third year of working via telehealth.

APPLICATION OF HART WITH PAULA

SHARM: Paula was at a transitional point in the session. We had closed one conversation and she was about to open another when I noticed that Paula appeared distracted. I reflected a change in her affect, and Paula began laughing. She shared that, out of the camera frame, her medium-sized dog, Parker, was trying to jump onto the guest bed. She said that he was struggling, but undeterred! Parker jumped again, and again, and again trying to land on the bed. Finally, Parker gave himself a little more space for a running start and sprang onto the bed! Paula laughed with delight and offered Parker an encouraging cheer!

HARP: I noted Paula's encouragement of Parker's efforts and her shared joy when he arrived onto the bed. Paula affirmed that she felt warm feelings when seeing Parker content on the bed after his heroic efforts. I took this opportunity to reflect frequent themes in our work together: perfectionism and self-compassion. I invited Paula to share what it was like for her to watch Parker try and miss and try again to land on the bed. Paula shared that she felt the tension of his struggle as she watched, but that she felt herself rooting for Parker to make it onto the bed. She described encouraging him internally without verbalizing it aloud. She expressed that she felt like his cheerleader in that moment! I then inquired about her own self-talk when she is on the path of accomplishing a goal but has not yet arrived. Paula referred back "my perfectionist part," which we had explored at length in previous sessions. She acknowledged that she would never say the things to Parker that she says to herself. Paula had previously explored family origin culture that validated outcome over effort. On this day, I took the opportunity to offer psych-education about "fixed vs. growth mindset" and then I used screen share to display a video explaining the terms (Dweck, 2006; https://www.youtube.com/watch?v=Yl9TVbAal5s).

HARTI: Paula expressed relief at understanding the difference between fixed and growth mindsets. She also realized that she had been raised with values consistent in having a fixed mindset. Paula was able to use the Parker metaphor as a tool to remind herself to honor her own efforts and return to a growth mindset when she noticed that she was criticizing herself. I invited her to experiment with using her cheerleader voice for herself when she is amidst struggle. Now when she hears her negative self-talk, she asks herself if she would talk to Parker the way she is talking to herself. If not, she practices shifting her language to the level of compassion that she would offer her sweet Parker.

TERMINATION ISSUES IN AAT

Termination of counseling services may occur for several reasons. Perhaps the client has completed therapy goals and no new goals have been established. Maybe the client wishes to take a vacation from therapy for a while. Perhaps the number of counseling sessions has been limited based on insurance reimbursements or agency policy. Or maybe new therapeutic client goals require a skill outside the competency area of the existing practitioner, so a referral is required.

There are standard steps to take in the termination process in counseling to promote effective and ethical practice (Cormier and Nurius, 2003). When the termination time approaches, it is important to prepare the client in advance before the last session arrives. The therapist should initiate a discussion with the client about terminating the therapy process at least 2 weeks ahead of time. The discussion should address the client's feelings about termination. Address the positive changes the client has made and give the client credit for the progress achieved. Assist the client in exploring how positive changes will be maintained and how to avoid sabotaging progress. Determine if the client desires a follow-up session to check on how they are doing. Provide the client with names of referral resources if the client wishes to continue therapy with another counselor or needs other types of services in the community.

It is likely that a client who has worked with a therapy animal will have established a strong relationship with that animal. Thus, in the termination process, the counselor needs to facilitate discussion regarding the client's feelings about having worked with the animal and about no longer having contact with the animal. Provide opportunity for the client to say goodbye to the therapy animal. Sometimes, when appropriate, the therapist can provide the client with a small token of remembrance of the therapy animal to help bring some closure to the relationship. For instance, when the participants completed the juvenile detention program where I volunteered and were leaving, I gave them a photocopy of a collage of photographs of my therapy dogs Rusty and Dolly, and my cat Snowflake with whom they had frequent contact during AAA or AAT. When participants completed the equine-assisted counseling program where I volunteered, they were given a certificate of completion with a photograph of themselves riding the therapy horse they had partnered with during counseling sessions.

DOCUMENTATION AND AAT

Counselors are required to complete thorough and comprehensive session reports for each client with whom they work. A popular model for documenting each counseling session is the four-part SOAP plan, which includes a description of: (1) the client's subjective presentation; (2) the counselor's objective observations and other facts about the client; (3) the counselor's assessment and conceptualization of the client; and (4) the counselor's action plan for the client (Cameron and Turtle-Song, 2002). At a minimum, I recommend that the counselor include in every counseling session report the following information:

- Name of the client (more thorough descriptive information about the client can be recorded on the client intake and initial interview form).
- Date, time, and location of the therapy session.
- Name of the counselor or counselors providing the therapy.
- Type of therapy (e.g., individual, couples, group, or family).
- Any relevant diagnosis and ongoing presenting problems of the client.
- Current functional status of the client (e.g., assessment of any crisis state).
- Client's presentation during the session of issues and concerns.
- Counselor's conceptualization of the client's presented issues and concerns.
- Counselor's goals and plans for the client in the session.
- Interventions used by the counselor during the session.
- Assessment of the outcome of applied interventions.
- Counselor's discussion of any progress (or lack of progress) observed in the client.
- Any recommendations made to the client for homework or referral.

If this is a termination session, then a termination summary report should also be completed that overviews the client's presenting problems, status, any observed progress across all sessions, the client's status at time of termination, the reason for termination, and recommendations or referrals made to the client at termination. If any standardized assessment instruments were used as part of the therapy process, then a brief session report should be written for inclusion in the client's file that interprets the results of the assessment.

When incorporating a therapy animal into the counseling process, the counselor must be sure to include relevant information about the therapy animal in the counseling session report. The name of the animal, its species and breed, and its credentials should be included. Describe in the session report specific decisions to include the therapy animal in the counseling session, and discuss in detail what client–therapy animal interactions took place and what AAIs were used during the session. Finally, the counselor should discuss in the session report his or her assessment of the value and outcome of the client–therapy animal interactions and interventions. The information regarding client–therapy animal interactions and interventions can be interwoven into the counselor's typical session report; thus, including information relative to AAT requires little additional effort on the part of the counselor.

PROGRAM EVALUATION AND AAT

An important consideration for validating the incorporation of AAT into counseling is evaluating the success of therapeutic intervention. Counseling program evaluation can be accomplished through qualitative or quantitative measures (Heppner, Kivlighan, and Wampold, 1999; Marshall and Rossman, 1999). Quantitative results are preferable over qualitative measures for obtaining measurable and replicable results. Sometimes it is difficult to achieve statistical significance in counseling research because in counseling interventions there is typically a small number of subjects involved, and some of the statistical variance analyses, such as analysis of variance (ANOVA), analysis of covariance (ANCOVA), or multivariate analysis of variance (MANOVA), lend themselves better to a large sample size to achieve statistical significance when only two data collection points are used, such as with the commonly used pre- versus post-test design.

In counseling research, it is better to consider using statistical strategies that are more appropriate for small sample research (Hoyle, 1999). Due to small subject samples typical of research studies in counseling, it is important to analyze clinical significance, or effect size, and not just statistical significance (Kramer and Rosenthal, 1999; Thompson, 2002). Analysis of effect size may produce clinical significance even if statistical significance is not found. Also, a researcher applying a simple pre- versus post-test comparison loses much information about potential client change with this type of two-data-collection-points design. A greater likelihood of measuring change is possible with an intensive design, also referred to as a multiple repeated-measures design, for data collection and analysis. The intensive design is a linear, individual growth trajectory model and provides more information for analysis, such as individual growth and individual differences in growth across time, compared with measuring individual change with simple observations limited to two time points, as in the pre- versus post-test design (Maxwell, 1998; Willett, 1989, 1994). However, an intensive multiple repeated-measures design does not provide significant benefit over a two-point design (pre- versus post-test) unless at least five to six data points can be obtained (Kraemer and Thiemann, 1989).

Gathering client data across time requires taking repeated periodic measures of the client's behavior. This is not always plausible if the researcher is using lengthy assessment tools or the assessments must be gathered from others who might observe the client, such as parents or teachers. Making video recordings of multiple sessions with the client's permission and having independent, trained judges view and rate the recordings for certain behaviors is one way to accomplish repeated measures, but achieving high inter-rater reliability is often difficult. Another way to gather client data on multiple occasions is to use a quantified client session form with a scale for measuring client change. One example of a session-to-session measure of client change is the Psychosocial Session Form (PSF) developed by Chandler (2005b); a copy is provided in Appendix C for your convenient use. A description of this instrument is provided in the following section.

Numerous social and psychological assessment measures are available that may be appropriate for assessment of client progress depending on a particular therapeutic focus. In my presentation in Chapter 2 of various research performed on AAT, I have included the names of many assessments utilized by researchers to evaluate the intervention program under study. Also, a useful resource for finding assessment measures is the *Buros Mental Measurements Yearbook* (available at a college or university library or from Buros Institute of Mental Measurements online at www.unl.edu/buros).

PSYCHOSOCIAL SESSION FORM (PSF)

The PSF (developed by Chandler, 2005b; see Appendix C) is used to effectively measure change occurring as a result of AAT and to determine human behaviors of two types: positive social behaviors and negative social behaviors. The PSF provides three scores: positive social behavior score, negative social behavior score, and a total (overall) behavior score. The test is designed to be completed on a client by a therapist or therapy team at the conclusion of each therapy session. It is a method for tracking client social behavior change across treatment sessions. The amount of a behavior present in a session is rated on a Likert-type scale: 0 (none), 1 (very low), 2 (low), 3 (medium), 4 (high), and 5 (very high).

A Rasch analysis was conducted on the PSF instrument (with data of 140 participants) evaluating its usability for creating a behavior variable (Trotter, 2006); the analysis clearly indicated that the rated items followed an expected pattern. The analysis supported the ordering (clustering) of rated items. The positive items grouped together along the continuum, and the negative items grouped together along the continuum. The Rasch test–retest internal-consistency reliability yielded values in the high 0.90s, indicating a high degree of score reliability or consistency. A test–retest Pearson correlation of logit score values also yielded reliability values in the high 0.90s. This indicated that the logit score responses were consistent or reproducible for each session (Trotter, 2006). The PSF demonstrated construct validity with trend analysis (ANOVA) of the negative behaviors scores and the positive behaviors scores—as positive behaviors significantly increased across 12 data points (12 sessions), negative behaviors significantly decreased (Trotter, 2006). Additionally, in the same study, the PSF demonstrated convergent validity by producing, with 12 data points, similar behavior change patterns as pre- and post-test (two-point) comparisons of the Behavior Assessment System for Children (BASC), Self- and Parent Reports (Trotter, 2006); that is, positive behaviors significantly increased and negative behaviors significantly decreased across time on the PSF, BASC Self-Report, and the BASC Parent Report (Trotter, 2006). While these validity and reliability measures on the PSF are significant and contribute to the establishment of the PSF as a valid and reliable instrument, these measures are limited to one sample (140 elementary and middle school children at risk for academic and social failure) and one study (equine-assisted counseling). In another study, Ryan (2010) effectively used the PSF to demonstrate positive change in at-risk youth participating in equine-assisted education and counseling at a secondary school (school years 10 and 11) in Bedford, UK. Additional studies with additional populations and different treatments would further establish the validity and reliability of the PSF.

9

Equine-Assisted Counseling

Equine-assisted counseling (EAC) is the incorporation of horses into the counseling process to facilitate therapeutic outcome. With EAC, both individuals and groups interact with horses to facilitate the prevention or resolution of emotional and behavioral difficulties with themselves and others (Beck, 2000; EAGALA, n.d.b). Research has demonstrated that mental health therapy with horses can assist participants in ways unique and superior to more passive counseling formats (Trotter et al., 2008). EAC provides a safe and secure environment that nurtures inner healing and encourages optimal growth and development. EAC can help individuals of all ages and backgrounds become stronger in communication, problem solving, self-confidence, conflict resolution, and relationships (Kersten and Thomas, 2004). O'Connor (2006) suggests:

> [I]t is the horse's differences to the socialized man that brings about the successes that the traditional therapist cannot achieve. Horses allow us to unite unconditionally with another living being. We can take our masks off without fear of rejection. The horse has no expectations, prejudices, or motives. All of these traits allow the patient to open up, reveal their selves, and receive feedback from the horse's responses. This is the key to healing: expressing true feelings and interactions with another being to develop a true self-concept.
>
> (p. 5)

Horses are well suited to their role as therapy animals as a result of their ability to perceive, evaluate, and respond to social behaviors—a necessary skill for survival as a prey animal and useful for coping in a herd with a competitive social order. This translates into an ability to detect and immediately respond to emotional and behavioral presentations by other animals as well as humans. A horse's ability to detect and quickly respond to social cues means that it can act as a mirror for a human participant in EAC, and the horse's behavior in response to the participant reinforces or confronts the participant's behavior (EAGALA, n.d.b). Horses are much more effective at confronting behaviors and attitudes than people due to their keen ability to detect and respond immediately and honestly to nonverbal and verbal communication (Irwin and Weber, 2001). Also, the opportunity to interact with such a majestic animal as a horse provides the client with unique opportunities to explore and address issues that are not possible with other animals or counseling experiences.

DOI: 10.4324/9781003260448-9

Horses signal their perceptions with vocalizations and nonverbal behaviors. Thus, understanding horse communication and behavior is very important to effectively facilitate EAC. In addition to information covered in Chapter 6, some helpful resources for understanding and interpreting horse communication include: *How Horses Feel and Think* by Marlitt Wendt (2011); *Trust Instead of Dominance* by Marlitt Wendt (2011); *Walking the Way of the Horse*: *Exploring the Power of the Horse–Human Relationship* by Leif Hallberg (2008); and *Equine Behavior* by Paul McGreevy (2012).

There are several approaches to EAC. Some programs involve a client working with a horse only on the ground, meaning the horse is not mounted. Other therapy programs have a mixture of some groundwork and some mounted activities. Some programs have clear, structured, and directed activities with a horse, while other programs are less directed, leaving plenty of space and opportunity for spontaneous relational engagement between client and horse. Some counseling programs have activities involving a variety of items to be used while engaging with a horse (for example different play therapy items), while other programs have very few items with which to engage a horse (maybe a halter, lead rope, or grooming brush only).

It is imperative that the EAC be provided by a well-trained and properly credentialed therapist. In addition to holding a professional degree and license as a mental health practitioner, one should have knowledge and certification in equine-assisted intervention (EAI). The two largest organizations that provide training and certification in this field are the Equine Growth and Learning Association (EAGALA; www.eagala.org) and the Professional Association for Therapeutic Horsemanship, International (PATH, Intl.; www.pathintl.org).

The following books present many ideas and techniques for equine-assisted interventions with various populations:

- *The Clinical Practice of Equine-Assisted Therapy: Including Horses in Human Healthcare*, Leif Hallberg (2017a).
- *The Equine-Assisted Therapy Workbook: A Learning Guide for Professionals and Students*, Leif Hallberg (2017b).
- *Harnessing the Power of Equine-Assisted Counseling*, Kay S. Trotter (Ed.) (2011).
- *Equine-Assisted Mental Health Interventions: Harnessing Solutions to Common Problems*, Kay S. Trotter and Jennifer Baggerly (Eds.) (2018a).
- *Equine-Assisted Mental Health for Healing Trauma*, Kay S. Trotter and Jennifer Baggerly (Eds.) (2018b).
- *Equine-Assisted Counseling and Psychotherapy*, Hallie Sheade (2020).

Leif Hallberg is an internationally acclaimed author, licensed mental health professional, educator, and avid lover of nature and animals. Her professional career and life's work have centered around researching the human–equine bond and studying the inclusion of horses in mental health and learning. Leif is considered one of the foremost leading experts in the equine-assisted mental health (EAMH) and equine-assisted learning (EAL) field. She has been involved with these fields since their inception in the early 1990s and has developed a reputation over the past 20 plus years for her broad-reaching and objective study. It has been Leif's goal to clarify, define, and objectively describe the complexity and diversity of the human–equine relationship and the professional applications of this relationship. Her books (2008, 2017a, and 2017b) are used by colleges and universities around the world and inform professionals and researchers about critical issues facing the industry. Leif offers a unique approach to EAMH and EAL called Embodied Awareness in Action™. This model combines an understanding of biophilic connections with mindfulness practices, principles of somatic (or embodied) awareness, and experiential learning—all within the context of safe,

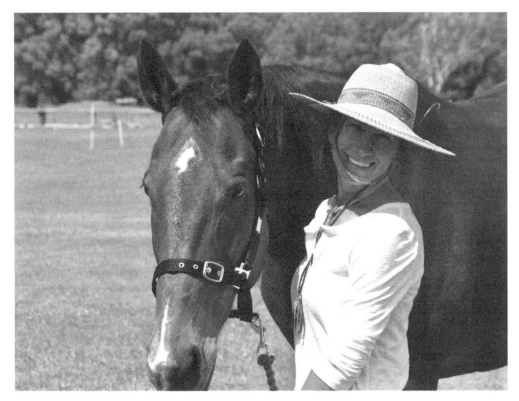

Figure 9.1 Leif Hallberg is a licensed mental health counselor and an internationally recognized author, consultant, and educator. Her professional career has centered on studying the human–equine bond and the practice of equine-assisted activities and therapy.

(*Source:* photo courtesy of Leif Hallberg.)

respectful, and relationally oriented equine and nature interactions. This approach offers students a complex and dynamic skill set that can be effectively applied to both clinical practice and learning environments with and without horses. As a riding instructor and horse trainer first, Leif relies upon both the science and study of horses and her practical experience to put understanding horses and equine welfare at the top of her priorities. Her training and professional development programs are also aligned with the American Counseling Association's *Animal-Assisted Therapy in Counseling Competencies* (Stewart et al., 2016) and champion the need for extensive competency especially in the areas of clinical intentionality and understanding each species as unique and different and every animal as his/her own individual being.

For safety and welfare considerations, it is recommended that EAC sessions involve at least two professionals to be present working as a team with a client and horse. The first professional is a credentialed counselor and the second professional is an equine specialist. An equine specialist should be competent in working with horses, especially knowledgeable of herd dynamics. Ideal characteristics of an equine specialist involved in EAC include: conveys genuineness, warmth, and empathy; is patient, open, and flexible; controls any desire to direct, probe, or teach so as not to affect the flow of a session being conducted by a counselor; and is fully alert and present during the session. The equine specialist is responsible for the physical and emotional safety of clients and horses; evaluating the area for potential stressors and safety issues; monitoring and managing equine stress levels; and overseeing the equine welfare and husbandry. Both the counselor and the equine specialist should be very familiar with how to communicate with a horse and reading horse body language. Some helpful information on these topics was provided in Chapter 6 of this book.

RESEARCH SUPPORTING THE EFFICACY OF EAC

EAI programs, including EAC and equine-assisted psychotherapy (EAP), are varied in their approach. Not all EAI programs involve counseling or psychotherapy yet can still show to be effective in assisting participants regarding emotional and relational issues. Some EAI programs involve mounted activities while others prefer all work to be done on the ground, that is, no mounting of the horse is involved. Research study of EAC and EAP is somewhat scarce, but there have been notable successes in demonstrating clinical efficacy. Bachi (2012) reviewed some existing research in EAI and concluded that "most of the research suffers from methodological problems that compromise its rigor" (p. 364). Bachi suggested that future research in EAI consider "methodological solutions to improve evaluation studies, use of grounded theory method to develop theory, as well as applying attachment theory to the human–horse context, which may offer insight about the underlying processes for change" (Bachi, 2012, p. 364).

Kendall et al. (2015) performed a systematic review of literature published between 2008 and 2012 involving the psychological effects of equine-assisted interventions or interactions. The researchers concluded that EAIs were very promising, especially in terms of child/adolescent social and behavioral issues, and perhaps adult affective disorders. However, the authors pointed to several methodological problems with the studies reviewed and concluded that more randomized controlled trials were greatly needed in this field.

Russell-Martin (2006) compared the effectiveness of equine-facilitated couples' therapy with that of solution-focused couples' therapy, as measured by relational adjustment scores on the Dyadic Adjustment Scale (DAS) developed by Spanier (1976). A total of ten couples participated in each group (Russell-Martin, 2006), either equine-facilitated therapy (EFT) or solution-focused therapy (SFT). The mean age of participants in each group was approximately 29 years. The DAS was administered three times: at pretest, after the third treatment session, and after the sixth and final treatment session. Treatment sessions were 1 hour in length for both groups and held once weekly for 6 weeks. The EFT consisted of the following couple activities: haltering a horse, horse billiards, obstacle course, and extended appendages.

The activity of haltering a horse involved providing each couple with a halter and lead rope and asking couple partners to catch and halter the horse to the best of their ability with no other direction or preparation. The horse billiards involved couples working together to move horses to areas of an arena designated by the therapist (like pockets on a billiards table) and to do so without using ropes, touching the horses, or bribing the horses. The obstacle course described by Russell-Martin was actually combining two exercises together: "Life's Little Obstacles" with "Give and Take." This activity involved couples being directed to: build an alleyway in an arena and fill it with a variety of obstacles (e.g., poles, hay bales, food, and jumps); pick a horse to work with; place the horse at the entrance to the obstacle course with a lightweight lead rope or string attached to each side of the halter that each partner of the couple holds at the extended end; and then guide the horse through the alley of obstacles (Life's Little Obstacles) by tugging and relaxing the lead rope (Give and Take). Too much pressure on the lead rope/string by either participant will cause it to break, and too little pressure will fail to lead the horse or allow the horse to go in the wrong direction. Finally, the activity of extended appendages involved having the couple link arms and, while using only the free arm and hand, to work together to halter and saddle a horse.

Russell-Martin (2006) used MANOVA to analyze data for the study as well as individual ANOVAs and chi-square tests. Results demonstrated that the first two administrations of the DAS did not yield significant differences between the EFT and SFT groups, but the third administration of the DAS (performed after the completion of all 6 weeks of treatment) did result in significant differences, with the EFT group scoring higher on relational adjustment of the DAS. Russell-Martin (2006) suggested that while both EFT and SFT were effective as treatment approaches, EFT was more effective for couples' relational adjustment, as measured by the DAS.

Another important study that demonstrated clinical efficacy of EAC was performed with 164 elementary- and middle school children at risk for academic and social failure (Trotter et al., 2008). This study demonstrated efficacy of EAC by comparing it with an established classroom-based counseling curriculum. Students identified as being at high risk for academic or social failure participated in 12 weekly counseling sessions. A comparison of within-group pre- and post-treatment scores on the Basic Assessment System for Children, Self-Report and Parent Report (Reynolds and Kamphaus, 1992) for externalizing, internalizing, maladaptive, and adaptive behaviors determined that the EAC made statistically significant improvements in 17 behavior areas, whereas the classroom-based group showed statistically significant improvement in only five areas, and four of these five were different areas. Between-group results additionally indicated the EAC treatment to be superior by showing more statistically significant improvement in seven areas when compared directly with classroom-based counseling. A repeated-measures analysis of the EAC participants' social behavior ratings on the Psychosocial Session Form (Chandler, 2005b) showed statistically significant improvement with increases in positive behaviors and decreases in negative behaviors. A more detailed description of results from this study (Trotter et al., 2008) is provided in the research chapter of this book (see Chapter 2).

Bachi, Terkel, and Teichman (2011) examined the effects of equine-facilitated psychotherapy (EFP) on at-risk adolescents at a residential treatment facility in Israel. Fourteen resident adolescents comprised the treatment group, and were compared with a matched group of 15 residents who did not receive EFP (control). The treatment comprised a weekly individual EFP session of 50 minutes each over a period of 7 months. Interventions included touching and grooming the horse to make a social connection and riding the horse for a physical dimension to facilitate the establishment of a healthy physical self-image and the healing of the damaged emotional and sensory motor elements. The study found a trend of positive change in all four research parameters within the treatment group: self-image, self-control, trust, and general life satisfaction (Bachi, Terkel, and Teichman, 2011).

Pendry and Roeter (2012) conducted a randomized controlled trial to determine if an 11-week equine-facilitated learning (EFL) program enhanced the social competence of school children in the fifth and eighth grades. There were 64 participants and sessions were conducted in a small group format. Sessions were 90 minutes in length, four times a week in the afternoon on weekdays. Participants received significantly higher post-test scores relative to pretest scores with moderate effect size. Activities included observing horses and herd dynamics, moving and leading horses, interpreting horse communication, riding and driving horses, horse massage, horsemanship, and obstacle courses. Program goals addressed leadership, respect, communication, trust, boundaries, overcoming challenges, enhancing self-regulation, and relaxation (Pendry and Roeter, 2012).

Pendry et al. (2014) performed a similar study of an 11-week EFL program to determine if there was improvement in social competence and behavior for school children in the fifth and eighth grades. Fifty-three children were in the EFL treatment group and 60 were in the waitlist control group. Sessions were once a week and 90 minutes long involving team-focused activities. EFL included observing horses and herd dynamics, moving horses, leading horses, driving horses, horse massage, horsemanship, riding, and moving a horse through an obstacle course. Results showed significant improvement in social competence with moderate treatment effects for the EFL group (Pendry et al., 2014).

Pendry, Smith, and Roeter (2014) investigated the effects of an 11-week EFL program on salivary cortisol levels of children. Fifty-three were in the equine intervention group and 60 were in the waitlist control group. The equine intervention was once a week, 90-minute sessions. Children in the equine intervention group had significantly lower afternoon cortisol and lower total cortisol concentration at post-test, compared with waitlist children (Pendry, Smith, and Roeter, 2014).

Bowers and MacDonald (2001) performed EAC with at-risk children and adolescents and found statistically significant decreases in depression following EAC; observations of participants also yielded increased like skills and improvements with communication, honesty, respect, awareness of power, and control struggles. Holmes et al. (2011) explored the benefits of equine-assisted activities (EAAs) for adolescents with emotional, behavioral, or learning difficulties. Ten adolescent males and one adolescent female attended a racehorse rehabilitation facility interacting with both live and model horses. A significant reduction in self-reported anxiety occurred but there was no significant improvement in measured self-esteem (Holmes et al., 2011).

Klontz et al. (2007) examined the effects of equine-assisted experiential therapy (EAET) on distress and psychological wellbeing for 31 adult participants enrolled in an experiential therapy program. EAET combines experiential therapy with specific equine activities to give clients the opportunity to work through unfinished business, relieve psychological distress, live more fully in the present, and change destructive patterns of behavior. In EAET, horses serve as catalysts and metaphors to allow clinical issues to surface. The core experiential treatment modality in EAET is based on the theory and techniques of psychodrama. Participants were involved in such activities as choosing a horse, horse grooming, mounted work, walking/trotting, lunging, and equine games that were combined with traditional experiential therapy tools of role-playing, sculpting, role reversal, mirroring, and gestalt techniques. The treatment program provided 28 hours of EAET in a group format (eight participants per group) across a 4.5-day residential program. Participants were assessed pre- and post-treatment and at a 6-month follow-up. Assessment instruments were the Brief Symptom Inventory (BSI) (Derogatis, 1993) and the Personal Orientation Inventory (POI) (Shostrom, 1974).

Using multivariate analysis of variance of results, participants showed reduction in psychological distress evidenced by significant decreases on the Global Severity Index Scale of the BSI from pre- to post-test to follow-up. Again, using multivariate analysis of variance, participants showed enhanced wellbeing evidenced by a significant increase on the POI from pre- to post-test and maintenance of the enhanced state at the 6-month follow-up. The researchers concluded that, as predicted, participants showed significant and stable reductions in overall psychological distress and enhancements in psychological wellbeing as a result of equine-assisted experiential group therapy. The study did not involve a control or comparison group; thus, it is difficult to ascertain how much improvement was a result of treatment effects. The promising results included participants reporting being: (1) more oriented in the present, (2) better able to live more fully in the here and now, (3) less burdened by regrets, guilt, and resentments, (4) less focused on fears related to the future, (5) more independent, and (6) more self-supportive (Klontz et al., 2007).

Lanning et al. (2014) investigated the effects of 9 weeks of participation in EAA on the behavior of children diagnosed with autism spectrum disorder. Of a total of 25 participants, 13 (aged 4–15 years) were in the EAA treatment group, and 12 (aged 5–14 years) were in the comparison group which was a nonequine intervention. Quantitative data were collected five times using two instruments, the Pediatric Quality of Life 4.0 Generic Core

Scales (PedsQL 4.0) (Varni, Seid, and Kurtin, 2001) and the Child Health Questionnaire (CHQ) (Raat et al., 2005). Parents of the children noted significant improvements in their child's physical, emotional, and social functioning following the first 6 weeks of EAA. The children participating in the nonequine program demonstrated improvement in behavior, but to a lesser degree (Lanning et al., 2014).

Memishevikj and Hodzhikj (2010) utilized EAI to improve psychosocial functioning of four children (two boys and two girls) who had autism: horsemanship activities, riding, and EAP. Sessions were once a week for 10 weeks. Each session was 30 minutes in length. Horsemanship activities were aimed at introducing and bonding children with horses through the grooming activities. These activities usually lasted for about 5–10 minutes. Riding and exercises included mounting the horse, riding for a couple of circles in the arena, and doing different kinds of exercises on the horses. This activity lasted for 10 minutes. EAP tasks were given to the children on the ground and included getting the horse from one side of the arena to the other and going with the horse across obstacles. The results of the study revealed that the therapy had positive effects for two of the four children. The improvement was reported in the domains of speech, socialization, sensory/cognitive awareness, and health/behavior (Memishevikj and Hodzhikj, 2010).

Signal et al. (2013) evaluated the efficacy of an adjunct EFT program run by a sexual assault referral center in Queensland, Australia. Their aim was to reduce depressive symptoms across three age groups: 15 children (aged 8–11 years), 15 adolescents (aged 12–17 years), and 14 adults (aged 19–50 years). Ten of the 44 participants identified as Indigenous Australians. Measures of depression, using the Child Depression Index or Beck Depression Inventory, were taken at three times; time of intake, after completion of in-clinic counseling but prior to commencing EFT, and after completion of EFT. Individual in-clinic counseling was once per week for an average of 6 weeks for children and adolescents. The adults participated in individual in-clinic counseling ranging from 2 weeks to more than 12 months. The EFT program was 90 minutes, once per week, for 9–10 weeks. EFT consisted of two therapists and four horses, and interventions were based on an EAGALA experiential model. EFT activities were all ground-based and included: basic horsemanship and communication, moving a horse in a circle, and moving a horse through an obstacle course.

> What emerges during these activities are patterns of thinking, reactions/responses to different situations and outcomes, and reactions to dynamics within the family group or within the group of participants. Each exercise is designed to address issues such as: trust, communication, boundaries, observation, body language, attitude and self-perception and all activities are dynamic, not static, to accommodate the needs of each group of participants, be it their age, developmental stage, disability, current mental health status or their cultural background.
>
> (Signal et al., 2013, p. 27)

Comparison of change scores showed EFT proved to result in greater decreases in depressive scores than that seen from time of intake to after in-clinic counseling (Signal et al., 2013).

Kemp et al. (2014) further investigated the efficacy of an adjunct EFT program run by a sexual assault referral center in Queensland, Australia. Their aim was to reduce psychological distress with two age groups: 15 children (aged 8–11 years) and 15 adolescents (aged 12–17 years). Several different measures were utilized: the Children's Depressive Inventory, the Child Behavior Checklist, the Trauma Symptom Checklist, the Beck Depression Inventory, and the Beck Anxiety Inventory. Measures were taken three times: at time of intake, after completion of in-clinic counseling but prior to commencing EFT, and after completion of EFT. The duration of the EFT program was 9–10 weeks. Significant improvements were found in functioning between in-clinic counseling and after completion of EFT across all psychometric measures and for both age groups. No or nonsignificant improvements were found between intake and completion of in-clinic counseling. Researchers concluded that overall, "results show that EFT proved an effective therapeutic approach for the children and adolescents referred to the service. Of particular note was the finding that efficacy was similar across gender, age and Indigenous/non-Indigenous status" (Kemp et al., 2014, p. 558).

Carlsson, Ranta, and Traeen (2014) conducted in-depth interviews with staff and clients who participated in an equine-assisted social work program in Sweden. The nine client participants were part of a residential program for young women with self-harm problems (aged 15–21 years). The content of the interviews revealed that both the staff members and clients had to become more aware of and regulate their emotions so as not to alienate the horse. Also, for clients there was decreased resistance to changing behavior. In conclusion:

> The horse seemed to set the framework for the interaction between the staff and young women. . . . A relationship based on empathy, trust, respect and negotiation, where clients shared private matters, resulted in the perception of a more authentic relationship.
> (Carlsson, Ranta, and Traeen, 2014, p. 19)

EAC TECHNIQUES

EAC programs may involve a mixture of both equine-based (horse directly involved) and nonequine-based (horse not directly involved) activities. Clinical processing after every EAC activity, whether it is with or without direct horse involvement, is critical to the counseling experience. Personal insight for participants can result in learning about their attitudes toward their temptations, addictions, or other destructive thought processes, and, as a result, they can identify thoughts, feelings, and behaviors that will assist them to either: (1) resist temptation or relapse, (2) cope with frustration or internalize low self-worth, (3) meet challenges or surrender to failures, and (4) conquer fears or avoid opportunities (Trotter et al., 2008). EAC lessons can focus on practicing healthy communication, forming healthy relationships, developing problem-solving skills, and searching for creative solutions. The skill of the process leaders is a key to the success of the program for the participants. Counseling processing techniques used by the counselor during or after every activity facilitate participants' ability to relate personal insight into their own lives.

Karol (2007) described six aspects of the equine-assisted experience conducive to psychotherapeutic work that included: (1) the existential or "actual" experience; (2) the unique experience of being in relationship with the horse; (3) the experience of the therapeutic relationship with the clinician; (4) nonverbal experiences in relation to communication with the horse; (5) preverbal/primitive experience such as contact comfort, touch, and rhythm; and (6) the therapeutic use of metaphor. Equine activities included grooming and riding around the arena while accompanied by the therapist. When opportunity presented, the therapist related the client's expressions and experiences to the struggles in the client's life (Karol, 2007).

Keren Bachi (2013) applies attachment theory to EFP. This work describes the fit between central features of EFP and several of the primary concepts of attachment-based psychotherapy, such as: secure base and haven of safety through the provision of a holding environment, affect mirroring, mentalizing and reflective functioning, and nonverbal communication and body experience (Bachi, 2012).

Tracie Faa-Thompson (2012) is a social worker who uses equine-assisted play therapy with children, adolescents, and adults in the UK, near the Scottish border. See Figures 9.2

through 9.5. She also frequently works in collaboration with Risë Van Fleet from the United States, and together they have developed a specialist training course for play therapists using dogs and horses as co-therapists. Faa-Thompson (2012) developed a safe touch program to teach sexually abused clients to value their body and themselves. This is an approximately ten-session model, where the first four sessions are spent on the ground and becoming familiar with the horse before progressing to riding; clients then work first with the saddle and then bareback so they can feel the horse skin to skin. Treatment goals are: (1) learn safe and appropriate touch; (2) gain an increased sense of self; (3) find the opportunity to experience close contact with others without having a sexual element; (4) experience feeling safe and trusting others, both human and animal; (5) increase the sense of acceptance by others; (6) experience being in control; and (7) have the courage to begin new relationships (Faa-Thompson, 2012, p. 55).

Hallie Sheade (2015, 2020, 2021) pioneered two innovative models for the practice of EAC: Relational Equine-Partnered Counseling (REPC) and Equine-Partnered Play Therapy (EPPT). Sheade founded her practice, Steps with Horses, in north Texas. She incorporates a variety of both full-size and miniature horses in her work. The EAIs used by Sheade and her staff encompass all groundwork, meaning participants do not mount the horse.

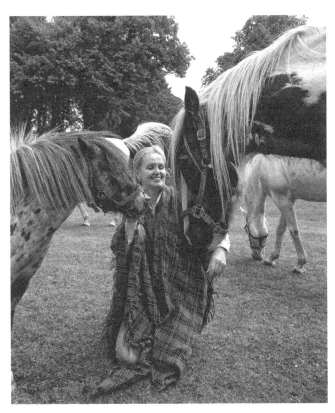

Figure 9.2 Tracie Faa-Thompson is a social worker and equine-assisted play therapist practicing in the UK.

(*Source:* photo courtesy of Tracie Faa-Thompson.)

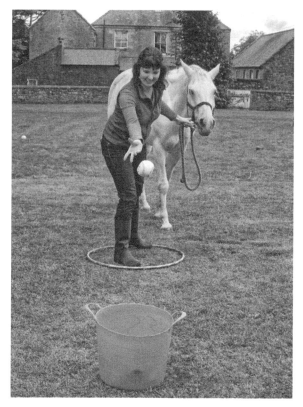

Figure 9.3 Equine-assisted adult play therapy: feelings bucket activity.

(*Source:* photo courtesy of Tracie Faa-Thompson and Risë Van Fleet.)

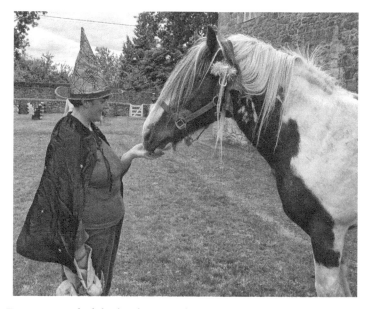

Figure 9.4 Equine-assisted adult play therapy: a horse is a majestic play companion in therapy.

(*Source:* photo courtesy of Tracie Faa-Thompson and Risë Van Fleet.)

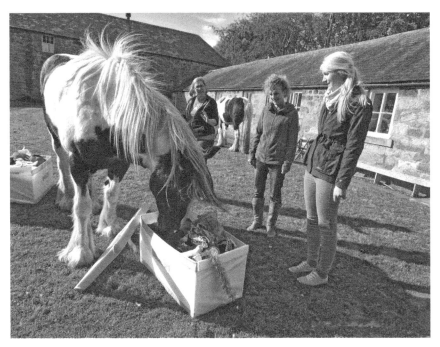

Figure 9.5 Equine-assisted adult play therapy: "Let's get some toys and clothes out and play."

(*Source:* photo courtesy of Tracie Faa-Thompson and Risë Van Fleet.)

Relational equine-partnered counseling (REPC) is an integrative, trans-theoretical approach, incorporating aspects of humanistic counseling with a focus on working within the relationship between participant and horse(s). The approach is developmental as the activities for each session are informed by progress made in the previous session and guided by the nature of the client's relationship with the horse(s) over time. REPC is a counseling approach facilitated by a counselor with the addition of horse(s) and an equine specialist. This approach has four domains: (a) experiential, (b) relational, (c) physiological, and (d) spiritual.

Activities may be used to target specific goals during the counseling session such as (a) relationship-building, (b) nurturing, (c) mastery and challenge, (d) self-regulation, stress inoculation, and mindfulness, and (e) creativity and free expression. These activities may include choosing a horse, haltering the horse, leading the horse, grooming the horse, being with the horse, moving the horse, bathing the horse, and stress inoculation or relaxation activities. Verbal responses from the treatment team include (a) tracking the client's work with the horse, (b) reflecting the client's feelings, (c) facilitating increased autonomy and decision-making, (d) utilizing immediacy, (e) providing psychoeducation [. . .], (f) using encouragement and esteem-building responses, (g) reflecting on the relationship between horse and client, (h) reflecting the horse's behaviors, (i) reflecting the horse's potential feelings and intentions, (j) expanding the meaning to outside the counseling session, and (k) facilitating relaxation and mindfulness techniques in partnership with the horse to provide feedback.

(Sheade, 2015, pp. 89 and 91)

In Hallie Sheade's performance of EPPT with children, she prefers to involve miniature horses rather than full-size horses (personal communication, July 2015). She recommends that a variety of miniature horses be involved of varied colors, genders, and personalities. Having multiple horses makes for varied interaction dynamics for a client and helps prevent burnout for the horses. She further recommends that the horses be thoroughly desensitized to all toys and in ways the toys may be played with before the horses participate in therapy. The play area should be: a warm atmosphere that appears friendly to the child; a clearly defined area in a location in which a child can make noise; and a space that is private from view and sound from parents and onlookers. It should have a place for toy storage and display, adequate flooring, and temperature control. The toys should represent multiple categories, such as real life, acting-out aggressive-release, and creative expression and emotional release. There should be an inclusion of additional horse-themed toys to provide further opportunities for a child to connect with a horse and project experiences onto the horse (H. Sheade, personal communication, July 2015). See Figures 9.6 and 9.7.

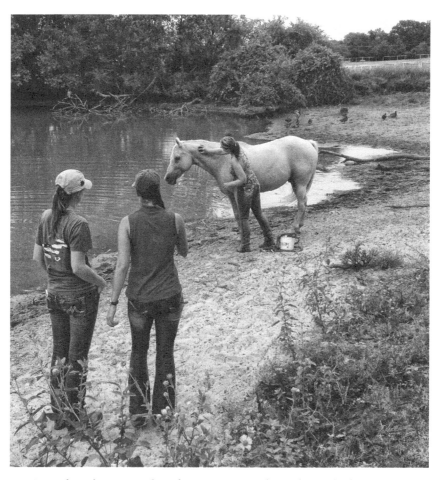

Figure 9.6 Counselors observe as a client forms a trusting relationship with a horse loose in a pasture.

(*Source:* photo courtesy of Hallie Sheade.)

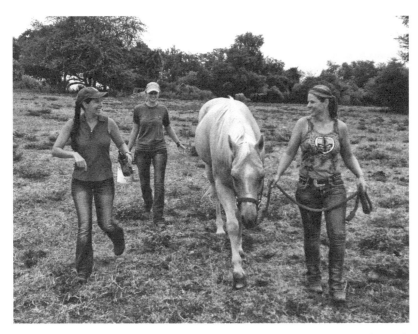

Figure 9.7 At an EAC intervention a client has successfully haltered and is leading a horse from pasture. Counselors: Hallie Sheade (*left*) and Lindsay Box (*center*); with a client (role played here by Brooke Knox).

(*Source:* photo courtesy of Hallie Sheade.)

There are a number of activities utilized in EAC but early in the treatment process it is always important to establish participants' expectations and discuss ways to be safe around horses. One way to accomplish this is with the "Five-Finger Contract" exercise where each finger of one hand represents an important safety rule for self and others (Trotter et al., 2008). The purpose of the five-finger contract is: (1) to understand and create safe and respectful behavioral norms under which to operate, (2) to gain a commitment to those norms by everyone in the group with a verbal and tactile agreement, and (3) to accept a shared responsibility for the maintenance of those norms. This is a simple way to establish and teach respectful behaviors expected of each participant, thereby creating an emotionally and physically safe environment supported by all. Along with safety issues, participants are introduced to the horse's world which covers topics such as the nature of horses, horse communication, horse body language, horse body parts, and in-depth horse safety. During activities on horse safety, participants are taught how to mount and dismount, including an emergency dismount, how to tie a safety knot to secure a horse to a rail, how to walk safely behind a horse, and about the "gas pedal and brake for a horse" (how to get a horse to stop and start) when one is mounted and when one is in an arena with horses who are moving about freely. "Horse Body Parts" (D. Goodwin-Bond, personal communication, April 2005; Trotter, 2012) is an exercise where participants work together to place small adhesive labels of horse body parts on the correct part of the horse using an anatomy guide. This exercise is educational and contributes to knowledge valuable for good horsemanship. When all of the labels have been applied, part of the discussion can be about functional (respectful) and dysfunctional (stereotyping) forms of labeling people.

An activity designed to be performed relatively early in the treatment protocol is "Building a Relationship With Your Horse" (D. Goodwin-Bond, personal communication, April 26, 2005), which allows participants to pick the horse they want to work with for the duration of the treatment regime for exercises that involve grooming, riding, or other human–horse pairing. For this exercise participants interact with all of the therapy horses that are loose in a small arena. Adequate time is allowed for the social mingle with no structure applied. It requires involvement and participation by both humans and horses. Getting close with their horses and learning about their horses' instinctual, natural, nonverbal cues can help participants understand their horses and generalize this to better understand themselves and other participants in the group. Group processing at the end of the exercise naturally leads to an exploration of how the basics of horse interactions can be translated into the basics of people interactions. For example, "Do you say what you mean and mean what you say?" The therapy team facilitates discussion of how the horse's actions and reactions can help the participant to recognize reinforcing cues and rewards that enhance relationship building, and also the behaviors that get in the way or interfere with relationship building. There ensues in-depth discussion around how, like people, horses treat you based on the way you communicate. Elements of communication that can be explored with the group include: (1) active listening with both the ears and the eyes, (2) attention to nonverbal cues regarding the horse's body language and the participant's body language, and (3) communicating to the horse that you are safe to be with or that you are not safe to be with (Trotter et al., 2008). The horse–human relationship has the opportunity to be strengthened during several interactive equine activities that take place over the course of treatment, and the relationship flourishes in an environment of support and honesty that benefits both the individual and the group. A common clinical observation from this exercise is that participants will often be drawn instinctively to a horse that has characteristics similar to their own and, as a result, the horse often dramatizes the participants' inner struggles and relationship issues by magnifying and mirroring what they need to recognize in themselves.

I volunteered as an assistant co-counselor for over 2 years at an EAC program in north Texas. One day, in the very early phase of treatment, EAC staff requested the group of adolescent male clients to spend time with each horse of a small group in a corral and decide which horse they wanted to partner up with for the remainder of the therapy program. Adolescents were instructed to keep their choice to themselves until instructed to share their choice in the group process so that choices would not be influenced by one another. The horses varied in size and personality, so it was informative to see which juvenile picked which horse.

In this group of six adolescents from the county juvenile detention center, there was one fellow we will call Sam who was much smaller than the others. Instead of choosing one of the full-sized horses to work with, he requested to be able to work with a small mule named Mabel that was watching the group from a nearby corral. Of the several groups of adolescents, male and female, that I worked with from the juvenile detention center, this was the first time one of the adolescents had requested to work with a mule instead of with a horse. The mule had been used before with smaller children from a local school, so the therapy staff agreed to let Sam work with her. It was fascinating to watch Sam as he led Mabel around the corral where the bigger horses were. The bigger horses would approach Mabel to try to bother her, and Sam would try to make himself as big as he could by standing tall, strutting with big steps, raising his shoulders, moving his arms out away from his body, and shooing the bigger horses away. When Sam was back at the juvenile facility and he was feeling intimidated or bullied by the bigger fellows, he took on this same posture. Thus, with Mabel, Sam was transferring that same behavior into his relationship with the small mule, except in this case he was acting as the mule's protector from the bigger horses. Sam had quickly transferred his issues of being small and maybe feeling somewhat inadequate onto the mule. He was obviously trying to work with these personal issues through his relationship with Mabel, and whether he was conscious of doing so is uncertain and not really pertinent one way or the other; the opportunity to face and work on the issues was the important thing. The therapy staff felt that this experience with Mabel would be very therapeutic for Sam but also recognized that in some ways working with a small mule did not challenge Sam to overcome the hesitation he may have to establish a trusting and positive relationship with someone or something much bigger than himself. Thus, one ultimate goal was to eventually move Sam to working with one of the bigger horses. In fact, this was accomplished by the midpoint of therapy when Sam agreed to mount a sorrel and white paint horse and soon achieved being comfortable with the larger horse and demonstrated confident competence in horsemanship. It is believed that Sam became ready to take on the challenge of interacting with and riding a horse after proving to himself that he could manage a larger animal by protecting his mule from the larger horses.

At the EAC program in north Texas where I volunteered as a co-counselor, I observed that participants often chose to partner with a therapy horse that was best suited to them, whether they realized it or not. For instance, in one group where I assisted, the two most stubborn and cantankerous adolescent females soon discovered they had chosen to work with the most stubborn and cantankerous horse. The therapy horses each had different and distinct personalities that became more obvious after one had a chance to spend more time with them. Some horses had more difficulty trusting new riders and were not very cooperative at first. Some horses were stubborn; on some days not wanting to be haltered or ridden. Some were very friendly from the onset but a bit mischievous, trying to steal hats off heads or nibbling at hair. Some of the horses tended to try to boss the other horses around. Whatever horse the adolescent chose, the desire to develop and maintain a positive relationship with a powerful being with an independent mind of its own was a very difficult yet important life lesson for an adolescent. In trying to establish a trusting relationship with a troubled adolescent without the presence of a therapy animal, a counselor is likely met with great resistance from the adolescent. Providing opportunity for a troubled adolescent to form a trusting relationship with a therapy horse first, a counselor is met with motivation to participate from the adolescent and a desire to change for success. Undoubtedly, some therapeutic tasks are more easily and quickly accomplished and better integrated with the assistance of a therapy horse.

During an EAC activity called "Catch and Release" (EAGALA, n.d.a), teams of two are handed a halter and lead rope and asked to go into the pasture and halter a horse to the best of their ability with little to no additional direction by the therapists. This exercise is utilized to further understanding of fostering a trusting relationship and the challenges that come with that—awareness of self in relation to others, including how one presents to others, and making adjustments that accommodate the comfort and safety needs of self and others. While the activity is ongoing, the treatment team observes and assesses participants' reactions. One assessment is to determine if a participant: (1) picks a horse that comes to them, meaning the horse initiated engagement; or (2) picks a horse that the participant goes up to, meaning the participant initiated engagement; or (3) was more fixated on doing the task the "the right way" than engaging in social interaction with a horse. Each of these possibilities is significant in contributing to an understanding of the participants' intrapersonal dynamics (Trotter et al., 2008). To assess participants' style of facing a challenge, therapists examined the following:

- Did participants use all of the resources available to them, such as asking members of the treatment team to assist them?
- What, if any, level of frustration was evoked by participants as a result of:
  — Not knowing "how to do it right."
  — Not asking for assistance.
  — Giving up on the task prematurely.
- Difficulty thinking "outside the box" (initiating creative solutions).

Therapists and participants process the experience immediately after the exercise. Participants share their experience while therapists share their observations. Therapists assist each individual and the group to translate their experience into enhanced self- and other awareness and an understanding of how this would help participants cope with other life challenges, such as with family members, peers, and achievement tasks. This includes processing of interpersonal dynamics (e.g., how this experience related to human-to-human interactions, like meeting someone for the first time, or interacting in a large group of strangers, or exploring how participants worked or did not work as a team) and defining and identifying various roles each participant may have assumed during the exercise (e.g., active or passive, leader or follower, and productive or counterproductive). This catch, halter, and release activity allows participants to improvise and to ask for what they need, but these actions need to be initiated by the participants; therapy team members, by not rescuing participants from their frustration, resist the temptation to enable helplessness. Providing support and encouragement while allowing participants to struggle through a challenging task provides a heightened sense of accomplishment for participants which may contribute to self-esteem (Trotter et al., 2008).

One day when I was volunteering as co-counselor at a therapy ranch for a group of adolescent boys, the therapy staff instructed the boys to go to the pasture and halter and bring in some horses—a task that none of these young men had ever done before. The one young fellow I was accompanying approached his horse with a gentle attitude, and the horse stayed in one place for him as he made several vain attempts to get the halter on. The horse was very patient with him. The young man got more and more frustrated with his failed attempts and soon said, "Okay, I give up," in an attempt to get someone to rescue him. I simply replied, "What if giving up was not an option? The horse is being very patient with you. You could keep trying. Take a deep breath and consider the benefit of continuing to try. And you might look across the pasture at some of your peers to see how the halters look on their horses' heads to help you have a mental picture of what you might need to do." He took a deep breath, smiled, and kept working at it because he wanted to head to the barn like his peers were doing and be able to spend time grooming and riding the horse. In another setting, this young man was prone to quit on himself, to give up quickly, but with an opportunity as unique as this one, he was motivated to give extra effort. This is one of the many reasons EAC can contribute to the efficacy of a juvenile rehabilitation program; that is, it increases juveniles' desire to persevere with a complex task. The young man did succeed with haltering his horse a few tries later and led his horse to the barn. He was quick to point out his success to staff at the barn and was all smiles as he told his story about not giving up on himself. He was proud that he had overcome his temptation to quit and recognized this as an important accomplishment for himself.

EAC activities can include participants learning how to groom a horse. Interacting with such a large and powerful animal potentially empowers the participant, increases self-esteem, and increases self-confidence. Through their experience with the horses, participants learn to observe and respond to behaviors presented by the horses in a fashion that results in success, and thus participants can become better at observing and responding to people in ways that promote positive outcomes instead of staying stuck in current patterns of negative behavior (Trotter et al., 2008). Courage to stay positively engaged with a powerful horse can generalize into courage to stay positively engaged with another person. Additionally, grooming a horse is a practice of caring for another being. Grooming a horse provides opportunity for making a social connection and exercising empathy and compassion.

In an equine activity called "Life's Little Obstacles" (EAGALA, n.d.a), participants are asked to work as a group to get a horse to go through, over, or around obstacles; for instance, to walk over a low jump placed in an arena, to go between two orange cones placed about

10 feet apart in the center of an arena, or to move the horse through or around a variety of objects. There are variations on this exercise. One approach involves the rule that, while engaging with the horse, there can be no physical touching of the horse, no halters or lead ropes used, no bribing the horse with food, and no verbal communication with each other. The group is allowed to verbally communicate with one another to form a plan before the task begins and during time-outs called by the therapists. Time-outs are called infrequently so as not to interrupt the participants' efforts and are used to allow the participants to briefly rest and process what is and is not working. There is no one "right" solution to this activity. It can be solved in any number of ways, but it is up to the participants to work together to come up with a creative solution. Many EAC activities are designed to symbolically recreate life situations in which participants may be struggling, and the rules for this exercise are designed to move the participants out of their comfort zone and help them become more aware of dysfunctional patterns of believing, communicating, and interacting, and then to discover new solutions with healthier ways of believing, communicating, and interacting. Completion times for this activity can vary depending on the interpersonal dynamics of the group. The therapeutic intent of the obstacle exercise is to: (1) allow the group to struggle, become frustrated, and then achieve success; (2) process after each attempt at the activity to discover what helped them be successful or not successful; and (3) relate what happened during the obstacle exercise with what happens at home, work, or at school (Trotter et al., 2008).

"Give and Take" (Tidmarsh and Tidmarsh, 2005) is an exercise that is designed to facilitate skill building in communication, cooperation, adaptation, and respect. A lightweight string of about 5 feet in length is tied to each side of the horse's bit and held at the end by one participant on each side of the horse. Using only the string as a communication and control device, the two participants guide the horse down a short path (about 9 feet) and weave the horse through a line of orange cones spaced close together on the ground. Too much pressure and the string breaks; too little and the horse goes the wrong way.

"Equine Billiards" (Kersten and Thomas, 2004) is an activity used as a team-building exercise and requires a group of participants to move three to four horses, which are loose in a small arena, to a designated spot in the arena for each horse, much like calling the pocket on a billiard table for a particular ball except the pockets and balls were preassigned by the therapy team. Participants are not allowed to touch or bribe the horses to get them to move. Creative solutions are allowed, and the more cooperative and creative the participants are with one another the quicker the exercise is completed. It is interesting to observe and worth noting during processing at the end of an equine activity how often members of a group jump to erroneous conclusions and impose rules on themselves that were not placed on them by the therapists. For instance, one group's success at "Equine Billiards" was significantly slowed by the self-imposed rule that once a horse was placed in a pocket it had to stay there while the other horses were directed to the other pockets; members dedicated to trying to keep a horse in a pocket were thus not available to help with the remaining horses. When self-defeating patterns, like rigidity of thinking and behaving, are revealed during equine activities, immediate opportunities are presented to enhance awareness of these patterns.

Nonequine Challenge-Based Techniques Used in EAC Programs

EAC treatment programs often incorporate some complementary team-building, challenge-based activities that do not directly involve a horse. These are designed to encourage creative thinking, cooperation, leadership, and integrity as well as to enhance communication and to build empathic responses. Following is a description of some of these activities that do not directly involve a horse.

"Horse and Rider" (D. Goodwin-Bond, personal communication, April 2005) is an exercise that emphasizes communication skills. One participant plays the role of a horse, and the other plays the role of a rider. The one playing the horse places a horse bridle around his or her own neck and holds the bit with both hands. The reins go back over each shoulder and are held by the rider standing behind. The rider uses the reins to direct the horse person to walk across the arena and around obstacles. Riders are not allowed to speak to the horse person, nor may they lead their horse person. Rider persons have to remain directly behind their horse person. Each rider has been confidentially instructed by the therapist to guide the horse person to perform specific tasks and a different instruction is assigned to each rider. The horse person is instructed to respond only to the rein commands and not to verbal commands. This exercise is designed to give participants a real-life experience of what it must be like to be a horse trying to understand what a rider is attempting to communicate and to be a rider who experiences the frustration of failed communication. Each participant has the opportunity to play both a rider and a horse. This activity serves to enhance communication and build empathic responses and is an effective way of teaching participants how difficult it is for a horse and rider to communicate. Therapist-facilitated, post-exercise processing assists to generalize the lesson to participants' other life experiences where a failure of communication resulted in a negative outcome. Clinical processing questions after this activity explores things such as, "What was more difficult—playing the horse or the rider?", "What was difficult about it?", "What did you like about what your partner did when he or she was the rider?", "What would you have liked your partner to do differently?", "How was playing the horse difficult?", "How did you feel about the way your rider treated you?", "What did you learn that you can apply when you are working with a horse?", "Can you think of other times in your life when you felt the same way you felt during this exercise?", and "What did you learn from this exercise that you can apply to other areas of your life?" (Trotter et al., 2008).

Another popular challenge activity that does not directly involve a horse is "Marshmallow River" (Rohnke and Butler, 1995). "Marshmallow River" requires a group of participants to form a mutually supportive plan to move each group member safely across an imaginary dangerous river that must be negotiated by stepping on imaginary giant marshmallow stones; members must be honest if they fall off and must submit to consequences, such as trying to cross again but the second time blindfolded and guided by a team member. "One True Path" (Cavert, 1999) is a choice challenge exercise where team members help one another step across a 10-foot square, flat grid maze with hidden safe and unsafe spaces. Only the therapist knows which spaces on the grid are safe and which are not. When one member uncovers a nonsafe space, this member has to go to the end of the line to try again. The team has to help one another remember which spaces are safe and which are not from attempts made by previous group members. The exercise is complete once all members of the team safely cross the grid. One of the more challenging activities that does not involve a horse but can be used in EAC programs is "Bull Ring" (Cain and Smith, 2006). This exercise requires a group to work with maximum cooperation to balance a small ball on a small ring supported by strings extending from the center out to the circle of group members who must move in unison to transfer the ball from one stand (an orange rubber cone) to another several feet away without the ball falling off the center ring. Any unbalanced tension on the string from any one group member will cause the ball to fall. The difficulty level of this exercise is very high, such that I frequently observed groups not be able to successfully complete the exercise even with multiple attempts. Though each of the challenge activities described is set up with the goal of trying to complete the exercise, the most meaningful aspect of these exercises is not necessarily the completion but rather the attempt and what that experience was like for each participant. As with all challenge exercises, during clinical processing the treatment team encourages participants to explore how to apply what they learned and experienced to problems, stressors, and issues in their everyday lives.

EAC usually takes place over a period of several weeks. It is often a very meaningful experience for participants. As a way for participants to review what they experienced and to further integrate personal gains from the treatment, it is beneficial to have participants engage in a closure activity. The "Horseshoe Closing Ritual" (D. Goodwin-Bond, personal communication, April 2005) is an effective last exercise of a treatment program. The purpose of the exercise is to bring closure to the experience by allowing participants to step back and view themselves and the group with objectivity and sensitivity. Horseshoes of various shapes and sizes are placed in the center of the group, and each participant is asked to choose a horseshoe. The therapeutic team guides the group in a discussion about each horseshoe being different and likewise everyone in the group being different, but this group experience having made everyone come together as one. As each group member guides a lanyard string through one of the holes of their horseshoe, they are asked to share their perception of enhanced personal awareness and growth for the individual and for the group as a whole. When all of the horseshoes are added, the ends of the string are connected to form a complete circle. This exercise allows participants to cognitively and emotionally integrate the experiences of the past weeks.

AN EXAMPLE EAC PROGRAM

Compared with my extensive experience counseling with canines as therapy animals, I have relatively little direct experience with horses. I performed EAC myself for a little over 2 years under the guidance and supervision of an experienced co-counselor and I have supervised the work of my students performing EAC for over 15 years. My direct practice of EAC was when I volunteered as an assistant co-counselor at an equine counseling program that was facilitated by three very experienced staff: one equine specialist, one challenge course expert, and one licensed counselor (who was also an equine specialist). From my time volunteering with this EAC program, located in north Texas, I was able to see first-hand the power of this counseling. Some of the basic activities of this EAC program included the following (D. Goodwin-Bond, personal communication, April 2005):

- Discuss horse safety.
- Discuss a horse's body language.
- Choose a horse to work with.
- Learn how to develop a relationship with a horse.
- Lead a horse with a lead rope.
- Learn about the "gas pedal and brake" on a horse.
- Get a horse to move in a corral without touching it.
- Learn to halter a horse.
- Learn to tie a quick-release safety knot.
- Learn to groom a horse.
- Learn an emergency dismount and horse safety while mounted.
- Walk in rhythm with a horse.
- Learn to walk-on, halt, and turn mounted bareback on a horse.
- Learn to saddle and bridle a horse.
- Practice riding with saddle and bridle on a horse.
- Ride around a simple obstacle course.
- Learn to trot, canter, and gallop on a horse.

The program was a successful integration of instruction and participation in equine expe-riential activities, cowboy challenge course games and activities, and group therapy pro-cesses. The purpose of this EAC program was to build group cohesion, to create a sense of community, to develop a safe environment to express oneself and be vulnerable to learn, to introduce problem solving, and to develop communication skills. Approximately six to ten children and adolescents participated in each group, ranging in age from 10–16 years. The children paired together and shared a horse through the duration of the program. Some common needs of participants included self-esteem enhancement, conduct or behavior remediation, academic development, social skill development, and grief resolution. Therapy horses were marvelous tools for facilitating growth and development in children in each of these life-skill areas. See Figures 9.8 through 9.12.

Additional equine activities used in the EAC program where I volunteered were described earlier in this chapter, including "Building a Relationship With Your Horse" (D. Goodwin-Bond, personal communication, April 26, 2005), "Horse Body Parts" (D. Goodwin-Bond, personal communication, April 2005), "Catch and Release" (EAGALA, n.d.a.), "Life's Little Obstacles" (EAGALA, n.d.a), "Give and Take" (Tid-marsh and Tidmarsh, 2005), and "Equine Billiards" (Kersten and Thomas, 2004). Several nonequine-assisted challenge exercises were also integrated, including "Marshmallow River" (Rohnke and Butler, 1995), "One True Path" (Cavert, 1999), "Bull Ring" (Cain and Smith, 2006), and the "Horseshoe Closing Ritual" (D. Goodwin-Bond, personal commu-nication, April 2005).

An early activity asked each participant to take on a self-chosen ranch name that reflects a positive attribute for that person. Sometimes other participants helped an individual to come up with a name, if assistance was requested. Example names were "Happy Hector," "Yan-kee Ken," "Jumping Jennifer," and "Dynamic Deb." One group of adolescents I was assisting helped me choose my ranch name: they called me "Changemaker Chandler" since I was instrumental in connecting this group with the EAC program and paid for their services via a research and service grant I had received. The adolescents gave my therapy dog Dolly her ranch name because they saw her as fearless, comfortable, and relaxed around the big horses; they called her "Daring Dolly."

As a trust-building exercise, participants led a blindfolded partner around obstacles. Counselors led participants through a life values auction exercise that aided in clarifying personal values. In addition, participants as a group were taught how to make a rope together for cohesion building and personalization of the experience. While making the rope, partic-ipants were asked to reflect on and share in turn what positive things they wanted in their life and send that energy into the rope. There was no limit to what thoughts and emotions I have heard projected into a rope by juveniles from detention—for example, courage, hope, strength, happiness, positive attitude, wisdom, appreciation for animals and nature, and love and appreciation for family members. All juveniles were allowed to take as many turns as they wanted to put good energy into the rope. The rope was put away and saved until group process on the last day of therapy. Then, on the last day, while reflecting on and sharing their entire experience, participants cut pieces of the rope to keep as a remembrance of their growth experience. All EAA activities and challenge games and activities were processed in depth in a group therapy format at the end of each session to assist participants in relating personal insights to their own life. The skill of the group process leaders was key to the suc-cess of the program for the participants. A final activity at the end of the last therapy session was a fun hot dog roast around a ranch campfire.

During my involvement with this north Texas EAC program, I observed highly troubled, at-risk children and adolescents reduce and eliminate manipulative behaviors, overcome fears, display courage, develop and practice stress management and anxiety-reduction skills,

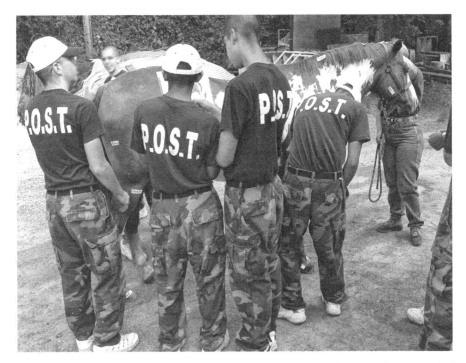

Figure 9.8 Juveniles from a detention facility exercise teamwork in learning the parts of a horse. Labeling a horse is educational and can lead to discussion about functional (respectful) and dysfunctional (stereotyping) forms of labeling people.

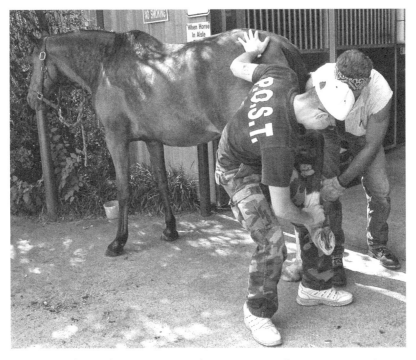

Figure 9.9 Juveniles from a detention center take part in an EAC program: exercising courage while learning to groom a horse.

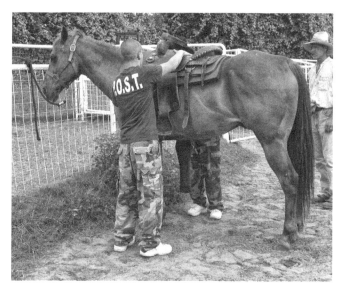

Figure 9.10 Engaging in a saddle lesson from an equine therapist—a lesson in preparation and attention to detail.

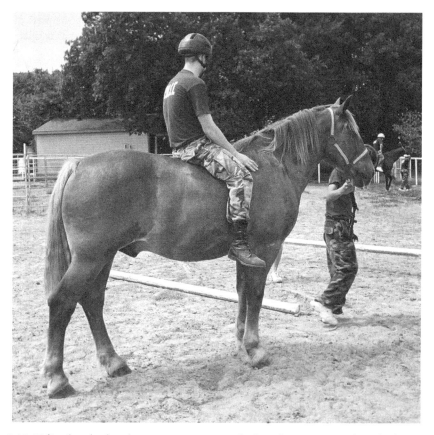

Figure 9.11 Riding bareback to learn sensitivity toward a horse's movement when the horse walks—an empathy-building exercise.

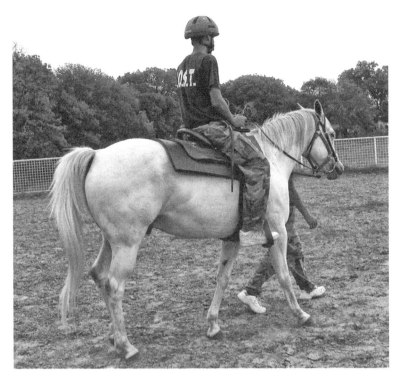

Figure 9.12 Riding tall in the saddle—achieving competency in riding skills boosts self-confidence.

become less self-focused and more other-focused, increase communication skills, and support, help, look out for, and encourage one another.

To demonstrate how EAC can benefit juveniles from a residential detention center, I will share some field notes from my 2 years at this north Texas EAC program. The names of the human participants have been changed to protect their identity.

At the Corral

In the first scenario, I describe adolescent girls working with a horse that they had not worked with before and trying to get the horse to follow them around a corral with only a rope loosely draped around the horse's neck. The horse had no halter, bridle, or saddle. The purpose of the exercise was to learn how to build a trusting relationship of mutual cooperation through the use of appropriate body language, the right attitude, and careful communication. We were working in a group format with six female adolescents who paired with one of three therapy horses.

Each pair of girls was given a rope and asked to go relate to their horse with speech and body language to get the horse to follow them around the corral. Each pair of girls draped the rope around their horse's neck and tried to get the horse to follow them. Kay and Sherry, who can be quite stubborn based on their prior history at the detention facility, tried physically pulling the horse named Oscar, but the horse would not move. These two girls had a body language that was not inviting to follow. They were the last pair to succeed of the three groups, but they eventually did get Oscar to walk with them a little toward the end. Kay and Sherry eventually succeeded with Oscar when they began talking nicely to the horse and became more gentle and inviting with soothing speech and relaxed body language as a result of intermittent coaching from the therapy staff.

The coaching from staff was only occasional and suggestive in that they asked the clients to look within themselves to decide what they needed to change in their attitude that would reflect body language telling the horse it could trust them, that is, to present to the horse with nonthreatening body language. The clients were allowed to struggle in their trial-and-error efforts to make interpersonal adjustments that were necessary to gain the horse's trust and cooperation. The goal of intermittent coaching and providing clues to clients is not for the ultimate purpose of achievement of task, although that is a welcome reward when it occurs. The ultimate purpose of counselor coaching is to provide encouragement to the client for self-exploration so the client may gain self-awareness and useful personal insights. It is imperative that a counselor does not rescue a client with step-by-step instructions as that limits opportunity for client self-discovery. The horse is a mirror to the client, reflecting how the client feels and presents him- or herself to the horse. The client learns to respect and honor what the horse's behavior is telling the client about him- or herself.

Another pair of adolescents, Janie and Denise, started out the exercise with gentle and calm speech and inviting body language with the horse named Stick, and he followed them all over the corral. They were the most successful of the three groups. Jackie and Heather had initial success with their horse named Dude, but a yard worker accidentally left a gate open to a small grassy lawn, and Dude slipped in there and got spooked when the group leaders herded him back into the corral. Now Dude was not so calm anymore. Jackie and Heather could not get near him without him running away and they became somewhat frantic too. So they asked for help. With brief coaching from therapy staff, they were reminded that they needed to observe and assess the horse's needs and reassure his safety. When Jackie and Heather slowed down and talked gently to the horse for a time, he let them pet him, and eventually he allowed them to lead him around again. Group process at the end of this activity centered on being aware of the body language of the horse and what it was saying it needed or what it was feeling and how to respond to the needs and feelings of a horse to foster a relationship. Also, discussion was about what messages the girls were sending to the horse through speech and body language that may cause the horse to resist or to cooperate. Although much frustration was exhibited by the girls during the difficult exercise, the girls did not give up but kept trying because they wanted to be successful with the horse. The attitude of the girls was very positive at the end of the session with each expressing gains in intrapersonal and interpersonal awareness.

At the Pasture and the Barn

On another day, two of the adolescents were especially challenged by a particularly stubborn horse, and the girls really had to exercise some frustration tolerance. It was a powerful lesson that might not otherwise have been accomplished were it not for the adolescents' strong desire to spend time with their therapy horse.

The horses were to be gathered from the pasture and brought to the barn to be groomed by the girls. The horse Oscar was reluctant to be approached and haltered in the pasture, but Kay and Sherry finally got him haltered when he paused to drink some water from a water bucket. Even after they got him haltered, he steadfastly refused to move. They requested assistance from a staff member who reminded them about presenting to the horse body language suggesting the horse could trust them, and to use signals the horse understood and felt comfortable with; such as to get him moving by having one person gently wave an arm behind the horse while the other led the horse. They finally got Oscar to the barn where he refused to lift his hooves for the girls to clean them. After many attempts by both Sherry and Kay, Kay had to walk away from Oscar and sit down for a few minutes and collect her emotions before going back and trying again to get him to lift his hoof for cleaning. She finally won him over with gentle speech and rubbing his neck. Each hoof after that came up easier. Kay and Sherry were persistent and patient with him, even though they were the last to get their horse groomed this day.

This experience challenged the girls to self-examine their tendency to be dominant and controlling, and provided immediate opportunity to make adjustments and practice more compassion and understanding in their social interaction with the horse.

At the Riding Practice Arena

Following is an excerpt from my field notes that describes some of the emotional and social benefits to be gained from learning to ride a horse.

> The girls practiced riding with saddles and bridles independently again today. Denise did very well with the riding today on Stick. She is looking very comfortable and confident up on her horse. She has progressed nicely in the last 2 days with her comfort level with riding and along with this she has maintained a much brighter mood. It is pleasant to see how her once depressed mood has been lifted over these past few weeks since she began the EAC. Janie is riding very well today on Stick. Her only expressed frustration was wanting the horse to go faster, demonstrating her increasing courage to face challenges, a favorable progression for her given she began the EAC with low confidence. After a few instructions from a staff member, she tried the instructions to trot and had good success. Her response was, "This is so cool!" Thus, her frustration turned into confidence and satisfaction. Janie is still relating well to all members of the group; it is nice to see her behavioral transformation since beginning EAC is showing some permanency.

> Heather got her horse Dude to start galloping today, but then she got scared and forgot how to stop her horse. While the horse was galloping, Heather repeatedly shouted, "Whoa!" and tried to pull the reins, but she was also tensing her legs from fear of falling off. This only encouraged the horse to keep going. Heather's eyes grew very big while the horse was galloping. The horse finally came to a gradual halt when it reached the far end of the arena. A staff member went down to the end of the arena on a horse to check on Heather, who was still in the saddle. The group leader led Heather on horseback to the near end of the arena and gave Heather the choice of continuing to ride or taking a break. Heather decided to dismount and collect herself because she was a bit shaken. Once off the horse, she began smiling and laughing with one of her peers, Sherry. When Heather was asked about the laughter, she said it was relief and humor about her situation. When Sherry was asked about the laughter, she said she wanted to laugh when she first saw Heather's horse was galloping and Heather was shouting but then quickly realized Heather was afraid. So,

she waited until Heather was safe on the ground and saw her smiling before she laughed, and then she laughed with Heather and not at her. This was a big step for Sherry because she has struggled in the detention center with her tendency to laugh at other people when they were in discomfort or pain.

When it was her partner's turn, Heather did lead the horse, named Dude, for her partner, Jackie, who was the only one still requiring a leader today because she is afraid of riding on her own. By her willingness to lead the horse for her partner, Heather was re-engaging quickly with the horse that had frightened her when it galloped with her a few minutes earlier. When her partner was done and everyone else had also finished, the group leader asked Heather if she wanted to remount and try again. Heather said yes. Then the staff and other girls gave her feedback and encouragement. Heather mounted the horse, named Dude, but the horse was a bit reluctant to be reined back out into the arena since it sensed the day of work was over. But with instruction from the group leader, Heather became appropriately assertive and got the horse to follow her directions. Heather became an appropriate leader for the horse and even got him to respond to a command to "back up," which is somewhat difficult for a novice rider. She performed great assertive communication with the horse. We were all so impressed with her we applauded. Having successfully re-engaged with the horse that had galloped with her earlier in the session, Heather dismounted her horse feeling confident and encouraged. Heather not only overcame the fear she experienced earlier in the session when the horse galloped with her, but she accepted and achieved an even greater challenge with this horse of learning to communicate a difficult "back-up" command. It is clear that the girls' motivation to spend time with the horses provides them with the additional motivation they need to challenge their growth.

> Jackie was so inspired by Heather's courage and accomplishment she asked if she could challenge herself further before the session ended. Jackie decided she wanted to try and ride on her own for the first time without her horse being led by a rope held by her partner. Jackie mounted the horse, named Dude, that Heather had just dismounted, the same one that had galloped with Heather astride earlier in the session. Jackie was doing better today with being calmer around the horses but she had never shown any confidence when interacting with a horse, and in this moment of trying to ride on her own the first time she still was not assertive with the horse. Sensing Jackie was not a leader to be trusted, with Jackie astride the horse, Dude decided he would be the decision maker and he kept going to the gate in an act of wanting to leave the arena and be done working for the day. After instruction and persistent encouragement from a counselor, Jackie finally got assertive with her horse and had a good response from him. Though startled by her success, her confidence shot really high from the experience. Jackie became noticeably different from that point forward.

Jackie's new confidence generalized to other areas. She lost her need and desire to bully others, which had been her way of compensating her personal insecurity. She made great progress in the detention facility after her success with the horse Dude and went from formerly lagging behind in her behavioral and emotional rehabilitation to surging ahead and being released ahead of schedule.

When the client Sherry started EAC she was quite the bully and frequently invasive of others' personal space. She was also very self-absorbed, with little demonstrated interest in others. When she began EAC she had a knowledge and comfort advantage over the other girls because Sherry had experience with horses. Unfortunately, in the early stages of EAC, she used that experience to dominate instead of cooperate. She presented as an obnoxious "know it all": but Sherry had been getting gradually better over the past few weeks and today she was better than I had seen her.

Sherry did not ride up too close on anyone today and looked very nice on her mount. She was relaxed and took it nice and slow around the arena. When off the horse and watching her partner, she was friendly with staff and watched her partner with interest. She has successfully adjusted to politely offering advice when asked, instead of making pronouncements of inadequacy about the other girls. Her behavior was very acceptable today. She has come a long way with improvements in her attitude toward others and in her ability and desire to be socially responsive and respectful.

Kay did well today. Kay learned to trot the horse today, as did her partner Janie, and looked great except for her tendency to lean forward in the saddle a little too much on the trot. Kay's confidence has come a long way since beginning the EAC. Sherry, who was watching Kay on her horse, noticed Kay was leaning too far forward in the saddle and was about to suggest an adjustment to Kay when a staff member beat her to it, and Sherry simply nodded her head in agreement. It was obvious Sherry just wanted Kay to be helped but had no investment in bossing Kay or showing off, which had been typical Sherry-like behaviors before she started the equine therapy.

After their time riding in the arena, the girls led the horses back to the barn. They removed the tack from the horses and returned everything to the tack room and their riding helmets to the helmet room (they are never allowed on a horse without a helmet). The girls led the horses to the pasture where they released them. All of the therapy horses decided to roll in the grass today right after being released, and the girls watched and laughed at this, a couple verbalizing, "Oh, how cool!" They had not seen their horses do this before today. It was a nice way to close out the day. Today was the first day we got a little break from the heat. The past five days of sessions have been miserably hot, which lends even greater credit to the girls who have been willing to come back each day in the heat and participate fully in the program.

On the Grassy Hill

This last set of field notes comprises observations on the girls describing the last day of therapy.

The juveniles had a final opportunity to ride. The girls were nervous about the challenge before them today but also excited at the opportunity to take their horsemanship to the next level. They were to ride outside of the arena today; there would be no fences to confine their horse. A staff member took the riders in a line, and they exited the arena onto the grassy, treed area on a hill. They rode amongst the trees and grass and felt the freedom and strength gifted them by their horse companion. All of the riders did very well. The horse Dude was a little troublesome as he wanted to graze instead of walk, but with corrections from his rider the horse went along. The riders rode back to the barn with a new spirit of accomplishment.

At the Barn and Pasture

The horses' tack was put away, and each pair of girls walked their horse to the pasture. They spent a few moments saying a final goodbye to their horses before releasing them. The girls all had tears coming back from the pasture.

At the Tree House

As we sat on the wooden planks of the giant tree house, the girls had tears when processing their day and how hard it was to say goodbye to their horses and to the staff. The girls thanked the staff, both counselors and equine specialists, for everything they had experienced and learned by taking part in the EAC program, and additionally thanked me for helping make the experience possible for them since I had made the arrangement and paid for their EAC with a grant. They thanked the juvenile detention staff who were present for being so supportive and trusting to allow them to come out to the therapy ranch. The girls were very sincere and emotional when conveying their remarks. The counselors passed out the rope the girls had made in an earlier session, and they each made a wish as they cut a piece to keep. They mostly wished for success through the detention program as well as in life after they had completed the detention program, and they also wished for happiness. Some also wished to be able to come back to the ranch to visit the horses and staff. The girls were asked to name one thing new they had learned about themselves from their equine experience. Denise said, "I learned that I could cry. Before, I had to make myself cry." Kay expressed, "I discovered I was a good person who people could respect." Janie said, "I found out I could have a positive relationship with more than one person." Heather said, "I learned I am a very brave person." Jackie articulated, "I discovered I have a sensitive side as well as a strong side." Sherry expressed, "I learned that I have good in me and can do good things and have positive relationships with people." The group leaders passed out certificates to the girls with photographs on them of the girls with their horse. Following this we moved over to the pavilion where there were some picnic tables and drinks.

Sitting at the Pavilion

We all sat under the shade of the pavilion and drank a cold soda and water, compliments of the staff. Typically, at this juncture, we would also build a fire in the fire pit and cook hot dogs but the searing heat of the day thwarted our desire to do that. Jackie came up with a spur-of-the-moment idea for the girls to march for the equine group leaders as a way to say thanks and to honor their total experience.

Marching in the Parking Lot

The girls demonstrated their graduation marching steps they learned and practiced at the detention center. It was meant as a gesture of honor and gratitude for the equine therapy staff, and staff did in fact feel honored. Permission was given by juvenile detention staff to exchange hugs. The girls loaded up in the van and drove away back to the juvenile detention center. It was clear from this experience that the adolescent girls were greatly impacted in positive ways from the EAC.

In this EAC program, multiple opportunities occurred for adolescents to enhance self-awareness, gain personal insights, boost self-confidence, strengthen self-concept, and make important attitudinal and interpersonal adjustments. Indeed, of the several groups of juvenile boys and girls from the post-adjudication juvenile detention program I observed complete this 12-session EAC program, I never saw any of them be uncooperative, belligerent, disrespectful, or choose not to participate or not to follow directions during the equine therapy. Most negative actions and attitudes that these kids may have chosen to exhibit while in the juvenile detention facility were not exhibited during equine therapy. Furthermore, such behaviors that may have existed at the juvenile facility before EAC were typically either significantly diminished or eliminated following completion of the EAC program. I firmly believe that equine therapy helped them to grow up a bit, to mature toward responsible adult character. The EAC presented the opportunity for participants to become more aware of their self-image and social deficits, and they were motivated to improve out of a desire to have a positive relationship with a horse.

OTHER EQUINE-ASSISTED THERAPY APPLICATIONS

Dance/Movement Therapy

Ford (2013) interviewed professionals who in their practice combine dance/movement therapy and EFP. From in-depth qualitative study of the interviews Ford ascertained significant evidence suggesting that dance/movement therapy can be effectively combined with EFP due to the natural fit of the two modalities. Major themes presented by interviewees were: the horses were impeccable reflectors and mirrors of clients' emotional state; the horses were mindful, intuitive, and powerful witnesses of what they perceived in clients; the horses facilitated nonverbal communication, embodiment, and congruence; the horses increased mindfulness in clients and cultivated awareness for clients of space, body, breath, movement, relationship, and community; and the horses increased opportunities for creative expression, touch, and support. Interviewees also stated the horses increased the breadth and depth of the therapeutic relationship (Ford, 2013).

Vaulting

Vidrine, Owen-Smith, and Faulkner (2002) presented a model for, and case examples of, equine-facilitated group psychotherapy using therapeutic vaulting. Therapeutic vaulting is the performance of gymnastics and acrobatics on a horse. While professional vaulting takes years of experience and training, introductory-level vaulting can be performed by beginners and thus can be useful with child, adolescent, and adult clients. Clients are highly motivated to participate in vaulting-assisted therapy, as exemplified by one adolescent who had previously been in a gang who said, "Vaulting is more fun than getting in trouble." The researchers report:

> Vaulting is a very structured experience, which helps many clients with organizational skills, spatial relations, and body awareness while satisfying the need for excitement.
> (Vidrine, Owen-Smith, and Faulkner, 2002, pp. 594–595)

A typical children's vaulting group described by these researchers included clients who were 7–10 years of age. The schedule for this age group was one 90-minute session per week for 8 to 10 weeks. The group was facilitated by a licensed psychotherapist with specially trained assistants. Types of group activities included: opening circle for roll call, announcements, sharing feelings, goal setting and planning, and snacks; tacking and grooming the horse; group members' stretching in a circle to warm up the body; learning new moves on the stationary barrel prior to performing on the horse; helping the horse warm up; taking turns practicing compulsory moves; and taking turns practicing freestyle moves. The children often saw their own lives, issues, and feelings reflected in the lives of their horse friends, and these reflections were included in group processing along with other issues related to clients' struggles and personal growth (Vidrine, Owen-Smith, and Faulkner, 2002). For more information on vaulting, see the organization Equestrian Vaulting USA (2023, https://equestrianvaulting.org/).

Eating Disorders

DeZutti (2013) is a nurse working in the realm of psychiatric/mental health and she describes her experiential approach utilizing horses to assist with the recovery of individuals or groups of adolescent and adult patients with eating disorders. She incorporates into treatment typical activities such as grooming, learning horse body language, petting and interacting with the horses, and guiding horses through an obstacle course. She describes how, even within the confines of one session, improvements can be observed in communication and cohesiveness within the group as well as improved individual sense of accomplishment and confidence. She encourages nurses and therapists working in the area of psychiatric/mental health with patients with eating disorders to consider equine therapy for their patients (DeZutti, 2013).

Trauma Recovery

Yorke, Adams, and Coady (2008) described the benefits of horse–human bonding for six people who had a previous bond with horses and who claimed this bond helped them in their recovery from trauma. Semi-structured interviews and video recordings of horse–rider interaction were used to describe the nature of the equine–human bond and its contribution to recovery for 18- to 51-year-olds (trauma had occurred 10 months to 11 years before the research interviews). Two participants had been injured in horse-related accidents, with one becoming paraplegic and the other brain injured. Two participants had been injured in car accidents, with both becoming paraplegic and one being brain injured. One participant was HIV positive, and one participant had experienced multiple physical and psychological traumas as well as abuse. All participants had been riding since childhood, and all had been in recovery from their traumas for at least 8 months before they returned to riding (and all participants had resumed riding at least 2 to 3 months before participating in the study). The physically disabled participants relied on assistance from others to mount and ride.

After data were coded and analyzed by the researchers, two broad categories emerged: (1) the nature of the equine–human bond, and (2) the therapeutic value of the equine–human bond. Each category had a number of components. Four main components of the nature of the equine–human bond were found: the intimacy–nurturing bond, the identity bond, the partnership bond, and the utility bond. The first two components were emotional and personal, whereas the last two components were more practical or task oriented. The second category, the therapeutic value of the equine–human bond, focused on aspects of the horse– human relationship that the riders identified as contributing to their healing and recovery. Three main components were found for the category therapeutic value of the equine–human bond: feelings, proximity or touch, and behaviors relevant to healing and recovery. The researchers concluded the results of this study suggested that the relationships participants had with their horses contributed significantly to their healing from trauma and that the findings suggested parallels between good equine–human relationships and good therapist–client relationships, both in terms of the nature of the bonds that were formed and their healing qualities. The researchers felt their results had two larger implications: they supported the general idea that human–animal relationships can be therapeutic, and they implied that equine–human relationships might have unique therapeutic aspects beyond those found in relationships either with small companion animals or with therapists (Yorke, Adams, and Coady, 2008).

Therapeutic Riding

Another field that incorporates work with therapy horses is called therapeutic riding. The premise behind therapeutic riding is that the act of riding a horse can have emotional and physical health benefits. Therapeutic riding involves the activities of horseback riding and sometimes horse grooming. Unlike EAC, therapeutic riding does not have to be directed or supervised by a licensed mental health professional or any other licensed health professional. It does not necessarily require individualized treatment plans or treatment goals, nor does it involve in-depth processing of human–horse interactions. However, I felt it was important to briefly include therapeutic riding here because there have been some measured health and mental health benefits, and because it is a popular application that incorporates therapy horses, although it should not be confused with EAC. For more information on therapeutic riding, see the following resources: *Special Needs, Special Horses* (Scott, 2005); *Therapeutic Riding I* (Engel, 1998); *Therapeutic Riding II*, revised (Engel, 2003); and *The Horse, the Handicapped, and the Riding Team in a Therapeutic Riding Program* (Engel et al., 2008).

Farias-Tomaszewski, Jenkins, and Keller (2001) evaluated the effect of a therapeutic horseback riding program for adults with physical impairments. A total of 22 adults with a variety of physical impairments participated in the 12-week program. A one-group pre- and post-test design was used to evaluate changes in levels of physical and global self-efficacy as well as self-confidence. Physical self-efficacy and behavioral self-confidence were found to increase from pre- to post-test, whereas global self-efficacy did not change over time. The researchers concluded the results provided evidence in support of the psychological value of therapeutic horseback riding for adults with physical impairments (Farias-Tomaszewski, Jenkins, and Keller, 2001).

Kaiser et al. (2004) investigated the effect of a 5-day therapeutic riding day camp on children's anger. A total of 16 children, ages 7–15 years with no known physical or psychological disability and no known history of psychotropic medications, participated in the study. Pre- and post-administration measures were obtained on the Children's Anger Inventory, Peds Quality of Life, and the Self-Perception Profile for Children. Results showed that after 5 days of therapeutic horseback riding the total score of the anger inventory and scores for all subscales except frustration decreased significantly, but no other differences were noted. The researchers concluded the decrease in children's anger was likely a result of the child's relationship with the horse, the social environment of camp, the horse and riding, increased contact with nature, or a combination of these factors (Kaiser et al., 2004).

Kesner and Pritzker (2008) performed therapeutic riding with children placed in the foster care system. A total of 14 children (eight boys and six girls), aged 5–17 years, participated in ten therapeutic horseback riding sessions 1 hour in length. Riding sessions focused on learning the basics of horse care, riding etiquette, and mastery of riding skills including maneuvering the horse. From interviews performed with the children, the researchers determined that positive behavioral and emotional changes in participants correlated with their completion of the therapeutic horseback-riding program. The participants described themselves as feeling happier, having more confidence, having improved behavior, having a desire to socialize with others, and having a greater sense of self-acceptance and responsibility:

> Some of the participants specifically identified their relationship with their horse as an important factor contributing to the positive changes they were experiencing.
>
> (Kesner and Pritzker, 2008, p. 84)

Lanning and Krenek (2013) performed an informal study of EAA with a small group of combat veterans to improve quality of life. This service was part of the Professional Association of Therapeutic Horsemanship, International (PATH, Intl.) Services for Heroes Program (formerly known as the Horses for Heroes Program), which is a broad-based program encompassing any number of different EAIs. The intervention in the Lanning and Krenek (2013) study was limited to therapeutic riding. The theme that emerged most was increased sociability in the participants. However, the results of their study cannot be generalized due to the small number of participants and lack of a control group (Lanning and Krenek, 2013).

Therapeutic horseback riding has been shown to be effective in the treatment of autism spectrum disorder (ASD). Bass, Duchowny, and Llabre (2009) studied the effects of horseback riding on social functioning of 34 children diagnosed with ASD. Compared with a waitlist control group, children exposed to the 12-week intervention "exhibited greater sensory seeking, sensory sensitivity, social motivation, and less inattention, distractability, and sedentary behaviors" (Bass, Duchowny, and Llabre, 2009, p. 1261).

Keino et al. (2009) applied a psychoeducational horseback riding program to the treatment of four Japanese children diagnosed with pervasive developmental disorders. The program was several months long. Children showed improvement in eye contact, verbal and nonverbal communication skills, and became more expressive in their emotional and empathetic interaction with their parents.

Gabriels et al. (2012) performed a study with 42 children and adolescents diagnosed with ASD participating in a 10-week horseback-riding program. Participants who completed the program demonstrated significant improvements on post-test measures, as compared with baseline measures, of irritability, lethargy, stereotypic behavior, hyperactivity, expressive language skills, motor skills, and verbal praxis/motor planning skills. When compared with the pre- and post-assessments of participants from the waitlist control condition, the therapeutic horseback riding group still showed significant improvements in self-regulation behaviors (Gabriels et al., 2012).

Hippotherapy

Another professional application that involves working with a therapy horse is called hippotherapy. Hippotherapy is a form of physical therapy or physical rehabilitation that occurs from horseback riding. Physical therapy is not the focus of this book but I mention hippotherapy because it is often confused with equine interventions for mental health application. Hippotherapy has a long history. The ancient Greek philosopher and physician Hippocrates was thought to be "the first to describe the benefits of the horse for rehabilitation purposes, calling horseback riding a universal exercise" (Macauley and Gutierrez, 2004):

> *Hippotherapy* is a specialization of EAT [equine-assisted therapy]. Hippotherapy means treatment with the help of a horse and is derived from the Greek word *hippos*, meaning "horse."
>
> (Macauley and Gutierrez, 2004, p. 205)

Horseback riding requires the use of muscles for balance and posture, and thus the act of riding can increase muscle flexibility, strength, and range of motion. Hippotherapy is performed or directed by a licensed therapist in a rehabilitation field, most typically from the fields of physical or occupational therapy and requires design and implementation of specific plans and goals for the treatment and rehabilitation of a specific condition of a human patient. Patient progress is periodically assessed and carefully documented. Macauley and Gutierrez (2004) described the effectiveness of hippotherapy for children with language-learning disabilities. The study compared traditional therapy for language-learning disabilities with hippotherapy for three boys, ages 9, 10, and 12 years. The results showed that both the children and their parents reported improvement in speech and language abilities after both traditional therapy and hippotherapy. However, "responses were noticeably higher following hippotherapy, with additional benefits of improved motivation and attention also reported" (Macauley and Gutierrez, 2004, p. 205). For more information on hippotherapy, see *Enhancing Human Occupation Through Hippotherapy* (Engel and MacKinnon, 2007).

From what we know about EAC, vaulting, therapeutic riding, and hippotherapy, it is clear that human–horse interaction offers great benefits for enhancing the health and wellbeing of humans.

10
A Variety of Animal-Assisted Therapy Applications

This chapter discusses a variety of animal-assisted therapy applications, including therapy zoo, therapy farm, therapy with dolphins, college and university applications, animal-assisted play therapy, and additional applications. Therapy zoo as a therapeutic environment provides opportunity for a client to interact with a variety of species they might not otherwise encounter. The novelty of this experience assists in bringing clients' issues to the surface where they can be processed for the benefit of the client. Therapy farm is typically an environment where all of the animals on the farm have sanctuary and are very well cared for by staff and children. AAT applications involving dolphins are popular and may involve playful interactions from outside the water, or swimming with dolphins. There are various types of AAT programs at colleges and universities. These most often involve the opportunity for students, staff, and faculty to interact with therapy dogs visiting campus or working with their handler in a student counseling center. The chapter also describes how play therapy and AAT are a natural fit, especially with dogs. Most dogs have a natural desire to play, so they feel right at home with a child playing in a therapy room.

THERAPY ZOO

AAT that involves interaction with farm animals, exotic animals, and sometimes even wild animals is referred to as therapeutic zoo. There are currently no guidelines for the choice of animals for this type of program. However, it is recommended that typically only domestically bred animals should be used, and no wild animals should be involved unless a wildlife care expert or wildlife rehabilitator is on staff. Following are example therapeutic zoo programs.

Companionable Zoo

An AAT program that involves interaction with farm animals, exotic animals, and sometimes even wild animals is the Companionable Zoo (Katcher and Wilkins, 2002). A sample list of animals found in this program includes chinchilla, canary, dove, gecko, miniature goat, guinea pig, hamster, hedgehog, miniature horse, iguana, parakeet, pot-bellied pig, and rabbit. Another program has a pasture of buffalo. The Companionable Zoo includes therapeutic education for children who face mental health issues and accompanying emotional and behavioral problems. Children involved in the Companionable Zoo program are held responsible for the care of the animals while learning about nature. The Companionable Zoo program "is an evolving product of therapeutic education that takes place at the junction between people,

DOI: 10.4324/9781003260448-10

animals, and nature" (Katcher and Wilkins, 2002, p. 2). The program uses the care of animals and contact with nature to help children, and sometimes adults, learn the rules of society:

> The Companionable Zoo is a moral therapy. The ways that animals are treated and the rules governing human–animal interactions are metaphors for how the children should be treated. Children learn about human morality by reflecting upon the moral principles inherent in the treatment of animals. Without an ethic of human–animal interaction, there is no therapy in the larger sense. In thinking through the animal care guidelines, the Zoo staff should see that they, as well as the actions that they imply, define the staff's humanity and signal how the children in their care will be treated.
>
> (Katcher and Wilkins, 2002, pp. 102–103)

Some of the therapeutic and learning goals of the Companionable Zoo program include (Katcher and Wilkins, 2002):

- Modulate arousal to the demands of the task.
- Experience sustained attention and comfort in a learning environment.
- Take responsibility for a meaningful task.
- Master fear and build confidence.
- Learn skills and build competence.
- Train in self-directed and other-directed speech.
- Receive social skills training.
- Train for positive attributions and expectations.
- Train in social perspective taking and empathic skills.
- Increase engagement with reading and writing tasks.
- Increase ability to work cooperatively at learning tasks.

The preferred design of a Companionable Zoo program is to provide natural habitat or pasture for a variety of animals. Gardens and fishponds are encouraged. Additional activities can include supervised trips to the woods or wilderness areas. Empirical studies of therapeutic zoo intervention:

> suggest that children, especially children who find it difficult to learn in a regular school setting, are more responsive to learning tasks as well as less symptomatic when they are participating in the care of animals and engaged in nature study.
>
> (Katcher, 2000a, p. 174)

The Small Zoo as Therapy

Utilizing a small zoo as a therapeutic environment provides opportunity for a client to interact with a variety of species they might not otherwise encounter. The novelty of this experience assists in bringing a client's issues to the surface where they can be processed for the benefit of the client. In December 2014, I traveled to Israel to view the work of a pioneer in animal-assisted psychotherapy, Efrat Maayan, who utilizes the small zoo as therapy. Maayan works with adults at a drug rehabilitation center as part of a recovery program and also with children and adults at her private practice where she has indoor and outdoor animal facilities, including a koi fish pond with waterfall. Maayan (2013) describes a small zoo facility as having a therapy room and therapy yard with cages and open areas. The types of animals involved in small therapy zoo include small rodents such as hamsters, laboratory rats, and gerbils; larger rodents such as rabbits and guinea pigs; various types of parrots; and to the extent that there is space and budget, goats, donkeys, ferrets, ducks, and other larger animals. According to Maayan (2013):

The therapy zoo contains a variety of animals that can be likened to "a rich and varied buffet" which offers the client possibilities to encounter various types of relationships that connect to the most basic element of human experiences ... the variety brings them in contact with many subjects that are relevant to their life and allows them to express that which they often cannot do in any other way [. . .]

Animals, too, can constitute a symbol. In general, one can relate to them as representing the instinctual level of the psyche—that is, the urges, drives, and the connection to the life forces and the healthy instincts of our psyche. Beyond the general symbolism of the animal world, each animal also possesses its own rich and unique symbolism, connected to its form, size, way of life, the environment in which it lives, and the cultural connections of the relationship with the animal, as well as through personal experiences.

(pp. 172 and 174)

When a therapy zoo is properly constructed it allows a client total severance from their experience of the norm, and movement into a kingdom where both treatment and therapy processes can occur (Maayan, 2013, p. 176). Maayan's perspective on the power of therapy zoo draws on Carl Jung's theoretical constructs regarding archetypes and symbolism. The animals and space of therapy zoo provide a private place that allows a client to differentiate the sacred from the profane (Maayan, 2013, p. 176). See Figures 10.1 through 10.6.

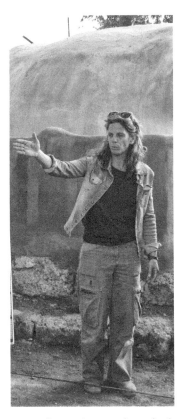

Figure 10.1 Efrat Maayan is a pioneer of animal-assisted psychotherapy in Israel and practitioner of the small zoo as therapy. She is standing among the natural-looking animal pens for the therapeutic small zoo at Retorno Jewish Center for Addictions in Israel.

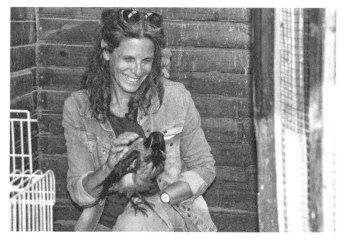

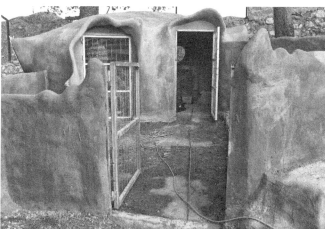

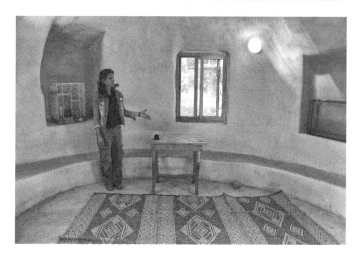

Figures 10.2–10.4 Retorno Jewish Center for Addictions in Israel: (*top*) Efrat Maayan with a bird in hand and one on the shoulder in the aviary—the birds are awaiting transfer to a new, more natural-looking habitat; (*center*) one section of the new natural-looking animal pens for the small zoo therapy program—this area is still under construction; (*bottom*) Efrat Maayan shows off the interior of the new counseling room set in the midst of the animal pens.

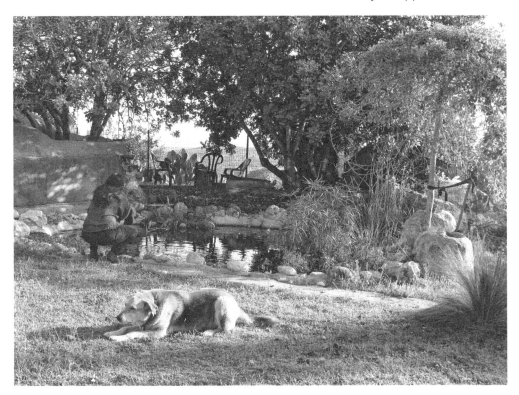

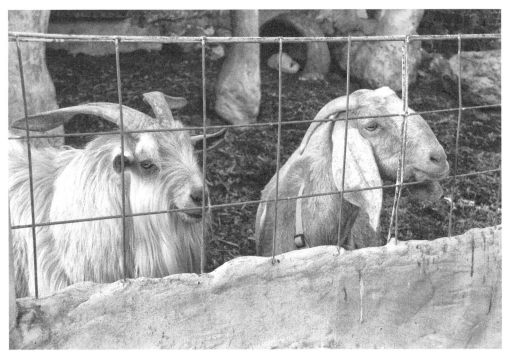

Figures 10.5 and 10.6 The small zoo psychotherapy private practice of Efrat Maayan in Israel: (*top*) a therapy dog is resting near the waterfall and koi fish pond in the outdoor therapy space; and (*bottom*) these goats are some of the animals at the small zoo.

THERAPY FARM

Green Chimneys of Brewster, New York has a very large therapy farm as part of the services provided to children who face mental health issues and the emotional and behavioral problems that accompany those issues. All of the animals on the farm have sanctuary and are very well cared for by staff and children. I visited Green Chimneys in the spring of 2015. The therapy farm has a greenhouse, an outdoor herb garden, and another very large garden where a variety of vegetables are grown. The farm has a wildlife center where several wild birds are provided care and rehabilitation and, if possible, released back into the wild. Also found on the farm is a dog kennel for rescued dogs and a dog run. There is a spacious barn with indoor and outdoor pens for small, medium, and large animals and a very large stable and spacious indoor riding arena for horses. Small-, medium-, and large-sized corrals and large fenced pastures provide ample room for a variety of animals. In residence, there are dogs, camels, llamas, sheep, goats, chickens, rabbits, pigs, cows, horses, mules, donkeys, emus, and peacocks; my apologies to any Green Chimneys animal I may have left off this list. The children have much opportunity to interact in the garden and with any of the animals. The children find the animals good companions in their growth and healing process and they gain in their capacity for empathy and compassion while interacting with and caring for the animals. See Figures 10.7 through 10.19.

In the Netherlands, there exist care farms (that may or may not be agriculturally productive), which offer care, a home, or reintegration work to clients with varying disabilities, for example clients with mental handicaps, psychiatric or addiction problems, (demented) elderly, and children and youngsters who need care or probationary work (Ferwerda-van Zonneveld, Oosting, and Kijlstra, 2012). The number of care farms in the Netherlands has increased rapidly from 75 in 1998, to 605 in 2007. In 2007, about one-third of all care farms were open to young people with autism spectrum disorder (ASD), and by 2010 this had already increased to almost two-thirds. Most care farms have animals on their premises. The bond with animals is used to improve the behavior of children with ASD using AAI. The communication of these children with animals reduces their feeling of anxiety and arousal and can act as a mediator to improve their social interactions with other humans. The interaction with the animals provides a feeling of safety, comfort, and entertainment, and allows the possibility of showing affection. Forming a relationship with animals helps the

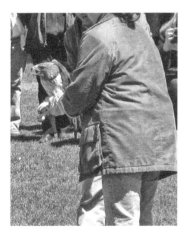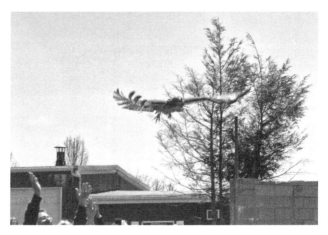

Figures 10.7 and 10.8 The Wildlife Center of Green Chimneys in New York releases hawks that have been rehabilitated back into the wild—a favorite event for children and staff.

(*Source:* photo 10.8 courtesy of Green Chimneys.)

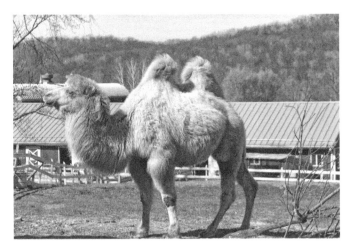

Figure 10.9 A camel provides unique human–animal interaction at Green Chimneys in New York.

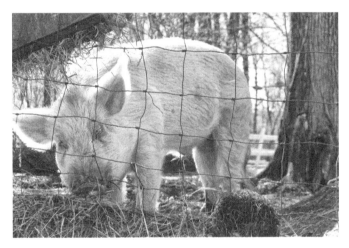

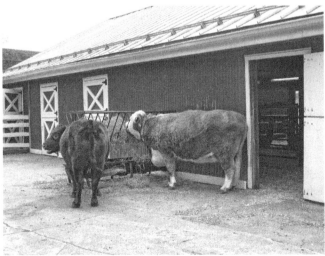

Figures 10.10 and 10.11 The therapy farm of Green Chimneys in New York offers sanctuary to animals; pigs and cows have a happy and safe home at the therapy farm.

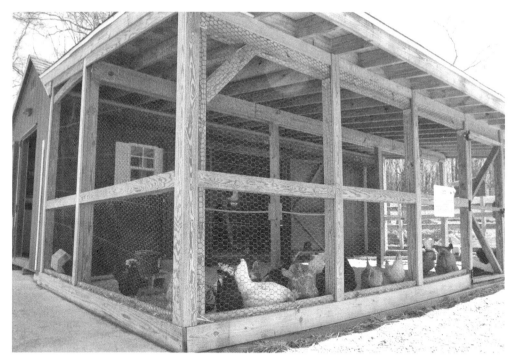

Figure 10.12 Chickens at Green Chimneys in New York: children and staff gather eggs, feed the chickens, and keep the pen clean daily.

children to develop a bond with other people and AAI helps to reduce the symptoms of ASD (Ferwerda-van Zonneveld, Oosting, and Kijlstra, 2012).

THERAPY WITH DOLPHINS

Health and mental health therapeutic applications involving dolphins as therapy animals are rising in popularity with the development of programs across the world. However, reports about this particular AAT application explain that it is still highly controversial for the following reasons: (1) most of the support for dolphin-assisted therapy is anecdotal or research without appropriate controls and thus there is relatively little scientific evidence to support this application; (2) the use of dolphins as therapy animals in many instances is considered inappropriate exploitation of a wild species; (3) AAT with dolphins can be harmful to the dolphin; (4) dolphin-assisted therapy is potentially harmful to the human participant in ways that outweigh its potential benefits to the human; and (5) dolphin-assisted therapy has not been found to be any more effective than other types of AAT, especially those that would put an animal or client at significantly less risk (*Science Daily*, 2007). Some of what has been reported about dolphin-assisted therapy is summarized as follows.

There are two primary types of dolphin-assisted therapy. One type is interaction with a dolphin in a tank of water while the human client remains outside of the water and situated on the edge of the water tank, such as petting or feeding the dolphin, tossing toys for the dolphin to fetch, or other types of similar interactions. Another type is interaction with a dolphin in the water while the human client is also in the water in the same enclosed area, such as swimming with the dolphin. The first type of interaction is much safer for both the

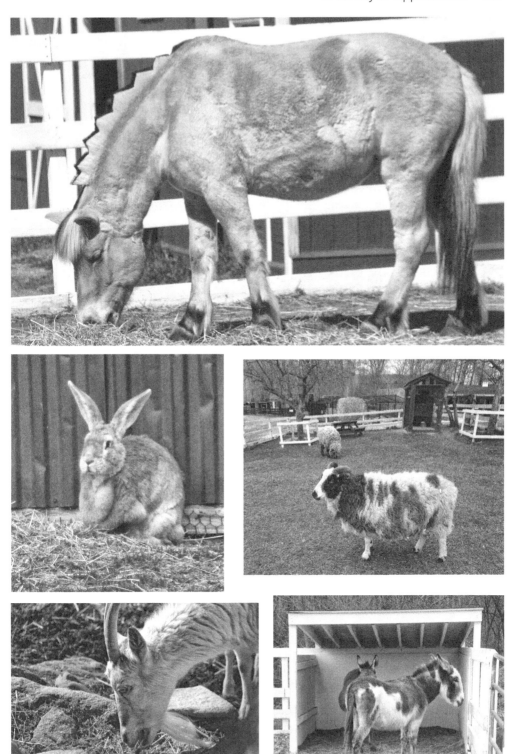

Figures 10.13–10.19 The therapy farm of Green Chimneys in New York has a wide variety of animals with which clients can interact: horses, rabbits, sheep, goats, donkeys, a peacock, and llamas.

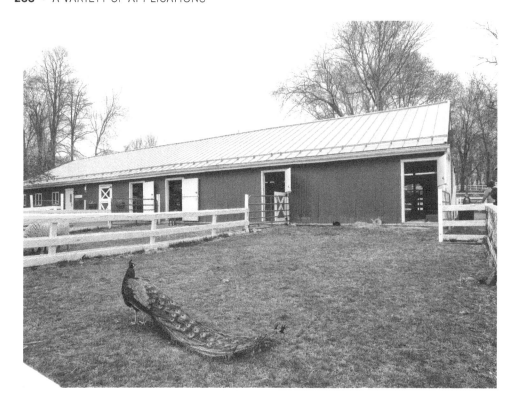

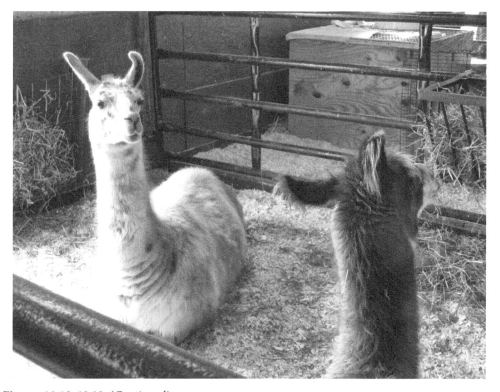

Figures 10.13–10.19 (Continued)

human and the dolphin, whereas the second type involves significantly more risks for injury and infection for both the animal and the human participants. The dolphins that are used in dolphin-assisted therapy include: (1) dolphins that have been bred in captivity, (2) wild dolphins that have been injured, rehabilitated, and can no longer fend for themselves in the wild and are thus having to live the remainder of their lives at an aquarium center, and (3) dolphins that are captured and removed from the wild against their will to participate in dolphin-assisted therapy. The third situation is considered unethical and even cruel for the animal (*Science Daily*, 2007).

Researchers demonstrated the short-term effectiveness of dolphin-assisted therapy with 47 children (20 females and 27 males) with severe disabilities (e.g., Angelman syndrome, autism, cerebral palsy, Cri-du-chat syndrome, Down syndrome, mental retardation, Rett syndrome, and tuberous sclerosis) (Nathanson et al., 1997). A 2-week dolphin-assisted therapy program called dolphin–human therapy was compared with 6 months of conventional physical and speech-language therapy. Following participation in conventional therapy, children received dolphin-assisted therapy for two consecutive 20-minute sessions (a total of 40 minutes) each day for 2 weeks. In each therapy session, children interacted in the water with dolphins as a reward for correct motor or cognitive responses. Following in-water reinforcement, the child and therapist returned to a floating dock for more work, with an increasing number and complexity of correct responses required prior to reinforcement. Standardized charting procedures were used to measure acquisition of independent motor and speech-language skills. Data were analyzed using t-tests for nonindependent samples and results indicated that, relative to the conventional long-term therapy, the dolphin-assisted therapy achieved positive results more quickly and was more cost effective (Nathanson et al., 1997).

Researchers have demonstrated long-term effectiveness of dolphin–human therapy (Nathanson, 1998). A survey questionnaire was completed by the parents of 71 children with severe disabilities who had completed the dolphin therapy program. The children were severely disabled due to genetic causes, brain damage, or unknown etiology. Each child had previously received at least nine therapy sessions in 1 week, although most received 17 therapy sessions in 2 weeks, and each child received dolphin therapy at least 12 months prior to gathering survey data. Parents reported that children maintained or improved skills acquired in therapy about 50 percent of the time even after 12 months away from therapy. It was also found that children who had received 2 weeks of therapy produced better long-term results than those who had received 1 week of therapy (Nathanson, 1998).

Lukina (1999) performed research involving 1,500 children who experienced dolphin-assisted therapy. The therapy was observed to have a positive influence on their autonomic homeostasis and psychoemotional status, which facilitated their psychophysiological rehabilitation. The research was conducted in the State Oceanarium in the aquatory of a Black Sea bay during the summer season. A biotechnical complex had been developed for the dolphin therapy sessions that included Black Sea Afalina dolphins specially trained according to the researcher's methods, including exercises that would stimulate a child to make contact with the dolphin. The patients would swim in the water with the dolphins and interact with the dolphins for 10–15 minutes. The complete set of procedures for each therapy session ranged from 30 minutes to 1.5 hours for each child. The treatment regimen was prescribed individually and consisted of an average of five to ten sessions. The treatment protocol followed these phases:

- Primary (percept-forming) psychotherapy.
- Primary psychophysiological control.
- Distant contact with the dolphin.

- Direct contact with the dolphin in the water.
- Consolidation of dolphin contact through "towing" (dolphin towed the child).
- Stabilization of effect through psychotherapy.
- Secondary psychophysiological control.
- Virtual psychotherapy.

Four groups of children participated in the program:

1. Children who were healthy but whose parents wanted them to improve their health by the dolphin therapy and learn how to swim.
2. Children with symptoms of phobia, enuresis, stammering, and other manifestations of infantile neurosis caused by psychotraumatic impacts of upbringing defects.
3. Children with developmental disability such as autism, mutism, or other speech disorders.
4. Children with weight-bearing and motor system disorders caused by a disease or post-traumatic syndrome.

The study demonstrated that the success of the dolphin therapy sessions depended on the primary psychotherapeutic preparation of the patients. To prepare patients for the dolphin interactions, the psychotherapy helped them to form a positive perception of the dolphins and used relaxation methods to improve their emotional state. As a result of the preliminary psychotherapeutic preparation, there was a positive reaction to the dolphin therapy procedures in almost all of the patients (Lukina, 1999). Regarding the first group of patients who were healthy but who wanted to improve their general health and learn to swim, the following was reported:

> The groupwise analysis of the results of the procedures showed that prior to the procedure, the healthy children felt nervous and many of them feared water and the dolphin. The verbal attitude formed in a child before the session, as well as the exercises with a dolphin in water, helped the children relax and begin to trust the attentive adults and friendly animal. The children's confidence in the animal helped the child to learn swimming. Playing with the dolphin and the resulting positive emotions were a reliable basis for achieving a fuller effect of the sea procedures. . . . Later on, the parents and pedagogues noted the emergence of new individual-personal qualities (kindness, attentiveness to the associates, self-control, and self-discipline) in the children who underwent the dolphin therapy sessions, which was exhibited on the child's family and social rating.
> (Lukina, 1999, p. 678)

For the second group of patients, at the end of the dolphin therapy the frequency and the manifestation of depression, night phobias, hysteria, and enuresis decreased by 50–70 percent on average and in some cases disappeared completely; the children became calmer and more controllable. For the third group of patients, at the end of the dolphin therapy 80 percent of the children were characterized by psychoemotional excitation; children made attempts to pronounce words and expressions, and their parents noted calm sleep patterns of normal duration. For the fourth group of patients, at the end of dolphin therapy 90 percent of patients reported improvements in sleep, general state of mind and body, and moods, as well as acquired confidence in their strength and abilities. The parents and pedagogues of the fourth group noted the appearance of the signs of sociopsychological activity and will (Lukina, 1999).

Research by Webb and Drummond (2001) showed that humans swimming with dolphins reported experiencing increased wellbeing and decreased anxiety. Participants were sampled from two marine areas with dolphin swim programs and included 74 females and 25 males aged between 13 and 65 years. In the wellbeing portion of the study, for each session four people swam with four captive bottlenose dolphins for 25 to 30 minutes. The swim area was approximately 3 meters deep and 200 meters in length and width. Before swimming, participants were given a short lesson in dolphin anatomy by a dolphin trainer, a brief outline on safety precautions while swimming, and instructions on the use of snorkels and flippers before entering the water. Participants completed a wellbeing questionnaire before and after the dolphin swim. For the anxiety part of the study, participants swam with wild dolphins who visited a beachfront area. Dolphins were present each day, and visits by the dolphins to the area were not contingent upon rewards of food. The frequent presence of dolphins at this beachfront meant that people often came to the area to swim and interact with the wild dolphins. Before and after they left the water, these participants filled out the "State" component of the State-Trait Anxiety Inventory. At each of the locations, people who were present but chose not to swim with the dolphins also completed the appropriate inventory. Wellbeing showed to be greater in participants who swam with dolphins than in those who swam without dolphins, both before and after the swim. However, wellbeing increased to the same extent in both swim groups. Thus, the results for wellbeing are inconclusive. In contrast, anxiety decreased for participants swimming with dolphins but not in those who swam without dolphins (Webb and Drummond, 2001).

A randomized controlled dolphin-assisted therapy experiment by Antonioli and Reveley (2005) demonstrated positive effects on depression with a small sample size, 25 adult participants, over a short duration of therapy, 2 weeks. The study showed significantly greater reduction in scores on the Hamilton Rating Scale for depression and on the Beck Depression Inventory for the dolphin-assisted therapy group than in the control group. Participants were adults who had been diagnosed with mild to moderate depression without psychotic features. The study took place at the Roatan Institute for Marine Sciences in the Bay Islands, Honduras. Each treatment session took about 1 hour a day. In the treatment group, participants were asked to perform a number of activities including playing, swimming, and taking care of the animals. In the control group, participants were assigned to an outdoor nature program featuring some similar water activities not involving dolphins. "To avoid disappointment," control group participants had a 1-day session with the dolphins after the final evaluation (Antonioli and Reveley, 2005).

Breitenbach et al. (2009) investigated the effect of dolphin-assisted therapy on changes in interaction and communication between children with severe disabilities and their caregivers. The experimental group included all three aspects of the therapeutic intervention: interaction with dolphins; parent counseling; and a curative, relaxing environment. Three control groups were used. Group 1 was limited to just interaction with the dolphins. In group 2, the parents were counseled after the children interacted with farm animals. Group 3 received no treatment. Pre- and post-evaluations were performed for all treatment and control group participants. Research instruments included questionnaires designed to assess communication and interaction (communication ability) and social–emotional behavior. Observations were taken from 20- to 30-minute video recordings of parent–child interactions carried out in each child's home. Multivariate analysis of variance and analysis of covariance were used to analyze the collected data. Parents of the dolphin-assisted experimental group and control group 1 reported stable and important functional therapy effects in verbal speech and nonverbal reactivity of the children. Furthermore, parents of the experimental group reported observing positive effects in social–emotional competence and self-confidence of their children. Observations of parent–child interaction from video recordings indicated that after treatment in the experimental group interactions of children could be interpreted more accurately by parents over the long term. It is important to note that the discovered therapeutic effects occurred regardless of whether the children were in the water during dolphin-assisted therapy (Breitenbach et al., 2009).

Stumpf and Breitenbach (2014) investigated the effects of a dolphin-assisted therapy program on the communication abilities of children with severe disabilities (Down syndrome, and physical or mental retardation) and their parents. The children participated in four therapeutic sessions of interaction with a dolphin with a focus on verbal and motor skill development; parents observed their children from an adjacent room. The results of the parental questionnaires showed positive, stable changes in children's communicative abilities and social–emotional behavior, as well as in parental quality of life, with mainly large effect sizes (Stumpf and Breitenbach, 2014).

There is much self-promotion by dolphin-assisted therapy programs of the positive impact of this modality on children with disabilities. Many of these programs claim that dolphins can sense and respond to children with needs. As an exploration of this premise, Brensing and Linke (2003) observed human–dolphin interactions in a fenced area in the Florida Keys in the United States to determine if dolphins had any type of preferences in their interactions. Based on their detailed observations of contact and distance behavior between dolphins and different groups of swimmers (adults, children, and children with mental and physical disabilities), they concluded that dolphins prefer children to adults. They also concluded that one female dolphin showed a clear preference toward children with mental and physical disabilities, as well as assisting behavior (Brensing and Linke, 2003). This observational study does not necessarily support a pattern, but it may be possible that dolphins are specially drawn to children and can sense a child in need.

Marino and Lilienfeld (2007) reviewed five peer-reviewed dolphin-assisted therapy studies published in the 8 years prior to their study and found that all five studies were methodologically flawed and plagued by several threats to both internal and construct validity. This review was conducted several years after their first such review of dolphin-assisted therapy studies (Marino and Lilienfeld, 1998). From both reviews, these researchers concluded there was no compelling evidence that dolphin-assisted therapy is a legitimate therapy or that it affords any more than fleeting improvements in mood. In reply to the first review, Nathanson (1998) accused Marino and Lilienfeld of being disingenuous with their positions on the flaws of dolphin-assisted therapy research. Nathanson argued that their criticisms do not have merit because: (1) the types of conditions treated could in fact be treated in a short period of time; (2) the lack of control and comparison groups, while presenting some methodological problems, does not necessarily make conclusions about outcomes premature; and (3) shortcomings in single subject research do not necessarily negate the clinical value of a treatment procedure.

According to Brensing (2005), dolphin-assisted therapy has been employed for about 20 years to help mentally and physically disabled people. She briefly describes a number of studies in support of the therapy, the first of which is a case study by Smith (1981), in which dolphins were used to motivate an autistic child to communicate. In another early study, Nathanson (1989) indicated that children learned two to ten times faster and with greater retention when working with dolphins. Nathanson and de Faria (1993) demonstrated significant improvements in hierarchical cognitive responses of mentally disabled children when they interacted with dolphins. Research performed by Salgueiro et al. (2012) examining the effects of dolphin interaction with children with autism spectrum disorders demonstrated small, but statistically significant, improvements in fine motor development, cognitive performance, and verbal development. Voorhees (1995) found that dolphin-assisted therapy demonstrated an improvement of the social situation in families with disabled children. Cole (1996) and Birch (1997) both reported that interaction with dolphins had a relaxing influence on humans. In addition, a study by Iikura et al. (2001) showed a reduction of anxiety in organized tourists' swimming groups interacting with dolphins in the wild. Aware of critical reviews of dolphin-assisted therapy by Marino and Lilienfeld (1998) and Humphries (2003), Brensing (2005, p. 3) summarized:

> Even if there are several criticisms which needs [sic] to be taken into consideration it could be concluded that the DAT [dolphin-assisted therapy] seems to be a successful animal-assisted therapy . . . However, until now no studies exist which prove or show any indications that DAT is more successful than other animal-assisted therapies.

Some advocates of dolphin-assisted therapy promote the idea that dolphins provide a unique type of therapy that justifies it as a therapeutic modality; that is, they propose that the ultrasound dolphins emit is therapeutic. However, Brensing, Linke, and Todt (2003) studied the ultrasound phenomena and concluded that there is no proof that dolphin ultrasound has an impact on therapy success; there are many good scientific reasons ultrasound should not have any impact under dolphin-assisted therapy conditions.

It seems that dolphin-assisted therapy may not be the best choice for treatment for most clients with physical, mental, or emotional disability for the following reasons:

- There is currently relatively little evidence to support the efficacy of dolphin-assisted therapy.
- Most of the existing evidence is inadequate.
- Dolphin-assisted therapy is very expensive, usually costing thousands of dollars.
- Dolphin-assisted therapy seems to be no more effective than other less expensive AATs.
- The risk of harm to both the dolphins and humans seems to make this a more high-risk therapy than other types of AAT (i.e., a higher risk for injury and infection for both dolphins and humans).

Since aggressive behavioral patterns have been observed in dolphins like hit, chase, ram, forceful push, or bites (Samuels and Spradlin, 1995; Frohoff and Packard, 1995), and water tanks involve additional serious risks of infections and parasitism (Geraci and Ridgway, 1991) for both humans and dolphins, we should strongly consider that dolphin-assisted therapy may pose more risks than benefits, especially since therapy with domesticated animals works just as well or better.

COLLEGE AND UNIVERSITY APPLICATIONS

There are various types of AAT programs at colleges and universities. Some institutions train students and sponsor them to participate in community visitation programs with their pets, such as the following:

- Colorado State University, Human–Animal Bond in Colorado (HABIC) program.
- Carroll College, Human–Animal Bond program.
- Cornell University, Cornell Companions program.
- Delaware University, Certificate in Animal Assisted Activities, Therapy and Education program.
- DePaul University in cooperation with the People, Animals and Nature (PAN, Inc.) program.
- North Georgia College and State University, Pets In Action program.
- Tuskegee University, Center for the Study of Human–Animal Interdependent Relationships.

- University of Tennessee, Human–Animal Bond in Tennessee (H.A.B.I.T.) program.
- Virginia Commonwealth University, School of Medicine, Center for Human–Animal Interaction, "Dogs on Call Program."

Additional college and university programs offer coursework and training in AAA and AAT, with some sponsoring their own animal visitation and therapy groups.

An important consideration for counselor training programs that permit students to perform AAT as part of their practicum or internship experiences is to ensure that the student can perform counseling skills adequately without the presence of a therapy animal before being allowed to integrate a therapy animal into his or her practice. AAT is a more advanced modality requiring more advanced skills than basic counseling skills, and only students who have demonstrated competency in their basic counseling skills should be allowed to incorporate AAT. Many colleges and universities have strict policies about animals, especially dogs, on campus. Thus, you should work with the institute's administration to formulate an institutional policy statement allowing for the presence of qualified therapy animals in classrooms and training labs and clinics. The institutional policy statement does not have to be long and complex; in fact it can be quite brief. However, such a statement should clearly define what is meant by a *qualified therapy animal* and where access is allowed for this animal and its human handler. In addition, the counselor training program faculty and staff need to establish program-level policies and procedures for the incorporation of AAT into their training program; see Appendix E for an example. Some training programs may prefer to limit the practice of AAT by students that occurs indoors (e.g., in the program's own classrooms, labs, and clinics) to certain species such as dogs and pocket pets (gerbils, guinea pigs, or hamsters) since these species are relatively easier to handle in an indoor training environment. In addition, it is very useful for a counselor training program to work with community practitioners and programs that offer AAT to broaden the educational and clinical training and practice of students in AAT, including equine-assisted therapy programs, llama-assisted programs, and therapy farms.

Some AAT or AAA applications at a college or university include one-time or intermittent community service projects, such as the one at Louisiana State University begun in 2009 (Looney, 2009). Initially, six students completed training in AAA that culminated in visits with residents at a Baton Rouge long-term care center. Since the students could not have their own dogs because they lived on campus, faculty and staff at the college volunteered to share their own dogs with the students for this AAA program. Both the students and the dogs had to pass a Delta Society Team Evaluation before they could participate in the visitations. A professor within the College of Agriculture, Catherine Williams, along with an associate dean of the college, Betsy Garrison, came up with the idea to institute the program as a way of creating a signature activity for the residential college, a 2-year "mini-campus" atmosphere offered to first-year students majoring in fields of study within the university's College of Agriculture. Since many of these students want to be veterinarians, it was thought that a program such as this gets the students involved with how animals can help people. Students were carefully selected to participate in this AAA program based on an application and questionnaire, a minimum grade point average of 3.25, and students' reliability and compassion for animals and people. The director of the program stated:

> This has been an excellent educational opportunity for the students, in terms of service they can do for the community with their animals as well as interacting with the residents [of the long-term care facility]. Many of [the students] have never been in a facility such as that, so it helps them to better relate to people in those situations.
>
> (Looney, 2009)

Oklahoma State University has an on-campus pet therapy program where students can receive stress reduction services from trained dog–handler teams (Raymond, 2016). Kent State University has a "Dogs on Campus" program (Raymond, 2016), which was begun after researchers determined that students had a high interest in being visited by dogs on campus as a way of relieving stress and loneliness and increasing social interaction (Adamle, Riley, and Carlson, 2009). The program has several dog teams that have completed training and evaluation. The AAA teams attend dog visitation sessions in the residence halls to help relieve stress and nurture other emotional concerns of students. The students can come into the visitation area, visit the dog teams, and leave. It is very much like what they would do at home (Raymond, 2016).

Gettysburg College in Pennsylvania has a fun AAA tradition that students and employees seem to love called "Dog Days." For the first 2 weeks of every semester, on Mondays and Thursdays from 5:15 to 6:15 p.m. outside the student union building, faculty and staff are invited to bring their dogs for play with students. "Students love seeing the pooches and really like getting to know faculty and staff in a non-stressful environment" (Dog Days, n.d.). This program allows students to meet faculty and staff in a fun environment while receiving some puppy love. The program is effective at increasing student interaction with college personnel and providing some relief from the stress of starting the school term.

Some college and university student counseling services have counselors who work with their pets to provide counseling and guidance services to students. Pam Flint is a psychologist who works with her blonde Labrador Retrievers at the University of North Texas (UNT) Student Counseling and Testing Center. The first therapy dog Dr. Flint worked with was named Roxy. After Dr. Flint and Roxy completed their Delta Society Pet Partners training and registration, Roxy began joining Dr. Flint at her place of employment at UNT. Roxy was welcomed with open arms by clients and staff. Staff often sought Roxy out for a hug or a pet to relieve job stress and requested her at staff meetings to relieve some of the tedium. This therapy team was so successful and so well received on campus that after only 1 year of service Dr. Flint and Roxy won the annual University Staff Service Recognition Award, the first-ever award to an animal at this university. Dr. Flint shared the following stories with me about her AAT work.

> Roxy was greeting one of my new clients during the intake. The client was a tall, muscular, athletic type. After several minutes I suggested that Roxy settle in on her bed because she seemed a little too enthusiastic with the client. The client immediately jumped in and said, "No, please, she is really helping me. I'm nervous telling my story." He continued petting Roxy throughout the interview and she offered him the comfort he needed in the session. He continued his therapy with Roxy and me. It seems that Roxy was more in tune with the client's needs than I was.
>
> On another day, I was working with a middle-aged African–American client. When I introduced the idea of AAT he was reluctant at first, but did agree to give it a try. Roxy won him over instantly by making him feel welcome. In subsequent sessions, when Roxy was at home, he would say how much he missed her. He recently returned to therapy after a protracted break and asked about Roxy. Roxy had since retired from therapy work, but the client formed a great relationship with my new dog, Dakota. The client reminded me how skeptical he was about animal assisted therapy in the beginning and how much he enjoys it now.
>
> (Pam Flint, personal communication, October 3, 2010)

A colleague of Dr. Flint, psychologist Mary K. "Kitty" Roberts, shared the following story with me about how Dr. Flint's dog Dakota has assisted her therapy work:

I am running a group in which group members are asked to recall painful memories regarding the trauma they experienced. They do not directly address the trauma, but how it continues to negatively affect their lives now. There are two individuals who see Pam Flint for individual therapy and know Dakota well. During our first group session, one of the individuals became very distressed. We discussed what might make her feel more comfortable and she suggested that we bring Dakota into our group the next week. The next week, Pam's other client was reading his homework to us. He was visibly distressed and covered his face with his hands. Dakota immediately went to his side and he started stroking Dakota's back. This calmed the client down and he was able to finish the task with less discomfort. I have also had Dakota in session with me for an individual client of mine and she seemed to be comforted by Dakota's presence.

(Mary K. Roberts, personal communication, September 30, 2010)

Another colleague of Dr. Flint, psychologist Martin Gieda, worked with Dr. Flint's dog Roxy and now works with her dog Dakota. He shared the following story with me:

One day I was running a mindfulness group and Dakota was sitting quietly in the therapy room with us. As part of an exercise, the clients and I got on the floor and lay down. At one point, while we were all lying there on the floor on our backs, tuning into our bodies to become more self-aware, I looked over at Dakota. There she was, lying peacefully on her back in the same position as the clients and myself. She had assumed the position all on her own without any prompting or direction. She was just lying there quietly in the same position as the rest of us. In her canine way, she was participating in the exercise like a regular member of the mindfulness group.

(Martin Gieda, personal communication, September 30, 2010)

Perhaps another application for AAT on a college or university campus would be a professor accompanied by his or her pet. Support for the potential benefits of this type of application is provided by Wells and Perrine (2001). In this study, 257 student participants were randomly assigned to view slides of an office and a professor with a pet dog, or a pet cat, or with no animal. The results showed that students perceived the office to be more comfortable and the professor to be friendlier when there was a dog in the office than when there was a cat or no animal in the office. Students also perceived the professor who occupied the office with a cat to be less busy than the professors who occupied the offices with a dog or with no animal. The researchers suggested the results imply that professors may be able to positively influence students' impressions of them by having their pet dog accompany them in their offices (Wells and Perrine, 2001).

While they are not AAT or AAA applications, some college programs allow students' pets to live in the same dormitory facility on campus. Stephens College, a private women's college in Missouri, has had this program since 2004 (Lou, 2010; Yang, 2010). There is a special dorm on campus called Pet Central that has a makeshift kennel, temporary boarding services, and a "doggie spa." Classrooms are pet-free zones so when students go to class their pets go to "Doggy Day Care." Students are monitored by dorm staff and if they are determined to not be taking proper care of their pets then the Pet Council may decide to revoke a student's pet privileges. College president Diane Lynch, who has three dogs and two cats, says,

We find that the students who bring dogs, cats, rabbits to campus are actually among our most responsible students. Part of it is time-management, part of it is responsibility and part of it is having somebody to come home to at night when you've had a tough day who loves you at face value no matter what.

(Yang, 2010)

One freshman student participating in the program said about her experience with her pet dog: "You realize you're away from home and this is it. Daisy was laying right next to me and just cuddling with me and I was like, 'I'm not alone, I'm going to be okay, I've got her'" (Yang, 2010).

Another college that allows pets to live with students on campus is Eckerd College in Florida, which has three residential halls designated as allowing pets along with staff housing. A variety of pets are allowed to live with their owners in the dormitory, including snakes as long as they are not venomous and are less than 6 feet long. Dogs allowed to live in the residence halls must not exceed 40 pounds, and certain "aggressive breeds" are not allowed. Eckerd College has posted on its website a detailed pet policy that may serve as a useful guideline for other colleges and universities wanting to establish a similar program (Eckerd College, n.d.). Some other colleges that allow students to have pets living on campus with them include Washington and Jefferson College in Pennsylvania (Niederberger, 2010; Peters, 2008); the Massachusetts Institute of Technology (Lou, 2010); State University of New York (Hogan, 2008); and Stetson University in Florida (StetsonU, 2010). While programs that allow pets to live on campus with their student owners are considered beneficial in enhancing the emotional wellbeing of the students, some major concerns must be addressed, including having sufficient monitoring of how well the pets are cared for, a possible need to require obedience training for the pets and handlers, and appropriate screening of pet temperament for the safety of other residents.

Cooke and colleagues (2023) performed a review of articles on performing animal-assisted interventions on college and university campuses. A total of 47 articles met the criteria for inclusion in their review, including 24 randomized controlled trials. The most favorable outcomes shown for AAI with college students and staff were for stress, anxiety, and mood. The researchers concluded, "These findings highlight that an AAI on campus could potentially provide a form of stress and anxiety relief, and could be a strategy for addressing rising levels of psychological stress and mental health issues among university students and staff" (p. 1).

ANIMAL-ASSISTED PLAY THERAPY

Different approaches to play therapy allow for a therapist's preferred counseling style; some are more nondirective, as in person-centered play therapy (Landreth, 2002), and others are more directive, as in Adlerian play therapy (Kottman, 2003). Recommended resources for learning about animal-assisted play therapy are VanFleet and Faa-Thompson (2010), Faa-Thompson (2012), and VanFleet (2008).

Play therapy and AAT are a natural fit, especially with dogs. Most dogs have a natural desire to play, so they will feel right at home with a child playing in a therapy room. The typical play therapy room requires some alterations to incorporate AAT. Even though the therapist will always be in the room with the animal, accidents can still happen. Very small toys that can be swallowed by a dog are a choking hazard and should be replaced with slightly larger objects. Sharp objects should also be removed as well as heavy tools that could hurt the therapy pet if used against it; for instance, a metal hammer. All products (e.g., paint, markers, or clay) in the animal-assisted play therapy room should be nontoxic if licked or eaten.

An item that is good to add to an animal-assisted play therapy room is a pet bed or mattress large enough for the pet and a small child to lie down on together. It should have a removable cover for cleaning. Among the standard play therapy toys should be an assortment of toys with animal themes such as dog and cat puppets, cat and dog face masks, and cat and dog action figures and dolls. There should also be toys for the pet to play with and for the pet and the child to play with together. All of the pet's toys should be grouped together on a shelf low enough for the child and the pet to reach. A small, soft-bristled grooming brush is a good item to have among the pet's toys in case the child wishes to brush the pet's fur. Good dog toys for a game of fetch in play therapy include a rubber ball (rubber can be cleaned more easily than a tennis ball) and a soft nylon cloth Frisbee (only if there is enough safe space to fetch and catch the Frisbee). The rubber ball should be textured and not be smooth or have a slick surface because these types of balls, especially handballs, can slip past the tongue and get stuck in a large dog's throat and choke it quickly. The ball should be large enough not to slip down the dog's throat but small enough for the dog to grasp. A nice alternative to the rubber ball is a sponge ball covered with tough canvas or nylon material, found in the toy section of any large department store, especially the ones that sell swimming pool toys. This type of ball will not hurt if it hits anyone and is very durable. It can also be washed easily. Tug-of-war toys should be avoided in AAT due to the high risk of a child getting a finger pinched by a dog trying to get a better grip. The therapy animal should be desensitized to all toys and other play objects in the play area prior to the animal's participation in a counseling session.

A double-safety dog leash should be included in animal-assisted play. This type of leash can be made by attaching a 3- to 4-foot leash to a 6-foot leash and attaching the 6-foot leash to the dog. If the child wants to walk the dog around the room, down the hall, or outside, then the child holds on to the shorter lead, and the therapist holds on to the longer lead that actually controls the dog. This procedure protects the dog from a child that may try to jerk it around on the leash and protects the child from a large dog that may move around and tangle the child in the leash if it is not guided by the therapist. Another safety technique is to attach the leash the client holds to a chest harness on the dog and attach the leash the therapist holds to the dog's neck collar. If the client tugs on the leash attached to the chest harness, it is less likely to cause discomfort for the dog than if the client were tugging on a leash attached to the dog's neck collar.

If the therapy pet is a cat, then the pet's toys should include those types that make for a good game of chase, such as feathers tied to a string. When working with a therapy cat, precautions should be taken to make sure the sand tray or sandbox of a play therapy room is covered at all times that a play session is not going on. The therapy cat will prefer to use its own litter box, hidden in a discreet place in the counseling facility; however, sand can be a tempting place to relieve itself. Though I have not heard of an instance when a therapy cat relieved itself in a therapy sand tray or box, why throw caution to the wind? Keep the sand tray or box covered in between play sessions with a therapy cat, never leave a cat alone in a play therapy room with an uncovered sand tray or box, and make sure the cat has sufficient access to its own litter box before and after a therapy session. A cat can be provided access to its own litter box during a play therapy session if this can be managed in a way that a child cannot access the cat's litter box, such as by placing the litter box in a locked closet where entry can be made only through a small cat-entry door.

Before therapy begins, a brief orientation about the therapy pet should be provided to children and their parent or guardian. This gives children the opportunity to meet and learn about the pet outside of the play therapy room. They will feel more comfortable with initiating interactions with the pet during play therapy if the therapist explains beforehand the types of activities they can do with the pet if they want to at some time, such as petting the animal, playing with toys with the pet, brushing the pet, talking to or about the pet, hugging or lying down with the pet, asking the pet to do tricks, and walking the pet. Emphasize to children that the choice to interact or not with the pet is entirely up to them. If children prefer not to interact with the therapy pet, the therapist can place the dog in a *down, stay* on its bed or mattress. This leaves the way open for the child to still initiate interaction with the therapy pet during a session if the child desires to. The pet's portable crate should also have a special place in the play therapy room in case the therapist needs to crate the pet for the comfort of the child or the pet gets tired and needs a break or a nap in the crate.

As children interact with the therapy pet, the therapist may need to use a limit-setting technique when necessary, for the protection of the pet—for instance, "Rusty the dog is not for hitting," or "Rusty the dog is not for painting." Any activity that in the therapist's judgment causes stress, discomfort, or danger for the therapy pet should not be allowed. Children should not be allowed to hit a pet or shoot a pet with a type of gun that projects objects, like a dart gun. Some play therapists believe a child should not point a toy gun at the therapist and pretend to shoot the therapist: "The therapist is not for shooting." These same therapists may feel that pointing a toy gun and pretending to shoot the therapy pet is not acceptable. While I am not willing to immerse myself in the "pretending to shoot the toy gun at the human or pet therapist" debate, I will recommend that therapists use their judgment given the circumstances. A common and fun trick that many dogs do well is play dead. Again, this trick can be avoided if a therapist judges it is not appropriate given the child and the circumstances.

If a child accidentally or purposefully pours paint onto a therapy animal, a therapist should treat the incident in the same way the therapist would if the child had poured paint onto another child. Together the therapist and child would wipe the animal's fur as clean and as soon as possible so the paint does not get in the pet's eyes or licked off by the pet and so it does not get further spattered. The paint should be nontoxic if ingested in case the pet

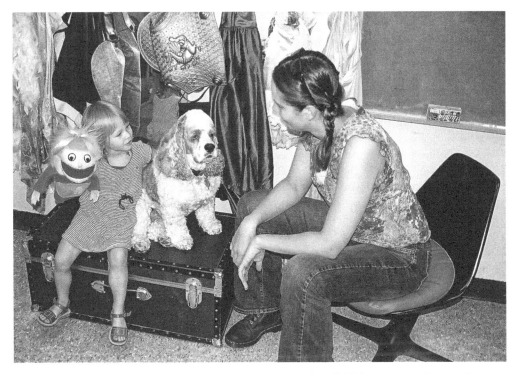

Figure 10.20 Therapy dog Rusty snuggles and interacts with a child during animal-assisted puppet play therapy.

does lick at it and water soluble so it washes out when you bathe the pet thoroughly when you get home. If a therapy animal will tolerate being dressed up by the child without being stressed, then this can be allowed. If a particular pet shies away from or is not comfortable being dressed up, then the counselor can simply reflect that the pet is not so sure about being dressed up or that the pet must not want to be dressed up or something similar that directs the child not to dress the pet up, such as, "This dog is not for dressing because he is not comfortable being dressed up."

During an animal-assisted play therapy session, it is very acceptable for the therapist to pet the therapy animal when the therapy animal seeks out affection from the therapist. This modeling behavior reinforces for the child that it is okay to pet the therapy animal if the client chooses to do so, and it also reassures the client somewhat that the therapist must be an okay person if the pet likes the therapist and likewise the therapist treats the pet nicely.

An exciting concept for animal-assisted play therapy is a play therapy yard. If you can create a small outside area near your counseling office, then a play yard can be used for more rambunctious play with a therapy dog. A play yard would allow a greater variety of activity for AAT, such as appropriate space for walking or running with the dog, to play a game of fetch, or to take the dog through agility obstacles. A play yard could incorporate many other aspects of nature therapy as well. You can add a small, shallow pond with fish and water plants and add a small waterfall. You can have feeders to attract neighborhood birds. You can plant a butterfly garden with plants to attract butterflies for laying their eggs, such as dill and fennel, and native nectar flowers for feeding the butterflies. A complete lifecycle butterfly garden is a unique opportunity to teach the cycle of life and instill hope and faith in the wonder of nature. A word of warning: place the bird feeders on the opposite side of the yard as the egg-laying plants that attract butterflies to give the poor caterpillars a fighting chance of survival from the birds, who find them a scrumptious delicacy. Once a caterpillar builds and submerses itself into its chrysalis it can be taken inside to a butterfly hatchery for safekeeping until it is time for the butterfly to emerge and be set free. As I write this piece, I am sitting out in my sunroom that looks out into my backyard and am watching a bright red, male cardinal feed two of its juveniles that have not yet learned to feed themselves. This is a common occurrence in my backyard that I have developed into a small "bird-scaped" sanctuary, yet each time I see this parental act of nature, I am deeply moved by it. Observations of nature help keep me grounded, reassured, and realistic. The therapeutic benefits of the observation of nature by clients are potentially vast.

Risë VanFleet (2008; http://risevanfleet.com/aapt/; www.playfulpooch.org) is a well-known practitioner of play therapy as well as animal-assisted play therapy in Pennsylvania. She teaches clients how to be around animals safely and facilitates a variety of human–animal interaction activities for clients and therapy animals to participate in together. Van-Fleet shares her views in an interview she gave (Ford Sori and Ciastko Hughes, 2014):

> The animals provide what's called a social lubricant effect, in that, if a client of any age finds it difficult to trust other humans, they might be able to relate to an animal more readily. Attachment theory is the primary underlying theory that I'm focused on when doing animal assisted play therapy. I'm really looking for how we create good relationships. . . . If we feel safe with the animals and are able to create some sort of connection with them, there are definitely indications that this carries over to human relationships. . . . There's something that happens when the animal is there; perhaps it creates an additional sense of safety, perhaps less focus on the child, less self-consciousness. . . . You might be the first person the child can trust

because you've shared your own animal with them. If they like the animal, they start liking you a little better; feeling more comfortable with you. That forms a bridge to improved human connections.

(Ford Sori and Ciastko Hughes, 2014, p. 351)

Nancy Parish-Plass (2008, 2013) works as an animal-assisted psychotherapist on a kibbutz in Israel and at a children's residential center. She presented a working model for integrating AAT into play therapy treatment of children suffering from insecure attachment due to abuse and neglect. Since an abused or neglected child may have a fear of adults, the presence of a therapy animal may assist with the child trusting the adult therapist. Parish-Plass integrated AAT into nondirective play sessions,

in which the child chooses the activities, materials, toys and themes, while the therapist flows with the child in an attentive and interactive manner. The therapist mirrors and reflects the child's actions, emotions and processes in order to encourage insight as well as further the development of themes within the play context. During the process of role play, the therapist may seek clarifications of the child's intentions and may request and/or receive instructions from the child as to how to act or react.

(Parish-Plass, 2008, p. 18)

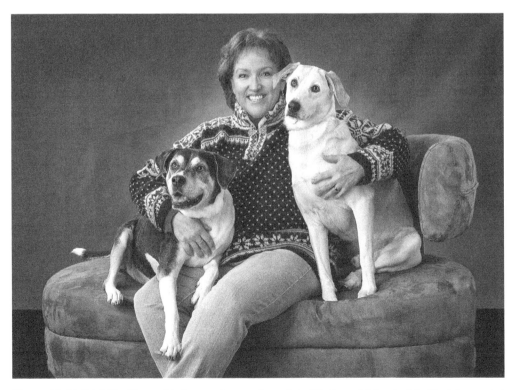

Figure 10.21 Risë VanFleet with her canine co-therapists, Kirrie and Murrie. VanFleet is a noted expert in animal-assisted play therapy.

(*Source:* photo courtesy of Risë VanFleet.)

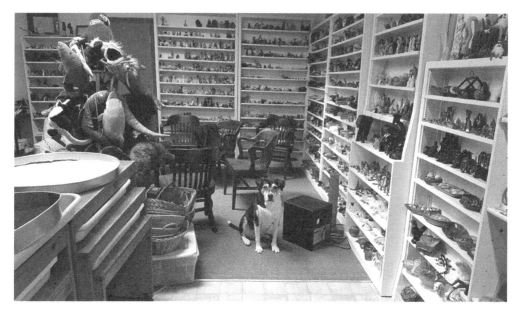

Figure 10.22 Therapy dog Kirrie in the play and sand tray room of therapist Risë VanFleet.

(*Source:* photo courtesy of Risë VanFleet.)

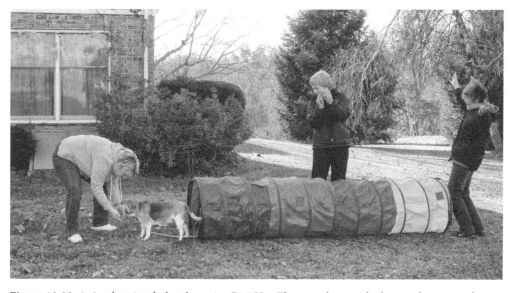

Figure 10.23 Animal-assisted play therapist, Risë Van Fleet, working with clients who are teaching a new agility skill to a dog as part of therapy.

(*Source:* photo courtesy of Risë VanFleet.)

The play therapy room contained the typical toys found in play therapy in addition to a number of well-socialized animals that were present. These therapy animals, which were the family pets of the therapist, included a dog, birds (cockatiels), rats, and hamsters. All of the animals were in cages at the beginning of the session except for the dog. The children decided which animals to take out and interact with and when. Based on several case examples presented by Parish-Plass (2008, pp. 13–15), ATT offered the following benefits to the treatment sessions of abused and neglected children:

- Enabling a social connection.
- Sense of normalcy, safety, and friendliness of the therapy setting.
- Acceptance from a social being.
- Reality at a safe psychological distance.
- Self-esteem from positive interactions with the therapy animal.
- The animal serving as a positively reinforcing attachment figure.
- Development of more adaptive representations and strategies.
- Empathy for the therapy animal.
- Fill a need for control of self, others, and the situation.
- Therapeutic touch.
- Reduce regression.
- Comfort from previous separation, loss, and bereavement.

Parish-Plass (2008, 2013) believed that the beneficial properties of AAT make it an effective method to lower the risk of intergenerational transmission of abuse, especially as a result of the positive nurturing relationship that can be formed between the child and the therapy animal and the way AAT can facilitate the formation of a positive relationship between the child and the therapist.

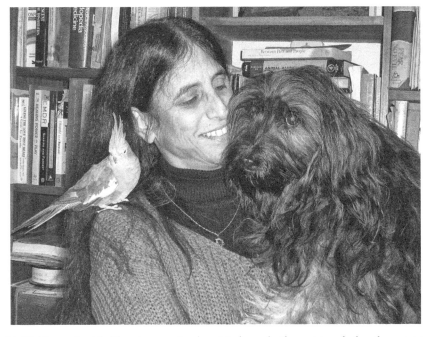

Figure 10.24 Nancy Parish-Plass is an animal-assisted psychotherapist and play therapist in Israel. She practiced on the kibbutz where she lived and at a residential children's center. She is seen here with her dog Mushu and pet cockatiel who work with her providing therapy.

(*Source:* photo courtesy of Nancy Parish-Plass.)

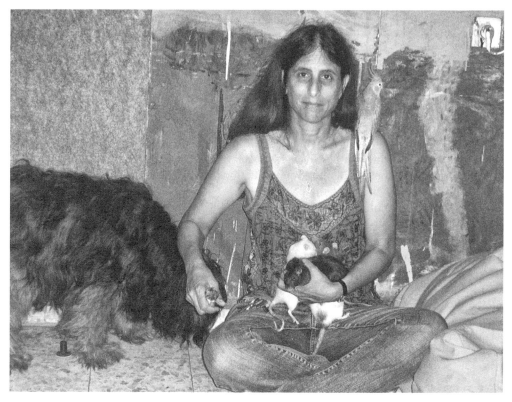

Figure 10.25 Nancy Parish-Plass in Israel performs animal-assisted play therapy with a variety of therapy animals: dog, cockatiel, rats, and hamsters.

(*Source:* photo courtesy of Nancy Parish-Plass.)

Reichert (1994) presented a model for animal-assisted group play therapy for sexually abused girls aged 9 to 13 years. The pet therapist in the intervention was a 4-year-old part Dachshund named Buster:

> The purpose of utilizing a pet in therapy was to build a bridge to ease tension and anxiety. The children had an option of disclosing their abuse into the pet's ear or to tell the group. Further the pet was used for playing, touching, and projecting their feelings. It was also effective as a means of gathering family histories and stories. The children would tell about their experiences with pets as well.
>
> (Reichert, 1994, p. 58)

Reichert (1994) used a variety of techniques such as nondirective play and some structured exercises to assist the girls in increasing an awareness of their feelings and to openly share their feelings. These exercises were often very creative, such as making a collage that represented inside versus outside feelings. The girls were encouraged to tell their sexual abuse stories, and some chose puppets for this outlet. Puppet theater was a useful medium for the therapist to convey metaphorical, therapeutic stories. The therapist led relaxation and guided imagery exercises to help children find a safe place in their mind. Empowerment exercises, including puppet theater activities and collage making, were incorporated to strengthen their inner resources. Throughout the sessions, the therapy dog was present. Sometimes the children would "hold the pet in order to ease tension, reflect anxiety, or for support" (Reichert, 1994, p. 60).

ADDITIONAL AAT APPLICATIONS

There are many possible applications for AAT in many different environments. Some practitioners and researchers have provided useful guidelines for these applications, some of which are briefly described below. The length and detail provided by the authors in the descriptions of their programs do not allow for an in-depth discussion of these program presentations here; thus, it is recommended that you obtain the cited work describing the program if you are interested in more information.

Sexual Abuse and Assault

Lefkowitz et al. (2005) recommended and described a session-by-session format for providing AAT to adult survivors of sexual assault suffering from post-traumatic stress disorder (PTSD). The authors described how AAT could be integrated into the prolonged exposure (PE) treatment approach for PTSD. The authors suggested that interactions with a therapy animal, such as petting and holding, during the PE treatment for PTSD, decreased anxiety, lowered physiological arousal, enhanced the therapeutic alliance, and promoted social interaction. In addition, the authors believed that AAT could decrease the number of sessions required for habituation to the traumatic experience (Lefkowitz et al., 2005).

Eggiman (2006) described a case study in which AAT was beneficial during cognitive-behavioral therapy with a 10-year-old girl with PTSD and a history of physical and sexual abuse. The girl's behaviors before the therapy animal was introduced into sessions included: constant body movements and walking around; constant talking with an inability to focus on one topic; difficulty following rules; difficulty remaining calm; could not identify feelings or show empathy for anyone she would hurt; appeared rough and uncaring; and did not respect boundaries or personal space. The girl's behaviors in the first and subsequent sessions where the therapy dog, a 3-year-old standard Poodle named Kotter, was present included the following: sat quietly on the floor with Kotter's head in her lap; listened to a therapeutic story and then drew a picture of her foster family; followed every rule with regard to Kotter, including petting rules; allowed her muscles to relax; shared thoughts and feelings about her mother; and showed a gentle and caring attitude toward Kotter. The therapist also shared that in subsequent sessions with Kotter the girl was able to disclose more memories of abuse in the safe and secure atmosphere. Also, her behavior at home and at school was reported to be improved (Eggiman, 2006).

Reichert (1998) described individual counseling with sexually abused children that included a role for therapy animals and story-telling. Some of the considerations and procedures she used are described briefly here. The therapist should allow time for the child to get acquainted with and become comfortable with the therapy animal so that the animal's presence can assist the child during other processes by serving as a friendly source of comfort. Indirect interviewing through the animal can be useful instead of directly asking questions to the child; for instance, "Buster [therapy dog] wants to know what your favorite game is," or "Buster would like to know how old you are." Initial discussion of the traumatizing event can occur when the child and therapist engage in a quiet, parallel activity, like side-by-side drawing or stroking and holding the animal. Incorporating the animal as the child's alter ego helps the child to express his or her feelings, for instance, telling a child, "Buster had a nightmare," and continuing, "The nightmare was about being afraid of getting hurt again by someone mean." This method allows children to indirectly express their feelings by projecting onto Buster. Story-telling by the therapist about the therapy animal can be used metaphorically to help children express their feelings and tell what happened to them. After the story the therapist can ask children questions about how they thought the dog felt during incidents in the story. The therapist can end the story processing by saying, "Bad things can happen to good little doggies like Buster, just as bad things can happen to good little kids." By integrating the animal into the story, the therapist "presents the child with the opportunity to identify with the animal and project her feelings onto the animal, thus facilitating disclosure and expression of feelings" (Reichert, 1998, pp. 182–184).

Anger Management

Hanselman (2002) provided a detailed framework for incorporating therapy dogs into a group-format anger management program with adolescents who have a history of aggression and abuse toward humans or animals. Some of the adolescent participants were court- mandated to participate. The therapy dogs were present for the adolescents to pet and interact with during the cognitive-behavioral treatment approach. The incorporation of the dogs was thought to be important as a stimulus for empathy development and attachment formation in the adolescents. The researcher documented client progress using standardized instruments and self-report mood logs. The results showed significant decreases in both emotional and behavioral anger for participants (Hanselman, 2002).

Autism

I described research studies of animal assisted treatment for autism in Chapter 2 of this book. In addition, some additional studies are presented in Chapter 9 on equine-assisted programs for the treatment of autism. Here I mention some related information on animal-assisted approaches to treating autism.

Silva et al. (2011) described how a 12-year-old boy diagnosed with ASD, who was living in Portugal, performed structured activities better with a therapist and therapy dog than with the therapist alone (no dog present). In the presence of the dog, the child exhibited more frequent and longer durations of positive behaviors, such as smiling and initiating physical contact, as well as less frequent and shorter durations of negative behaviors, such as aggressive manifestations. They concluded that interactions with a therapy dog may "prime" a child with autism for treatment (Silva et al., 2011).

Obrusnikova et al. (2012) described a program for integrating therapy dog teams in a physical activity program for children with ASD. The therapy dog-assisted activities provided physical, social, and emotional benefits for the children. Obrusnikova et al. (2012) explained how to: partner with a therapy dog organization, screen and choose therapy dog teams, screen and select child participants, run and evaluate the program, and keep contact after the program.

11

Sensitivity to Cultural Differences and Populations with Special Needs

The clients you provide services for may have a different opinion from you about animals. Thus, it is important to be sensitive to varying attitudes about animals by clients that might be a result of differences in cultural background or prior experiences. A client may have a family history that considers pets to be outside animals only and may not feel comfortable with an animal indoors. A client may be afraid of large dogs, having only limited exposure to them as aggressive guard dogs or unfortunate victims of organized dog fighting. A client may originate from a country that does not generally view animals as pets but rather as food or as laborers. A client may not have had many or any opportunities to be around certain types of animals, especially farm animals or horses, and therefore might be uncomfortable around them. A client may have once had a bad or overly sad experience with a pet and thus may find it difficult to be around a similar type of pet. Thus, to be better prepared for the initial session with a client, it is important for the therapist to include in the client-screening process for AAT an inquiry about the client's previous exposure to or attitude about animals or pets (see the Client Screening Form for Animal-Assisted Therapy provided in Appendix B).

To minimize anticipatory anxiety or discomfort about interacting with a therapy animal, the therapist should provide clients with an explanation for the animal's purpose and expected types of interactions the pet may engage in with the client. A description of potential benefits to be gained by working with a therapy animal can be described to the client. Clarification as to how and when a client can typically engage with a therapy animal can also be given. Also, a therapist can initiate some animal behaviors at a distance from the client to help the client warm up to the idea of being around the therapy animal. A common technique I use to demonstrate that the therapy pet is not a threat is to ask one of my therapy dogs to do a trick or a series of tricks for the client. This usually gets the client smiling or laughing and helps to relieve the initial fear or distrust the client had toward the animal. Then, I invite the client to ask the dog to repeat one of the tricks at the client's request. This almost always results in the client moving in much closer to the dog and speaking to it. Once the dog has performed the trick for the client and is happily wagging its tail afterward in anticipation of a treat or pet on the head, the once uncertain client then may even reach out and pet the dog. This slow initiation technique is very useful with clients in whom you sense an uneasiness about being around the therapy animal, which occurs especially for small children.

Always respect a client's desire not to work with a therapy animal. Provide a safe and comfortable place for the therapy animal to rest during the counseling session with that client. One possibility is to place the therapy pet on a bed or in a crate the animal is familiar with in a corner of the therapy room away from the client or in another room nearby. Occasionally invite the client to spend time with the therapy pet without pressuring or coercing the client to do so. If the client does choose to spend time with the therapy pet, let the client set the distance parameters for the client's own comfort level.

In my volunteer therapy work at a juvenile facility, I experienced that about one in every ten of the adolescents was afraid of being around my therapy dog the first time they met the dog. This ratio was high because many of these juveniles came from a severely dysfunctional home, and it was not uncommon for highly dysfunctional families to also have a dysfunctional relationship with a dog or not to have a dog at all. Adolescents afraid of the therapy dogs typically had or knew dogs that were not properly socialized and trained and therefore the dogs were unruly or aggressive. Sometimes the dogs they had known were trained to be aggressive, such as guard or fighting dogs. Either way, the adolescents afraid of dogs usually had a negative or absent history with them. Over the many years that I performed AAT with the kids at the juvenile detention center almost all of the adolescents who were originally afraid of the therapy dog overcame their fears and apprehension over a period of several sessions and engaged in frequent touching and playing with the dog. In addition, these adolescents commonly described their ability to overcome their fears with pride as they shared their animal therapy experiences with counselors, case workers, and family members.

At the graduation ceremony, held when the juvenile is ultimately released from custody after having completed the residential rehabilitation program, the adolescents often sought me out to introduce me and the therapy dog to family members, and the family members commented on how remarkable it was that their child overcame their strong fear of dogs and how proud they were of their child for this accomplishment. Also, these adolescents commented on how their work with the therapy dog helped them to be less anxious around other dogs that they could now more objectively judge as presenting no threat to them. I believe the original fear of the therapy dogs subsided quickly with these adolescents because they had multiple opportunities to observe from a comfortable distance all of the other adolescents interacting with the dog in a fun and playful manner. They could then slowly move toward or away from the animal at their choosing to test their sense of safety and comfort until they could remain close to and interact with the therapy dog without being inhibited by their fear. They were motivated to try to move closer because they saw how much fun the other kids were having, and they wanted to experience the same enjoyment. Motivation to participate is a key to any desensitization therapy, as is having a sense of control over the situation.

CULTURAL DIFFERENCES IN ATTITUDES ABOUT ANIMALS

While it is important not to stereotype individuals based on the culture or ethnic group with which they affiliate, it is important to be aware of potential cultural differences in how people view animals. There is relatively little published on the subject of cultural comfort with AAT or culturally sensitive applications of AAT. This is an area where research is much needed. From existing literature, mostly on pet ownership, we can discern some idea as to how to be more culturally aware and sensitive when considering AAT with members of different cultures.

Caucasians

Caucasians, that is non-Hispanic white people, were estimated in 2022 to make up 58.9 percent of the U.S. population at over 194 million (U.S. Census Bureau, 2023a). Taken as a cultural group, Caucasians in general are more likely to have and value companion animals than most other cultural groups, considering them to be sources of emotional support, unconditional love, and viewing these animals as family members (Risley-Curtiss, Holley, and Wolf, 2006). Thus, Caucasians may be more likely to be accepting of AAT and to feel very comfortable with companion animal interaction. However, counselors must not erroneously assume that all Caucasians feel comfortable with companion animals. Some people may have had little contact with certain species of companion animals or may have had a negative experience with a particular type of companion animal (Sheade and Chandler, 2014).

Caucasian Europeans and Caucasian Americans have incorporated cats and dogs and other animals as pets into the family system for centuries, and the concept of the household pet is very common. Caucasian Europeans and Caucasian Americans traditionally take individual or family ownership of a pet and assume private responsibility for the feeding, training, and care of a pet; neutering or spaying the pet; and typically confining the pet to the owner's home or property when the pet is not accompanying the owner on a leash or riding with the owner in a vehicle.

Native Americans, First Nations, and Indigenous Peoples

American Indian or Alaska Native is defined by the U.S. Census Bureau as a person having origins in any of the original peoples of North and South America (including Central America) and who maintains tribal affiliation or community attachment (U.S. Census Bureau, 2023a). In 2022, the nation's population of Native American Indians was estimated to be 6.79 million, which is about 2.09 percent of the entire population (U.S. Census Bureau, 2023a). There are about 574 federally recognized tribes, and 15 states have populations over 100,000. Native Americans, First Nations, and indigenous peoples may have some of the strongest human–animal relationships and are more likely to have companion animals than most other ethnic groups (Risley-Curtiss, Holley, and Wolf, 2006; Robinson, 1999). These groups often focus on the equality and interdependence of all creatures and see opportunities for health and healing through relationships with animals (Kesner and Pritzker, 2008). Dell and colleagues created a culturally sensitive model for building resiliency in First Nations youth struggling with solvent abuse by adding an equine-assisted learning component based on the horse's profound sacredness to this tribe and the belief that the horse will lead one in the right direction (Dell et al., 2008). From a study of this program, it was concluded:

> [Y]ouths' healing was aided through the availability of a culturally-relevant space; from within an Aboriginal worldview this understanding of space is central to individual and communal well-being. This was conveyed in three key themes that emerged from the data: spiritual exchange, complementary communication, and authentic occurrence. This understanding provides insight into the dynamics of healing for Aboriginal youth who abuse solvents, and may be applicable to other programming and populations.
> (Dell et al., 2011, p. 319)

Although incorporating animals into counseling can be very effective for Native American clients, practitioners must remember that each tribe has its own customs and traditions associated with animals and the human–animal relationship (Risley-Curtiss et al., 2006). On some Native American reservations, individuals do not own dogs and cats, but rather prefer to allow these animals to roam freely; in contrast, personal pet ownership of dogs and cats is more common among Native Americans who live off of a reservation (Munro, 2004). Large numbers of dogs and cats can be found running loose on some Native American reservations. The tribe shares in the feeding and care of the reservation dogs and cats. Few of these reservation animals, if any, are ever spayed or neutered. Native Americans have a special respect for an animal's spirit and purpose, and tradition and culture impose an informal noninterference policy of sorts for these animals:

> David Ortiz is a writer and anthropologist based in Flagstaff, Arizona. His work has taken him to the heart of the Navajo population—a patriarchal culture where elders still pass down traditions and customs, and shape the attitudes of younger generations. "Many older people on the reservation lands were brought up with the idea that animals are a resource," says Ortiz. "Dogs guard the hogan or house and herd sheep and goats. A cat's job is to kill mice and other smaller animals. When animal welfare people show up and start talking about altering the animals to control the population, they just can't relate to it. They feel in part that dogs and cats need to reproduce to provide food for coyotes and other predators. They're part of the cycle of life".
>
> (Munro, 2004, p. 14)

The cost of taking care of an animal also prohibits the idea of a family pet for many Native Americans:

> Many tribes are excessively poor, and some of the most basic human needs—food, medical care, and adequate housing—are not met. And that's often the biggest stumbling block when trying to change attitudes about animals. Add to that the belief that all of life will begin and end as it is intended, as part of the natural world, and the resistance to animal welfare is understandable.
>
> (Munro, 2004, p. 14)

Latinos and Hispanics

Latino refers to being from a Latin American family of origin, while Hispanic refers to being from a Spanish-speaking family of origin (Pittman, 2015). While the two groups greatly overlap, they are still considered different groups. The U.S. Census Bureau reports statistics for Hispanics with no separate category for Latinos. In 2022, Hispanics were estimated to be 17.8 percent of the entire U.S. population at 47.7 million (U.S. Census Bureau, 2023a).

Latino and Hispanic individuals are more likely to have companion animals than most other minority groups in the United States, but are less likely to have cats as pets than either Caucasians or Native Americans (Risley-Curtiss, Holley, and Wolf, 2006). Latino and Hispanic clients are much more likely to have dogs than other animals (Risley-Curtiss, Holley, and Wolf, 2006). Members of the Latino and Hispanic cultural group do tend to see their animals similarly to Caucasian clients in their view of them as sources of support and companionship, and as members of the family (Faver and Cavazos, 2008; Johnson and Meadows, 2002; Schoenfeld-Tacher, Kogan, and Wright, 2010). Members of the Latino and Hispanic cultures form strong human–animal bonds and place a higher degree of emphasis on the animal's ability to provide a sense of safety than Caucasian clients (Risley-Curtiss, Holley, and Wolf, 2006; Schoenfeld-Tacher, Kogan, and Wright, 2010). Clients who have immigrated from Central and South America may see animals, especially dogs, differently from Latino and Hispanic clients who have lived in the United States or Europe. In Peru, dogs may serve a more utilitarian purpose as herding and work animals (Walsh, 2009). Central and South American clients are often not used to having private companion animals but may have formed relationships with free-roaming community dogs in the village. These animals were valued as pest control and working animals that were often fed by many, but belonged to no one:

> The concept of the "community dog" is at the heart of Latino custom. Few people would have a personal pet but all would interact with the dogs and cats who lived

within the village. Animals who were prized were the working animals who could help a family survive economically. In poor villages, stray dogs were often fed by many but belonged to none.

(Richard, 2004, p. 12)

Depending upon a client's environment, some Latino and Hispanic clients may dislike and even fear dogs. Latino and Hispanic residents born in the United States, as opposed to Mexico, reported less fear of dogs. Poss and Bader (2007) found that most residents of colonias saw free-roaming dogs as a problem and feared going outside. Colonias are low-income, mostly Hispanic, communities located primarily along the United States and Mexico border. Colonias can be found in Texas, New Mexico, Arizona, and California, but Texas has both the largest number of colonias and the largest colonia population—there are more than 2,294 Texas colonias along the 1,248-mile border (Texas Secretary of State, 2016). Approximately 400,000 Texans live in colonias. Overall, the colonia population is predominately Hispanic; 64.4 percent of all colonia residents and 85 percent of those residents under 18 were born in the United States.

It is important for counselors to consider the unique context of a Latino or Hispanic client in determining the appropriateness of AAT. In a study on interpersonal violence, Schultz, Remick-Barlow, and Robbins (2007) found that in a mixed sample of Hispanic and Caucasian children, both groups received therapeutic benefits following animal-assisted psychotherapy, indicating that members of this population can equally benefit from AAI. Risley-Curtiss, Holley, and Wolf (2006) recommended that working with dogs as co-therapists could benefit Latino and Hispanic clients.

African–Americans

An African–American is defined by the U.S. Census Bureau as a person having origins in any of the Black racial groups of Africa (U.S. Census Bureau, 2023a). Black persons in the United States in 2023 represented 13.6 percent of the entire population at about 47.2 million (U.S. Census Bureau, 2023a). There is scarce information regarding the African–American population and the human–animal relationship. In comparing Caucasian and African–American veterinary students, Brown (2002) found several differences between the two groups. Brown found African–American students to hold more utilitarian and negative views toward animals and to demonstrate less attachment to their companion animals than Caucasian students. Brown offered several hypotheses for this phenomenon, such as differences in values, socioeconomic status, and cultural norms.

In considering these differences, it is especially important for a counselor to thoroughly explore an African–American client's perceptions of and prior experiences with animals before introducing a therapy animal as these clients may be less receptive toward forming a therapeutic relationship with an animal. However, Brown (2002) reported that African–American students acknowledged the health benefits of having a companion animal. Researchers have reported benefits such as feelings of acceptance and loyalty by animals in AAT with African–American children (Greenwald, 2000; Mallon, 1994a).

Asians

In 2022 the Asian population in the United States was estimated to be 6.3 percent, this was over 21 million people (U.S. Census Bureau, 2023a). More than 60 percent of this growth in the Asian population came from international migration.

Some researchers have reported success utilizing AAI with Asian populations in their native country. Yeh (2008) found that incorporating dogs into work with children with autism facilitated the development of social skills in Taiwan. Keino et al. (2009) successfully applied a psychoeducational horseback riding program to the treatment of four Japanese children diagnosed with pervasive developmental disorders which resulted in enhanced social and interaction behaviors by the children. In their investigation of patients with schizophrenia in Japan, Iwahashi, Waga, and Ohta (2007) found most patients wanted contact with animals and that they liked animals, with their favorite animals being dogs and cats.

Animals hold a powerful symbolic place in some Asian cultures, such as the Chinese emphasis on the animal associated with one's birth year. However, a symbolic reverence for animals does not always translate into personal comfort with a companion animal. Risley-Curtiss, Holley, and Wolf (2006) found Asian people to be the least likely to have companion animals. Many Asian people may consider dogs and other animals to be unclean or a nuisance, thus providing a potential barrier to an Asian client's ability to form a relationship with a therapy animal (Matuszek, 2010). Koreans may see some animals, such as dogs, as a source of food and not appropriate for working in a professional role (Chandler, 2012). Some clients may fear dogs, having only experienced them as aggressive guard dogs (Chandler, 2012). Even in contemporary, modern Asian cultures, such as in Hong Kong and South Korea, many people do not have pets because historically animals were not kept as pets and a lack of space and finances does not allow for the adequate care of pets (Chandler, 2012). Although AAT may potentially provide many benefits for Asian clients, counselors must consider an individual's possible discomfort with animals or prior negative beliefs or experiences that may hinder the client's ability to benefit from AAT.

Middle Easterners

According to the U.S. Census Bureau (2023b), Middle Easterners are considered to be those of Arab or North African (MENA) descent and there were 3.5 million MENA persons living in the United States in 2020. The Census Bureau's classification of the MENA population is geographically based and includes Arab-speaking groups, such as Egyptian and Jordanian, and non-Arab speaking groups, such as Iranian and Israeli. It also includes ethnic and transnational groups from the region, such as Assyrian and Kurdish. Regarding Middle Eastern people, there is very little literature about AAT or pet ownership with this population. People from certain regions have a fear of dogs that is part of their culture. A student enrolled in our counselor training program at the university, who was from Kuwait, jumped away in fear when she entered our office suite and saw me standing there with my dog Rusty, who was on a leash. I immediately acknowledged her reaction and reassured her that the dog was safe to be around. She politely requested I remove the dog, and out of respect for her wishes I took the dog back to my office and rejoined her in the office waiting area. She explained to me that in Kuwait many packs of wild dogs roam free and that she was always taught to fear dogs out of self-preservation. She said that many people from the Middle East have this same fear because free-roaming wild dogs are very common there. Sensitivity to people's fear of animals is very important to consider while being accompanied by a therapy animal.

Middle Eastern people may view dogs and other animals as unclean or a nuisance, thus impeding the animal's ability to be therapeutic (Matuszek, 2010). It is also important to be sensitive to religious views about animals. According to Sheikh Ahmad Kutty, a senior lecturer and Islamic scholar at the Islamic Institute of Toronto, Canada, the teachings of Islam consider a dog unclean, and therefore people who follow this religion may not keep dogs as pets or may not desire to have interaction with dogs (Kutty, 2010). However, there are instances where dogs may be kept and interaction with dogs is permissible in this religious culture, such as a trained dog for hunting, a trained dog that provides service for persons with a disability, a dog trained for police duties, a guard dog for houses or property, or dogs who work with farmers to shepherd cattle and sheep (Kutty, 2010). One should be respectful of individuals who hold a religious view that does not condone contact with certain animals, and one should not take offense at their request to not have contact with a therapy animal.

Some Middle Eastern people may benefit from working with animals in therapy. In her study on animal-assisted play therapy, Parish-Plass (2008, 2013) incorporated a variety of animals into her practice with Israeli children who suffered from attachment issues and intergenerational abuse and neglect. Parish-Plass found that, with animal interaction, the children showed improvement and positive outcomes through therapy. There are several psychotherapists who practice AAT in Israel and some universities with comprehensive training programs on animal-assisted psychotherapy. There has been great success with practice of therapeutic zoo in Israel for both adults and children (Maayan, 2013). Of all the Middle Eastern countries, Israel may be considered the most ethnically integrated with many family origins being from America, Europe, and other parts of the Middle East. This may be why people in Israel are more comfortable with the concept of animals as pets and with the idea of AAT.

Religion

Many spiritual traditions honor the human–animal relationship; for example, various scriptures in Judaism, Christianity, and Islam indicate that the life of animals is valuable to God, not for food, but for instruction, joy, and companionship (Walsh, 2009). In addition, these scriptures have teachings to honor animals for their ability to teach humans about the world and God (Kesner and Pritzker, 2008; Skeen, 2011). Christian practitioners have incorporated EAI into Christian and Biblical counseling, using the human–horse relationship as a metaphor for the client's struggles and belief system (Christian, 2005). Eastern religions, such as Hinduism and Buddhism, often emphasize the interdependence of all species. Hindu teachings encourage interaction with the universe in order to stay balanced (Kesner and Pritzker, 2008). However, interactions with animals may not always be welcomed in counseling. Despite Islamic teachings to honor and be kind to animals, followers of Islam may also consider dogs to be unclean and therefore refrain from interacting with or keeping dogs as pets (Matuszek, 2010). Certain Christian beliefs may place humans on a higher moral plane than animals, in that animals do not have souls or go to heaven (Lawrence, 1995). Clients who hold these beliefs may have little faith in an animal's ability to be therapeutic, and thus experience more difficulty in forming a relationship with an animal co-therapist.

DEMOGRAPHIC DIFFERENCES IN ATTITUDES ABOUT ANIMALS

Socioeconomic Class

Few researchers have attended to socioeconomic diversity in AAT. Historically, possession of animals often indicated high social status (Blazina, Boyraz, and Shen-Miller, 2011). In Asian countries, the wealthy often owned purebred dogs, and in Europe, lap dogs were seen as a status symbol (Walsh, 2009). Horses historically have been, and continue to be, a symbol of the wealthy (Robinson, 1999). There is a continuous trend for members of higher socioeconomic classes to be much more likely to report having companion animals (Pew Research Center, 2006). This phenomenon may be partly explained by Risley-Curtiss, Holley, and Wolf's (2006) observation that people who live in a more stressful environment may be less inclined to have companion animals as caring for animals may result in added stress. As clients of lower socioeconomic classes may have had less exposure to and positive interactions with animals, these clients may be fearful or uncomfortable with a therapy animal. This fear may be especially pronounced for clients living in low-income communities where the police may utilize dogs to intimidate or apprehend the residents (Walsh, 2009). In contrast, clients in higher socioeconomic classes may welcome an animal as part of the counseling process. As the middle class is a prominent populace, their favorable cultural beliefs and positive attitudes toward animals may influence members of other cultural groups' attitudes toward animals (Pew Research Center, 2006; Risley-Curtiss, Holley, and Wolf, 2006), and thereby assist in making AAT more acceptable.

Gender

Gender is one of the most important demographic influences on attitudes toward animals (Kellert and Berry, 1987). Overall, females have demonstrated more humanistic and moralistic attitudes towards animals, whereas men often have a more utilitarian view of animals (Herzog, Betchart, and Pittman, 1991; Kellert and Berry, 1987). Therefore, AAT may be more effective with females than with males, as females may have a stronger tendency toward forming a therapeutic relationship with a therapy animal. Parshall (2003) recounted the observations of a grief counselor who witnessed that women tended to stroke and hold a therapy dog for comfort, whereas men often played more aggressively with the dog and used the animal as a diversion from pain.

Although women may show higher levels of positive behavior toward animals, they also may have more fear of them (Herzog, 2007; Kellert and Berry, 1987; Poss and Bader, 2007). In working with horses, female clients may feel intimidated, resulting in nonassertive behavior and dangerous situations (Taylor, 2001). In contrast, men may have difficulty relinquishing control in work with horses and may also create dangerous situations while trying to aggressively assert themselves (Taylor, 2001). Finally, men may be more resistant to certain AAIs that they perceive as female activities, such as horseback riding (Robinson, 1999).

It is important that counselors consider a client's unique experience with animals. Although some women may find forming a relationship with an animal easy, other women may experience a great amount of fear and anxiety (Kellert and Berry, 1987). Despite the potential challenges of conducting AAT with male clients, facilitating the development of a relationship between a male client and an animal can become very therapeutic and powerful. Through the relationship with the animal, a male client may be able to practice social and relational skills, as well as become more self-aware.

AAT WITH ELDERLY CLIENTS

Elderly clients may have special needs that must be considered when engaging in AAT. Many seniors may not see or hear as well as they used to. It is therefore important, when counseling someone with sensory disability, that you explain right away that a therapy animal is present and the role and purpose of the animal. Otherwise, if the animal is not expected by the client and cannot be seen or heard, contact or interaction with the animal may startle the client. A visually impaired client who wishes to touch or pet a therapy animal may need assistance. Always receive permission before touching a client, but having received such permission you might need to take the hand of a visually impaired client and guide it to the pet. An elderly client may not be agile and may even be in a wheelchair, so reaching down or over to pet a therapy animal may be physically difficult. A small pet may be placed in the lap of elderly clients with their permission. If you will be placing a therapy pet in a client's lap, you might first want to place on the lap a clean towel or cushion the pet is familiar with to minimize the amount of fur that gets onto the client's clothing. A thick foam cushion is usually best because it is light and also firm enough to provide a soft yet sturdy platform for the small pet to keep it from sliding between the client's legs or off the side of the client's lap. A medium-sized therapy animal like my Cocker Spaniels, Rusty and Dolly, is too big for a client's lap but too small to be reached from the floor. A medium-sized therapy animal can be placed on a couch with a client to sit or lie next to the client or may be placed in a steady chair next to the client so it is easier for the client to reach the pet. Make sure the chair on which you place the therapy animal does not have wheels; if it does have wheels, hang on tightly to the chair and keep it steady for the animal's safety. Usually, large therapy animals, like large dogs, can still be easily reached even when they are sitting on the floor. I highly discourage placing a large dog on a bed with any client since the weight of the dog may injure the client.

Dementia is common in older seniors; thus, extra supervision may be required to ensure the safety of a therapy animal around these clients. Dementia clients prone to aggression should probably not be considered for AAT. Memory impairments from dementia or aging memory processes are common in older seniors, so counselors need to be prepared to reintroduce themselves and the therapy animal many times. The presence of a therapy pet in the room may serve as a source of comfort for elderly clients, who may wish to pet the therapy animal, and the therapy animal may be effective in enhancing their focus and attention during a counseling session and may encourage them to be more expressive. Some animal-assisted structured interventions may be helpful for elderly clients. Walking, petting, grooming, and interactive play with the therapy animal can be performed during a counseling session to help stimulate clients' physical and neurological pathways. The animal's presence may encourage elderly clients to recall personal life stories about previous pets. Life story-telling has the therapeutic benefits of enhancing elderly clients' mood and reinforcing a sense of self-worth. Sharing photographs of the therapist's pets with elderly clients may also encourage them to tell life stories.

Many elderly people no longer have opportunities to provide something meaningful to others, which can damage their self-worth. Thus, they may want to give something to the therapy animal to make it feel good. Provide healthy treats for clients to share with your therapy pet. Also offer a soft grooming brush that is easy for clients to grip and hence brush the animal. Describe for clients the animal's favorite spots to be petted or massaged. The ability to do something meaningful for someone else reinforces in clients that they still have positive value.

Gammonley and Yates (1991) presented their recommendations for developing and providing AAT to residents in nursing homes. Through case examples, the authors described how the therapy animals provided entertainment for residents and, more importantly, assisted many residents to accomplish desired health and behavioral responses and goals (Gammonley and Yates, 1991).

Elderly Residents in Long-Term Care Facilities

Many elderly clients reside in a nursing home or assisted-living facility. These types of facilities may have a residential therapy animal that freely roams the facility during the day and goes home with its owner, a member of the staff, at night. In some facilities, accommodations are made for the animal to stay in the facility at night, especially if the animal is a bird or fish. It is imperative that a staff member is designated to have primary responsibility for the care of a residential therapy animal, whether the animal is present only during daytime or also stays at the facility at night. A useful resource for designing and implementing a therapy animal program at a residential facility is the book *Animals in Residential Facilities* (Appel et al., 2003). If you and your pet are planning to provide therapy services at a facility that has an existing therapy pet in residence, be sure that the pet you bring with you to your therapy sessions gets along with the residential therapy animal.

Kogan (2000) delineated steps needed to successfully introduce "live-in" (residential) animals, visiting animals, and human–animal team intervention programs in long-term care residential facilities for the elderly. She provided practical advice for staff and care-takers in residential settings "to help promote positive, smooth transitions" toward more animal- friendly facilities. Kogan included case examples to demonstrate the practicality of recommended applications. Lee et al. (1983) provide comprehensive recommendations on integrating residential pets into a nursing home, including details on the evaluation and selection of animals as residential pets.

Katsinas (2000) presented detailed treatment plans and intervention goals developed and used for a canine companion therapeutic day program for nursing home residents with dementia. For 2 full days a week, the dog was allowed to wander freely through the facility off lead to visit with residents; the exceptions to this were when residents walked the dog on a leash, when staff took the dog on a leash to visit certain residents to facilitate socialization, or during group activities occurring elsewhere on the large campus. The dog was allowed time to rest during the day when it became tired. This canine companion program was described as being successful at achieving the prescribed goals: (1) maintaining a program with a free-roaming dog that was safe and effective for both humans and the animal, (2) promoting appropriate social interaction between the animal and the residents and between residents about the dog, and (3) orientation of individuals to the present in the presence of the dog. The objectives for the second and third goals involved individual-initiated cross-species socialization from both verbal and nonverbal cues:

> When a group member called the dog, even when the wrong name was used, it came unless it was already engaged in socializing with another resident. The dog also responded to nonverbal invitations to socialize. When an individual whistled, clapped their hands, snapped their fingers, or used other nonverbal cues to entice the dog to socialize, the dog came.
>
> (Katsinas, 2000, p. 22)

Filan and Llewellyn-Jones (2006) performed a review of literature, published in the years 1960 to 2005, on AAT applications for dementia in long-term care facilities for the elderly. Based on their review of controlled-trial studies that measured the effect of AAT for dementia, the authors concluded that whereas AAT seemed to ameliorate some symptoms of dementia, the duration of the beneficial effect was not explored. Also, the relative benefits of resident versus visiting dogs were unclear and confounded by the positive effect of pet inter-action on staff and caregivers. The authors therefore recommend that the potential benefits of AAT for dementia patients be explored with further research, particularly since most of the studies included only a small sample size (Filan and Llewellyn-Jones, 2006).

Behling, Haefner, and Stowe (2011) performed a follow-up of a 1990 exploratory and descriptive study of animal programs and AAT in Illinois long-term care facilities. Data were collected using a self-administered questionnaire. They discovered that: (1) favorable feel-ings concerning the utilization of animals rose from 84 percent in 1990 to 95 percent in 2010; (2) nonscheduled animal visits, scheduled animal visits, resident animals, and AAT are occurring in approximately the same percentage of facilities in 2010 as in 1990; (3) there was a significant increase in the number of requests from staff for animal programs; (4) animal programs continue to be perceived as having significant psychological and physical benefits for residents; and (5) there was a significant increase in the number of facilities that have formal policies and procedures for animal programs (Behling, Haefner, and Stowe, 2011). One can conclude that animal therapy programs in long-term care facilities continued to be popular over the span of years studied, 1990 to 2010.

AAT WITH HOSPITALIZED CLIENTS

> A small pet is often an excellent companion for the sick, for long chronic cases especially.
> (Florence Nightingale, *Notes on Nursing*, 1859)

Clients with a serious illness requiring lengthy hospitalization are isolated from the rest of the world. A counseling session or even a brief visit involving a therapy animal offers a warm and inviting interaction that is very different from the sterile hospital atmosphere. The therapy animal may brighten clients' mood, making them more receptive to counseling, and possibly carrying over improved mood long after the counseling session is finished. Clients in a hospital for a long time may miss their pet at home, and time spent with a therapy animal may provide a type of substitute. Having contact with a therapy animal may even encourage them to talk not only about their own pets but also about how they miss home and how they are experiencing the difficulties of hospitalization or struggles with their illness. Pleasure experienced from interacting with a therapy animal may actually help to counteract some of the physical pain or discomfort resulting from clients' illness. Playing with a therapy animal or walking a therapy animal may assist in getting or keeping clients mobile if that is deemed a healthy element for recovery.

Research supports the benefits of AAT in a hospital setting. In one study in which hospitalized patients received brief visits from a therapy dog and were compared with a control group that did not receive such visits, researchers concluded that AAT improves cardiopulmonary pressures, neurohormone levels, and anxiety in patients hospitalized with heart failure (Cole et al., 2007). Harper et al. (2015) found that the inclusion of AAT during the immediate postoperative period following total joint anthroplasty resulted in substantial improvement in pain scores of patients, as compared with patients in the control group who did not receive AAT. Havey et al. (2015) found that, after joint replacement surgery, hospitalized patients who received AAT visits from a handler with a therapy dog used significantly less pain medication than patients who did not receive these AAT visits. In another study, researchers concluded that pet visits with hospitalized children and members of their family relieved stress, normalized the hospital milieu, and improved patient and parent morale; also, the benefit received by the participants correlated with the amount of physical contact and rapport developed with the visiting animal (Wu et al., 2002). Sobo, Eng, and Kassity-Krich (2006) found that hospitalized children's visits with a therapy dog provided distraction from the pain or situation, eased the pain, brought pleasure/happiness, and were calming. The researchers concluded that canine visits may be a useful adjunct to traditional pain management for children and that nurses may better serve their patients when canine visitation is an option (Sobo, Eng, and Kassity-Krich, 2006). Coakley and Mahoney (2009) discovered that therapy pet visits with patients in hospitals resulted in significant decreases in pain, respiratory rate and negative mood state, and a significant increase in perceived energy level for patients. Quantitative and qualitative findings provided support for decreased tension/anxiety and fatigue/inertia and improved overall mood. Their conclusions were that pet therapy is a low-tech, low-cost therapy that improved mood and was meaningful to hospitalized patients (Coakley and Mahoney, 2009).

Jalongo, Astorino, and Bomboy (2004) presented case examples and made useful recommendations for canines to visit young children in classrooms and hospitals, including:

- Work exclusively with registered therapy animals.
- Prepare children for the canine visitors.
- Assess individual children's suitability for interaction with the dogs.
- Consider the dog's safety and wellbeing.

The authors also discussed how to address common issues and concerns for children interacting with a therapy dog, such as possible injury, infection, allergies, fear of dogs, and cultural differences (Jalongo, Astorino, and Bomboy, 2004). A useful resource for AAT in a hospital environment is a publication by Tucker (2002) titled *Visiting Hospitalized Children*.

Many hospitals encourage hospital staff and volunteers to utilize scripted communication to organize interactions with patients. A popular form of scripted communication for hospital service is referred to as AIDET: A = Acknowledge, I = Introduce, D = Duration, E = Explanation, and T = Thank You (Studer, Robinson, and Cook, 2010). The AIDET model of scripted communication with hospital patients has been shown to be effective at reducing patient anxiety, increasing patient satisfaction, and recommending the hospital to others (Cook, 2013). I have created an example of how the AIDET model (Rubin, 2014, p. 1) can be incorporated into communication during an AAT interaction in a hospital (words in brackets and example dialogue were added by me):

- *A = Acknowledge*. Acknowledge the patient. Make eye contact, smile, and acknowledge everyone in the room (patient and families). Example dialogue: "Hello." [This greeting should occur a safe distance from the people in the room, i.e., near the doorway, so you can first discern their comfort level with you and the therapy dog before moving closer.]
- *I = Introduce*. Introduce yourself, your skill set, your credentials, and experience. Example dialogue: "My name is Cynthia, and this is therapy dog Jesse. She and I are a registered therapy team who have been providing animal-assisted therapy to patients at this hospital for 2 years."
- *D = Duration*. Give an accurate time expectation. Example dialogue: "We would like to invite you to visit with and pet Jesse for a few minutes. Would you like to pet Jesse?"
- *E = Explanation*. If the patient says yes, explain step by step what will happen, and answer questions. Use language a patient can understand. Example dialogue: "Since Jesse is small, I can place her on a clean towel next to you in your bed, or I can place her on a chair next to your bed. Or, if you prefer I can have her sit on the floor. What is your preference today?" [During the AAT interaction you can interpret the dog's behaviors, "Jesse really likes having her back rubbed, that's why she turned around and snuggled her back against you just now." You can answer any questions the patient may have about your dog or AAT service, engage patients in talking about a pet if they have one or have had one, and engage in polite small talk such as telling funny stories about your dog. Do not ask patients about their health condition as that is private information. If a patient volunteers information about their condition, give simple reflections like "I hope you feel better." Attend to verbal and nonverbal signals from patients regarding their comfort in interacting with the animal, and look for signals when the patient is ready for you and the dog to leave—for instance, they stop touching the dog or say things like, "Thank you for coming," that suggest they are finished with the visit. Typically you would stay no more than 5 minutes, unless circumstances suggest a briefer visit or allow for a somewhat longer visit requested by the patient, if you deem it appropriate. Remember to invite others who may be in the room visiting the patient to pet the therapy dog.]
- *T = Thank You*. You may thank the patient for allowing you to serve them. Example dialogue: "Thank you for visiting with Jesse and me today. She really enjoyed being petted by you."

Many hospital programs incorporate AAA/AAT as part of patients' recovery process. Three well-known hospital AAA/AAT programs involving Pet Partners teams are the National Institutes of Health in Washington, D.C., Warm Springs Rehabilitation Hospital in San

Antonio, Texas, and Summa Health Systems in Akron, Ohio (Ptak and Howie, 2004). The popularity of hospital AAT visitation programs in the United States and around the world is continuing to rise.

While I do not provide counseling services at a hospital, I do volunteer with my dog Jesse at three hospitals in the county where I reside. Jesse and I began our hospital volunteer work in 2012. As a registered Pet Partners handler–animal team, Jesse and I provide nonprofessional, volunteer social visits with patients, visitors, and staff. Visits with staff are quite brief, yet much appreciated as a stress reliever. Visits with patients and visitors are usually a few minutes in length and serve to brighten mood, nurture, and soothe anxiety of patients and visitors. Jesse and I visit patients in physical rehabilitation units, pediatric units, surgical units, and so forth. Patients are screened in advance of our visit either by nursing staff or volunteer staff, depending on the particular procedure set up by the hospital AAT program. From screening, patient preference for a therapy dog visit is noted as well as whether the patient's condition is conducive to a visit from a handler–animal team. During the screening, permission for a visit from a handler–animal team is obtained from the patient. For two hospitals where I volunteer, the patient's file or door is marked with a paw print that signals the desire and appropriateness for a visit. The system works well, but because staff can fall behind, I always check with the nursing staff for each unit to clarify the screenings and permissions are up to date. At another hospital where I volunteer, a hospital general volunteer asks each patient if they would like a visit from a therapy dog while showing a photograph of the animal. This occurs the day before the therapy animal visits are scheduled. Permission is obtained and a list is compiled and provided to the handler–animal team the next day when they arrive. This is my favorite system for obtaining patient permission for a visit with a therapy animal because it is done the day before the visit and, thus, is very up to date. It is important to note that patient status can change. So all AAT volunteers must be aware of notices on doors for "no contact" or "infection risk" or "no visitors" and avoid entering those rooms. I keep a log of each visit with each patient and rate my assessment of how the visit went. The original log is filed with the volunteer coordinator of the hospital and I keep a copy of the log. As a member of Pet Partners, I also log the visit with that organization. I have met many people and had many wonderful interactions with patients at hospitals. There are too many great stories to tell all here, but I will share a couple.

Jesse and I were requested to visit a 4-year-old boy in the pediatric unit. We were informed that just before we arrived the nurses and the boy's mother were attempting to get him to comply with a procedure flushing his intravenous line, but the boy had been throwing a temper tantrum and would not let anyone touch his arm. Upon seeing my dog Jesse, the boy became positively excited and trotted over to the dog. He added his little hand to the leash, behind mine so I could maintain control of the dog, and together we walked Jesse up and down the hallway. The boy giggled, laughed, and jumped up and down out of glee. After a 10-minute visit with Jesse, which included some hugs and petting, the boy was compliant and the nurse easily flushed his line.

On one of our weekly visits to a hospital, as usual Jesse and I enjoyed visiting with several patients, visitors, and staff, and happily responding to patients' requests to have their photograph taken with Jesse. During our volunteer rounds, we received a request by a nurse to assist with an elderly woman who wanted to see therapy dog Jesse but could not move any of her limbs. When we arrived in the room the patient quietly verbalized that she wanted Jesse to sit next to her on her bed. While Jesse lay snuggled next to the patient, the nurse gently lifted the patient's arm and moved the patient's hand across Jesse's fur. The patient gave a small smile and seemed to very much enjoy this assisted petting. Then the nurse was called away briefly. While the nurse was out of the room, Jesse stayed snuggled against the patient's side and the patient continued to gaze at Jesse and talk softly to her. I noticed the patient was

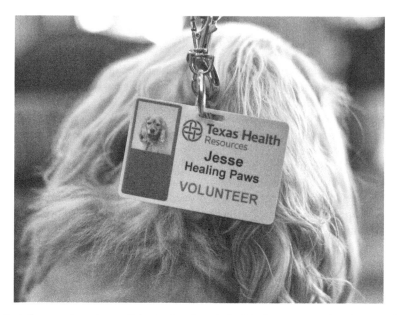

Figure 11.1 A therapy dog who participates in a hospital visitation program has its own official hospital volunteer badge.

(*Source:* photo courtesy of Kristen Watson and the *Denton Record Chronicle.*)

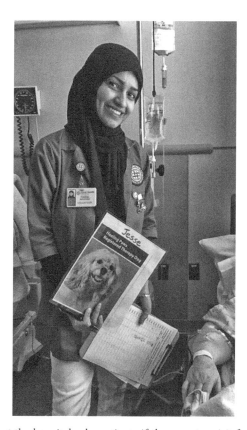

Figure 11.2 A volunteer at the hospital asks patients if they want a visit from a therapy dog the day before the visit.

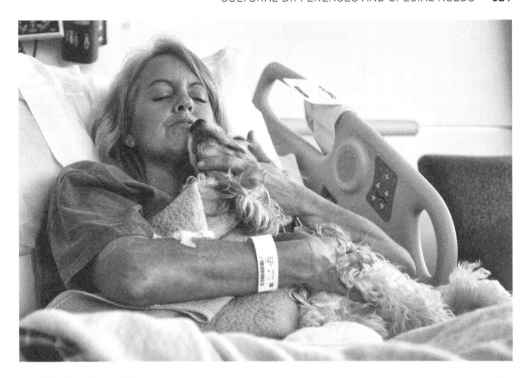

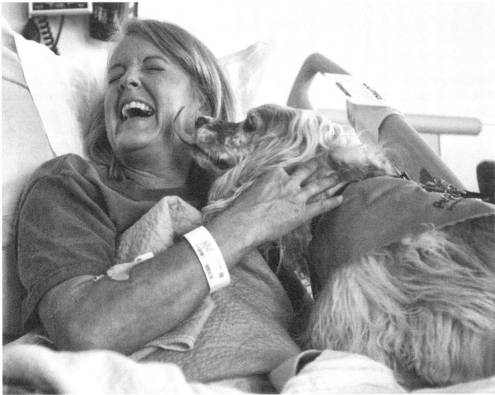

Figures 11.3 and 11.4 Therapy dog Jesse is a comfort for patients in a hospital. Her silken fur and lovable personality provide much healing nurturance and brighten the mood of patients.

(*Source:* photos courtesy of Kristen Watson and the Denton Record Chronicle.)

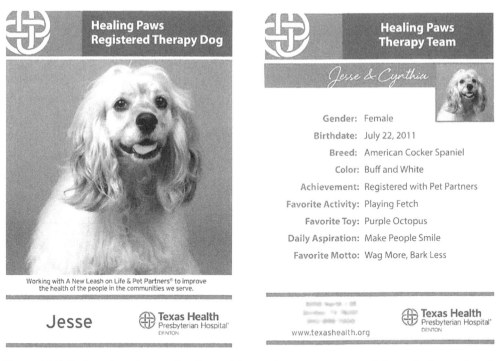

Figure 11.5 Each patient therapy dog Jesse visits receives a visitation card from the hospital with Jesse's photograph on the front and some information about her on the back (you can have a card designed for your dog at www.custom-tradingcards.com).

struggling to move her arm and hand toward Jesse on her own initiative. Just as I noticed this, the nurse re-entered the patient's room and saw what was happening and remarked about it. She was very pleased and excited to see the patient initiating these movements. To help the patient, I moved Jesse about 2 inches from the patient's fingers. With our encouragement, the patient navigated the distance and gently rubbed the fur on the dog's leg between her thumb and forefinger and then gently squeezed Jesse's paw two or three times. The nurse was once again very pleased and excited and exclaimed that the patient's physical and occupational therapists were going to be very happy that the patient had finally moved her arm, hand, and fingers. The immobile patient's desire to pet Jesse was the motivating force for her to initiate movement; an important first step on her road to recovery.

AAT WITH HOSPICE AND PALLIATIVE CARE CLIENTS

Hospice clients are terminally ill and often are provided end-of-life care at home by qualified health professionals. Counseling clients in the final stages of their lives is indeed a special type of counseling. A therapist must help the client maintain the highest possible quality of life during this final journey. Therapy animals bring an exuberant energy into what could be a gloomy environment for a client who is dying. Therapy animals are playful, funny, and entertaining. They offer genuine and endless affection and nurturance, all of which are much needed by a hospice client. A therapy animal can also offer relief for visitors and family members of the hospice client as well as other health professionals assisting a terminally ill client.

Hospice and Palliative Care of Louisville, Kentucky, provide hospice care and bereavement services to approximately 2,500 patients and their families annually (Ptak and Howie,

2005). In 2001, this agency formally added AAA and AAT to its services by partnering with Pet Partners affiliate WAGS (Wonderful Animals Giving Support) to provide a visiting animal program. The AAA and AAT program involves a variety of options, including regularly scheduled visits with individual hospice patients in their homes, regularly scheduled visits at inpatient or nursing home settings, visits with social workers to children, visits to patients' children and grandchildren, and involvement with bereavement groups (Ptak and Howie, 2005).

Pet Partners' Douglas Gray and his Bernese Swiss mountain dog named Bart began providing AAA at Bailey-Boushay House in 1995 (Ptak and Howie, 2005). Bailey-Boushay House in Seattle provide inpatient services with their 35-bed residential facility, and outpatient services through their Adult Day Health program. All of the clients in the Adult Day Health program and 70–75 percent in the residential facility are living with HIV/AIDS (Ptak and Howie, 2005).

Zia Hospice in New Mexico serves hospice patients who are either living on their own in their homes, living with a caregiver, or residing in a nursing home or assisted-living facility (Ptak and Howie, 2005). Student volunteers in the community partnered with Zia and Pet Partners to start an AAA program in 2003. Zia requires that all volunteers complete their training sessions, which consist of several modules over several weeks. Volunteers in training accompany others on AAA visits and view videos provided by Zia. The Zia volunteer coordinator said of the new AAA program:

> During the first visit I did with a Pet Partners team I was amazed by the response. You could see patients' eyes and faces light up. For many I believe it brought back memories, maybe of their childhood or a pet that they once had; it took them back to a place where they may have many happy memories. Some of the patients began to talk about the pet they had. One common theme was about the pet being a part of their family.
>
> (Ptak and Howie, 2005, p. 6)

A list of several hospice programs that include AAA or AAT in their services can be found in Ptak and Howie (2005).

A therapist for a hospice client can assist by providing counseling sessions that include a therapy animal as well as other types of animal-related services. For example, the therapist can guide the development of a bird-feeding center outside a window or in an accessible garden. A butterfly garden can be planted with nectar flowers to attract butterflies to feed on and garden plants such as passion vine, dill, and fennel for the butterflies to lay eggs on. The therapist can help the client harvest a caterpillar chrysalis and create a butterfly hatchery in the home of the client, and arrange a counseling session with the client centered on the actual release of the hatched butterfly. The butterfly and caterpillar transformation life cycle is a powerful metaphor for a client who is dying and may be thinking about a hereafter. The therapist working with hospice clients may also assist them in making provisions for the transfer of care of their pet once they are too ill to take care of it, and in setting up adoption procedures for their pet once they have died.

A therapist who is providing AAT in a hospital or hospice environment must be especially careful to follow established policies and procedures for infection control to protect both the client and the therapy animal. In addition, the therapy animal must be healthy, without open wounds, and parasite free. The animal must be clean, and bathed and groomed within 24 hours of the counseling session. Be sure the animal's claws are clipped and filed to a dull state. Be careful the animal does not come into contact with any body fluids of a client with a contagious illness. Make sure all items that may have contacted body fluid are not in reach of the animal, such as tissues, bed clothing, undergarments, eating utensils, and leftover food. Also, have clients wash their hands with an antibacterial soap or gel before and after visiting with the therapy animal. Make sure any pet items the client may interact with are clean before you begin the therapy session (e.g., collar, leash, toys, and pet cushion). When you get home, carefully clean all pet items to remove any potential germs they may have accumulated. Be sure to disinfect the pet items with substances nontoxic to your therapy pet and clients you may work with next.

Jesse and I have never worked in a formal hospice program outside of a hospital setting, but sometimes family members ask us to come by the room of a patient who is receiving care at the hospital during the patient's final days of life. One day when therapy dog Jesse and I arrived at the hospital for our volunteer service we were informed that a family with a member in the intensive care unit, a unit we typically do not visit, requested that Jesse and I visit. A nurse manager escorted us to the patient's room. A young man lay comatose on the bed surrounded by his mother and two adult sisters. One sister explained that her brother loved dogs, and that his favorite dog was a Cocker Spaniel named Misty. Though her brother was nonresponsive and not likely to awaken before death, the family wanted him to be able to pet a dog before he passed away, preferably a Cocker Spaniel like my dog Jesse. I held Jesse up next to the patient's bed near his arm while the patient's sister gently moved the patient's hand over Jesse's soft and silky fur. Jesse remained relaxed and calm. Each time the assisted petting paused, Jesse stretched her nose forward and gently nuzzled the patient's hand. We were all brought to tears; that is, I with the family and the several nurses who had come to the room to witness the pet visit. Even now when I recall the event I have tears running down my cheeks. After a few moments the sister next to the bed thanked me and I took this as a sign the family was ready for our visit to end. We will never know if the man knew of Jesse's presence or if the tactile stimulation helped him recall or dream of his own dogs; but it is certain Jesse's visit provided compassion and comfort for the family and for staff who were caring for the man in his final days.

On one afternoon visit we were informed that an elderly woman was in the hospital for hospice care during the final days of her life. Though the elderly patient was now comatose and nonresponsive, the family had requested a therapy dog visit because the patient had loved dogs her whole life. When Jesse and I visited the patient, her family was not present that day. A nurse who was providing care for the patient expressed that she was very glad we had come. She described the patient as having become very unsettled in her sleep and breathing the last few days. The nurse was hoping the visit with the dog would calm the patient and hopefully make it easier for her to pass away. The nurse went with Jesse and me to the patient's room. The woman was covered with her favorite quilt the family had brought from home. I gently placed Jesse on the patient's bed and she snuggled in next to the patient. Fulfilling an earlier bequest from the family, the nurse took a photograph of the patient with Jesse to send to the family as an aid in the comfort of their grief. Then the nurse moved over next to Jesse and me, and she gently moved the patient's hand over Jesse's back. After a few strokes, the patient's breathing began to slow. With each stroke of Jesse's fur the patient's breathing became slower and steadier. The nurse commented on the profound effect the assisted petting was having, remarking on how simple human touch had not had the same positive effect. The nurse, who had developed an emotional connection with the patient, allowed tears to flow down her cheeks. Jesse's visit was providing the nurse with much needed comfort. After a few minutes I felt it was time for Jesse and me to end the visit—but Jesse had something to say about that. Usually, when I say, "Jesse, let's go," at the end of a visit, she sits up and reaches her paws toward me in anticipation of being lifted off the bed and onto the ground. Yet this time, when I said, "Jesse, let's go," and reached out for her she moved away from my arms and leaned in closer to the patient. So I reached underneath Jesse to pick her up, but she scooted away from my hands and even closer to the patient, where she could lay her head on the patient's chest. I turned to the nurse and said, "Wow, this is really not typical, Jesse is trying to tell us something. I think she is telling us she is not ready to go yet, that she needs a little more time." The nurse had interpreted Jesse's behavior the same way. So we sat next to the patient's bed and let Jesse have some more time with the patient who was sleeping and breathing easily. The nurse and I had tears streaming down our faces as we sat there next to the bed watching this gentle dog administer peace to the patient. Jesse lay very still gazing at the face of the patient, her head gently moving ever so slightly up and down with each of the patient's breaths. After about 5 minutes, Jesse lifted her head from the patient's chest, sat up in the bed, turned to me and raised a paw, signaling me to lift her off of the bed. For Jesse, it was now time to go. She had done what she needed to do. The nurse told me the patient passed away peacefully that evening.

One day a nurse manager specifically requested that Jesse and I visit an elderly woman who was chronically depressed in the palliative care unit of a hospital. The woman broke a big smile as soon as she saw Jesse and me enter the room. She hugged and petted Jesse. She laughed and told stories of her pets. It was an uplifting experience even for me. When it was time to go, as is typical at the end of all of our visits, I gave her one of Jesse's visit cards that contained Jesse's photo and a brief description of Jesse. The next week, the nurse manager told me that the woman kept the card handy and showed it to everyone who entered her room and with a big smile told about her special visit from Jesse. The nurse manager explained how important this behavior was because before the visit with Jesse the woman had been crying and moaning loudly. The nurse said the patient had smiled for the very first time since entering the unit only when she met therapy dog Jesse. Also, she was no longer prone to crying and moaning, she was more compliant, and her mood was much better for the entire week since our previous visit.

When working with the chronically ill or involved with end-of-life care, a client may request assistance in saying goodbye to the people in the client's life who are important to the client. Sometimes the counselor and the therapy animal are included in this group of significant others. Thus, the counselor must be aware of offering an opportunity for the client to achieve some emotional closure on the therapeutic relationship with the counselor and the counselor's pet practitioner. When working with the chronically or terminally ill, sometimes other people involved in providing care for the patient also become attached to the therapy animal. Thus, remember friends, family members, and medical staff when the life of the patient nears an end and allow time for these significant others in the patient's life to say goodbye to you and the therapy pet.

AAT WITH CLIENTS IN PRISONS AND JUVENILE DETENTION CENTERS

Sometimes it is difficult to gain the trust of a client confined in a prison or detention center. Detainees are suspicious of all authority figures and are hesitant to express themselves honestly and sincerely for fear of repercussions. It may be easier for this type of client to trust a counselor working with a therapy animal because the client can judge the counselor based on observing the positive and trusting relationship between the therapy animal and the counselor. Detained clients typically do not get opportunities to interact with animals, so being able to spend time with a therapy animal can motivate them to attend counseling sessions as well as maintaining good behavior to be allowed to continue to interact with the therapy animal. Detainees will positively view structured time to pet, interact with, and play with the therapy animal. They also have limited opportunity to be outdoors, so they usually appreciate the counselor gaining permission to spend some sessions with them outside in a secure recreational area. As with all clients, detainees should never be left alone with the therapist's animal. Detainee clients who participate in AAT should be carefully screened for aggressive tendencies, as some may not be appropriate for this type of therapy due to aggression. Also, the counselor working in a prison or detention facility must be very aware of and carefully follow security procedures as well as maintain a constant awareness of where security personnel are and how to contact them in case of an emergency.

There are several types of AAT programs in prisons and detention centers in the United States and around the world. Many of these programs are not necessarily counseling programs but do have positive emotional and behavioral benefits for inmates. For example, inmates have helped rescue organizations to domesticate and train wild horses for adoption, and to train unruly dogs so the dogs could be more easily adopted by approved families, as well as raising and training dogs for preparation as service animals to help the disabled. Detainees have worked with animals to learn vocational skills that may be helpful once the inmates are released, such as veterinarian technician skills, grooming and bathing of dogs and horses, and exercising and training dogs and horses. In many of these instances, the dogs in these programs are housed in kennels on site at the facility, or some even live with the detainees in their cells. When keeping therapy animals on site, extensive monitoring and supervision measures must be in place to ensure the safety of the animals at all times. The goal of residential-type AAT programs at prisons and detention centers is to provide mutual assistance for the therapy animal and the detainee. Residential AAT program goals to assist detainees include decreasing behavior problems, manipulative behaviors, and the frequency of conflicts between detainees. Meanwhile, program goals aim to increase detainees' attention to task, life skill development, and positive attitudes, as well as increasing the frequency of prosocial behaviors like cooperation and sharing, and positive interactions between detainees and facility staff. Finally, residential AAT programs aim to enhance the mood of detainees.

AAT Programs in Prisons

Pet therapy programs in prison have been shown to uplift the spirits of detainees and reduce violence in the facility (Haynes, 1991). Pet therapy programs in correctional facilities can be a mutually beneficial coalition between humans and animals who need the type of assistance that each can offer the other:

> Taffy is just days away from euthanasia. The young Heeler/Beagle mix needs obedience training and socialization, and his luck is running out. A few days later, Taffy is relaxing in the cell of Eric Roberson, an inmate at the Mansfield Correctional Institution, a maximum security prison in Ohio. Taffy and Roberson are one of 30 inmate/shelter dog pairs participating in the Tender Loving Dog Care program at Mansfield. The program provides the inmates with the opportunity to train and socialize otherwise doomed dogs, who are then adopted into good homes. Roberson, who is serving 24 years for a 1992 murder conviction, has given a new life to 22 dogs; an additional 200 have also been saved [since the program began in 1998].
>
> (Rhoades, 2001, p. 24)

A television channel called Animal Planet broadcasted in 2004 a program series called *Cell Dogs* that demonstrated the benefits of animals interacting positively with inmates in prisons. One particular story was especially touching. A local humane society in Nevada brought several dogs to the Warm Springs Correctional Center for the male inmates to assist. Some were adult dogs that had been neglected by their owners and were never properly socialized, trained, or housebroken. Some of the dogs had been badly abused by previous owners and were so afraid they would just cower in a corner and shake. Two litters of puppies too young to be kept at the humane society shelter were also included in this group. Inmates kept the dogs for 6 weeks and spent time providing affection and nurturance for all of the dogs and training for the adult dogs. The dogs stayed in the inmates' cells with them so they were together for 24 hours a day. The outcome of the program was delightful. The little puppies that had been on the edge of survival at the time they arrived became healthy and robust balls of bouncing fur. The adult dogs became happy, friendly, and obedient animals. Two of the dogs were socialized and trained around prison horses that had been rescued from the wild and were undergoing training and socialization by prisoners so the horses could go to a good home; both dogs were adopted by local ranchers. All of the puppies and dogs were adopted by the time the program ended after several weeks, and many of the dogs were actually adopted by facility staff. A father of one of the inmates visited with the inmate and with the puppies in the inmate's care. When the father lost his own dog from age-related illness, he adopted one of those puppies. It seemed to mean a great deal to the inmate and to the father because the inmate could provide something very meaningful to his father that he and his father could connect with for many years to come. At the conclusion of the program, the inmates described the experience as very positive, feeling as though they had done something very worthwhile.

There are several animal welfare and rehabilitation programs in correctional facilities in the United States. The Ohio Reformatory for Women in Marysville and the Marion Correctional Institution for Men work in cooperation with the Ohio Wildlife Center (Rhoades, 2001). The wildlife center was finding it difficult to care for over 4,000 sick, injured, or orphaned wild animals per year. Then they set up branch programs within the two correctional facilities. The inmates are trained by wildlife rehabilitators to provide 24-hour nursing care for a variety of wildlife, including hand-feeding mealworms to birds and tube-feeding baby opossums. Once rehabilitated, the animals are returned to the wild. The effects of the program are reflected by one inmate, Sharon Young, who is serving time for aggravated murder:

> Our goal is to get as many animals healthy and back into their natural habitats as we can. . . . It's difficult to see them go, but it makes you feel proud to know that you've done something good and really miraculous.
>
> (Rhoades, 2001, p. 25)

Animal care programs in correctional facilities provide many useful services for both the inmates and the animals (Rhoades, 2001). Dog grooming is taught in a number of prison programs including the Women's Correctional Institute in Purdy, Washington. The Hutchison and El Dorado facilities in Kansas serve as foster facilities for greyhounds that were destined to be euthanized after being retired from racing. The Hutchison correctional facility also works with the National Wild Horse and Burro program by gentling and socializing wild horses to be adopted by the public. The Animal Cruelty unit of the Maricopa County Sheriff's Office in Phoenix, Arizona, works with inmates to rehabilitate animals rescued by the unit so the animals can be adopted by the public; inmates learn basic animal first-aid and veterinary skills as well as animal socializing and obedience training as a by-product of this program (Rhoades, 2001).

There are numerous prison programs involving horses. The Thoroughbred Retirement Foundation was founded in 1982 in the State of New York by Monique Koehler to provide a safe home for racehorses after finishing their racing career; the first location was established at the Wallkill Correctional Facility in upstate New York with its 72-acre farmland (Strimple, 2003). In 1999, the Kentucky Thoroughbred Retirement Foundation opened its program at Blackburn, a correctional facility in Lexington, Kentucky (Strimple, 2003). The Pulaski State

Prison for women in Georgia started the state's first horse rescue program for neglected, abused, or abandoned horses impounded by Georgia's Department of Agriculture (Wallace, 2012; Stoker, 2011). The inmates at Pulaski help to care for and train the horses, and once the horses are rehabilitated they are put up for sale and adoption. The prison in Canon City, Colorado, teamed with the U.S. Bureau of Land Management to develop a rehabilitation and adoption program for wild horses. The program was started in the 1970s by Ron Zaidlicz and his nonprofit foundation, the National Organization for Wild American Horses. The program gives the inmates responsibility and changes attitudes in positive ways (Associated Press, 1987, 2009). The Wyoming Honor Farm Inmate/Wild Horse Program (n.d.) started in 1988 in Riverton; their Wild Horse program assists in teaching inmates new job skills and improving their social and daily living habits. The inmates work with the horses to gentle them for sale and adoption. Warm Springs Correctional Center (n.d.) near Carson City, Nevada, has a wild horse gentling program and works in cooperation with the U.S. Bureau of Land Management to rehabilitate and train wild horses for sale and adoption (Bureau of Land Management, n.d.). Some of these rehabilitated horses from Warm Springs have made their way to a horse drill team. The Cowgirl Way Equestrian Drill Team of Norco, California heard about the training at Warm Springs and started out by adopting ten mustangs to form an all-mustang drill team to promote the breed. The drill team performs at numerous drill performances and parades (Bureau of Land Management, 2005; *Horse and Man*, 2010). Cushing and Williams (1995) performed a study of the Wild Mustang Program at the Southern New Mexico Correctional Facility located west of the city of Las Cruces. The program was associated with a reduction of disciplinary reports, particularly for those who simultaneously participated in substance abuse counseling and for violent offenders. Additionally, their findings suggested that inmate and staff perceptions about the success of the program exceeded statistical evidence (Cushing and Williams, 1995).

The Pocahontas Correctional Unit in Chesterfield, Virginia is home to the prison's Pen Pals program in which trusted female inmates help socialize abandoned cats until they are ready for adoption (Associated Press, 2005). One inmate was working with a kitten named Scarlett that was so traumatized she would not let anyone touch her. After the inmate had provided love and patience for many months, Scarlett began trusting the inmate, and the two often cuddle up together. Of this experience the inmate says, "When I look at her, I see that after all this time, I'm not so wild anymore—and she's not so wild anymore." This Virginia Pen Pals program also became a shelter for some of the cats rescued by the Jackson County Alabama Animal Shelter in the aftermath of Hurricane Katrina, which devastated the Gulf Coast region in August 2005. From Alabama,

> The animals arrived agitated and scared, many suffering from respiratory illnesses due to the stress of a long truck ride in a plastic carrier and weeks of cramped shelter. The inmates started giving them food, medicine, love and—of course—hurricane-appropriate names.
>
> (Associated Press, 2005).

The names given to a litter of six frisky black kittens include VooDoo, Gumbo, and the Ragin' Cajuns. Of the opportunity to help the cats rescued from Hurricane Katrina one inmate said,

> It makes us feel like we can be a part of something—to be a part of the storm—to help out. We are so secluded from the world and there's somebody waiting on their pets. And while I might never meet them, I took care of them while they're getting their life together.
>
> (Associated Press, 2005)

Another program that cares for rescued kittens and cats and prepares them for adoption into homes is the Nine Lives Program at Pendleton Correctional Facility in Madison County, Indiana (Binette, 2015; and Mackin, 2014). The Anderson Animal Care and Control Unit has limited space and thus partners with the Pendleton Correctional Facility to save cats that would otherwise be marked for death. In June 2009 the Pendleton program was caring for 59 cats and kittens, which were getting more love and attention in the program than the felines could receive in an overcrowded animal shelter environment. Six inmates are chosen to care for the cats in 8-hour shifts. One inmate serving time for manslaughter says of the program, "It makes me feel better about myself: something to care about" (Longnecker, 2009, p. 1). A staff member described the benefits of the program as,

> If you come in here and you make the choice that you want to walk a different path and you are trying to be different, I do believe they should have a chance to be different and I do believe that animals can help them be that way.
>
> (Longnecker, 2009, p. 1).

Shelter officials say of the program,

> It's a win–win solution because the extra attention the cats receive from the prisoners will result in better socialization, alleviating the stress and depression they often develop while in cages. The offenders get the chance to give back to society.
>
> (Longnecker, 2009, p. 1)

The Pendleton Correctional Facility had already benefited both humans and dogs with their ongoing successful Fido program, where inmates train and foster dogs for adoption (Longnecker, 2009).

The Washington State Correctional Center for Women in Gig Harbor established a program in 1981 called Prison Pet Partnership, where inmates help others by training dogs that will assist a disabled person (Prison Pet Partnership Program, n.d.). This is a cooperative effort among Washington State University, Tacoma Community College, and the Washington State Department of Corrections. Volunteers teach inmates how to train, groom, and board dogs within the prison walls. The program reports that more than 500 dogs have been placed with individuals who have disabilities since the program began. Dogs that do not have the necessary temperament to be placed as service animals are trained in obedience so they can be adopted into homes as pets. The Prison Pup Program at Bland Correctional Center in Virginia also trains puppies to be future service dogs (Deaton, 2005). After a year of training at this medium-security facility, the dogs are given to the St. Francis of Assisi Service Dog Foundation in Roanoke. In 2001, the Pen Pals program began at the James River Correctional Center in Virginia; this program is designed to train shelter dogs to make them more adoptable (Deaton, 2005). The Second Chance Prison Canine Program, founded by Gayle Woods, started a prison program to train service dogs in 2003 at the Florence Correctional Center in Arizona, a privately operated medium-security prison (Deaton, 2005).

The Hounds of Prison Education (HOPE) program was launched at the Correctional Institute at Camp Hill in cooperation with the Central Pennsylvania Animal Alliance (HOPE, n.d.). The inmates work together with a professional dog trainer in providing rescued shelter dogs with socialization, behavior modification, and nurturance so they may be adopted into new homes. The inmates and dogs live together in the cell and attend weekly training sessions. The Puppies Behind Bars program (Puppies Behind Bars, n.d.) is facilitated in three women's and three men's correctional facilities in New York State. In this program, carefully screened inmates raise puppies to become working dogs to assist disabled persons, and dogs that do not have the right temperament to be a working dog are adopted as pets. A similar program began in 1999 in the Downeast Correctional Facility, a medium-security prison in Maine. In this program, puppies donated by breeders spend about a year in training performed by male inmates, and after graduation the dogs are placed with a disabled person in the community by the National Education for Assistance to Dogs Service (Deaton, 2005). The Wisconsin Correctional Liberty Dog Program (n.d.) also helps to meet the needs of physically challenged individuals by training service dogs for placement with persons who are disabled. Another similar program is the Prison PUP Program (n.d.) at the North Central Correctional Institute in Massachusetts, which began in 1998 as a partnership between the Massachusetts Department of Corrections and the National Education for Assistance Dog Services organization. In this program inmates are taught how to teach dogs basic obedience skills and other skills necessary to prepare them for a life as service dogs for the physically disabled. The dog training program Pen Pals: A New Leash on Life (n.d.), at the CCA-Davis Correctional Facility in Holdenville, Oklahoma, began in 2004 to train rescued shelter dogs in obedience and social skills so they can be adopted into homes. The program claims important benefits.

> The Pen Pals Prison Program teaches inmates at CCA-Davis Correctional Facility in Holdenville, Oklahoma to train shelter dogs into well-mannered companion dogs, who are then adopted by people in the community. Research shows the inmates benefit as much as the dogs and their new owners. The inmates become more patient, tolerant, learn a skill and the value of community service. Their increased confidence, empathy and ability to share emotions with the dogs open new ways of thinking and relating to others, making a significant difference in their lives and the lives of families, staff and other inmates.
>
> (Pen Pals: A New Leash on Life, n.d., p. 1)

The People, Animals and Love (PAL) program was begun in 1983 at the Lorton Correctional Facility in Lorton, Virginia. Carefully screened inmates in this program were taught how to care for companion animals that lived with them as pets. The program was first evaluated in 1989 by Katcher, Beck, and Levine. These researchers found that the pet program provided valuable recreation for the prisoners but had "only small and inconsistent effects on antisocial behavior as defined by the prison staff" (Katcher, Beck, and Levine, 1989, p. 175). The program was evaluated again in 1991 by Moneymaker and Strimple. The researchers reported the following findings:

> The men who have completed this program have for the most part shown considerable change in their outlook toward others and their sense of self-worth, as well as their sense of achieving a better goal in life. . . . This is largely due in part to their own admission that the animal they owned instilled in them compassion, love and responsibility to another living creature.
>
> (Moneymaker and Strimple, 1991, pp. 149–150)

The Saxierriet Correctional Facility for men in eastern Switzerland is a semi-open facility for about 130 inmates who mainly work in the fields and on the farm with cows, pigs, and with the breeding of horses (Nef, 2004). The facility began a new program in the mid-1980s that involved allowing inmates to have their own cat as a pet with very strict regulations concerning the wellbeing of the animal. A primary purpose for the program is "to give the participants the opportunity to make decisions and take responsibility on their own to learn to care for the welfare of another being" (Nef, 2004, p. 1). Open-ended, structured interviews were conducted with inmates who had a cat, with inmates who did not have a cat, and with staff who were responsible for and involved in the program, and positive results were reported with all three groups (Nef, 2004). For the cat owners, the pet was a means of coping with loneliness, a generally accepted way of giving and receiving beneficial affection, and for some a reason to go on living while incarcerated. For inmates without a cat, they appreciated the presence of the cats in the environment though they did not want the responsibility of caring for the cat themselves. For the staff involved with the program, they were satisfied that the program met their objectives including teaching the inmates how to take responsibility and increasing self-esteem and self-confidence in the inmates with the cats, which was considered an "important step for resocialization in view of their lives after prison" (Nef, 2004, p. 1).

Fournier, Geller, and Fortney (2007) investigated the impact of a human–animal interaction program in a U.S. prison setting on criminal behavior, treatment progress, and social skills. A total of 48 male inmates allowed researchers to access their institutional files and completed self-report measures. The human–animal interaction program was an existing Pen Pals program; a dog training program in which dogs are selected from local shelters and trained by volunteer inmates in prison for 8–10 weeks. During that time, dogs live with selected inmates who are educated in dog training skills. The inmates provide for the dogs' basic needs (i.e., food, shelter, and grooming) and train them in basic obedience. After the training period, the dog is adopted by individuals in the community, and the inmates begin the process again with a new shelter dog. The control group for the study was inmates who applied and met criteria to work in the program but who remained on the waiting list during the research period. The dependent measures included the frequency of institutional infractions, inmate treatment level within the prison's therapeutic community, and social skills. Frequency of infractions was obtained from inmates' institutional files. Treatment level was obtained via self-report. The Human–Animal Interaction Scale was used to measure self-reported interactions of inmates with the animals. The Social Skills Inventory was used to assess basic social and emotional communication skills. Analysis of variance was used to compare pre- and post-test scores. Pre-test measures were obtained before treatment-group participants were involved with the human–animal interaction program. Post-test measures were obtained after treatment-group participants were involved with the program for 2 weeks. Results indicated that the treatment group, those inmates participating in the program, showed statistically significant improvements in all of the dependent measures compared with the control group. The researchers suggested this study has important implications that support rehabilitation of inmates through involvement in human–animal interaction programs (Fournier, Geller, and Fortney, 2007).

Strimple (2003) described some successful inmate–animal interaction programs in prisons. The Southeastern Guide Dogs, Inc. brought dogs to the federal prison facility Coleman Federal Complex, a minimum-security work camp for women located in Coleman, Florida. Once the women were trained as dog handlers, the inmates housebroke and socialized the dogs, after which the dogs were returned to Southeastern Guide Dogs for 6 months of advanced training before being given to individuals with impaired vision. At two U.S. Army federal prisons the Animals in the Military Helping Individuals (AIMHI) programs involve inmates as dog trainers: one program is at Fort Leavenworth, Kansas (begun in 2000) and another at Fort Knox, Kentucky (begun in 1994). In the AIMHI programs, the dogs are trained as service dogs, hearing dogs, or social therapy dogs, and prisoners receive instructions on dog training, animal husbandry, and human and animal behavior. The AIMHI program "provides vocational training and helps the men in their transition back to civilian life" (Strimple, 2003, p. 74). According to Strimple, the state of Ohio has been exemplary in introducing dog training programs in 26 state and two private prisons. These dog training programs in Ohio prisons contribute significantly to fulfilling the governor's mandate in

1991 that prisoners in Ohio be "good citizens" in the communities where they exist and that all inmates partake in community service: "Dogs are trained to assist people with visual deficits; mobility problems; and hearing, neurological, and emotional problems" (Strimple, 2003, p. 75).

In 2002, the Missouri Department of Corrections partnered with C.H.A.M.P. (Canine Helpers Allow More Possibilities) Assistance Dogs to start a C.H.A.M.P. Prison Dogs program at the Women's Eastern Reception, Diagnostic, and Correctional Center in Vandalia, Missouri (Miller, 2008). The program was evaluated by a team of researchers from the University of Missouri–St. Louis, led by Jody Miller. The researchers reported the following findings based on interviews of inmate participants and facility staff. Inmate motivations to join the program predominantly involved a desire to develop a relationship with a dog and the sense of family that came from sharing this experience with other inmates participating in the program. A desire for emotional and behavioral change was also identified as a motivator to join the program. One inmate dog trainer stated in an interview, "It makes me feel responsible. It gives me a sense of accomplishment, even in a place like this." Another stated, "C.H.A.M.P. gives you something to be proud of" (Miller, 2008, p. 23). Regarding the impact on relationships between inmate participants and staff,

> Respect was a consistent theme that emerged independently in interviews conducted with inmate trainers and volunteers, and correctional staff. Most importantly, both groups report that such respect is mutually experienced—with inmates showing respect for staff, and staff likewise showing respect for inmates who participate in C.H.A.M.P.
> (Miller, 2008, p. 37)

The researchers also discovered that inmates developed new skills from participation in the program: assuming responsibility, people and social skills, decision making and problem solving, teamwork, and leadership. Additionally, inmates experienced emotional growth as well as enhanced life skills and relationships. Regarding the effect of the program on the prison atmosphere, the researchers reported the C.H.A.M.P. wing was considered a very "quiet" and "peaceful" wing (Miller, 2008, p. 67). The dogs were reported by the inmates to "calm the nerves" and provide "an overall lightening of the atmosphere" (Miller, 2008).

Furst (2006) performed a national survey of state prison-based animal programs. The survey was sent to the top administrator of each state's Department of Correction. A total of 46 of 50 states returned surveys; the four states that did not respond were Illinois, Iowa, Louisiana, and Texas. Of the states that participated, ten reported having no prison animal program: Arizona, Arkansas, Delaware, Hawaii, Maine, Minnesota, Mississippi, New Hampshire, Rhode Island, and Utah. A total of 36 states reported on 71 designs, or models, of prison animal programs at 159 sites throughout the country. Furst summarized the survey results as showing that prison animal programs are in most states, are most commonly of a community service design that uses dogs, are more likely to involve male than female participants, and were mostly established after 2000. Further, Furst suggested that livestock care and prison farms emerge as a unique type of prison animal program.

Each of the inmate–animal interaction programs described in this chapter has, in its own way, benefited both human and animal participants and served to further humanize the correctional institutions. It is also clear that inmate–animal interaction programs are beneficial for the communities where they exist because they save pets from euthanasia by training them to be adoptable; in addition, they provide training for dogs to become service animals for disabled persons.

Mulcahy and McLaughlin (2013) reviewed prison animal programs (PAPs) and determined that, while there were many anecdotes supporting the value of these programs, there was insufficient research to support the efficacy of PAP programs. They made the following suggestions regarding the need for more research to measure the efficacy of prison programs that incorporate animals:

> To encourage further research and build the body of knowledge surrounding PAPs, all new and existing PAPs should incorporate an evaluative component into the existing design. For new PAPs, a baseline measure of participants and the general prison population would be particularly advantageous. Programs that aim to produce well-trained animals and measure their success on adoption or placement rates will require different evaluative processes from those that focus on the therapeutic benefits for prisoners and may well target a different type of offender. Where prisoner variables are targeted, measures of psychosocial outcomes are recommended to complement measures of recidivism in identifying meaningful change. These evaluations should also include both quantitative and qualitative measures, if prisoner well-being, prison culture or personal change is a desirable outcome.
>
> (Mulcahy and McLaughlin, 2013, p. 377)

Juvenile Detention Programs with AAT

At the invitation of the director of the residential post-adjudication program, I began the AAT program at the Juvenile Detention Center of Denton County, Texas. All of the juveniles in the post-adjudication program were repeat offenders with theft and drug possession as common offenses. For 7 years, I went to the facility almost every week with some combination of my two dogs and cat so the juveniles could have group social visits with my pets. I was assisted by trained graduate students so we could maintain the ratio of one trained animal handler per pet. Over this same period, I volunteered my services as a professional counselor with one of my therapy animals, providing weekly individual or group counseling to the juveniles in the facility. Prior to my starting the AAT programs there, the Denton County Juvenile Detention Center Post-Adjudication Program had already made opportunities for the juveniles to go on supervised trips to local horse ranches for horse-riding lessons in exchange for community service at the ranches. Thus, when I proposed that I would seek funding to provide an opportunity for the juveniles to receive formal EAC, the post-adjudication program director was very enthusiastic. I submitted and received a moderate-sized grant to pay for the services of two groups of juveniles (eight males in one group and eight females in another group) to participate in an EAC program. The effects of the program were so successful that the County Board of Directors agreed to fund the program themselves the following year. Case workers reported that the AAT benefited the juveniles greatly in progressing through their rehabilitation program. The coping and social skills taught as a basic part of post-adjudication rehabilitation were reinforced by the juveniles' participation in the various AAT programs. In addition to opportunities to build and reinforce self-confidence and self-esteem, the AAT provided opportunities to practice teamwork, leadership, communication, and appropriate socialization. The therapy animals were also highly valued as a source of affection and comfort for the juveniles.

A juvenile detention AAT program in Dallas County, Texas, sponsored by the Dallas Society for the Prevention of Cruelty to Animals (SPCA), is most beneficial for the adolescents in the program as well as for the dogs that participate. Some of the dogs at the SPCA shelter are unruly and thus have difficulty being adopted. Volunteers transport these selected dogs to the juvenile facility once a week for a 2-hour training session by the adolescents in residence there. The dogs have previously been evaluated as not being aggressive, so they are safe to work with the juveniles. The adolescents at the detention facility teach the dogs basic obedience commands and introduce the dogs to agility training. The volunteers who train and supervise the juveniles with the dogs are experienced dog trainers. At the completion of the several-week program, the juveniles present their dog at a graduation ceremony in front of a large group of facility staff and other juveniles. The presentation includes an introduction and description of the dog, a history of its breed, what the dog was like when it began the training program, and a demonstration of what the dog can do now. Then the juvenile hands the dog over to a new owner who is adopting the trained dog from the SPCA. This last process is especially moving to observe. Juveniles are given an opportunity to say goodbye to the dog with which they have worked for several weeks and see it placed with a new owner. Most of the dogs find new owners to adopt them after they graduate from the juvenile training program because the program is so successful in training the dogs to be good companions. In my observation of this program, I overheard juveniles talk about how they related to the dog and felt they were helping the dog have a better chance in life by training it. The dogs were locked up like they were and needed help to be able to function better in society so they could be free again. Rehabilitating these unruly dogs so they could be adopted was a powerful metaphor for the juveniles to work hard in their own rehabilitation, and they seemed to truly understand this about their participation.

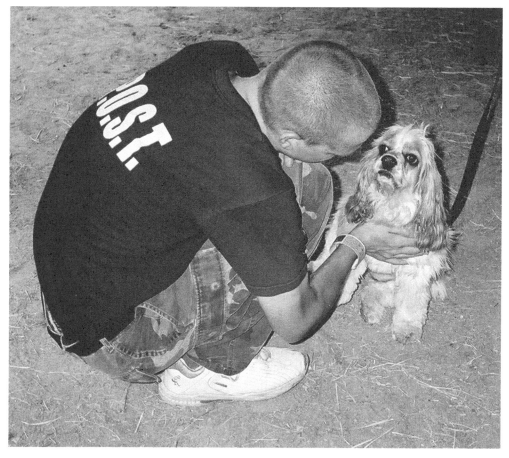

Figure 11.6 My therapy dog Dolly is a comfort for juveniles in a detention facility. Her quiet and affectionate personality has a calming influence.

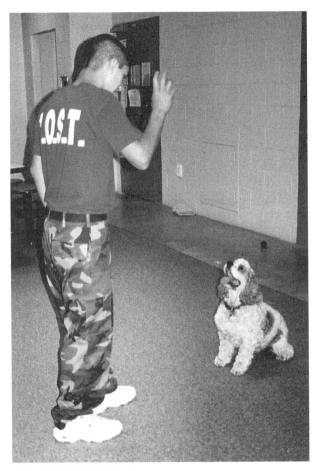

Figure 11.7 My therapy dog Rusty patiently waits for a ball to be tossed by an adolescent at a juvenile detention facility. Adolescents looked forward to their time with Rusty, who loved to play fetch.

Equine therapy programs have been designed to assist troubled teens. The Charles H. Hickey School in Baltimore, Maryland, a residential institution for young men, paired troubled students with Thoroughbreds; the program was begun in 1991 with the assistance of the Thoroughbred Retirement Foundation (Strimple, 2003). The students are responsible for all aspects of care for the farm's many horses, including grooming, feeding, exercise, first aid, and studying about horse physiology and horsemanship (Rhoades, 2001). The effects of the program were reflected by the comments of two 16-year-old participants in the program:

Samuel: "When I came here, I had an anger problem.... Working with horses has really helped me out. It's given me a good perspective on animals, on how to treat them properly."
   Allen: "You really want to go out there and work. I'd never been around an adult horse before. I like working with them."

(Rhoades, 2001, p. 25)

Ocean County Department of Juvenile Services in New Jersey began the Pet Therapy Program (n.d.) in 2002 in which a volunteer visited the facility twice a week with her therapy dogs, Rottweilers named Duffy and Pippin, to interact with the residents. The dogs do tricks for the juveniles and, on nice days, go outside and play "keep away" on the basketball court or fetch with the juvenile residents: "The dogs seem to be able to sense when a juvenile is upset and will cuddle or lick him/her until their anxieties lessen." This program was so successful that in 2007 a new program was added called the Saturday Therapy Dog Program. The curriculum for this new program permits the children to experience different types of dogs, along with the expertise and knowledge of their handlers. The Saturday Therapy Dog Program courses for the juveniles consist of the following elements to teach the juveniles the basics about dogs: doggie etiquette; the origin of dogs; grooming, healthcare, and nutrition; and training (*sit, stay, down, leave it*, and *heel*). The goal for the program is to teach the juveniles to care for and train their own pets when they return to their homes and in their future lives.

The Juvenile Detention Center in Calcasieu Parish works in partnership with the Humane Society of Southwest Louisiana to provide the New Leash on Life Project (n.d.). The program teaches the juveniles how to obedience train dogs during an intensive 4-week course. The juveniles volunteer and are carefully screened and selected to participate in this project; participation is a privilege that must be constantly earned. The dogs live at the Juvenile Detention Center and the juveniles must care for them 24 hours a day while learning how to train the dogs in basic and advanced obedience so the dogs can be adopted into good homes. The purpose of the project is to rehabilitate both the juveniles and the rescued dogs:

[The project] provides the juveniles with positive responsibility: the life of these dogs is in their hands, and the dogs will give back unconditional love for their effort. In return, the juveniles will provide the community with dogs that are ready to be wonderful family members and invaluable service animals.

(New Leash on Life Project, n.d.)

One of the first programs to bring incarcerated juveniles together with abandoned and abused dogs was Project POOCH, started by Joan Dalton in 1993 at MacLaren Juvenile Correctional Facility in Woodburn, Oregon, where she was the principal of the resident high school (Merriam-Arduini, 2000). At the time of its founding in 1993, it was believed to be "the only canine-based training program for incarcerated juveniles in a secure, closed facility" (p. 25). The youth who participated in the program were between the ages of 15 and 25 years:

They are youth that have been through a system that has given them every opportunity to change. No particular training or treatment has been effective enough to keep them from being locked up in a high security institutional environment, enclosed with barbed and razor wire. . . . Human–animal interaction is used to assist and augment behavioral, social, cognitive and affective attributes provided in the classroom. At its core, the program brings abandoned, abused or unwanted shelter dogs that would normally be put to death (sentenced to death row), to the MacLaren facility and allows incarcerated youth to care for and train them. The youths care for every need of the dogs and then adopt the dogs back into the community.

(Merriam-Arduini, 2000, p. 26)

The juveniles in the Project POOCH program learn real-life skills involving dog grooming and dog training, study the health needs of animals, and learn to run a boarding kennel:

The dogs are housed in specially constructed, professional kennels within the campus of MacLaren. There is a "clean room" for training and demonstrations, a regular classroom, lecture room and special area for grooming and cleaning. Project POOCH adheres to veterinary standards of care. The health, welfare, and training advancement of the dog are the scope and subset of the formal curriculum.

(Merriam-Arduini, 2000, p. 30)

"Participation in the program is selective" and considered "an honor and a privilege that carries great prestige" (Merriam-Arduini, 2000, p. 29). It could take up to 1 year from the point of application for a juvenile candidate to be accepted for participation in the Project POOCH program. The Project POOCH program requires participants to write in journals every day, and the journals are collected each Friday. The rule for journaling is to reflect on the week of classroom and hands-on experiences using both statements and questions. The following Monday, time is set aside for "voluntary oral presentations, for the student to interview and be interviewed, emphasizing the reflections and questions the student raised while writing on Friday" (Merriam-Arduini, 2000, p. 32). Merriam-Arduini evaluated Project POOCH from the period of 1993 to 1999 and reported the following positive effects of the program in her dissertation. The findings indicated a zero recidivism rate for those juveniles participating in the program and the program assisted to meet judicial orders and educational expectations for juveniles with high percentages. Adult survey respondents reported marked behavior improvements for the juvenile participants in the Project POOCH program, most especially in the areas of respect for authority, social interactions, and leadership. The juvenile participants described their change and growth in the areas of honesty, empathy, nurturing, social growth, understanding, confidence level, and pride of accomplishment.

Human–animal interaction assisted the youth to learn patience, tolerance, trust for animals and caring for people and animals.

(Merriam-Arduini, 2000, p. 88)

The Animal Humane Association of New Mexico teamed with the Youth Diagnostic and Development Center of New Mexico to teach incarcerated youth how to train shelter dogs so the dogs could be adopted as pets (Harbolt and Ward, 2001). Each of the shelter dogs was at moderate risk for euthanasia. The dogs were housed in kennels on the campus of the youth center, and only the participants were permitted to visit the dogs, visiting two to three times a day. During a 3-week training program, the dogs were taught basic obedience such as *sit*, *stay*, *come*, and *heel*. In addition, the young people received a basic course in dog grooming by a local dog trainer. The participants were required to keep the dogs' kennel areas clean, walk the dogs three times a day, and spend 2 hours in the afternoons training, grooming, and socializing. The youths were incarcerated for a variety of reasons: gang involvement, drugs, prostitution, or sexual offenses such as having an underage girlfriend. A few had committed more violent crimes. At the end of the 3-week training program the dogs were returned to the animal shelter for adoption. At this time the participants were given a certificate showing they had completed the program with a dog and asked to write a letter to the potential adopter of the animal they had trained. Excerpts from these letters demonstrated the youths' empathy and compassion for the dogs they had trained. For instance, one youth wrote about the dog, named Stuckers, he had paired with in the training program:

Stuckers is a very loving dog. He will always sit by your side and is well trained. I think Stuckers once had a family, but they abandoned him and all he needs is some attention and love. . . . Whoever adopts Stuckers is very lucky to have such a well-behaved dog. I took very good care of Stuckers, and whoever adopts him, I hope will do the same.

(Harbolt and Ward, 2001, p. 179)

12

Crisis and Disaster Response Counseling with Therapy Animals

Search-and-rescue dog teams have been working for many years in crisis and disaster situations all over the world. They assist in the recovery of lost persons and even bodies. These brave and dedicated animals risk their own lives working long hours in all types of weather, terrain, and dangerous environments to provide a valuable service to the human community. The success of search-and-rescue dogs has more than proven the ability of dogs to provide invaluable aid in the face of tragedy.

Working as a handler–animal team for crisis or disaster response is not as rigorous as search-and-rescue work, but it can be quite stressful and demanding. I classify animal-assisted crisis and disaster response in two ways: comforting and counseling. Crisis and disaster response animal-assisted comforting can be performed by nonprofessional volunteers and involves presenting the animal for clients to visit, pet, and hug for temporary relief from pain, stress, and grief. Crisis and disaster response animal-assisted counseling is performed by a professional counselor, who may also be donating their time as a volunteer, and activities for clients with the therapy animal include comforting but also include the professional performance by the counselor of interventions used in a crisis or disaster response setting. Sometimes, when a counselor has no qualified therapy pet of their own, the counselor may wish to invite into the counseling session a volunteer with a qualified therapy pet to assist the counselor with clients. Clients may find it easier to participate in the counseling session when a therapy animal is present.

There are well-known instances of therapy dogs assisting with crisis and disaster response comforting or counseling in the aftermath of great tragedy in the United States. Cindy Ehlers and her dog, Bear, of Eugene, Oregon, worked with students traumatized by the May 21, 1998 shootings at Thurston High School in Springfield, Oregon; and Cindy and Bear also assisted with crisis response following the violence on April 20, 1999 at Columbine High School in Littleton, Colorado (Rea, 2000). Numerous therapy dog teams volunteered disaster response services through the American Red Cross in New York providing comfort and stress relief to victims and families following the World Trade Center terrorist attack of September 11, 2001 (Teal, 2002; Shubert, 2012). Therapy dog teams assisted counselors with their counseling of children traumatized by the Sandy Hook Elementary School shooting that occurred on December 14, 2012 in Newton, Connecticut (Betker, 2014). K-9 Comfort Dog teams, sponsored by the Lutheran Church Charities, were flown in from Chicago to Boston to comfort persons following the Boston Marathon bombings that occurred on April 15, 2013 (*Huffington Post*, 2013). Hope Animal-Assisted Crisis Response (HOPE AACR) teams provided

DOI: 10.4324/9781003260448-12

comfort to those affected by the Navy Yard shootings in Washington, D.C. that occurred on September 16, 2013 (Gordon, 2013). K-9 Comfort Dogs, a team of 12 Golden Retrievers with their handlers, tended to the grieving at memorial services, churches, and hospitals following the shooting on June 12, 2016 of 102 persons, 49 of whom perished, at a primarily gay bar in Orlando, Florida (Bromwich, 2016). In 2005, I was able to provide disaster response comforting and counseling for victims of Hurricane Katrina.

DISASTER RESPONSE FOR HURRICANE KATRINA

On August 29, 2005, Hurricane Katrina passed east of New Orleans, Louisiana. Winds were in the category 4–5 range, and the tidal surge was category 5. The storm surge caused levee breaches in New Orleans, resulting in the worst engineering disaster in U.S. history. By August 31, most of the city's levees were breached, and 80 percent of New Orleans was flooded. These breaches were responsible for at least two-thirds of the flooding in the city. A total of 90 percent of the residents of southeast Louisiana were evacuated (CNN.com, 2005). In the immediate aftermath of Hurricane Katrina, survivors from the city of New Orleans and surrounding area were displaced to temporary shelters across the United States far from their homes. Prior to their arrival in the shelters, survivors had experienced intense life-threatening trauma and tragic loss. This mass displacement of disaster victims was unlike anything experienced before in the United States. Mental health providers responded by volunteering services to the displaced survivors at local shelters.

Following is a description of services I provided as a mental health worker responding to the needs of Hurricane Katrina survivors at two north Texas shelters (Chandler, 2008). The services I provided included working both with and without the assistance of a therapy dog across a span of 2 weeks. Animal-assisted disaster response was especially effective in this tragedy and, in many instances, observed to be clinically superior to nonanimal-assisted mental health intervention. When compared with nonanimal-assisted disaster response, response with animals was observed to be more effective in initiating client participation in interactions, relieving client tension and anxiety, facilitating client sharing of emotional responses and personal stories, and providing appropriate comfort and nurturance. In addition to working with survivors, the therapy dogs attracted almost as many professional disaster responders who were seeking relief from the stress of the event including doctors, nurses, police officers, and National Guard members.

An integral requirement for crisis and disaster response counseling is to be trained and registered in advance for this type of work; these counselors become the first responders to a disaster. As a registered American Red Cross crisis and disaster response mental health counselor, I began volunteering on the first day evacuees arrived at the Dallas Reunion Arena. For the first 2 days I volunteered, no therapy dogs were present, because the American Red Cross director was delayed in gaining permission to allow therapy dogs into shelters by the Dallas city manager, who initially did not understand the concept of therapy dogs. No professional therapy dogs had been previously involved in this type of response in the Dallas area. By the third day, therapy dogs Rusty and Dolly, red and white American Cocker Spaniels, were allowed to assist me in the counseling process within the shelters. The dogs took turns working with me on alternate days, and both worked side-by-side on one day when a trained graduate assistant joined us. Though the delay in getting approval for the therapy dogs' assistance in response to the Hurricane Katrina disaster was an initial nuisance, in hindsight it resulted in an opportunity to compare disaster response counseling first without and then with the assistance of therapy dogs.

Over the course of the first 2 days, mental health counselors universally shared a mutual frustration—the shelter evacuees did not approach the counselors for assistance. Even when the counselors went out among the hundreds of cots that lay across the floor to make contact and encourage individuals to share their thoughts and feelings, evacuees did not want to share personal stories with the counselors. While polite, survivors said few words, if any, about their experience or their emotional needs. Certainly, cultural barriers may have contributed to evacuees' hesitancy to speak with counselors about their trauma. The majority of evacuees were African–American, and almost all of the counselors were Caucasian. The evacuees were in a strange city a very long way from their beloved New Orleans and probably did not relate to the people of Dallas. Even though the evacuees expressed grateful appreciation for all that was being provided in the way of food and shelter, it was very difficult for the evacuees to trust their personal tragedy to a stranger many miles from their own home and very different from themselves.

On the third day, the therapy dogs were allowed into the Dallas shelters to assist me with my disaster response counseling. Both Rusty and Dolly were registered through the national organization Pet Partners at the highest rating of Complex Environment work, and they had already been assisting me for several years in the counselor training program at the university where I worked and with my volunteer counseling at a county juvenile detention center. Thus, I felt confident they would be an asset at the shelters with the hurricane evacuees. I did not know what to expect with the dogs assisting me at the shelters as this was the first disaster response counseling I had participated in either with or without my therapy dogs. As it turned out, the disaster response counseling with the therapy dogs was a very different experience compared with the previous 2 days of counseling at the shelters without the dogs. The time the evacuees had been at the shelters can be ruled out as a reason for the difference because new evacuees were arriving at the shelters every day. The difference was clearly as a result of the dogs. The first day the therapy dogs assisted with the Hurricane Katrina effort was at the Dallas Convention Center shelter. Dolly, Rusty, me, and a graduate student trained in AAT techniques worked side-by-side as a team.

The first noticeable difference in working with the therapy dogs was that it took much longer to get into the facility with the dogs, not because security was suspicious but because they wanted to pet and visit with the dogs. The first line of security was the National Guard around the perimeter of the convention center. When the two nearest guards saw us coming with the happy-faced dogs they broke into broad smiles and asked to pet the dogs. As they petted my dog Rusty, one guard spent several minutes discussing how much he missed his Golden Retriever and was looking forward to getting back home to his dog. The next line of security was a police officer just inside the main entrance. She saw us come through the door, gave us a stereotypical security-like sizing up as we approached, and when we got within a few feet she got down on her knees and started laughing and hugging on the tail-wagging canines. She shared how stressed out she was and how nice it was to love on a dog. After several minutes we proceeded with the dogs to the volunteer check-in table near the entrance. While we signed in under our shift time, the volunteers at the table were petting Dolly, who had stretched the limits of her 6-foot leash to greet the people on the other side of the table.

Leaving smiling check-in volunteers behind us we finally entered the facility where hundreds of evacuees were sitting on cots or standing in lines for clothes and supplies. Our plan was to walk down the aisles separating the groups of cots and invite people to pet the dogs as a way to relieve their stress. Based on my previous experience over the past 2 days when not working with the dogs, I expected that people would not seek us out and that we instead would have to approach people and that people still may not want to visit much. Yet much to my surprise, something very different happened. As soon as people heard the jingle noise of the dogs' tags, they looked up to locate the source. When they saw the jolly, freckle-faced Cockers coming, people sitting on their cots smiled. Many got up off their cot and came over to greet us partway. This was the case for adults and children alike. Shocked, grief-stricken faces gave way to pleasant grins and laughs upon seeing the dogs. Each person who wanted to interact with the dogs spent several minutes petting them, and, unlike in the nonanimal-assisted disaster response counseling, almost every evacuee we encountered spoke with the counselors at length while petting the dogs. An extraordinary, persistent pattern of interaction emerged with the animal-assisted disaster response counseling.

This frequent communication pattern was completely spontaneous and occurred with no prompting or direction from the counselors. First, evacuees asked numerous questions about the pets, such as name, gender, age, breed, and "Are they twins?" Second, evacuees shared their worries over the pets they left behind, and some shed tears at this time. And third, evacuees segued right into discussing details about their Hurricane Katrina trauma, loss, and evacuation. The presence of the therapy dogs had removed many of the social barriers that had been impeding the sharing process by evacuees, which had been mutually discussed by many frustrated counselors working at the shelters over the previous 2 days. The dogs were a catalyst for making a social connection with the evacuees. I was pleasantly amazed; it seemed as though the dogs were a bridge of commonality that united strangers in a strange environment. Over 100 evacuees gave and received canine hugs that day and walked away a little happier and lighter in mood. The children were especially impacted by the dogs. After visiting with the dogs and counselors, many of the children continued to accompany us as we moved down the aisles separating the cots. To the delight of all, two of the children spontaneously took over my role of introducing the dogs and explaining their role and function to each person we greeted. Several times we had to stop and sit down with children when the tag-a-long group had grown too large to get down an aisle; this allowed us to do spontaneous, brief group counseling with the children, who shared their feelings and traumatic experiences while petting and hugging the dogs.

The evacuees in the shelters were very thankful for the therapy dogs. One middle-aged woman said she had to leave behind two dogs—Missy, a very smart dog who would knock on the door with her tail when she wanted out, and a mother dog with nine puppies. "I'm just looking to see how pretty these dogs are," she said. "Truly, I miss mine. They were my babies. My children are grown and gone, but my dogs kept us safe, and we had to leave them. These babies here [Rusty and Dolly] are just so pretty, so pretty. I just love dogs." Another woman, a young adult, said, "I started to smile the minute I saw the dogs," as she petted Rusty while he turned over on his back for a belly rub. "I miss my dog so much. She was so spoiled. We were all crying when we left her behind. We left her in a second-floor room with a lot of food and water. I hope somebody kicks in the door and finds her." One 8-year-old girl said, "I think Dolly's precious. I have two cats, but dogs are smarter than cats." Her 8-year old cousin added, "This dog's smarter than two cats. I think they're fun and smarter than cats; they work hard, playing with people." In another interaction, "I felt like I'd seen everything in the way of kindness here in Texas, but these dogs just put it over the top," said a middle-aged woman, wiping away a tear after petting Dolly in silence for a minute.

The therapy dogs helped people release emotions and receive healing nurturance. Evacuees shared with the therapy dog team many stories of tragedy. Many had lost loved ones to death, both humans and pets. While petting Dolly, a young adult woman told of her harrowing rescue by helicopter after spending hours stranded atop her roof with her husband, surrounded by flood waters. She and her husband were separated during the rescue and ended up in shelters in different cities—she in Dallas and he in Houston. Many people became separated in the evacuation process, and many had not been able to locate loved ones. Two children petted the dogs while sharing a story of watching a dead body float by while their parents trudged through murky flood waters navigating a floating mattress supporting the young girl and her little brother.

One 9-year-old boy told the following heartbreaking story. When the hurricane winds subsided, his father went down the street to check on his grandmother who lived in the neighborhood. While he was gone, water began coming down the street. His mother rushed down the street to get his father. No one knew just how fast the water was going to rise. With his parents gone and the water rising fast and starting to come into the house, the little boy lifted his little brother onto the kitchen table. He lifted up his dog with her litter of puppies and joined them on top of the table—but the water kept rising fast. He could see the tall porch on the house across the street through the window and decided to get his brother and dogs to higher ground. He helped his little brother out of the house as they waded through water that came up to his chest and up to the chin of his little brother. When they stepped off the curb the water went up to his chin and over his brother's head. He proudly claimed that he had learned how to swim last summer, but his brother didn't know how yet. So while bouncing off his tiptoes and swimming halfway, he kept his brother's head above the water until they both arrived safely on the steps of the tall porch of the house across the street. He turned to go back for his dog and her puppies, but it was too late. The water had risen over the top of the front door of his house. He was overcome with guilt and grief from not being able to save his dog and her puppies from drowning and cried and petted my dog Rusty when telling about his experience. His little brother sat patting the back of his big brother and nodding and petting Rusty while the counselors listened compassionately and acknowledged the little boy's pain of having to make a difficult life-and-death choice. Thankfully, the father and mother made their way back to the boys through the muddy water and were with them at the shelter in Dallas.

It was apparent that the dogs put evacuees at ease and helped them feel safe enough to share personal information with the counselors. Animal-assisted counseling for this disaster was much more effective than nonanimal-assisted counseling in several significant ways including providing comfort and nurturance, relieving anxiety and tension, and facilitating the sharing of emotional responses. Interacting with approximately 100 highly stressed adults and children a day was exhausting. To help manage the stress of the disaster response counseling, the therapy dogs were provided multiple rest and water-break times. The dogs were monitored closely, and each animal received a nurturing massage at the day's end. The dogs' attitude remained jolly, and their temperament calm throughout their disaster work; however, they became visibly fatigued as the day progressed. Thus, their disaster response work was limited to no more than 4 hours a day. It is important to note that organizations such as Pet Partners (2014) recommend that therapy animals in any situation work no more than 2 consecutive hours at a time, and even less if the animal becomes stressed or fatigued.

THERAPY DOGS ARE BEST FOR CRISIS AND DISASTER RESPONSE

Therapy dogs can be especially helpful as part of a crisis and disaster response team. They offer a sense of normalcy to a very abnormal situation. Seeing and interacting with something familiar like a dog can provide some reassurance that although the world has been turned upside down, somehow things are going to be okay. Thus, the therapy dog is a powerful grounding mechanism for a client in crisis. The therapy dog can provide safe, nurturing touch and affection at a time when it is needed the most to comfort victims and survivors of tragedy. Being social animals, dogs have a fairly constant natural smile and tail wag that are universally known by all as friendly canine gestures; these gestures can relieve tension in the observer. Several studies have shown that the presence of a dog or another type of companion animal can help reduce the physiological stress response and alleviate anxiety and distress; thus, petting a therapy dog can soothe rattled nerves (Barker and Dawson, 1998; Friedmann et al., 1983; Friedmann, Locker, and Lockwood, 1993; Hansen et al., 1999; Katcher, 1985; Nagengast et al., 1997; Odendaal, 2000; Robin and ten Bensel, 1985).

I recommend the use of therapy dogs over other types of companion animals for work in a crisis or disaster response situation. Dogs have a calmer demeanor and more predictable behavior than other animals. Canines are more easily trained to obey direction and commands, imperative when in the center of disorganization and chaos that may erupt after a tragedy has occurred. Dogs can be trained and socialized to accept hurried crowds, intense emotions, loud noises, large equipment, blaring sirens, fast-moving emergency vehicles, and disrupted physical environments. Many medium- to large-sized dogs are robust and can sustain long and stressful working hours if they are in good physical condition.

THE NATURE OF CRISIS AND DISASTER

The National Organization for Victim Assistance (NOVA, 2004) describes in its *Community Crisis Response Team Training Manual* a number of characteristics of a crisis. Crises are typically caused by three categories of disaster:

- Naturally occurring: tornadoes, floods, hurricanes, lightning-instigated fires, and earthquakes.
- Human made: terrorist attacks, suicide, or homicide.
- Technologically based: train wrecks, building collapses, chemical spills.

The reactions to a crisis are both physical and emotional. Physical reactions include immobilization (frozen by fear), mobilization (fight, flight, or adapt), and exhaustion. Emotional reactions include shock, disbelief, denial, and emotional numbness. A cataclysm of emotion may occur that involves anger, fear, confusion, frustration, shame, humiliation, and grief. It is important to note that persons in crisis are trying to reconstruct some sort of equilibrium after their world has been plummeted into turmoil.

NOVA (2004) describes three stages of crisis intervention. The first stage is safety and security. The crisis response team must help the client experience physical safety and emotional security. The second stage of crisis intervention is ventilation and validation. The crisis response personnel validate for the client the client's crisis reactions. It is important that the client feel as normal as possible in this abnormal situation. Crisis and disaster response personnel must be caring and compassionate listeners. The third stage of crisis intervention is prediction and preparation. The crisis response team must help the client anticipate the future and prepare to cope with the impact of the tragedy on the client's life.

CRISIS AND DISASTER RESPONSE SAFETY

Special precautions must be undertaken to ensure the health and safety of the therapy dog in a crisis or disaster situation. Given the intensity and duration of such a situation, the dog may need more short breaks during the working day such as brief walks away from the crisis or disaster scene if possible and brief naps. During a crisis or disaster event, the dog may tend to change its eating and sleeping habits or get an upset stomach as a response to stress. Thus, pay special attention to the dog's nutrition and digestive responses. Make sure the dog gets lots of water and positive praise and affection from its handler. Give the dog a daily massage to help it relax after a hard day's work involving crisis and disaster counseling. Be careful when working in the aftermath of an event that has destroyed buildings (e.g., fires, tornadoes, or explosions) because dust particles released into the air when a structure was damaged can be toxic for the therapy dog. Also remember, after the crisis or disaster has passed, your dog and you will both still be significantly impacted by the stress from having worked in a crisis or disaster situation, so take good care of yourself and your dog; eat well and take a long rest.

It is vitally important to carry a doggy care bag with you when you and your dog are working as a crisis and disaster response team. Include fresh, bottled water; clean containers for food and water; dog food or snacks; a blanket, bed, or crate the dog is familiar with for resting and naps; a dog first-aid kit; supplies to clean up after the dog goes to the bathroom; a dog toy for play breaks; and a dog chew toy to use during breaks for the dog's stress relief. Include cloths or antibacterial wipes to wipe the dog's fur in between visits with each client to minimize cross-contamination of infectious germs and to help keep the dog's fur clean. Include a spare leash and collar for your dog in case the original ones choose this time to wear out.

For animal-assisted crisis and disaster response counseling, I also recommend carrying a crisis and disaster response bag for the therapist, meaning the dog's owner or handler. You will want snacks for yourself, bottled water, and antibacterial wipes to clean your hands and for clients to clean their hands before and after visits with the dog. Include a lint brush to keep fur off your clothing and for clients to remove fur from their clothing after visiting with your dog. You may not mind fur on your clothing, but others might be put off by it. You may want to include a first aid kit for yourself for minor injuries that may occur to you or your dog. Do not offer medical treatment to your clients unless you are a trained medical professional and are acting in an officially recognized capacity to provide such aid. It is best that if your client needs medical attention you seek that for them by finding the nearest medical care provider on the scene or by asking for assistance from a police officer or firefighter. Include in your crisis and disaster response bag for yourself at least a one-day change of clothes, in case you get caught on the scene for a long time or your clothes get soiled, plus any medication or hygiene toiletries you may need for a 24-hour period. A cell phone and battery charger, flashlight with extra batteries, and money or a telephone service card for a paid landline telephone (because cell phone service may get too busy to access during a crisis) are useful. You might also want to place a book to read in your bag because there may be long waiting periods at a crisis scene before you are called in to perform your counseling services. You may want to include rain gear and a weatherproof jacket or maybe a blanket for yourself in case the weather turns cold or you have to sleep in your car or stay in a community shelter overnight. Be sure to include a writing pen and paper for taking notes that may be necessary for a report later on. Add to the bag any small counseling tools that you may need, such as dog puppets or dog toys for the children to use to interact with the therapy dog during counseling sessions. You may even want to give the children you counsel in a crisis response session a small, inexpensive, stuffed dog toy to keep and take away with them after the session as a continued source of comfort. All of this is a lot to pack, so the real trick will be configuring the dog's care bag and your care bag so that they can be toted around easily. Also, a lightweight, collapsible dog crate is much easier to travel with than a heavy, bulky metal crate. Technology has advanced such that some dog crates fold up quite small and are extremely light, weighing only a few pounds.

When working in a crisis and disaster response situation, wear comfortable clothing appropriate for the environment or scene where you will be providing the crisis counseling with your pet. Also, you and the therapy dog should both wear visible identification that clarifies your role as a crisis and disaster response counseling team. This will reduce the likelihood of being confused with curious bystanders, who may be shooed away by security. Remember, though, you are in fact no more than a bystander unless you have been officially invited to the scene to provide crisis or disaster response counseling with your pet. Thus, let us examine some ways to become officially involved in animal-assisted crisis and disaster response counseling.

BECOMING A RESPONSE TEAM WITH YOUR PET

If you have not had formal training in crisis and disaster response counseling, then before becoming involved as a crisis and disaster response counselor you should pursue crisis and disaster response training at a local, state, or national conference or continuing education seminar. If you have not had crisis and disaster response training for many years, you might want to get some current training in this area. Crisis and disaster response training is provided by the American Red Cross (n.d.) and NOVA (2004). I recommend *Psychological First Aid*, 2nd edition, by the National Child Traumatic Stress Network and the National Center for PTSD (2006) as an educational resource. Other informative publications in crisis response include *Terrorism, Trauma and Tragedies*, 3rd edition (Webber and Mascari, 2010), *A Practical Guide for Crisis Response in Our Schools*, 5th edition (Lerner, Volpe, and Lindell, 2004a), *A Practical Guide for University Crisis Response* (Lerner, Volpe, and Lindell, 2004b), and *Acute Traumatic Stress Management* (Lerner, Shelton, and Crawford, 2001). Opportunity to become part of a crisis or disaster response team is offered by K-9 Disaster Relief (n.d.), a nonprofit humanitarian foundation; by Hope Animal-Assisted Crisis Response (HOPE AACR) (n.d.), a nonprofit organization; and by LCC K-9 Comfort Dog Ministry (n.d.), a service of Lutheran Church Charities.

In the case of a community tragedy, the American Red Cross organization is often a primary respondent. Thus, many community crisis and disaster response service providers coordinate their efforts through the American Red Cross response structure. To become a crisis and disaster response service provider for the American Red Cross, you must take their standardized training and then register with your local American Red Cross chapter as a crisis and disaster response counselor with your therapy pet. In the instance of a local school tragedy, many schools have in place their own existing crisis and disaster response team. Contact your local school district office to find out how to become part of the school district's crisis and disaster response counseling team. Whether you are a crisis and disaster response counselor for the American Red Cross or a local school district, you may need to check in from time to time to make sure you are still listed as an active service provider and to keep your telephone numbers and other contact information current. In the time of a real tragedy, things will need to happen quickly, so advance preparedness is the best approach. Many well-meaning people will want to help out in a crisis or disaster, but the fact is that you will most likely only get in the way unless you are part of an established response structure with a clearly identified chain of command. You must know whom to contact to obtain your crisis or disaster response counseling assignment, including names and contact information of back-up supervisors if you cannot reach your assigned supervisor.

THE NATURE OF CRISIS AND DISASTER RESPONSE COUNSELING

The immediate aftermath of a crisis or disaster is not the time to do in-depth, insight- oriented counseling. Crisis and disaster response counseling is very different from traditional talk therapy. Crisis and disaster response counseling is briefer and focuses mostly on helping the recipient to feel safe. Crisis and disaster response counseling is considered band-aid therapy—sufficient to aid the survivor through the initial stages of the crisis and, if necessary, provide referral to other resources to satisfy more long-term needs. Crisis and disaster survivors are often in shock and confused. They may be overcome with worry and grief over loss. In a crisis or disaster, counselors focus on calming people, helping them to feel safe, and assisting them to obtain their most immediate needs. It is vital that counselors be caring and compassionate listeners. If survivors need to tell their story in the immediate aftermath of a crisis or disaster, a counselor should be supportive and reflect their thoughts and feelings. Crisis and disaster counselors must listen with a caring attitude. How effectively a counselor can assist a survivor in the immediate aftermath of a crisis or disaster may have a direct impact on how well a person copes with the crisis or disaster, both in the short term and in the long term. If opportunity presents itself, a counselor can prepare a survivor for reactions they may experience in the coming hours, days, and weeks after a crisis or disaster and encourage a client to seek additional assistance if necessary. These reactions may include flashbacks of the event, insomnia, heightened startle reflex, feeling jumpy and irritable, short-tempered, angry, sad, and depressed. Providing a handout explaining these possible reactions can be useful in reassuring a client that these uncomfortable experiences are common after a crisis or disaster event. Providing a handout with contact information on community resources can be very useful for survivors, such as where to receive follow-up counseling or medical care, and assistance in finding housing and gaining financial support.

I observed that all the mental health professionals performed in excellent fashion at the two Dallas shelters where I volunteered. Disaster response counseling with Hurricane Katrina survivors involved a great amount of assessment, triage, and information provision. Liaison with the onsite psychiatrist and medical staff was vital. Evacuees demonstrated heightened anxiety as a result of the disaster and displacement. Many individuals who had been stranded in the New Orleans Convention Center or Superdome for over a week prior to evacuation had been without medication, including psychotropic medication, for many days, and a large number did not remember the name of their medication. Counselors gathered detailed descriptions of the evacuees' lost medication and self-reported symptoms to assist an onsite psychiatrist in writing new prescriptions. Emotionally and mentally disabled persons had been separated from caretakers in the chaotic departure from New Orleans and needed assessment and placement with local agencies. Counselors assisted evacuees in making important contacts. Hundreds of evacuees were separated from loved ones and were desperate to find them. Many were trying to contact friends and family who were not affected by the hurricane so they would not have to remain long at the temporary Dallas shelter. Survivors were anxious to contact state and federal agencies to report the loss of property and change of address. Many survivors were not computer literate and needed assistance with the Internet service that was provided for reporting lost property and applying for disaster relief and aid.

Many professionals responded to the disaster response effort in Dallas, including social workers, counselors, psychologists, and psychiatrists. While many volunteered, there were often not enough mental health providers to cover every shift. Disaster response counseling for Hurricane Katrina required the ability to make some independent decisions because, due to other responsibilities, there often was no supervisor available to direct decisions. As is typical in disaster response, the atmosphere at the Dallas shelters was one where chaos often ruled and communication was very poor. Disaster counselors had to be able to size up a situation very quickly and then act where needed. To be an effective crisis and disaster response counselor one must handle stress well, be capable of some necessary independent decision making, be willing to exercise appropriate assertive responsibility, and to liaise well with other responders including mental health, medical, and rescue personnel. A crisis and disaster response counselor needs to contribute calm and order to a stressful and confusing atmosphere.

Victims and survivors of tragedy experience and display an array of emotions. Each child and adult will deal with the crisis in a unique way, but some common experiences help us to prepare as professionals to provide counseling services in response to a crisis and disaster. Victims and survivors of tragedy are likely experiencing some form of emotional shock. This may be exhibited as a sense of disorientation and confusion, difficulty with communication, difficulty focusing attention or concentrating, and trouble making decisions. Some clients will be very quiet, and some will be very emotional and talkative. Demonstrating empathy, immediacy, and sincerity while listening attentively or sitting quietly with clients can be comforting for them. Despair, sadness, and anger are common emotions expressed in a crisis situation. Sometimes client anger may be directed at service personnel, so it is important not to take things said to you personally. All clients in a crisis or disaster situation are likely experiencing some level of anxiety. Their psychophysiological stress level will be significantly aroused. Thus, strategies to help calm a client can be implemented.

Lerner, Shelton, and Crawford (2001) describe four categories of responses commonly experienced by persons who have been exposed to a traumatic event: emotional responses, cognitive responses, behavioral responses, and physiological responses. A number and variety of emotions are possible; some examples for each category of response are listed as follows (Lerner, Shelton, and Crawford, 2001):

- Emotional Responses:

  — Shock and numbness
  — Fear and terror
  — Anxiety
  — Anger
  — Grief and guilt
  — Uncertainty
  — Irritability
  — Sadness or depression.

- Cognitive Responses:

  — Difficulty concentrating
  — Confusion and disorientation
  — Difficulty with decision making
  — Short attention span
  — Suggestibility
  — Vulnerability
  — Blaming self or others
  — Forgetfulness.

- Behavioral Responses:

  — Withdrawal and isolation
  — Impulsivity
  — Inability to stay still
  — Exaggerated startle response.

- Physiological Responses:

  — Rapid heartbeat and elevated blood pressure
  — Difficulty breathing
  — Chest pains
  — Muscle tension and pains
  — Fatigue
  — Hyperventilation
  — Headaches
  — Increased sweating, thirst, and dizziness.

Clients perceived as needing medical attention (e.g., those disoriented, experiencing chest pains or who have difficulty breathing, or injury) should be assisted immediately by locating a nearby, onsite medical emergency provider.

A crisis and disaster response counselor must attend to the many needs of a client that are unique to a crisis and disaster response situation. It is important to help clients feel that they are currently safe by reassuring them that the immediate tragic event is over. The crisis and disaster response counselor must be able to listen effectively to clients who desire to express emotions and talk about how they feel and how they have been impacted by the event. If someone has died, processing the shock and grief of the death may be important for the client. Processing the loss of property and pets is also very meaningful for the client. A client may not be thinking clearly, and so a crisis counselor may need to assist the client through some imminent decision-making process appropriate to the situation, although significant life-changing decisions should be postponed if possible until the client is thinking more clearly. Guiding the client through some brief relaxation exercises can calm the client's nerves. These exercises take only a few seconds each but can have significant positive impact. They can be practiced several times a day every day to alleviate stress. Following are some brief relaxation responses that are helpful to teach a client:

- *Deep breathing.* Have clients place their hands on their stomach just above their belly button and take slow deep breaths while focusing on how their hands gradually rise and fall as they breathe. Also, have clients imagine inflating an imaginary balloon inside their stomachs beginning with filling up the bottom near the belly button and finishing with the top near the chest. Then deflate the imaginary balloon by reversing the process. Coach the client to take smooth, easy breaths and to not hold their breath, especially in between inhales and exhales. Proper diaphragmatic breathing is key to good health. The entire body responds positively to it. The blood is oxygenated, feeding the vital organs, muscles, and brain, which aids in clearer thinking and more energy and health. Dogs have a nice natural diaphragmatic breathing process. So to facilitate the slow-breathing exercise for a client, I had my dog Rusty lie down with his belly showing. I taught Rusty to respond to the word *relax* during our daily massage time so he could relax on command in most situations, having associated the word with relaxation. I would tell Rusty to relax, and as he would lie there calmly, breathing slowly and deeply, I asked clients to put their hands on Rusty's warm belly, breathe deeply, and count how many of Rusty's breaths they can fit into one inhale and one exhale of their own, because dogs have faster breathing patterns than humans. I instructed clients to sense the warmth of the skin and relaxation of the stomach muscles on Rusty's tummy while doing this exercise.
- *Shoulder shrug.* Have clients reach for their ears with the tops of their shoulders while taking a long, deep breath and then drop and relax the shoulders on the exhale. This will aid in releasing tension that inevitably builds up in the shoulder region at times of stress.
- *Shoulder roll.* Have clients slowly roll the shoulders backward and forward to release tension.
- *Slow neck stretch.* Have clients slowly let the head fall to one side down toward the top of the shoulder without raising the shoulder to meet it, gradually stretching the neck muscles while taking deep breaths. Then repeat on the other side.
- *Relax the dog.* After clients had practiced the aforementioned exercises, I asked them to continue their slow breathing and release as much of any remaining tension in their bodies as they can while they slowly pet Rusty, thereby trying to get Rusty as still and relaxed as possible. I told clients that the dog could pick up on their emotional and physical stress so they have to relax themselves to get the dog to relax.
- *Humor the dog (or funny face).* The point of this exercise is to have clients stretch their facial muscles to help tight muscles relax. I asked clients to stretch their facial muscles by making as funny a face as they can, without touching their faces, to see if they could

get my dog Rusty to respond to their funny faces in a positive way, such as giving a responsive tail wag or walking over to the client and sniffing or licking their faces.

Extreme or constant psychophysiological arousal is very detrimental to emotional and physical wellbeing. When a threat is perceived, a chain of events occurs that sends a variety of stress-related hormones cascading into the bloodstream. In response, the heart rate increases, blood pressure rises, muscles become tense, and digestive processes are interrupted. The stress hormones, such as cortisol, have toxic effects on the immune system, thereby making us more susceptible to illness. Even after the tragic event is over, the client's rumination on the event continues the re-experiencing of it and thus maintains psychophysiological arousal. Visiting with an animal can interrupt the rumination process and lower anxiety in a client. The presence of a therapy dog has been found to counter the stress response by reducing the amount of stress hormones released, such as cortisol and adrenalin, and increasing the release of health-inducing hormones, such as endorphins and oxytocin (Odendaal, 2000). Helping a client to manage and control the stress response as part of the crisis or disaster recovery process is vitally important. It is believed that the likelihood for developing post-traumatic stress disorder (PTSD) is significantly increased when levels of adrenalin are sustained in the system; thus, interaction with a therapy pet soon after an event can perhaps decrease the chance for someone developing PTSD. Simply petting or playing with the therapy dog can help a client to relax and feel better. Holding or hugging a friendly therapy pet can make the client feel more secure and grounded as a result of the familiarity that a therapy pet presents to an otherwise strange and upsetting situation.

Frank Shane of K-9 Disaster Relief (Shane, 2004) has written heartrending stories that epitomize the value of making it possible for a client to pet or hug a therapy pet during a crisis response situation. A brief reiteration of two of these stories follows.

A woman and her child were seeking financial assistance from the Red Cross disaster headquarters after the woman lost her husband in the World Trade Center attack on September 11, 2001. The woman was visibly emotional upon seeing a therapy dog, saying that she missed her dog very much that had died of cancer a few months before September 11. The woman requested to pet the therapy dog. The animal's handler, who was a mental health provider trained in AAT, facilitated an interaction between the woman and the dog. The woman petted the therapy dog and talked about her own pet loss, the dog, which her husband had named Ginger. She went on to process her grief from losing her husband. Then the woman's child spent time with the therapy dog and handler while the mother went to complete the forms for gaining financial assistance. The therapy dog lay underneath the table near the child as the child drew pictures of the former family dog, Ginger, playing ball with the child's now-deceased father.

In a second incident described by Shane (2004), a volunteer AAT team was working just outside the World Trade Center disaster site, very near Ground Zero. Several exhausted firefighters and other rescue personnel were resting in this area. At one point, a firefighter knelt down next to the therapy dog and started crying. The firefighter spent nearly half an hour with the therapy dog. He told the dog's handler that the dog's reddish hair was the same color as that of a young man he had just taken out of a building. The firefighter spent time processing with the animal's handler the many terrible days working in the aftermath of the September 11 terrorist attack. The firefighter then asked the handler to come back the next day so he could give the dog something special.

FORMING A MULTI-MEMBER RESPONSE TEAM

If your local school or community does not have a crisis and disaster response counseling team, then you may want to form one to include several therapists working with their therapy animals as part of the team. Form your crisis and disaster response counseling team in coop-eration with local school districts and community emergency management officials such as police, fire, and medical personnel. Make sure crisis and disaster response counseling team members receive or have had crisis and disaster response training, such as may be provided by the American Red Cross organization or NOVA. Also, only therapy animals (preferably therapy dogs) that have been evaluated as being appropriate for crisis and disaster response work should be allowed to be part of the crisis and disaster response team. A crisis and dis-aster response therapy animal needs to have a high tolerance for stress, have a very even tem-perament, be very well behaved, demonstrate very predictable behaviors, and have a quick and efficient response to commands.

The NOVA (2004) *Community Crisis Response Team Training Manual* suggests guidelines for establishing a crisis response team. Based on NOVA guidelines, following is a step-by-step procedure for establishing an animal-assisted crisis and disaster response counseling team. Step 1 is to develop (a) a contract of agreement, and (b) a policy and procedures manual for each team member outlining responsibilities, duties, and obligations. Include in the contract and the policies and procedures information that clarifies the increased potential risk of injury and stress involved with crisis and disaster response counseling for both the counselor and the therapy pet. State clearly in the policies and procedures the chain of command for community contact of the team, including back-up contacts, procedures for disseminating crisis and disaster response assignments, procedures for onsite supervision of crisis and dis-aster response counseling team members, procedures for recording and reporting activities performed during the crisis and disaster response counseling, and procedures for debriefing and processing after the crisis and disaster has passed.

Step 2 for developing an animal-assisted crisis and disaster response team is to designate at least two coordinators who will serve as initial contact persons for your response team. Two coordinators are necessary so that one coordinator is always available locally to be con-tacted by school or community emergency response supervisors in the event of a disaster. These coordinators will provide to school and community emergency response management supervisors and to other appropriate emergency response personnel a description of the ser-vice your team offers and contact information for the two designated coordinators of the response team. The response team coordinators will be the initial persons contacted when the school or community emergency management system supervisor calls upon the services of your crisis and disaster response counseling team. In fact, it might be a good idea to have a team coordinator on 24-hour call at all times as it is never known when disaster may occur. Make sure school or community emergency management supervisors continue to be aware of your team and of how to contact the team coordinators, and when to call upon the team's service. Periodic communication with school and community emergency managers will more likely assure that your crisis and disaster response team will be used even though a certain amount of disorganization and chaos rules the aftermath of a tragedy. Your crisis and disaster response team coordinators will contact team members to organize a response to the tragedy, oversee the response, and organize a process and debriefing session regarding the crisis and disaster response once the crisis and disaster is over. Also, response team coordi-nators will be the designated contact persons for crisis and disaster response team members to check in with after a tragedy has occurred to find out if their services will be called upon. The response team coordinators serve as group communication personnel, directing com-munication among response team members during a crisis as well as coordinating commu-nication with outside agencies, organizations, and facilities. The designated response team coordinator must not provide direct client services with or without their pets during a crisis because they will be busy coordinating and communicating the response effort. Response team coordinators can also organize crisis and disaster response training for potential new members and coordinate community outreach activities between team members and the community for education about the service the team provides.

Step 3 is to designate at least one team member as a team assessor who is an onsite supervisor of all the crisis and disaster response team members. This assessor will not provide direct services to clients and will not work with his or her pets but will supervise the services of the active team members with their pets. The team assessor oversees the services being provided at the crisis or disaster site and serves as a feedback resource to both the crisis and disaster response counseling team coordinator and to the school or community emergency management supervisor. The team assessor is often the person who initially evaluates team members with their pets to approve them as crisis and disaster response team members. Thus, it is most helpful if the team assessor is a counselor and a trained animal evaluator. All response teams must, with their animals, check in with the team assessor once they reach the crisis or disaster response site. The team assessor screens team members at the crisis or disaster site in advance of the team reporting for duty and continuously monitors each team's capacity to cope with a specific population, trauma, or environment. If a team becomes overwhelmed or fatigued, the assessor makes recommendations to remove the team from the site. The team assessor can cooperate with the team coordinator to provide ongoing emotional support for team members who respond to crisis or disaster. The team assessor should definitely be an important participant at the debriefing and processing session or sessions that are organized by the team coordinator after the crisis or disaster has passed, and that all response team members must attend.

Step 4 for developing an animal-assisted crisis and disaster response counseling team is to designate at least one team member whose role will be to locate and alert an on-call veterinarian in case his or her services will be needed by the responding therapy animals. Step 5 is to develop and maintain an up-to-date resource directory of approved team members and their approved therapy pets with names and contact information with multiple phone numbers for each team member. Designate in the directory at least two coordinators who will serve as the initial contact persons for community emergency managers who wish to call on the response team for services. All key personnel for the response team should be designated in the directory. Step 6 is to choose a recognizable team name that can easily become familiar to emergency management personnel. Step 7 is to develop and distribute recognized identification badges and clothing for team members to wear at the crisis site. The therapy pets should all wear visible identification, such as a neck scarf or vest of the same colored material and team markings, to clearly identify the animal as a crisis response team therapy animal. Human team members should also wear recognizable clothing, such as a team vest or jacket. All human team members should also wear a laminated team identification badge with the name of the crisis and disaster response team or organization or institution affiliation, the names of the therapist and the therapy pet, and a photograph of both the human and animal team member on it. In a crisis or disaster situation, it is the duty of onsite security to make sure you belong there. You must be cordial and cooperative with any and all requests to check your identification.

Keys to effective crisis and disaster response counseling include preparation and organization as well as ongoing coordination and supervision. In most instances, a crisis or disaster cannot be predicted, and sometimes the best-laid plans can have hitches given the chaotic nature of a disaster. Following the terrorist attack on the World Trade Center of New York on September 11, 2001, the American Red Cross was contacted by hundreds of personnel wanting to donate their services. One enthusiastic response team was a group of faculty and student play therapists from our graduate program in counseling at the University of North Texas. Upon their return the therapists described the designated site in New York for counseling services as a hastily created, large common area where families and individuals would come for free counseling services. The manner in which it was arranged was chaotic and intrusive with a significant lack of privacy for the client and multiple impositions upon the therapists. Professionals readily invaded the space of other professionals, while volunteers stumbled into counseling sessions interrupting therapeutic process. As it was described to me, in one instance a play therapist was working with a child using a portable play therapy kit when a volunteer with a therapy dog walked over, interrupting the play therapy session and inviting the child to play with or pet the dog. This happened on multiple occasions. In another instance, a play therapist was working with a child using play therapy and a psychologist walked over, interrupted the counseling session, and started directing the child to respond to the psychologist's inquiries. It seems obvious that both the volunteer with the therapy dog and the psychologist neither recognized nor acknowledged the potential benefit of the child's engagement in the play therapy. It is easy to understand how a nonprofessional community volunteer might make such an error, but even professionals were stumbling over one another. The well-meaning volunteers and professionals may have been more effective had there been better coordination of facilities and services in this situation.

CRISIS AND DISASTER RESPONSE IS NOT FOR EVERY COUNSELOR OR EVERY DOG

The experiences I had working with my therapy dogs providing counseling services for survivors of Hurricane Katrina were among the most meaningful experiences of my professional career. I would do it again without hesitation. However, it was also some of the most difficult work I have ever done. I am very glad the therapy dogs were there to help because they made the experience more tolerable for me and those that we served. Crisis and disaster response work can involve continuous engagement with a large number of people who are experiencing a great deal of stress; this includes both survivors and responders. In a crisis and disaster situation, a large number of people have a great deal of need in an environment where there is a great amount of chaos. One of the counselor's roles is to help everyone stay calm and another is to assist everyone in getting what they need. A crisis and disaster response counselor can fulfill many roles and be involved wherever appropriate. At a crisis or disaster scene a counselor can be a human traffic director, an information provider, a liaison between medical personnel and victims or their families, a diffuser of spontaneous conflicts, a soother of emotional crises, and a compassionate listener. A crisis and disaster response counselor must have a high tolerance for compounded stress, very sound assertiveness skills, very good organizational skills, work very well with other professionals providing services at the scene, and capacity for independent decision making when needed. There is a great need for mental health professionals to serve communities at times of crisis and disaster, so if you think you can do it, I encourage you to contact your local chapter of the American Red Cross and become a crisis and disaster mental health responder for your community. You must have a license or certification to practice as a professional mental health provider in order to be an American Red Cross mental health crisis and disaster responder. Also important to note is that not all therapy dogs are capable of being crisis and disaster response dogs. Therapy dogs should not be brought to crisis and disaster scenes unless they have a high tolerance for stress, chaos, and noise; a consistent and reliable response to commands; and a highly sociable attitude toward all types of people.

13

Establishing a School-Based Program for Animal-Assisted Counseling and Education

There is much anecdotal information about pets being at school such as in ways teachers, librarians, counselors, and occupational therapists incorporate animals for children's comfort as well as to enhance learning. There has also been research about animals assisting in schools. This chapter presents ideas about how animals are helpful in the education setting.

RESEARCH SUPPORT FOR THE BENEFITS OF THERAPY ANIMALS AT SCHOOL

Rud and Beck (2003) performed a descriptive study to examine the presence of pets in classrooms by surveying a convenience sample of teachers at rural, suburban, and urban elementary schools in Indiana. Over a 3-year period, surveys were sent to 2,149 teachers at 115 schools, and 431 teachers who were contacted returned the mailed survey instrument. Over a quarter of those who returned the survey (26.1 percent) had pets in the classrooms; animals were significantly more common in suburban and rural schools than in cities. The presence of classroom animals was not associated with the size of the school, and there was a surprising variety of animals kept in the classroom: fish (27.5 percent); mammals, including gerbils, guinea pigs, hamsters, and rabbits (26.3 percent); amphibians/reptiles (22.1 percent); insects/spiders (11.7 percent); invertebrates/others, including worms, crabs, and snails (10.8 percent); and birds (1.6 percent). Nearly half (46 percent) of the teachers who did not have classroom pets allowed students to bring animals in as "visitors." Animal visitors were not simply an alternative to classroom animals because significantly more classrooms that also had classroom animals had visiting animals. Reasons given for bringing animals to class included "enjoyment" (37.4 percent), "hands-on teaching" (22.8 percent), and "psychological well-being" (22.1 percent) (Rud and Beck, 2003).

Several studies have demonstrated that the presence of a therapy dog can contribute to social and educational gains for children. One research study demonstrated that the presence of a dog in a classroom had beneficial effects such as improving social competence and empathy in children in the first grade (Hergovich et al., 2002). The participants were 46 first graders (43 of them were immigrants) who were divided into two classes: one class served as a control group, and the other as the experimental group. In the experimental group a dog was present in the classroom for 3 months. According to the researchers, the presence of the therapy dog "fostered the development of autonomous functioning and better segregation of self/non-self, which is the foundation of sensitivity towards the needs and moods of

DOI: 10.4324/9781003260448-13

other people" (Hergovich et al., 2002, p. 37). Additionally, based on the view of the teachers, the children who were in the class with the dog exhibited higher social integration and less aggression compared with the children who were not with the dog. The authors concluded that a dog can be an important factor in the social and cognitive development of children (Hergovich et al., 2002).

Another research study demonstrated that the presence of a dog improved the emotional stability of six children with severe emotional disorders (Anderson and Olson, 2006). Over an 8-week period, the following data were collected: observations of children, interviews with parents, and behavioral data when children went into emotional crisis. Based on a qualitative analysis of the data, researchers concluded that the dog's presence in the classroom contributed to students' overall stability evidenced by prevention and de-escalation of episodes of emotional crisis. Furthermore, the dog's presence improved students' attitudes toward school and facilitated students' learning lessons in responsibility, respect, and empathy (Anderson and Olson, 2006).

Kotrschal and Ortbauer (2003) tested the behavioral effects of the presence of a dog in a classroom. One of three dogs was introduced alternately into a class at an elementary school in Vienna, Austria, attended by 24 children (14 boys and 10 girls; mean age of 6.7 years). The group of children was multiethnic in background, and most of the children came from first-generation immigrant families. The dogs in the study were a male Retriever, a female Husky, and a female cross-breed. They were all owned by the main classroom teacher and were all registered therapy dogs. The dogs were:

> gentle and friendly with the children who were allowed to interact with the dogs in a respectful way at any time. It was only when the dog was on its mat that the children were asked to leave the dog alone. At the start of the project, children were instructed about the dogs' needs and were shown how to care for and handle the dogs.
> (Kotrschal and Ortbauer, 2003, p. 150)

The researchers explain that the children's behavior was recorded on video for 2 hours every week, during "open teaching situations," first during a 1-month control period in the absence of dogs, followed by an experimental period of similar duration, when a dog was present in the classroom: "frequency and duration of all observable behaviors of individuals and their interactions were coded from these tapes" (Kotrschal and Ortbauer, 2003, p. 147). Significant positive effects were found from the presence of the dog in the classroom. The group became socially more homogenous due to decreased behavioral extremes, such as aggressiveness and hyperactivity; and formerly withdrawn individuals became socially more integrated. The researchers found these effects to be more pronounced for the boys than the girls. Also, even though the children spent considerable time watching and making contact with the dog, they also paid more attention to the teacher. The researchers concluded that the presence of a dog in the classroom positively stimulated social cohesion and improved teaching conditions (Kotrschal and Ortbauer, 2003).

The presence of a dog has increased children's motivation to complete motor skills tasks for language-impaired and typical preschool children (Gee, Harris, and Johnson, 2007). A total of 14 children, males and females between the ages of 4 and 6 years, performed ten gross motor skills tasks (e.g., long jump/high jump) either in the presence of a therapy dog (a miniature Poodle) or in the absence of a therapy dog. In the dog-present condition the dog either performed the task immediately prior to or at the same time as the child. As predicted by the researchers, the children completed the tasks faster when the dog was present than when the dog was absent. The researchers concluded that the presence of the therapy dog served as an effective motivator for the children, who performed faster but without compromising accuracy, in all tasks but one. Based on these results the authors recommended a role for therapy dogs in speech and language development programs for preschool children (Gee, Harris, and Johnson, 2007). Another study demonstrated that when a dog serves as a model for the execution of gross motor skills tasks, language-impaired and typical preschool children ($n = 11$) are more likely to adhere to instructions than if a human or a toy dog modeled the same tasks (Gee et al., 2009).

Research has shown that preschoolers make fewer errors on an object categorization task in the presence of a dog (Gee, Church, and Altobelli, 2010). Three conditions were applied: a real dog (a black miniature Poodle named Louie), a toy dog, or a human. The dependent variable was completion of a match-to-sample task in which 12 children were asked to choose a picture of an object that goes with another. Three different categories of stimuli were used in the experiment: taxonomic, thematic, and irrelevant. The presence of the real dog resulted in significantly fewer irrelevant choices than either the toy dog or the human conditions. The researchers concluded that fewer errors made in the presence of the miniature Poodle indicated that the presence of the real dog had a positive impact on performance of this cognitive task (Gee, Church, and Altobelli, 2010).

It has been demonstrated that preschool children require fewer instructional prompts to perform a memory task in the presence of a dog (Gee, Crist, and Carr, 2010). A total of twelve 3- to 5-year-old preschool children (six boys and six girls) participated in the study. There were three different conditions presented involving: (1) a real dog (the dog sat near the child with a human assistant holding the dog's leash and the child was allowed to touch or pet the dog during the exercise); (2) a stuffed toy dog (the same human assistant manipulated a stuffed dog to sit near the child—the stuffed dog was similar in size, shape, and color as the real dog and was named Kory); and (3) a human confederate (the same human assistant sat near the child). The real dog was a black miniature Poodle named Louie. Louie was registered as a therapy dog with Therapy Dogs International. Louie wore a collar and a 6-foot leash while participating in the experiment. The researchers recorded the number and type of prompts that each child required for the execution of an object-recognition task. A "general prompt" was a general instruction aimed at keeping the child in the proper location to perform the task (e.g., facing forward). A "task specific prompt" was a prompt required to keep the child focused on executing specific aspects of the task (e.g., picking one of the objects). Two object-recognition experiments were performed, one with three-dimensional objects and one with pictures of three-dimensional objects. For both types of experiments, the real-dog condition required the fewest prompts, followed by the stuffed-dog condition, and the human condition required the greatest number of prompts. The researchers concluded that the results of their experiments indicated that the presence of a well-trained dog reduces the need for instructional prompts in a traditional cognitive task. The researchers further stated:

> The common assumption that the presence of a dog can be distracting for children during the execution of cognitive tasks appears to be false.
>
> (Gee, Crist, and Carr, 2010, p. 173)

Research has shown that the presence of a dog had beneficial effects for developmentally disabled children by increasing positively initiated behaviors, decreasing negatively initiated behaviors, and improving social responsiveness (Walters Esteves and Stokes, 2008). The effects of the presence of an obedience-trained dog, a German Shepherd/Labrador Retriever mix, on social interactions among three children (ages 5–9 years) with developmental disabilities and their teacher at an elementary school were analyzed. Interactions were examined during morning sessions using reliable direct observation interval recording procedures. All of the children demonstrated an increase in overall positive behaviors, both verbal and nonverbal, toward the teacher and the dog. Additionally, the children showed an overall decrease in negative initiated behaviors. Further, observational ratings showed positive generalization of improved social responsiveness in the classroom by the children even after the treatment sessions (Walters Esteves and Stokes, 2008).

Interactions with dogs as part of a school-based violence prevention and intervention and character education program significantly altered beliefs about aggression and levels of empathy in elementary and middle school children (Sprinkle, 2008). Interactions with rescued shelter dogs were used to teach antiviolence and prosocial messages to the children. Data collected before and after the intervention program included student self-report, disciplinary data, and teacher observational data. The researchers concluded that receiving the program significantly altered students' normative beliefs about aggression, levels of empathy, and displays of violent and aggressive behaviors (Sprinkle, 2008).

Zasloff, Hart, and Melrod Weiss (2003) offered a humane education program at an inner-city school in Los Angeles targeting at-risk seventh-grade children in an attempt to teach empathy and gentleness with animals. The intervention was called the Teaching Love and Compassion (TLC) program. It was offered to groups of 10–12 students during their 3-week vacation from year-round school. The study assessed four successive sessions of TLC with an experimental group of 41 children. There was also a control group (no TLC program) of 42 children. In morning sessions, the experimental group had discussions focusing on interpersonal issues and conflict management. In the afternoons they were taught the proper care and obedience training of shelter dogs. Pre-test, post-test, and follow-up measures were taken to assess the children's knowledge of animal care, conflict management skills, attitudes toward self and others, and fear of dogs. According to the reported results, members of the experimental group increased their understanding of pet care and the needs of animals and retained this information more than did the control group for all four TLC sessions, both at post-testing and follow-up testing. At post-testing, the experimental group showed a trend toward decreased fear of dogs, and this result was significant at follow-up testing. The researchers suggested this program was effective at teaching humane attitudes and behaviors to children who are exposed to daily violence and aggression toward people and animals in the surrounding community (Zasloff, Hart, and Melrod Weiss, 2003).

Researchers have found that reading to dogs helped children improve their fluency (Paddock, 2010). Researchers from the University of California–Davis School of Veterinary Medicine studied participants in the already established AAT program called All Ears Reading Program. The third-grade children visited the veterinary school campus every week for 10 weeks and regularly read out loud for 15–20 minutes to one of three shelter-rescued dogs named Molly, Digory, and Lollipop. Lead researcher Martin Smith reported that reading fluency went up 12 percent in the school-based students and 30 percent in the home-schooled students. Also, reading speeds increased by up to 30 words per minute. Researchers feel these results are because the dogs helped the children to feel accepted and more relaxed while reading. One child told the researchers, "I feel relaxed when I am reading to a dog because I am having fun," and another child said, "The dogs don't care if you read really, really bad so you just keep going" (Paddock, 2010, p. 1). After the study, 75 percent of parents reported that their child was now reading aloud more frequently and with more confidence (Paddock, 2010).

Ryan (2010) performed a pilot study with four children who participated in equine-assisted education at a secondary school (school years 10 and 11) in Bedford, UK. One student had a little experience with horses, and the other three had no previous experience. The horses were brought to the school, and the intervention was performed in an appropriate area on the school grounds. The school was located in a neighborhood subject to socio-economic deprivation, and the proportion of students eligible for free school meals was well above average. Students at the school were ethnically diverse with English as a second language proportionately higher than at most other schools. Ryan provided parents, students, and school staff with a booklet she had prepared explaining the project, the potential benefits of working with horses, and the educational learning outcomes:

> Students will learn to care for and handle a horse. On completion of the course they will be able to demonstrate the following:
>
> - How to safely approach a horse.
> - Knowledge of the evolution of the horse.
> - How to groom a horse.
> - How to measure and weigh a horse.
> - An understanding of equine anatomy.
> - How to guide and control a horse in hand.

Ryan (2010) described the aims of the study:

> It was hoped that engagement with equine partners would reengage the students as active learners. Using these interventions to raise their self-esteem, it could reasonably be expected that any positive change would be observable back in the classroom.
>
> (p. 11)

The sessions were for 2 hours per week over 6 weeks. Trained to work with horses and as a counselor, Ryan designed, directed, and performed the intervention. She was assisted by two school staff members—one knowledgeable about horses and one who was skilled in working with young people. Two horses were used for the intervention: Shonty, a 15-hands high Piebald mare; and Tregoyd Alias (nicknamed Shiloh), a 16.3-hands high Cleveland bay gelding. Using the Psychosocial Session Form developed by Chandler (2005b), baseline and weekly assessments were made of each student, based on observations of the students in a typical classroom setting. One student dropped out of Ryan's study after 2 weeks because the family moved away. For the three remaining students, total scores on the Psychosocial Session Form increased for all three students across each week of the study, indicating positive alteration in social behaviors. The end of the equine-assisted course was marked with a presentation of certificates by the head teacher. One of the support staff was able to arrange an opportunity to visit Holme Park Stud facility, where the students were given a guided tour. They were able to learn about the breeding and training of the Trakehner horse and to see the stallions, mares, and foals (Ryan, 2010, pp. 14–15). At the conclusion of the study, the school planned to run the equine-assisted education intervention again and the students were already asking when that would be (Ryan, 2010).

These research results are strongly suggestive that animals in an educational environment can have beneficial effects for children. Support was provided for the premises that having therapy animals at school can greatly enhance children's motivation, tasks performance, and socialization.

ANECDOTAL SUPPORT FOR THE BENEFITS OF THERAPY ANIMALS AT SCHOOL

Following are some anecdotal reports supporting the benefits of having therapy animals at school.

Counseling with Pocket Pets

Pocket pets are small animals such as hamsters, gerbils, and guinea pigs. In Wisconsin, Barbara Flom (2005) works with hamsters in both her counseling and classroom curricula in an elementary school. When children returned to school after the summer break, they learned that the hamster, Harry, had died, and Flom used lessons on grief resolution that were especially helpful for two brothers still grieving over the loss of their pet. In getting to know the new hamster, Ginger, Flom facilitated the children she worked with in learning about responsibility by encouraging them to assist with Ginger's daily feeding and care. With Flom's facilitation, Ginger assisted children in learning about how to calm their selves to calm the hamster adjusting to a new environment; this resulted in improved social skills and reduced aggression in the children. Ginger is helpful to the children in gaining self-insight about their own feelings and learning and practicing new, more productive behaviors, especially self-calming and impulse control. Flom reports:

> Ginger and his predecessors have given my students and me hours of pleasure and countless life lessons. An effective adjunct, the animals have supplemented the bibliotherapy, behavior management plans, expressive art techniques, and group counseling strategies I continue to use.
>
> (Flom, 2005, p. 471)

According to Flom, the pocket pets she works with "add richness, depth, and an element of the unexpected to the counselor's toolbox" (Flom, 2005, p. 471).

A Llama at School

Mona Sams is an occupational therapist who works with a variety of animals in seven different schools in Roanoke, Virginia, providing therapy services to a case load of 35 children consisting primarily of 5- to 16-year-olds with autism and multiple handicaps (Marmer, 1997). The therapy animals assist Sams with virtually all therapeutic goals—from cognition and communication to perceptual skills and motor planning. The animals also benefit in the ways the students are involved in the caring for the animals, such as grooming, feeding, walking, and petting, which further teaches the students about responsibility and nurturing and the good feelings that come with those accomplishments. Sams works with many types of therapy animals who assist her in providing the children's services; including rabbits, sheep, goats, dogs, ducks, and even llamas. All animals are kept on leads while they are in the school, and no animal is ever left unattended. In addition to making sure the children are safe, Sams makes sure that the animals are also always safe. Strict hand-washing policies are designed to eliminate the chance of germ contamination between children and the animals. Also, children are properly screened for allergies and parental permission is obtained before the children are allowed to interact with the animals (Marmer, 1997).

A Dog at School

Lucy, a black standard Poodle, has for many years been going to work with her owner, Robert Vitalo, headmaster of the Berkeley Carroll School in Brooklyn, New York (McDonough, 2009). Lucy either sits with Vitalo in his office or accompanies him as he moves about the building. Of Lucy, Vitalo says, "Her presence helps humanize me with the students. She makes me seem more approachable and less intimidating" (McDonough, 2009, p. 1). Lucy visits the upper and middle schools (grades 5–12) and holds "near movie-star status" in the eyes of the students. Some of the remarks by students about Lucy are, "I love Lucy. She's sweet and playful and whenever I see her it makes me happy," and, "She makes the school feel more like a family" (McDonough, 2009, p. 1).

Dogs at the Library

At a branch of the New York Library, a Border Collie–Greyhound mix named Theo helps children to practice their reading (Brundige, 2009). The New York Library started a reading assistance dog program in 2004. About a dozen dog–handler teams visit library branches once a month giving children a chance to choose a book and read to the dog and the handler. The children are motivated to participate in the reading practice program for a chance to spend time with the dog and the additional practice the children receive improves their reading skills. The dogs help the children feel less anxious and more relaxed while they are practicing their reading (Brundige, 2009).

Dogs in the Classroom

Lucy and Dottie are top dogs in the classroom—literally (Tarrant, 2000). Lucy is a 9-year-old black and white Australian Shepherd and mother of Dottie, a 3-year-old red and white Australian Shepherd. Both dogs are extremely well behaved and do exactly what the teacher wants them to do: "No bones about it—Lucy and Dottie are the teacher's pets" (Tarrant, 2000, p. 1C). They belong to Tracy Roberts, who brings her pets with her to work as her teacher's aides at the Canterbury Episcopal School in DeSoto, Texas, where she teaches fourth and fifth grades. The dogs are the most popular members of the class, getting hugs throughout the day, and they especially like being scratched behind the ears.

> Lucy and Dottie have no specific role in class, and yet all the kids consider the dogs vital for their calming and soothing influence. "Sometimes, the dogs will figure out who's upset and go sit by that child," Ms. Roberts says [. . .]
> Dunman Foster has experienced the dogs' healing powers. An energetic child with eager blue eyes who loves to answer questions in class, Dunman doesn't seem as if he would ever find himself in low spirits. But three years ago, the fourth-grader's best friend died during heart surgery. Sometimes the memory of his friend will overwhelm Dunman, "and I'll be sad and can't focus, and it makes me upset," he says. At such times, one of the dogs will come and sit by him. "And you just hug them. They're like a big pillow," Dunman says. The dogs have helped calm many of the kids' fears of school and meeting new people. They have given students a sense of connection as well as affection. They've even won over children who were afraid of dogs.
>
> (Tarrant, 2000, p. 3C)

As teacher's aides, the dogs are able to reach children in ways that adults cannot, and without judgment. As Joe Parnes, aged 9 and a new student, put in a letter to Dottie and Lucy: "You made me feel welcomed and not so worried when I didn't know what to do" (Tarrant, 2000, p. 3C).

History Is More Fun with Animals

One day my therapy dog Rusty and I were visiting with some adolescents during their recreational break at a juvenile detention center in Denton, Texas. The children were discussing how boring their history class was and how much they dreaded the history paper they had to write. I asked them what they were studying, and they explained it was the Lewis and Clark expedition. I am a lover of history, and I wanted to find a way for the students to find history lessons more interesting. So, with their teacher's permission, the following week when I met with the students I shared with them some stories about the dog Seaman, a big-hearted Newfoundland that accompanied the Lewis and Clark expedition and was mentioned favorably and often by the biographer of the expedition (Pringle and Henderson, 2004). As I had hoped, the information about Seaman brightened the attitude of the students, and they became excited about what they were studying when they imagined what it must have been like for the dog during the expedition. With their teacher's permission, I encouraged the students to look up the role animals played in significant historical events and include them in an upcoming educational lesson. Both the teacher and the students said it was one of the most fun and interesting history lessons they had experienced due to the incorporation of the study of significant roles that animals served throughout history.

AGE-OLD WISDOM REGARDING THE EDUCATIONAL VALUE OF CHILD-ANIMAL INTERACTION

Philosophers and poets have long recognized the educational value of child–animal interaction in promoting development of valuable social abilities such as empathy, kindness, and responsibility. The educational value of children interacting with animals was recognized by English philosopher John Locke, of the seventeenth century, who recommended giving children "dogs, squirrels, birds or any such things" to look after as a means of encouraging the development of tender feelings and a sense of responsibility. John Locke's thoughts concerning the education of character included the following:

> I cannot but commend both the kindness and prudence of a mother I knew, who was wont always to indulge her daughters when any of them desired dogs, squirrels, birds or any such things as young girls use to be delighted with; but then, when they had them, they must be sure to keep them well and look diligently after them, that they wanted nothing or were not ill used. For if they were negligent in their care for them, it was counted a great fault which often forfeited their possession, or at least they failed not to be rebuked for it; whereby they were early taught diligence and good nature. And indeed, I think people should be accustomed from their cradles to be tender to all sensible creatures.
>
> (Locke, 1699, p. 154)

Age-old wisdom regarding child–animal interactions at school is provided in a familiar children's poem. According to the Center for Children's Literature and Culture at the University of Florida (Smith, 2003), the well-known rhyme "Mary's Lamb," better known today as "Mary Had a Little Lamb," is attributed to author Sarah Josepha Hale and was published in the September–October 1830 issue of *Juvenile Miscellany*. The message of the poem speaks well of the potential benefits and lessons from having animals at school:

> Mary had a little lamb
> Its fleece was white as snow,
> And everywhere that Mary went
> The lamb was sure to go.
>
> It followed her to school one day,
> That was against the rule;
> It made the children laugh and play
> To see a lamb at school.

And so the Teacher turned him out,
But still he lingered near,
And waited patiently about
Till Mary did appear:

And then he ran to her, and laid
His head upon her arm,
As if he said, "I'm not afraid,
You'll save me from all harm."

"What makes the lamb love Mary so?"
The little children cry—
"O Mary loves the lamb, you know,"
The teacher did reply:

"And you each gentle animal
In confidence may bind,
And make them follow at your call,
If you are always kind."

Simple yet profound wisdom, such as that of John Locke and Sarah Josepha Hale about care, compassion, and companionship, reflects the social and educational value that animals provide in their interactions with children. As social companions in an educational environment, animals can support a vast array of educational goals.

GENERAL ASSUMPTIONS UNDERLYING AAT IN SCHOOLS

According to Walters Esteves and Stokes (2008), AAT encourages positive social interaction among students and between students and their teacher. Therapy dogs can:

> be used as an assistant in the classroom in teaching a specific task such as daily living skills, or as part of a curriculum such as reading, writing, story time, circle time, etc. A dog can act as the subject for creative writing, for reading stories about dogs, or can participate with children in group activities, with the dog being counted as a member of the group. This may increase participation for the children in some activities. It may not be beneficial to have the dog present throughout the school day, however, as this would be exhausting for the dog and disruptive for the children. It should also be noted that some cultural customs and some children's experiences may preclude them from being participants who may benefit from these procedures.
>
> (Walters Esteves and Stokes, 2008, p. 14)

Regarding the welfare of the animal and the learning environment, it would be advisable to have periods during the day where AAT was not a part of activities—during which the therapy animal would not play an active role and would be provided with a quiet place to rest and relax without interruption. This too would be educational since children would have an opportunity to learn lessons on respecting personal space and would gain appreciation for honoring personal boundaries during these times when the therapy animal was quietly resting without being disturbed.

Friesen (2010) reviewed literature on school-based AAT programs and made the following conclusions. With social engagement and verbal communication being desirable in both classroom and therapeutic settings, interaction with therapy dogs may support and encourage social risk taking in these environments, particularly for children who are otherwise unwilling or reluctant to engage socially. Also, the therapy dog's interactive nature may have a profound calming effect on children perceived to be under stress. Children seem to perceive therapy dogs as a neutral or nonjudgmental participant in the therapeutic or classroom environment, and thus the therapy dogs serve in a supporting role for social, emotional, and academic achievements by the children. Since the applications of AAT in a school environment go much further than assisting with maladjustment issues, perhaps a more appropriate term for school applications of AAT would be "animal-assisted learning" (Friesen, 2010).

Many schoolteachers and school counselors across the United States work successfully with their pets at their schools. Following, I describe some recommended procedures for establishing such a program. The recommendations can apply whether it is just one professional who wishes to work with a pet or an entire group of professionals or volunteers with their pets.

GUIDELINES FOR SCHOOL-BASED AAT PROGRAM DEVELOPMENT

The first step is to develop a proposal that clearly outlines the program you wish to establish. The proposal should include the following:

- A program mission statement and educational or therapeutic objectives.
- Expected benefits of the program.
- Any potential risks of the program and how they will be prevented and managed.
- The adults and animals that will participate in the AAT program.
- The students who will participate in the AAT program.
- Types of activities expected to take place in the program.
- The training, evaluation, and credentials of the persons and animals providing the AAT.
- The exact location of the AAIs.
- All relevant persons who will be consulted about the development of the AAT program (e.g., school nurse, custodial services, facilities management, grounds maintenance, other teachers, other counselors, other administrators, and parents).
- An intent to develop a set of policies and procedures for the AAT program with consultation with relevant school personnel.

It is imperative that there be a consultation with all relevant personnel that may be impacted by the program. The persons left out of the information loop will inevitably be those who complain about the program or try to sabotage the program. This is usually because they do not understand the program's implications and fear it will interfere with their work or add to their workload. Also, consulting with them may make them feel more a part of the program, thereby adding to its chances for success.

Policies and procedures for the developing AAT program should be as comprehensive as necessary. Recommendations for items to include are as follows:

- Procedures for obtaining informed consent to participate from parents and informed assent from students.
- Procedures for keeping the environment clean: cleaning up and disposing of animal excrement; cleaning up animal fur from the floor, furniture, and participants; and making available safe, nontoxic cleaning materials in case of an accident (e.g., the animal poops or vomits indoors).
- Procedures for injury prevention for human and animal participants.
- Procedures for handling and reporting injuries to humans and animals.
- Procedures for infection prevention for humans and animals.
- Dress code for human participants and grooming code for animal participants.
- An appropriate behavior code for human and animal participants.

If you write a proposal to begin an AAT program at school, present the proposal at a meeting with the school principal or headmaster, or other appropriate administrator. Briefly explain in person the basics of the program you wish to offer, answer any questions, and share the written proposal for the administrator to read. Handlers should initially invite school administrators and other appropriate staff to meet animals that would be participating in the proposed program. It is important that all AAT teams have proper training and evaluation prior to offering AAT services in a school; that is, complete handler training and handler–animal team evaluation from an organization such as the Pet Partners program.

TYPES OF AAT SCHOOL-BASED PROGRAMS

A common simple application of AAT in the school is the school counselor who brings a pet to work. Children can appreciate the novelty of the pet's presence and can use it as an excuse to drop by and visit with the counselor without feeling awkward. A child who needs some nurturing touch or affection can safely get that by hugging or petting a therapy animal. Children who feel dejected can feel affirmed by the way the therapy animal responds positively to them. Children who may have difficulty expressing their needs or hurts may find it easy to talk to the therapy animal or may find it therapeutic to just spend time quietly petting the therapy animal. An abundance of school counselors work with their pets in the Fort Worth–Dallas–Denton metro area. They have communicated to me that their therapy pets become popular, unofficial mascots for the school children, teachers, and staff. The presence of the therapy animal lifts the spirit of the school. Many teachers and administrators also drop by for a moment's visit with a therapy animal at the school to lift their mood.

Another popular school-based program is AAT for classroom and instructional enhancement. Math and reading teachers have shared with me that having a dog in the classroom seems to have a calming effect on the students. The students seem to have fewer behavior problems and pay greater attention to the lesson when the teacher's therapy dog is in attendance. In addition, students who are otherwise anxious to read out loud seem more motivated to participate and less anxious when they can pet the therapy dog while engaged in the exercise. Having animals in the classroom to facilitate the educational process for students is a growing interest across the United States.

Therapy pets can aid in vocational training for students. Participants can learn skills in, for example, grooming, obedience training, agility training, and tracking. Community professionals can volunteer to teach these skills to the students with their pets. Getting students involved with existing dog training and performance groups in the community can provide a healthy outlet for recreation. In addition, students can become trained to provide community service with their pet by completing training like the Pet Partners program. Then, under adult supervision, student Pet Partners teams can visit nursing homes, hospitals, and younger students at the school. Providing community service can teach a student the benefits of community caring and involvement. It can enhance the student's relationship skills and contribute to teaching and reinforcing moral and humane values. Volunteer work at the local animal shelter or animal rescue facility can contribute to the education and development of the student and could save the life of many animals. Some dogs are difficult to place because they lack obedience training or are hard to handle. As long as the dogs have been evaluated to be nonaggressive, student training groups can work with these unruly dogs and teach them in a matter of weeks to be obedient and socially responsive, and thus they will be more attractive for adoption.

A school can also partner with an existing AAT program. For instance, students can attend a nearby equine facility to learn horsemanship and enhance social skills through human–horse interactions. Another fun school program idea that involves animals is a nature or wilderness study program. Supervised field trips to bird sanctuaries, wild game preserves, and wildlife and wilderness areas can help students to get in touch with nature and engage in science lessons. Students can participate in the annual Audubon Society bird count. This is a fun one-day activity held once per year that contributes to an important database for tracking birds and determining whether they are endangered. Our environment is facing ever increasing pollution and global warming, and sensitizing students at an early age about nature preservation is of vital importance for current and future generations.

Useful resources for learning about school-based AAT programs are *Canines in the Classroom* (Rivera, 2004) and *Pet Assisted Therapy* (Salotto, 2001). Another very useful resource for understanding how to use AAT in a classroom setting is a large collection of reprinted articles and other materials found in *Animals in the Classroom* (Delta Society, 2005).

HOW TO REPORT ON THE PROGRESS OF YOUR AAT PROGRAM

Once you have your program up and running, it is useful to complete periodic progress reports. These reports should be done at least once per year. Basic components typically included in a program progress report are as follows:

- Name and title of your program.
- Your contact information.
- An introduction and brief description of the program.
- Program goals that have been established.
- Goals that have been completed.
- Outcome measures and results and any adjustments to program services or goals based on these outcome measures.
- Goals in progress and their current status.
- Any future goals.

For reportable outcome measures, it is very useful to conduct statistical analysis on the collected data. If you are not interested in doing this yourself, you can probably hire someone to do it for you, such as a professor or a graduate student from a local college or university.

Once you have collected sufficient data and analyzed it, you might want to publish your results. There are many professional journals available for this. A visit with a college or university librarian can point you in the right direction. Guidelines for submission are usually printed in the back or front of the journal, but not necessarily in each volume, so you may have to look through several copies before you find them. Also, guidelines for submission are usually posted on the journal's website. Many journals now provide articles online so you may conveniently peruse the contents on your computer to examine the format and content that is common to the journal. In most cases, you will receive no money for publishing work in a professional journal. However, it is nice to be a published author, and you perform a great service by sharing the success of your program with the rest of the world.

I highly encourage you to present your program description at a regional, state, or national conference in your field. Your own professional organization probably has an annual meeting, and you can submit a presentation proposal for the meeting or conference program board to review. Most organizations that sponsor conferences these days have a website with downloadable conference program proposals, so you can do the whole submission online. Usually, program presentation proposals must be received months in advance of the actual conference date. Typically, one does not receive any money for presenting at these conferences, but it is a great opportunity to share information and network with those with similar interests.

14

International Considerations and Applications of Animal-Assisted Therapy

The human–animal social connection construct embraces the ideology of mutual companionship, assistance, and affection between humans and domesticated animals; and as the ruling species humans have an obligation to demonstrate infinite compassion and appropriate protection for all animals. The human–animal social connection is different from the construct of human dependence on animals. Human dependence encompasses the use of animals for protection, labor, food, and shelter; and exploitation for experimentation and entertainment. The human–animal social connection is interaction that benefits both humans and animals with an emphasis on safety and welfare for both.

The United States has a long history of human dependence on animals. For many centuries, the Native Americans shared their camps with dogs that provided early warning for danger in exchange for food scraps. Native Americans and immigrants to the United States used horses for transportation that were brought over from other continents and left by early European explorers. Native Americans and immigrant settlers relied on native buffalo, antelope, and other animals of the wilderness as sources for food and clothing. The use of animals for food and shelter in pretechnological eras is viewed as justifiable; however, today with many more options available to people for meeting basic survival needs, the essentiality of human dependence on animals becomes more difficult to defend.

COMPANION ANIMAL WELFARE: INTERNATIONAL CONCERNS

The evolved concept of human–animal social connection in the United States was inherited from the European immigrants of the seventeenth and eighteenth centuries. By the time the United States declared its independence from England in 1776, the concept of the family household pet with access to home and hearth was firmly established in Western society (Adams, 1999; Blaisdell, 1999; Fogle, 1999). Today, the cultural attitude toward animals in the United States is by no means a paragon. There remain incidents of animal cruelty or neglect that are still too prevalent; far too many stray pets are euthanized for failure to find them good homes, and many animals are victims of the controversial practice of experimentation. Historically, the United States made significant progress in the twentieth century in complying with an ethical duty as a compassionate protector of animals. States enacted and enforced laws against animal cruelty, including the outlawing of dog fighting and rooster fighting (Animal Legal and Historical Center, n.d.). Laws were passed to protect the sanctity of the household pet, primarily the dog and the cat. Thanks to the work of advocates like

Temple Grandin (Grandin, 1993; Grandin and Smith, 2004), various regulations incorporated more humane ways of raising and killing farm animals prior to meat processing. Today, numerous volunteer groups rescue stray animals and find them loving homes. Although experimentation on animals for research purposes continues, there is an increase in efforts to raise general public consciousness about this concern. Although not completely satisfied with ourselves, most U.S. citizens are fairly comfortable with the state of the cultural position on animals in the United States, and view existing laws and ethical standards as mostly sufficient for handling failures to meet humane obligations. However, many would agree that there is still much room for improvement.

An area of human action toward animals that currently has international heightened sensitivity is unnecessary cosmetic surgery for dogs, such as ear and tail docking, prescribed for certain breeds by breed clubs and organizations. These types of procedures are painful for the animal and the intensity or duration of the pain is difficult to quantify (American Veterinary Medical Association (AVMA), n.d.). Veterinary associations in several countries have spoken out against the practice, including the American Veterinary Medical Association. The primary reason for tail and ear docking is the maintenance of a distinctive appearance for a particular breed and to take part in an ongoing tradition. There is no substantive reason for ear and tail docking other than to please the human eye. The only argument with any merit is that tail docking prevents later tail injury for working dogs, but this reason does not seem to justify the act: "Tail injuries generally have a low rate of occurrence and many working breeds tails go undocked" (AVMA, n.d.). As of now, ear and tail docking is legal in the United States and is promoted by individual breed clubs as well as the prestigious American Kennel Club. However, cosmetic surgery for dogs for any reason other than for veterinary purposes, such as to benefit a dog's health, is considered by many to be cruel for the animal, so the act has been banned in many countries. The essential question that should be posed regarding procedures such as ear and tail docking is whether there is sufficient justification for performing the procedure:

> Performing a procedure for cosmetic purposes (i.e., for the sake of appearance) implies the procedure is not medically indicated. Because dogs have not been shown to derive self-esteem or pride in appearance from having their tails docked (common reasons for performing cosmetic procedures on people), there is no obvious benefit to our patients in performing this procedure. The only benefit that appears to be derived from cosmetic tail docking of dogs is the owner's impression of a pleasing appearance. In the opinion of the AVMA, this is insufficient justification for performing a surgical procedure.
>
> (AVMA, n.d.)

The World Small Animal Veterinary Association unanimously endorsed the following position in August 2001 regarding dog tail docking (Broughton, 2003):

- The WSAVA considers amputation of dogs' tails to be an unnecessary surgical procedure and contrary to the welfare of the dog.
- The WSAVA recommends that all canine organizations phase out any recommendations for tail amputation (docking) from their breed standards.
- The WSAVA recommends that the docking of dogs' tails be made illegal except for professionally diagnosed therapeutic reasons, and only then by suitably qualified persons, such as registered veterinarians, under conditions of anesthesia that minimize pain and stress.

Countries that have banned tail docking and other unnecessary cosmetic surgery include Norway, Sweden, Switzerland, Finland, Germany, Denmark, Great Britain (and the devolved assembly of Wales) and parts of Australia. Several European countries have ratified a European Convention that prohibits unnecessary cosmetic surgery including Cyprus, Greece, Luxembourg, Switzerland, and Austria (Royal Society for the Prevention of Cruelty to Animals (RSPCA), 2005–2006).

A related area of concern regarding humane responsibility toward companion animals that currently has heightened international sensitivity is purposely breeding animals with deformities and disabilities to conform to breed standards, even though the physical characteristic can cause the dog to suffer and be uncomfortable and can even be dangerous for the animal. An example of this is breeding for a flat nose, in breeds such as Pug dogs, that impairs breathing and causes respiratory disorders for the dog. Many believe that breeding dogs for cosmetic reasons instead of health and welfare reasons is an act of cruelty that should be prohibited (RSPCA, 2005–2006).

Working with companion animals as partners in AAT requires that we advocate for the safety and welfare of companion animals in the same way we advocate for humans. As practitioners of AAT, social advocacy for humans and companion animals is a professional responsibility, and acting on this responsibility will not only improve the quality of life for persons and companion animals but will also preserve and enhance the acceptance and practice of AAT.

SOUTH KOREA: SAMSUNG AAA AND AAT PROGRAMS

Animals have a long history as beasts of burden and a food source in South Korea. With little concern for animal cruelty, the generally accepted idea of companion animal, or family pet, is yet to evolve there (Shin, 2003). Conversations with various South Korean officials revealed an abundance of concerns regarding the current cultural position on the human–animal connection (Y. Kim, D. H. Lee, J. Lee, and S. Lee, personal communications, November 2–12, 2003).

Only a small handful of pet dogs can be seen walking with their owners, and the uniqueness of this draws a good deal of attention from passersby. Pet dogs are typically purchased from privately owned pet stores that line up in groups of about four or five, side-by-side along a busy city street—it looks like puppy row. Small pet dogs are the most popular in South Korea, especially the American Cocker Spaniel, Cavalier Spaniel, Yorkshire Terrier, Boston Terrier, Pomeranian, and miniature Poodle. South Korean pet owners have a high incidence of quickly giving pet dogs to shelters after discovering that dog ownership requires more than they expected. Due to an ever increasing population and absence of space, most people in major cities in South Korea live in a conglomeration of apartment skyscrapers (referred to by locals as "apartment forests"), and this makes exercising pets inconvenient. Animal shelters in South Korea are typically not very sanitary and are overcrowded, and many are privately owned. Most pet owners do not train or socialize their dogs very well, or at all, which further adds to the lack of attraction for them as pets. Most of those who do have trained dogs have sent the dog away to training school and thus have little understanding of continuing training or reinforcing what the pet has learned. Typical South Korean pet owners do not pick up after their dogs relieve themselves, and city officials are hesitant to pass laws compelling them to do so. As a result, city officials ban dogs from many parks where they could meet people and other dogs and exercise. Some large dogs have historically been used as guard dogs, and most South Koreans are afraid of large dogs as a result. Other types of large dogs are still raised as a food source, and the killing of such animals is done in cruel ways. Cats are not a popular choice as pets, and the very few cats visible in South Korea run wild in the streets. The most common horse in South Korea is the native, small JeJu pony, which was frequently observed to have good physical health but whose role was mostly relegated to giving pony rides around a very small arena or being mounted for brief photograph opportunities for tourists.

The enactment of laws to protect animals from cruelty in South Korea is new to the current generation and is met with reluctance from older generations. Common companion dog activities in the United States, such as obedience training and trials, agility and fly ball trials, and work by service and therapy animals for the emotionally and physically challenged, are extremely new to South Korea and very rare. In fact, community acceptance and employment of disabled persons is a relatively new concept in South Korea. Public service announcements on television are frequent right now in South Korea and encourage the acceptance and employment of disabled persons. Numerous animal activity and animal education television programs discuss proper care for pets. It is interesting how increased attention to and advocacy for these two diverse groups—disabled persons and animals—seem to parallel one another in this country at this time.

Various South Korean organizations promote animal protection and humane education. Such organizations have campaigned worldwide to educate the international community about the difficult conditions for dogs and cats in South Korea. A major victory came in 2007 with the revision and strengthening of South Korea's 1991 Animal Protection law, which animal welfare organizations in South Korea had long campaigned and petitioned to improve (International Aid for Korean Animals, n.d.). The Korean Animal Protection and Education Society (KAPES) was founded in 2007 as a response to the newly strengthened Animal Protection law to educate the public and create greater empathy for animals, and to counter the impact of potential protests about animal welfare and protection by those who trade in dog and cat meat. KAPES strives to teach South Koreans about the humane treatment of animals and to instill in them a deep compassion for dogs and cats.

> With the new Animal Protection law in place, KAPES seeks to work in partnership with the government to successfully affect positive change in Korean society. It seems that the time is finally right to eliminate the plight of Korea's dogs and cats.
> (International Aid for Korean Animals, n.d.)

In 2003 I had the opportunity to present at the First International Symposium on the Human–Animal Bond held in South Korea, where I exchanged information with a number of officials interested in animal welfare and AAT. I was invited to South Korea by Samsung Corporation to present at the symposium and additionally to train their AAT program staff in AAT techniques across several days. Samsung Corporation has been actively engaged in numerous activities in South Korea to promote the welfare of animals (Choi, 2003). A description of Samsung's intent is as follows:

> Since the late 1980s Samsung has been working towards creating a society of harmony and love where all life forms are respected. Samsung continues to work domestically as well as internationally to promote positive awareness of human animal relationships and to change the negative perceptions of Korea. Because Samsung believes that a society which protects and cares for its animals in effect enhances the quality of life for its people.
>
> (Samsung, 2003)

What is significant about the Samsung Corporation animal programs is that there is virtually nothing else like them in the rest of South Korea at this time. Residents in this country are solely reliant on Samsung for many animal-related services. Samsung's interest in animal activity and welfare began in 1988 when Samsung built a modern, state-of-the-art equestrian facility in South Korea and imported top-breed horses to participate in equine sports. Samsung equestrian teams have been winning numerous honors and are rapidly gaining a well-respected international reputation. Samsung also built a state-of-the-art dog kennel, dog training, and animal care facility, and an animal hospital nestled among the heavily wooded slopes at Samsung Everland (an animal preserve and entertainment park). Samsung Corporation began a Responsible Pet Ownership Program in 1992. Dogs raised in the kennel or rescued from shelters are provided to Samsung employees, and the welfare of the pet is tracked so that if proper care is not provided the animal is withdrawn from the owner for better placement. The Samsung Guide Dogs for the Blind Program began in 1993. These dogs, mostly Labrador Retrievers, are imported by Samsung from other countries, trained by Samsung professional staff, and donated to visually impaired persons of South Korea. The Samsung Search and Rescue Dogs Program began in 1995. German Shepherds are trained at spacious indoor and outdoor facilities to track and find lost persons and buried victims. These dog teams have received international honors for their response to tragedies, such as a devastating earthquake in Taiwan. The Samsung AAA and AAT programs using a variety of dogs began in 1995. These AAT and AAA programs involve mostly social visits with therapy dogs at nursing homes, schools, and juvenile detention centers. The Samsung Riding for the Disabled Program was begun at the Samsung equestrian facility in 2001. The Samsung Hearing Dogs for the Deaf Program began in 2002. Samsung hearing-assistance dogs are typically small-breed dogs that will be easily integrated into the typical South Korean small-sized residence of the recipient of the donated dog. Samsung recently completed in 2003 at Samsung Everland a state-of-the-art training facility for the hearing dog program that includes apartments for the recipients of the dogs to stay in during the last training and owner transition days of the hearing dog. Typically known more for their electronic products, Samsung Corporation has significantly contributed to efforts to bring South Korea into the modern age regarding the culture of the human–animal social connection.

While in South Korea I was invited to speak at Cheju National University in JeJu on AAT applications in the United States. With a translator's assistance, I spoke to a class of about 100 veterinary medical students and a handful of professors. I also gave a demonstration of a typical Pet Partners standardized handler–animal team evaluation in front of this very large crowd. Afterward, a private lunch was hosted by the dean of the College of Natural Sciences of Cheju National University, Dr. Young-Oh Yang. In the afternoon, I evaluated a second handler–animal team who shared the same dog as the first team that morning. From the morning and afternoon evaluations were born the first two Delta Society Pet Partners teams in South Korea; first was Dr. Yang Soon (Angela) Kim with a Cavalier Spaniel named Lulu and then Ju-yeon (Queenie) Lee with the same dog. Ju-yeon (Queenie) Lee flew down to JeJu that day for the animal evaluation because, although Ms. Lee works at Samsung Everland near Seoul, she also had the opportunity to work with Lulu on occasion. After the evaluations, I was invited to observe an animal-assisted play therapy session by Dr. Kim with an autistic child. Dr. Kim was the first mental health professional in South Korea to practice animal-assisted play therapy. She established a training program in this area of study at Cheju National University in JeJu.

HONG KONG: ANIMALS ASIA'S DR. DOG AND PROFESSOR PAWS PROGRAMS

I was invited to present a paper titled, "Working in Harmony with Animals: Animal-assisted Therapy, Theory and Applications," at the International Conference on Social Work and Counseling Practice held at City University in Hong Kong in June 2009. While in Hong

Kong I networked for 3 days with the staff of Animals Asia, a not-for-profit animal welfare organization that advocates for the humane treatment of animals in China and Hong Kong, and most especially lobbies for an end to the farming of moon bear for their bile and torturing, killing, and eating dogs and cats. Animals Asia is also the parent organization for the Dr. Dog and Professor Paws programs (Animals Asia, n.d.). Dr. Dog and Professor Paws are teams of volunteer animal owners in Hong Kong who, with their dogs, visit patients in hospitals to lift spirits, and provide educational programs to schoolchildren on the proper care and treatment of dogs. Most children in Hong Kong do not have a pet of their own because most families live in an apartment and most apartments do not allow pets. Thus, the work of the Professor Paws program is vitally important. It hopes that by exposing schoolchildren to the love and nurturance of dogs it is moving the cultural attitude toward animals in a more humane direction. I was privileged to accompany the Dr. Dog and Professor Paws AAT and AAA teams on two separate days and observed the educational and emotional benefits of these programs.

In 2015, I returned to Hong Kong to serve as a featured speaker at a conference focused on AAT sponsored by the social work and social administration department of Hong Kong University and coordinated by Professor Paul Wong. At the conference there were many presentations, and I was pleased to see how AAT was now being integrated into the professional social work of a few private agencies providing services for special populations (especially because there were no existing government agencies in Hong Kong that were providing animal-assisted service). One successful program that was described at the conference was performed by the Chinese Evangelical Zion Church, Social Service Division. They used interaction with dogs and pet grooming instruction to assist more than 200 people with social inhibitions beginning in 2010. The program was designed to assist reclusive persons to become more social and to develop confidence and relationship skills that would help them get into the workforce. A study of 68 participants of this program by Hong Kong University showed that the employment rate of participants in this animal-assisted group rose from 7 percent to 55 percent. The therapy lasted about a year before participants were confident enough to enter the workforce. Of participants in the program, 80 percent either went back to work or back to school. According to psychiatrist Dr. William Fan, interactions with the dogs made participants more willing to talk to counselors so they could get the assistance they needed.

The animal-assisted service providers in Hong Kong have several obstacles to overcome. Availability of therapy pets is limited. Having a pet in Hong Kong is not as commonplace as having a pet in the United States because in Hong Kong there is little space for a pet and many people live in small apartments. Transporting a pet to a therapy site is also problematic because pets are not allowed on public transportation. The most common form of transportation for people in Hong Kong is by metro-subway or taxi service, neither of which allows pets.

INDIA: ANIMAL ANGELS FOUNDATION AAA AND AAT PROGRAMS

Several years ago I was pleased to assist Minal Lonkar Kavishwar by providing her and some of her colleagues training in AAT through my distance learning program I offered through the Consortium for Animal Assisted Therapy at the University of North Texas. Minal Kavishwar and therapy dog Kutty were India's first registered team with the Pet Partners organization (the organization's former name was Delta Society's Pet Partners). Minal and Kutty were winners of the prestigious Pet Partners "Beyond Limits Award" in 2007 for the professional practice of AAT. Minal Kavishwar is the founder of the Animal Angels Foundation in India. Animal Angels Foundation is India's first organization consisting of mental health

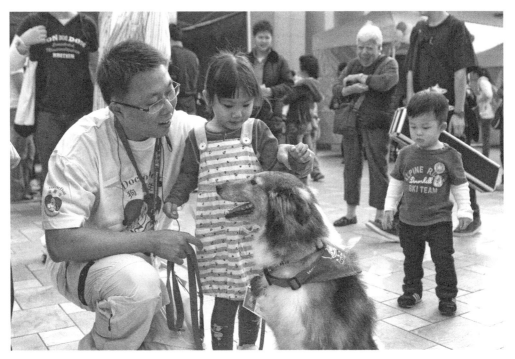

Figure 14.1 The Dr. Dog program in Hong Kong.

(*Source:* photo courtesy of Animals Asia, Hong Kong.)

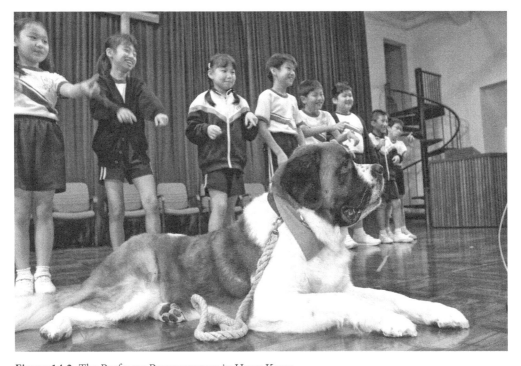

Figure 14.2 The Professor Paws program in Hong Kong.

(*Source:* photo courtesy of Animals Asia, Hong Kong.)

professionals trained in AAT. The goal of this AAT program is to enhance the quality of human life through interaction with animals. Animal Angels Foundation is currently working with special needs children in schools and institutes. It also works in psychiatric settings in hospitals and institutes for children. Additionally, the Animal Angels Foundation is active in crisis and disaster response in India. On December 21, 2009, the Animal Angels Team conducted an awareness campaign of AAA for post-trauma stress after the November 26 Mumbai terror attacks. Therapy dogs Goldie (a Golden Retriever) and Onit (a St. Bernard) comforted people present at the program and demonstrated how animals can help to heal the emotional trauma after a disaster (Animal Angels Foundation, n.d.). Some of the other accomplishments of the Animal Angels Foundation include the following (Minal Kavishwar, personal communication, October 3, 2010):

- Research on benefits of AAT for mentally challenged children at Anand Dighe Jidda School.
- Research on the effects of AAT on the emotional expression in children with autism at the Prasanna Autism Center in Pune.
- Setting up aquariums to give emotional support to cancer patients at Cipla Cancer Centre.
- AAT for orphan children with HIV at the Manavya AIDS orphanage.
- AAT and AAA at multiple schools and education centers including: Jidd School, Thane, Mumbai with a Labrador Retriever named Kutty; ICMH's Skills and Ability School, Nerul, Navi Mumbai; Prasanna Autism Centre with a Labrador Retriever named Sophie; Pune Sevasadan Society's Dilaasa Kenra (for mentally challenged children) with a therapy cat; Shri Ma Snehadeep, Hiranandani (for special needs children), Thane, with a therapy dog named Goldie; and Sapling School, Mumbai for slow learners with a Labrador Retriever therapy dog named Coco.
- AAT for disabled children at Bal Kalyan Sanstha.
- AAA for children with hearing and speech impairment at Mookdhwani Vidyalay, Vile, Parle, Mumbai.
- AAT for children with special needs at Dinaz Wadia's Disha.
- AAT for women cancer patients with therapy dog Kiara in association with the Cancer Patients Aid Association.

In 2015 I was fortunate to travel to India and spend considerable time with Minal Kavishwar and the Animal Angels Foundation teams in both Pune and Mumbai. It was wonderful to see the great work they are doing in India. Minal explained the difficulties they still face in getting acceptance for their program at many places due to the general cultural attitude toward dogs. There is a negative and dismissive attitude toward dogs in India. There are thousands of individual dogs and hundreds of packs of dogs that have no owners that freely roam the streets of a city in India such as Mumbai. They live on the streets, interact with people, and survive from handouts. The dogs are not dangerous, but they are dirty, untrained, and unruly and thus many people think of dogs as an annoyance and as having little value. This stigma of dogs having little value and being dirty and unruly is the first thing that must be overcome in establishing an AAT program at a school, hospital, or agency in India. Furthermore, pets are not allowed on public transportation (such as trains, taxis, or rickshaws); thus, one must be able to afford a car in India to transport a therapy animal. The dense, and I mean very dense, traffic in India, means that people prefer to travel by motorcycle rather than car, so many people do not have access to a car. Dogs that are properly trained and socialized serve as therapy pets for the Animal Angels Foundation program but there are more therapists than there are pets available for service provision.

Dogs who qualify are limited and not all of the therapists own a pet. Animal Angels Foundation partners select pet owners in the community who are willing to loan out their pet to a trained therapist for a few hours. This is done after the pet has been evaluated as appropriate and the therapist who will be paired with the pet spends time with and befriends the animal. Then the therapist must coordinate their schedule with that of the pet owner so the dog is available to be picked up, transported to a site, provide a service for a few hours, and taken back home. Despite the obstacles, the Animal Angels Foundation is making a big difference for the people they serve in India and is helping to effect a change in attitude about the benefits of interacting with a companion dog.

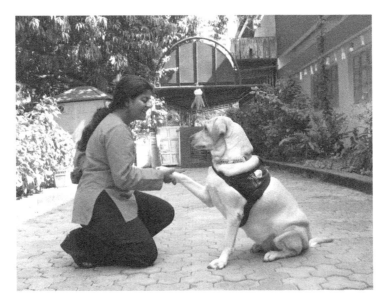

Figure 14.3 Minal Kavishwar with Kutty, an award-winning therapy team.

(*Source:* photo courtesy of Animal Angels Foundation, India.)

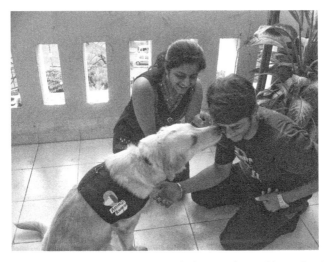

Figures 14.4 Minal Kavishwar providing therapy, with therapy dog Goldie and a client.

(*Source:* photos courtesy of Animal Angels Foundation, India.)

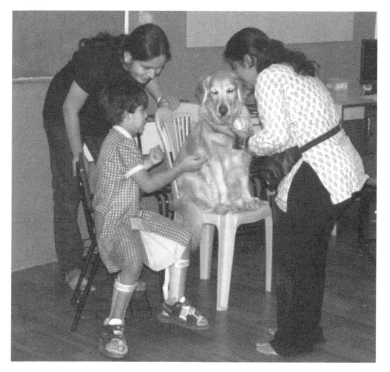

Figure 14.5 Minal Kavishwar providing therapy, with therapy dog Mimi and a child client.

(*Source:* photo courtesy of Animal Angels Foundation, India).

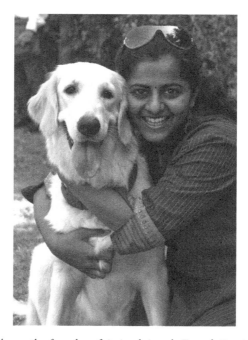

Figure 14.6 Minal Kavishwar, the founder of Animal Angels Foundation in India, with therapy dog Kiara.

(*Source:* photo courtesy of Animal Angels Foundation, India).

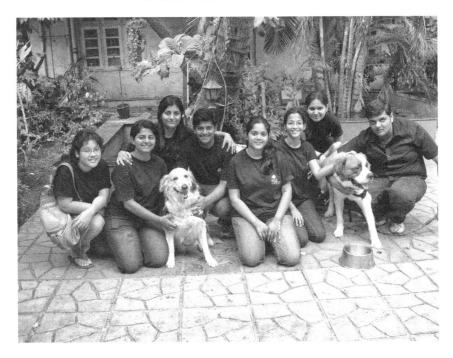

Figure 14.7 Team Animal Angels 2010 with therapy dogs Goldie, the Golden Retriever, and Onit, the St. Bernard.

(*Source:* photo courtesy of Animal Angels Foundation, India.)

The work of Minal Kavishwar includes training many volunteers and professionals to practice AAT. Some of her students go on to work in other agencies both in India and other countries. One of Minal's former students, Zahra Poonawala, flew all the way from Dubai to India to meet me when I visited. The former student was now a practicing professional at an animal therapy center in the United Arab Emirates called the Al Tamini Stables in Sharjah, Dubai. Al Tamini Stables is a 12-acre animal education and petting farm with over 500 animals of different species, including dogs, horses, donkeys, cats, goats, a cockatoo, guinea pigs, rabbits, cows, ducks, and chickens (Ghazal, 2014) (see also: www.tamimistables.com/). AAA and AAT services were provided at the stables through a program called Sense and included therapists working onsite and traveling to locations to provide professional services at homes, schools, special needs centers, or residential facilities for the elderly. The Sense program only lasted from 2014 to 2016, but Al Tamini Stables is still offering some AAA and AAT services onsite.

Many countries have AAT and AAA programs with which I am not personally familiar, but are surely doing wonderful work in providing education, nurturance, and healing to many people. For example, Dr. Philip Tedeschi of the Institute for Human–Animal Connection at the University of Denver (www.du.edu/humananimalconnection/) told me of an international alumni's program in Heredia, Costa Rico, Centro de Intervenciones Asistidas con Animales (n.d.). This organization provides AAA, AAT, animal-assisted psychotherapy, and animal-assisted play therapy services. There are likely thousands of these programs in existence across the world. I encourage you to do your own investigation of these programs and take the opportunity to become familiar with their services and accomplishments.

References

Adamle, K. N., Riley, T. A., and Carlson, T. (2009). Evaluating college student interest in pet therapy. *Journal of American College Health*, *57*(*5*), 545–548. doi: 10.3200/JACH.57.5.545-548

Adams, M. (1999). Emily Dickinson had a dog: An interpretation of the human–dog bond. *Anthrozoös*, *12*(*3*), 132–137.

Agnes, M. (Ed.). (2002). *Webster's New World Dictionary* (4th ed.). Cleveland, OH: Wiley.

Albuquerque, N., Guo, K., Wilkinson, A., Savalli, C., Otta, E., and Mills, D. (2016). Dogs recognize dog and human emotions. *Biology Letters*, *12*, 20150883. doi: 10.1098/rsbl.2015.0883

Alderton, D. (2000a). *Dogs*. London: Dorling Kindersley.

Alderton, D. (2000b). *Cats*. London: Dorling Kindersley.

American Counseling Association (ACA). (n.d.). ACA Community website: Retrieved on June 8, 2022: https://www.counseling.org/aca-community/aca-connect/interest-networks

American Counseling Association (ACA). (2014). *ACA Code of Ethics*. Alexandria, VA: Author. Retrieved on July 25, 2023: www.counseling.org/knowledge-center/ethics

American Kennel Club (AKC). (2023a). Canine Good Citizen test procedures. Retrieved on March 1, 2023: https://www.akc.org/products-services/training-programs/canine-good-citizen/canine-good-citizen-test-items/

American Kennel Club (AKC). (2023b). Therapy dog program. Retrieved on March 1, 2023: https://www.akc.org/sports/title-recognition-program/therapy-dog-program/

American Psychiatric Association. (1994). *Diagnostic and Statistical Manual for Mental Disorders* (4th ed.). Arlington, VA: Author.

American Psychological Association (APA). (2010). Ethical principles of psychologists and code of conduct. Retrieved on July 25, 2023: www.apa.org/ethics/code/index.aspx

American Red Cross. (n.d.) Take a class. Retrieved on July 25, 2023: www.redcross.org/en/takeaclass

American Veterinary Medical Association (AVMA). (n.d.). Ear cropping and tail docking of dogs. Retrieved on July 25, 2023: www.avma.org/KB/Policies/Pages/Ear-Cropping-and-Tail-Docking-of-Dogs.aspx

Anderson, D., White, S. H., Ohm, R., Brown, S., and Poggio, J. P. (2021). The effect of animal-assisted therapy on nursing student anxiety: A randomized controlled trial. *Nurse Education in Practice*, *52*. doi: 10.1016/j.nepr.2021.103068

Anderson, K. L., and Olson, M. R. (2006). The value of a dog in a classroom of children with severe emotional disorders. *Anthrozoös*, *19*(*1*), 35–49. doi: 10.2752/089279306785593919

Andics, A., Gábor, A., Gácsi, M., Faragó, T., Szabó, D., and Miklósi, A. (2016). Neural mechanism for lexical processing in dogs. *Science*, *353*(*6303*), 1030–1032. doi: 10.1126/scienceaaf377

Animal Angels Foundation. (n.d.). Animal angels. Retrieved on July 25, 2023: www.animalangels.org.in

Animal-Assisted Intervention International (AAII). (n.d.). About AAII. Retrieved on July 25, 2023: www.aai-int.org/

Animal Legal and Historical Center (ALHC). (n.d.). Michigan State University, College of Law. Retrieved on July 25, 2023: www.animallaw.info

Animals Asia. (n.d.). Dr. Dog and Professor Paws programs. Retrieved on July 25, 2023: www.animalsasia.org

Antonioli, C., and Reveley, M. A. (2005). Randomised controlled trial of animal facilitated therapy with dolphins in the treatment of depression. *British Medical Journal (BMJ)*, November 26. doi: 10.1136/bmj:331.7527.1231. Retrieved on October 14, 2016: www.bmj.com/cgi/content/full/331/7527/1231

Appel, D., Dapper, N., Elcock, M., et al. (2003). *Animals in Residential Facilities: Guidelines and resources for success.* Bellevue, WA: Delta Society (name changed to Pet Partners).

Asay, T. P., and Lambert, M. J. (1999). The empirical case for the common factors in therapy: Quantitative findings. In M. A. Hubble, S. D. Miller, and B. L. Duncan (Eds.), *The Heart and Soul of Change: What works in therapy* (pp. 33–55). Washington, D.C.: American Psychological Association.

Associated Press. (1987, August 26). Rehabilitating horses and prisoners. *New York Times.* Retrieved on July 25, 2023: www.nytimes.com/1987/08/26/us/rehabilitating-horses-and-prisoners.html

Associated Press. (1999, October 31). Therapy dogs have time for pupils. *Denton Record Chronicle*, p. A26.

Associated Press. (2005, October 19). Inmates welcome cats orphaned by Katrina. *NBCNews.com.* Retrieved on July 25, 2023: www.nbcnews.com/id/9755228/us_news-katrina_the_long_road_back/t/inmates-welcome-cats-orphaned-katrina/#.WA_PAjUbi2E

Associated Press. (2009, March 12). At Colorado prison, wild horses tame inmates. *Today.* Retrieved on July 25, 2023: https://www.today.com/news/colorado-prison-wild-horses-tame-inmates-wbna29657460

Association of Animal-Assisted Intervention Professionals (AAAIP) (n.d.). Home page: Who we are. Retrieved on August 6, 2022: https://www.aaaiponline.org.

Association for Multicultural Counseling and Development (AMCD). (2015). AMCD Multicultural and Social Justice Counseling Competencies. Retrieved on July 25, 2023: www.counseling.org/knowledge-center/competencies

Attractions Magazine. (2012, April 19). Cheetah and dog friends celebrate anniversary together at Busch Gardens Tampa. Retrieved on July 30, 2022: www.youtube.com/watch?v=Ndlf5_L5gsE

Bachi, K. (2012). Equine-facilitated psychotherapy: The gap between practice and knowledge. *Society and Animals, 20*, 364–380. doi: 10.1163/15685306-12341242

Bachi, K. (2013). Application of attachment theory to equine-facilitated psychotherapy. *Journal of Contemporary Psychotherapy, 43*, 187–196. doi: 10.1007/s10879-013-9232-1

Bachi, K., Terkel, J., and Teichman, M. (2011). Equine-facilitated psychotherapy for at-risk adolescents: The influence on self-image, self-control and trust. *Clinical Child Psychology and Psychiatry, 17(2)*, 298–312. doi: 10.1177/1359104511404177

Balluerka, N., Muela, A., Amiano, N., and Caldentey, M. (2014). Influence of animal-assisted therapy (AAT) on the attachment representations of youth in residential care. *Children and Youth Services Review, 42*, 103–109. doi: 10.1016/j.childyouth.2014.04.007

Bandler, R., and Grinder, J. (1975). *Patterns of the Hypnotic Techniques of Milton H. Erickson, M.D.* (Vol. *1*). Cupertino, CA: Meta Publications.

Banks, M. R., and Banks, W. A. (2002). The effects of animal-assisted therapy on loneliness in an elderly population in long-term care facilities. *Journal of Gerontology, 57A(7)*, M428–M432. doi: 10.1093/gerona/57.7.m428

Banks, M. R., and Banks, W. A. (2005). The effects of group and individual animal-assisted therapy on loneliness in residents of long-term care facilities. *Anthrozoös, 18(4)*, 396–408. doi: 10.1093/gerona/57.7.m428

Barak, Y., Savorai, O., Mavashev, S., and Beni, A. (2001). Animal-assisted therapy for elderly schizophrenic patients: A one-year controlled trial. *American Journal of Geriatric Psychiatry, 9(4)*, 439–442.

Barker, S., and Dawson, K. (1998). The effects of animal-assisted therapy on anxiety ratings of hospitalized psychiatric patients. *Psychiatric Services, 49(6)*, 797–801. doi: 10.1176/ps.49.6.797

Barker, S., Knisely, J., McCain, N., and Best, A. (2005). Measuring stress and immune response in healthcare professionals following interaction with a therapy dog: A pilot study. *Psychological Reports, 96*, 713–729. doi: 10.2466/pr0.96.3.713-729.

Barker, S. B., Knisely, J. S., McCain, N. L., Schubert, C. M., and Pandurangi, A. K. (2010). Exploratory study of stress-buffering response patterns from interaction with a therapy dog. *Anthrozoös, 23(1)*, 79–91. doi: 10.2752/175303710X12627079939341

Barol, B. (2002, May 13). Listen, Spot. *Time*, p. F14. Retrieved on July 26, 2023: https://content.time.com/time/magazine/article/0,9171,235437,00.html

Bass, M. M., Duchowny, C. A., and Llabre, M. M. (2009). The effect of therapeutic horseback riding on social functioning of children with autism. *Journal of Autism and Developmental Disorders*, *39*, 1261–1267. doi: 10.1007/s10803-009-0734-3

Batson, K., McCabe, B., Baun, M., and Wilson, C. (1998). The effect of a therapy dog on socialization and physiological indicators of stress in persons diagnosed with Alzheimer's disease. In C. Wilson and D. Turner (Eds.), *Companion Animals in Human Health* (pp. 203–215). Thousand Oaks, CA: Sage.

Baun, M. M., Bergstrom, N., Langston, N. F., and Thoma, L. (1984). Physiological effects of human/companion animal bonding. *Nursing Research*, *16*(3), 126–129.

Beck, A. M. (2000). The use of animals to benefit humans: Animal-assisted therapy. In A. Fine (Ed.), *Handbook on Animal-Assisted Therapy* (pp. 21–40). San Diego, CA: Academic Press.

Beck, A. M., Seraydarian, L., and Hunter, G. F. (1986). Use of animals in the rehabilitation of psychiatric in patients. *Psychological Reports*, *58*, 63–66.

Beck, A. T., and Steer, R. A. (1987). *Manual for the Beck Depression Inventory*. San Antonio, TX: The Psychological Corporation.

Beetz, A., Kotrschal, K., Turner, D., Hediger, K., Uvnäs-Moberg, K., and Julius, H. (2011). The effect of a real dog, toy dog and friendly person on insecurely attached children during a stressful task: An exploratory study. *Anthrozoös*, *24*(4), 349–368. doi: 10.2752/175303711X13159027359746

Behling, R. J., Haefner, J., and Stowe, M. (2011). Animal programs and animal-assisted therapy in Illinois long-term care facilities twenty years later (1990–2010). *Academy of Health Care Management Journal*, *7*(2), 109–117.

Benjamin, C. L. (1985). *Mother Knows Best: The natural way to train your dog*. New York: Howell.

Berget, B., Ekeberg, Ø., and Braastad, B. O. (2008a). Attitudes to animal-assisted therapy with farm animals among health staff and farmers. *Journal of Psychiatric and Mental Health Nursing*, *15*, 576–581. doi: 10.1111/j.1365-2850.2008.01268.x

Berget, B., Ekeberg, Ø., and Braastad, B. O. (2008b). Animal-assisted therapy with farm animals for persons with psychiatric disorders: Effects on self-efficacy, coping ability and quality of life, a randomized controlled trial. *Clinical Practice and Epidemiology in Mental Health*, *4*(9). doi: 10.1186/1745-0179-4-9

Bernstein, B. E., and Hartsell, T. L. (1998). *The Portable Lawyer for Mental Health Professionals: An A–Z guide to protecting your clients, your practice, and yourself*. New York: John Wiley and Sons.

Bernstein, P. L., Friedmann, E., and Malaspina, A. (2000). Animal-assisted therapy enhances resident social interaction and initiation in long-term care facilities. *Anthrozoös*, *13*(4), 213–224. doi: 10.2752/089279300786999743

Bessant, C. (2001). *The Cat Whisperer*. London: John Blake.

Betker, K. (2014, Winter). Human+animal interactions help healing begin at Sandy Hook. *Interactions Magazine*, 2–3.

Binette, K. H. (2015, April 10). Prisoners and shelter cats benefit from rescue program. *Life with Cats*. Retrieved on July 25, 2023: https://www.lifewithcats.tv/prisoners-and-shelter-cats-benefit-from-prison-program/

Binfet, J-T., Green, F., and Draper, Z. (2022). The importance of client–canine contact in canine-assisted interventions: A randomized controlled trial. *Anthrozoös*, *35*(1), 1–22. doi: 10.1080/08927936.2021.1944558

Binfet, J-T., Tardif-Williams, C., Draper, Z. A., Green, F., Singal, A., Rousseau, C., and Roma, R. (2022). Virtual canine comfort: A randomized controlled trial of the effects of a canine-assisted intervention supporting undergraduate wellbeing. *Anthrozoös*, *35*(6), 809–832. doi: 10.1080/08927936.2022.2062866

Birch, S. (1997). *Dolphin–Human Interaction Effects*. Unpublished dissertation. Monash University, Caulfield Campus, Australia Department of Electrical and Computer Systems Engineering.

Birke, L. (2007). "Learning to speak horse": The culture of "natural horsemanship." *Society and Animals*, *15*(3), 217–239. doi: 10.1163/156853007X217177

Blaisdell, J. D. (1999). The rise of man's best friend: The popularity of dogs as companion animals in late eighteenth-century London as reflected by the dog tax of 1796. *Anthrozoös*, *12*(2), 76–87.

Blazina, C., Boyraz, G., and Shen-Miller, D. (2011). Introduction: Using context to inform clinical practice and research. In C. Blazina, G. Boyraz, and D. Shen-Miller (Eds.), *The Psychology of the Human–Animal Bond*. New York: Springer.

Blum, N., and Fee, E. (2008). Howard A. Rusk (1901–1989): From military medicine to comprehensive rehabilitation. *American Journal of Public Health*, 98(2), 256–257. doi: 10.2105/AJPH.2007.120220

Bowers, M. J., and MacDonald, P. M. (2001). The effectiveness of equine-facilitated psychotherapy with at-risk adolescents. *Journal of Psychology and the Behavioral Sciences*, 15, 62–76.

Brandt, K. (2004). A language of their own: An interactionist approach to human–horse communication. *Society and Animals*, 12(4), 299–316.

Breitenbach, E., Stumpf, E., Fersen, L., and Ebert, H. (2009). Dolphin-assisted therapy: Changes in interaction and communication between children with severe disabilities and their caregivers. *Anthrozoös*, 22(3), 277–289. doi: 10.2752/175303709X457612

Brensing, K. (2005, May). Expert statement on "Swim with the dolphin programs and dolphin-assisted therapy." Third meeting of the scientific committee of the Agreement on the Conservation of Cetaceans of the Black Sea, Mediterranean Sea, and contiguous Atlantic Area, Cairo. Retrieved on July 25, 2023: https://www.accobams.org/wp-content/uploads/2016/06/SC3_Final_Report.pdf

Brensing, K., and Linke, K. (2003). Behavior of dolphins towards adults and children during swim-with-dolphin programs and towards children with disabilities during therapy sessions. *Anthrozoös*, 16(4), 315–331. doi: 10.2752/089279303786992035

Brensing, K., Linke, K., Busch, M., Matthes, I., and Eke van der Woude, S. (2005). Impact of different groups of swimmers on dolphins in swim-with-the-dolphin programs in two settings. *Anthrozoös*, 18(4), 409–429. doi:10.2752/089279305785593956

Brensing, K., Linke, K., and Todt, D. (2003). Can dolphins heal by ultrasound? *Journal of Theoretical Biology*, 225(1), 99–105. doi: 10.1016/s0022-5193(03)00225-x

Brickel, C. M. (1984). Depression in the nursing home: A pilot study using pet-facilitated psychotherapy. In R. K. Anderson and B. L. Hart (Eds.), *The Pet Connection: Its influence on our health and quality of life* (pp. 407–415). Minneapolis: Center to Study Human–Animal Relationships and Environments, University of Minnesota.

Briere, J. (1996). *Trauma Symptom Checklist for Children: Professional manual*. Odessa, FL: Psychological Assessment Resources.

Briggs, K. (2013, December 11). Equine sense of smell. Retrieved on July 25, 2023: www.thehorse.com/articles/10055/equine-sense-of-smell

Bromwich, J. E. (2016, June 16). In Shaken Orlando, comfort dogs arrive with "unconditional love." *The New York Times*. Retrieved on July 25, 2023: http://mobile.nytimes.com/2016/06/17/us/in-a-shaken-orlando-comfort-dogs-arrive-with-unconditional-love.html?_r=0&referer=

Broome, M. E., Lillis, P. P., McGahee, T. W., and Bates, T. A. (1992). The use of distraction and imagery with children during painful procedures. *Oncology Nursing Forum*, 19, 499–502.

Broughton, A. L. (2003). Cropping and docking: A discussion of the controversy and the role of law in preventing unnecessary cosmetic surgery on dogs. *Animal Legal and Historical Center, Michigan State University, College of Law*. Retrieved on July 25, 2023: www.animallaw.info/article/cropping-and-docking-discussion-controversy-and-role-law-preventing-unnecessary-cosmetic

Brown, S. (2002). Ethnic variations in pet attachment among students at an American school of veterinary medicine. *Society and Animals*, 10, 249–266. doi: 10.1163/156853002320770065

Brown, S. W., and Goldstein, L. H. (2011). Can seizure-alert dogs predict seizures? *Epilepsy Research*, 97(3), 236–242. doi: 10.1016/j.eplepsyres.2011.10.019

Brundige, W. (2009, August 16). Reading to dogs helps kids build literacy skills. *ABC News*. Retrieved on July 25, 2023: http://abcnews.go.com/GMA/Weekend/story?id=8339031

Burch, M. R. (1996). *Volunteering With Your Pet: How to get involved in animal-assisted therapy with any kind of pet*. New York: Howell.

Burch, M. R. (2003). *Wanted! Animal Volunteers*. New York: Howell.

Bureau of Land Management. (n.d.). Saddle-trained wild horse and burro inmate training program. Retrieved on July 25, 2023: https://www.blm.gov/programs/wild-horse-and-burro/adoptions-and-sales/adoption-centers/northern-nevada-correctional-center-horse-facility

Bureau of Land Management. (2005, November 1). World's highest-ranking law enforcement camel visits wild horse and burro adoption. *News Bytes*, issue 204. Retrieved on October 24, 2016: www.blm.gov/ca/news/newsbytes/xtra-05/204-xtra_whb_norco.html

Burger, E., Stetina, B. U., Turner, K., Lederman Maman, T., Handlos, U., and Kryspin-Exner, I. (2009). Changes in emotion regulation and emotion recognition in adolescents: Improvements during animal-assisted training. *Journal of Veterinary Behavior*, 4(2), 92–93. doi: 10.1016/J.JVEB.2008.09.056

Burrows, K., Adams, C., and Spiers, J. (2008). Sentinels of safety: Service dogs ensure safety and enhance freedom and well-being for families with autistic children. *Qualitative Health Research*, 18(12), 1642–1649. doi: 10.1177/1049732308327088

Bustad, L. K. (1980). *Animals, Aging, and the Aged*. Minneapolis: University of Minnesota Press.

Cain, J., and Smith, T. (2006). *The Revised and Expanded Book of Raccoon Circles: A facilitator's guide to building unity, community, connection, and teamwork through active learning*. Dubuque, IA: Kendall/Hunt Publishing Co.

Cameron, S., and Turtle-Song, I. (2002). Learning to write case notes using the SOAP format. *Journal of Counseling and Development, 80*, 286–292. doi: 10.1002/j.1556-6678.2002.tb00193.x

Carlson, J., Watts, R. E., and Maniacci, M. (2005). *Adlerian Therapy: Theory and practice*. Washington, D.C.: American Psychological Association.

Carlsson, C., Ranta, D., and Traen, B. (2014). Equine-assisted social work as a mean for authentic relations between clients and staff. *Human–Animal Interaction Bulletin, 2(1)*, 19–38. doi: 10.1079/hai.2014.0004

Cavert, C. (1999). *Affordable Portables: A working book of initiative activities and problem solving element* (revised and expanded version). Oklahoma City, OK: Wood 'N' Barnes Publishing.

Center for the Human-Animal Bond (n.d.). History and Mission. Retrieved on July 26, 2023: https://vet.purdue.edu/chab/

Centro de Intervenciones Asistidas con Animales. (n.d.). Retrieved on July 25, 2023: https://www.facebook.com/centroiaacr/?locale=es_LA

Chamove, A. S., Crawley-Hartrick, O. J. E., and Stafford, K. J. (2002). Horse reactions to human attitudes and behavior. *Anthrozoös, 15(4)*, 323–331. doi: 10.2752/089279302786992423

Chandler, C. K. (2005a). *Animal-Assisted Therapy in Counseling*. New York, NY: Routledge.

Chandler, C. K. (2005b). Psychosocial Session Form. In *Animal-Assisted Therapy in Counseling* (pp. 181–184). New York: Routledge.

Chandler, C. K. (2008, March). Animal-assisted therapy with Hurricane Katrina survivors. Presented at the annual meeting of the American Counseling Association. Honolulu, HI.

Chandler, C. K. (2009). Animal-assisted therapy. In *American Counseling Association, The ACA Encyclopedia of Counseling* (pp. 24–25). Alexandria, VA: American Counseling Association.

Chandler, C. K. (2012). *Animal-Assisted Therapy in Counseling* (2nd ed.). New York, NY: Routledge.

Chandler, C. K. (2015, April 20). Confirming the benefits of emotional support animals. *Counseling Today Online Exclusives*. Retrieved on July 25, 2023: http://ct.counseling.org/2015/04/confirming-the-benefits-of-emotional-support-animals/

Chandler, C. K. (2015b, March). Animal-assisted therapy interventions. Presentation at Animal Angels Foundation Professional Meeting. Mumbai, India.

Chandler, C. K. (2015c, June). Animal-assisted therapy in practice: Post conference workshop. Presentation at Animal-Assisted Therapy Conference, Department of Social Work, University of Hong Kong. Hong Kong, China.

Chandler, C. K. (2017). *Animal-Assisted Therapy in Counseling* (3rd ed.). New York, NY: Routledge.

Chandler, C. K. (2018). Human–animal relational theory: A guide for animal-assisted counseling. *Journal of creativity in mental health, 13(4)*, 429–444. doi: 10.1080/15401383.2018.1486258

Chandler, C. K. (2019, February). Is there an epidemic of emotional support animals? *Counseling Today*. Retrieved July 25, 2023: https://ct.counseling.org/2019/02/is-there-an-epidemic-of-emotional-support-animals/

Chandler, C. K., Fernando, D. M., Barrio Minton, C. A., and Portrie-Bethke, T. (2015). Eight domains of pet–owner wellness: Valuing the owner–pet relationship in the counseling process. *Journal of Mental Health Counseling, 37(3)*, 268–282. doi: 10.17744/mehc.37.3.06

Chandler, C. K., and Johnson, A. (2009, May). Petition for the Establishment of the American Counseling Association Animal-Assisted Therapy in Mental Health (AATMH) Interest Network. Unpublished document presented to the ACA Governing Council. American Counseling Association, Alexandria, VA.

Chandler, C. K., and Otting, T. L. (Eds.). (2018). *Animal-Assisted Interventions for Emotional and Mental Health: Conversations with pioneers of the field*. New York: Routledge.

Chandler, C. K., Portrie-Bethke, T. L., Barrio Minton, C. A., Fernando, D. M., and O'Callaghan, D. M. (2010). Matching animal-assisted therapy techniques and intentions with counseling guiding theories. *Journal of Mental Health Counseling, 32(4)*, 354–374. doi: 10.17744/mehc.32.4.u72lt21740103538

Chen, C., Hung, C., Lee, Y., Tseng, W., Chen, M., Chen, T. (2022). Animal-assisted therapy on middle-aged and older adults with schizophrenia. *International Journal of Environmental Research and Public Health, 19(6270)*. doi: 10.3390/ijerph19106270

Choi, Y. (2003, November). History of the human–animal bond in Korea. Paper presented at the First International Symposium on the Human–Animal Bond, Samsung Everland, South Korea.

Christian, J. E. (2005). All creatures great and small: Utilizing equine-assisted therapy to treat eating disorders. *Journal of Psychology and Christianity*, *24*(*1*), 65–67.

Christie, S. (2002). Standards of strength: Proportionate, powerful and agile, bully breeds share common physical traits and ancestry. *Popular Dogs Series: Bully Breeds*, *21*, 19–33.

Cirelli, A. Jr., and Cloud, B. (n.d.). Horse handling and riding guidelines part I: Equine senses. Fact sheet 98–29. *Cooperative Extension*, University of Nevada, Reno. Retrieved on September 27, 2016: www.unce.unr.edu/publications/files/ag/other/fs9829.pdf

Clothier, S. (1996). *Understanding Puppy Testing.* St. Johnsville, NY: Flying Dog Press.

CNN.com. (2005). Hurricane Katrina. Retrieved on July 26, 2023: www.cnn.com/SPECIALS/2005/katrina

Coakley, A. B., and Mahoney, E. K. (2009). Creating a therapeutic and healing environment with a pet therapy program. *Complementary therapies in clinical practice*, *15*(3), 141–146. doi: 10.1016/j.ctcp.2009.05.004

Coetzee, N., Beukes, J., and Lynch, I. (2013). Substance abuse inpatients' experience of animal-assisted therapy. *Journal of Psychology in Africa*, *23*(3), 477–480. doi: 10.1080/14330237.2013.10820654

Coile, D. C. (1998). *Encyclopedia of Dog Breeds.* Hauppauge, NY: Barron's.

Cole, D. M. (1996). Phenomenological effect of dolphin interaction on humans. Paper presented at the International Symposium on Dolphin Healing. Co-hosted by the Aqua Thought Foundation. Cancun, Mexico.

Cole, K. M., Gawlinski, A., Steers, N., and Kotlerman, J. (2007). Animal-assisted therapy in patients hospitalized with heart failure. *American Journal of Critical Care*, *16*(6), 575–585.

Commings, K. (n.d.). Understanding your cat's senses. *PetPlace.com*. Retrieved on July 30, 2022: www.petplace.com/cats/understanding-your-cat-s-senses/page1.aspx

Consortium for Animal Assisted Therapy (CAAT). (n.d.) Retrieved on July 26, 2023: www.coe.unt.edu/consortium-animal-assisted-therapy

Cook, S. L. (2013, August 7). *Scripted Communication.* Unpublished dissertation. Regis University, Denver, Colorado. Retrieved on July 25, 2023: http://epublications.regis.edu/cgi/viewcontent.cgi?article=1196&context=theses

Cooke, E., Henderson-Wilson, C., Warner, E., and LaMontagne, A. (2023). Animal-assisted interventions in universities: a scoping review of implementation and associated outcomes. *Health Promotion International*, *38*(3), daac001, 1–27. doi: 10.1093/heapro/daac001

Cooper, M. (2003). *Existential Therapies.* Thousand Oaks, CA: Sage.

Cormier, S., and Nurius, P. (2003). *Interviewing and Change Strategies for Helpers: Fundamental skills and cognitive behavioral interventions.* Pacific Grove, CA: Brooks/Cole.

Cornu, J-N., Cancel-Tassin, G., Ondet, V., Girardet, C., and Cussenot, O. (2011). Olfactory detection of prostate cancer by dogs sniffing urine: a step forward in diagnosis. *European Urology*, *59*(2), 197–201. doi: 10.1016/j.eururo.2010.10.006

Correa, J. E. (2011, June). The dog's sense of smell. Alabama Cooperative Extension System, Alabama A and M and Auburn Universities, document UNP-66. Retrieved on July 25, 2023: https://www.yumpu.com/en/document/read/8514905/the-dogs-sense-of-smell-alabama-cooperative-extension-system

Corson, S. A., Corson, E., Gwynne, P. H., and Arnold, L. E. (1975). Pet-facilitated psychotherapy in a hospital setting. *Current Psychiatric Therapies*, *15*, 277–286.

Costa, P. T. Jr., and McCrae, R. R. (1992). *Revised NEO Personality Inventory (NEO-PI-R) and NEO Five Factor Inventory (NEO-FFI) Professional Manual.* Odessa, FL: Psychological Assessment Resources.

Coto, J. A., Ohlendorf, E. K., Cinnamon, A. E., Ellis, T. L., Ondrey, M. A. and Bartuch, P. (2022). A correlational study exploring nurse-work anxiety and animal-assisted therapy. *The Journal of Nursing Administration*, *52*(9), 498–501. doi: 10.1097/NNA.0000000000001188

Craig, E. A. (2020). Equine-assisted psychotherapy among adolescents with ACEs: Cultivating altercentrism, expressiveness, communication composure, and interaction management. *Child and Adolescent Social Work Journal*, *37*(6), 643–656. doi: 10.1007/s10550-020-00694-0

Cushing, J. L., and Williams, J. D. (1995). The Wild Mustang Program: A case study in facilitated inmate therapy. *Journal of Offender Rehabilitation*, *22*(3–4), 95–112. doi: 10.1300/J076v22n03_08

D'Amore, A. R. T. (1976). Introduction. In *William Alanson White: The Washington years 1903–1937* (pp. 1–12). Washington, D.C.: U.S. Department of Health, Education, and Welfare, Public Health Service.

Daley Olmert, M. (2009). *Made For Each Other: The biology of the human–animal bond.* Philadelphia, PA: Da Capo Press.

Deaton, C. (2005). Humanizing prisons with animals: A closer look at "cell dogs" and horse programs in correctional institutions. *Journal of Correctional Education, 56*(1), 46–62. doi: 10.1177/0032885516671919

DeCourcey, M., Russell, A. C., and Keister, K. J. (2010). Animal-assisted therapy: Evaluation and implementation of a complementary therapy to improve the psychological and physiological health of critically ill patients. *Dimensions of Critical Care Nursing, 29*(5), 211–214. doi: 10.1097/DCC.obo13e3181e6c71a

Dell, C. A., Chalmers, D., Bresette, N., Swain, S., Rankin, D., and Hopkins, C. (2011). A healing space: The experiences of First Nations and Inuit youth with equine-assisted learning (EAL). *Child Youth Care Forum, 40*, 319–336. doi: 10.1007/s10566-011-9140-z

Dell, C. A., Chalmers, D., Dell, D., Sauve, E., and MacKinnon, T. (2008). Horse as healer: An examination of equine-assisted learning in the healing of First Nations youth from solvent abuse. *Pimatisiwin: A Journal of Aboriginal and Indigenous Community Health, 6*(1), 81–106.

Delta Society. (1997). *Animals in Institutions*. Renton, WA: Author. (Delta Society is now Pet Partners.)

Delta Society. (2000). *Pet Partners Team Training Course Manual* (5th ed.). Renton, WA: Author.

Delta Society. (2002). Introduction to horse behavior. *Team Evaluator Course* (supplemental material). Bellevue, WA: Author.

Delta Society. (2003). Pet Partners program. Retrieved on September 27, 2016: www.deltasociety.org

Delta Society. (2004). *Pet Partners Team Training Course Manual* (6th ed.). Renton, WA: Author.

Delta Society. (2005). *Animals in the Classroom*. Bellevue, WA: Author.

Demiralay, S., and Keser, I. (2022). The effect of pet therapy on the stress and social anxiety levels of disabled children: *A randomized controlled trial. Complementary Therapies in Clinical Practice, 48.* doi: 10.1016/j.ctcp.2022.101574

Deneen, S. (2002). Extraordinary bullys: Meet seven talented and athletic emissaries for their breeds. *Popular Dogs Series: Bully Breeds, 21*, 52–59. Irvine, CA: Fancy Publications.

DePrekel, M., and Welsch, T. (2000a). *Animal-assisted Therapeutic Interventions*. Unpublished manuscript.

DePrekel, M., and Welsch, T. (2000b). *Hands-on Animal-assisted Therapy and Education Activities*. Unpublished manuscript.

Derogatis, L. R. (1993). *Brief Symptom Inventory (BSI): Administration, scoring and procedures manual*. Minneapolis, MN: NCS Pearson.

DeZutti, J. (2013). Eating disorders and equine therapy. *Journal of Psychosocial Nursing, 51*(9), 24–31. doi: 10.3928/02793695-20130612-01

Dictionary.com. (n.d.). Online dictionary. Retrieved on October 9, 2016: www.dictionary.com

Dietz, T. J., Davis, D., and Pennings, J. (2012). Evaluating animal-assisted therapy in group treatment for child sexual abuse. *Journal of Child Sexual Abuse, 21*, 665–683. doi: 10.1080/10538712.2012.726700

Dog Days. (n.d.). Gettysburg program brings freshmen, dogs together for orientation. Retrieved on October 14, 2016: www.gettysburg.edu/about/offices/college_life/counseling/dog_days/

Doolittle, H. (1956). *Tribute to Freud*. New York: Pantheon.

Dreikurs, R. (1950). *Fundamentals of Adlerian Psychology*. Chicago, IL: Alfred Adler Institute.

Dweck, C. (2006). *RSA Animate: How to help every child fulfil their potential*. Retrieved on June 17, 2023: https://www.youtube.com/watch?v=Yl9TVbAaI5s

Earles, J. L., Vernon, L. L., and Yetz, J. P. (2015). Equine-assisted therapy for anxiety and posttraumatic stress symptoms. *Journal of Traumatic Stress, 28*, 149–152. doi: 10.1002/jts.21990

Eckerd College. (n.d.). *Pet Policy*. Retrieved on July 25, 2023: www.eckerd.edu/housing/pet-life/policy/

Eggiman, J. (2006). Cognitive-behavioral therapy: A case report—Animal-assisted therapy. *Topics in Advanced Practice Nursing eJournal, 6*(3). Retrieved on July 25, 2023: www.medscape.com/viewarticle/545439

Encyclopedia.com (n.d.). Website: www.encyclopedia.com/topic/mammal.aspx, retrieved on November 11, 2016.

Engel, B. T. (1998). *Therapeutic Riding I: Strategies for instruction*. Durango, CO: Barbara Engel Therapy Services.

Engel, B. T. (2003). *Therapeutic Riding II: Strategies for rehabilitation, revised* (3rd ed.). Durango, CO: Barbara Engel Therapy Services.

Engel, B. T., Galloway, M., Bull, M., and Harvey, M. (2008). *The Horse, the Handicapped, and the Riding Team in a Therapeutic Riding Program: A training manual for volunteers* (revised ed.). Durango, CO: Barbara Engel Therapy Services.

Engel, B. T., and MacKinnon, J. R. (2007). *Enhancing Human Occupation Through Hippo-therapy: A guide for occupational therapy*. Bethesda, MD: AOTA Press.

Engel, G. L. (1980). The clinical application of the biopsychosocial model. *American Journal of Psychiatry, 137*(5), 535–544. doi: 10.1176/ajp.137.5.535

Epilepsy Foundation (2007). Seizure-alert dogs: Just the facts, hold the media hype. Retrieved on July 25, 2023: https://www.epilepsy.com/stories/seizure-alert-dogs-just-facts-hold-media-hype

Equestrian Vaulting USA. (2023). Home page. Retrieved on July 25, 2023: www.equestrianvaulting.org.

Equine Assisted Growth and Learning, Association (EAGALA). (n.d.a). Home page. Retrieved on July 25, 2023: http://eagala.org/

Equine Assisted Growth and Learning, Association (EAGALA). (n.d.b). About EAGALA. Retrieved on July 25, 2023: www.eagala.org/

Equine Assisted Growth and Learning, Association (EAGALA). (n.d.c). EAGALA Code of Ethics. Retrieved on July 25, 2023: http://eagala.org/

Faa-Thompson, T. (2012). Safe touch using horses to teach sexually abused clients to value their bodies and themselves. In K. S. Trotter (Ed.), *Harnessing the Power of Equine-Assisted Counseling* (pp. 53–58). New York: Routledge.

Fadiga, L., Fogassi, L., Pavesi, G., and Rizzolatti, G. (1995). Motor facilitation during action observation: A magnetic stimulation study. *Journal of Neurophysiology, 73*(6), 2608–2611. doi: 10.1152/jn.1995.73.6.2608

Farias-Tomaszewski, S., Jenkins, S. R., and Keller, J. (2001). An evaluation of therapeutic horseback riding programs for adults with physical impairments. *Therapeutic Recreation Journal, 35*(3), 250–257.

Faver, C. A., and Cavazos, A. M. (2008). Love, safety, and companionship: The human–animal bond and Latino families. *Journal of Family Social Work, 11*(3), 254–271. doi: 10.1080/10522150802292350

Fawcett, N., and Gullone, E. (2001). Cute and cuddly and a whole lot more? A call for empirical investigation into the therapeutic benefits of human–animal interaction for children. *Behaviour Change, 18*(2), 124–133. doi: 10.1375/bech.18.2.124

Ferwerda-van Zonneveld, R. T., Oosting, S. J., and Kijlstra, A. (2012). Care farms as a short-break service for children with Autism Spectrum Disorders. *NJAS—Wageningen Journal of Life Sciences, 59*(1–2), 35–40. doi: 10.1016/j.njas.2012.01.001

Fick, K. (1993). The influence of an animal on social interactions of nursing home residents in a group setting. *American Journal of Occupational Therapy, 47*(6), 529–534. doi: 10.5014/ajot.47.6.529

Filan, S. L., and Llewellyn-Jones, R. H. (2006). Animal-assisted therapy for dementia: A review of literature. *International Psychogeriatrics, 18*(4), 597–611. doi: 10.1017/S1041610206003322

Filiatre, J. C., Millot, J. L., and Eckerlin, A. (1991). Behavioural variability of olfactory exploration of the pet dog in relation to human adults. *Applied Animal Behaviour Science, 30*, 341–350. doi: 10.1016/0168-1591(91)90139-O

Fine, A. H. (Ed.). (2000a). *Handbook on Animal-Assisted Therapy: Theoretical foundations and guidelines for practice.* San Diego, CA: Academic Press.

Fine, A. H. (2000b). Animals and therapists: Incorporating animals in outpatient psychotherapy. In A. H. Fine (Ed.), *Handbook on Animal-Assisted Therapy: Theoretical foundations and guidelines for practice* (pp. 179–211). San Diego, CA: Academic Press.

Fine, A. H. (Ed.). (2015). *Handbook on Animal-Assisted Therapy: Theoretical foundations and guidelines for practice* (4th ed.). San Diego, CA: Academic Press.

Fine, A. H. (Ed.). (2019). *Handbook on Animal-Assisted Therapy: Theoretical foundations and guidelines for practice* (5th ed.). San Diego, CA: Academic Press.

Firstscience TV. (2007). Polar bears and dogs playing. *YouTube.* Retrieved on July 25, 2023: www.youtube.com/watch?v=JE-Nyt4Bmi8

Fleischer, J., Breer, H., and Strotmann, J. (2009). Mammalian olfactory receptors. *Frontiers in Cellular Neuroscience, 3*(9), 1–10. doi: 10.3389/neuro.03.009.2009

Flynn, E., Roguski, J., Wolf, J., Trujillo, K., Tedeschi, P., and Morris, K. (2018). A randomized controlled trial of animal-assisted therapy as an adjunct to intensive family preservation services. *Child Maltreatment, 24*(2), 161–168. doi: 10.1177/1077559518817678

Flom, B. L. (2005, June). Counseling with pocket pets: Using small animals in elementary counseling programs. *Professional School Counseling, 8*(5), 469–471.

Fogle, B. (1999). The changing roles of animals in Western society: Influences upon and from the veterinary profession. *Anthrozoös, 12*(4), 234–239. doi: 10.2752/089279399787000084

Fogle, B. (2000). *Cats: Portraits of over 70 pedigrees.* New York: Dorling Kindersley.

Folse, E. B., Minder, C. C., Aycock, M. J., and Santana, R. T. (1994). Animal-assisted therapy and depression in adult college students. *Anthrozoös, 7*(3), 188–194. doi: 10.2752/089279394787001880

Ford, C. (2013). Dancing with horses: Combining dance/movement therapy and equine-facilitated psychotherapy. *American Journal of Dance Therapy, 35*, 93–117. doi: 10.1007/s10465-013-9156-z

Ford Sori, C., and Ciastko Hughes, J. (2014). Animal-assisted play therapy: An interview with Risë VanFleet. *The Family Journal, 22*(3), 350–356. doi: 10.1177/1066480714534394

Fournier, A., Geller, E. S., and Fortney, E. V. (2007). Human–animal interaction in a prison setting: Impact on criminal behavior, treatment progress, and social skills. *Behavior and Social Issues, 16*(1), 89–104. doi: 10.5210/bsi.v16i1.385

Freud, M. (1983). *Sigmund Freud: Man and father.* New York: Jason Aronson.

Freud, S. (1992). *The Diary of Sigmund Freud 1929–1939: A record of the final decade* (translated and annotated by M. Molnar). New York: Charles Scribner's Sons.

Friedmann, E., Galik, E., Thomas, S., Hall, S., Cheon, J., Han, N., Kim, H. J., McAtee, S., and Gee, N. R. (2019). Relationship of behavioral interactions during an animal-assisted intervention in assisted living to health-related outcomes. *Anthrozoös, 32*(2), 221–238. doi: 10.1080/08927936.2019.1569905

Friedmann, E., Katcher, A., Lynch, J., and Thomas, S. (1980). Animal companions and one-year survival of patients after discharge from a coronary unit. *Public Health Reports, 95*, 307–312.

Friedmann, E., Katcher, A., Thomas, S., Lynch, J., and Messent, P. (1983). Social interaction and blood pressure: Influence of animal companions. *Journal of Nervous and Mental Disease, 171*, 461–465. doi: 10.1097/00005053-198308000-00002

Friedmann, E., Locker, B., and Lockwood, R. (1993). Perception of animals and cardiovascular responses during verbalization with an animal present. *Anthrozoös, 6*(2), 115–133. doi: 10.2752/089279393787002303

Friedmann, E., and Thomas, S. (1995). Pet ownership, social support, and one-year survival after acute myocardial infarction in the Cardiac Arrhythmia Suppression Trial (CAST). *American Journal of Cardiology, 76*, 1213–1217. doi: 10.1016/s0002-9149(99)80343-9

Friedmann, E., Thomas, S. A., Cook, L. K., Tsai, C., and Picot, S. J. (2007). A friendly dog as potential moderator of cardiovascular response to speech in older hypertensives. *Anthrozoös, 20*(1), 51–63. doi: 10.2752/089279307780216605

Friesen, L. (2010). Exploring animal-assisted programs with children in school and therapeutic contexts. *Early Childhood Education Journal, 37*, 261–267. doi: 10.1007/s10643-009-0349-5

Frohoff, T. G., and Packard, J. M. (1995). Human interactions with free-ranging and captive bottlenose dolphins. *Anthrozoös, 8*(1), 44–53. doi: 10.2752/089279395787156527

Fung, S., and Leung, A. S. (2014). Pilot study investigating the role of therapy dogs in facilitating social interaction among children with autism. *Journal of Contemporary Psychotherapy, 44*, 253–262. doi: 10.1007/s10879-014-9274-z

Furst, G. (2006). Prison-based animal programs. *Prison Journal, 86*(4), 407–430.

Gabriels, R. L., Agnew, J. A., Holt, K. D., Shoffner, A., Zhaoxing, P., Ruzzano, S., Clayton, G., and Mesibov, G. (2012). Pilot study measuring the effects of therapeutic horseback riding on school-age children and adolescents with autism spectrum disorders. *Research in Autism Spectrum Disorders, 6*(2), 578–588. doi: 10.1016/j.rasd.2011.09.007

Gammonley, J., Howie, A. R., Jackson, B., Kaufman, M., Kirwin, S., Morgan, L., et al. (2003). *AAT Applications I: Student guide.* Renton, WA: Delta Society. (Delta Society is now Pet Partners.)

Gammonley, J., Howie, A. R., Jackson, B., Kaufmann, M., Kirwin, S., Morgan, L., et al. (2007). *Animal-Assisted Therapy (AAT) Applications I: Student guide.* Bellevue, WA: Delta Society.

Gammonley, J., Howie, A. R., Kirwin, S., Zapf, S. A., Frye, J., Freeman, G., et al. (1997). *Animal-Assisted Therapy: Therapeutic interventions.* Renton, WA: Delta Society.

Gammonley, J., and Yates, J. (1991). Pet projects: Animal-assisted therapy in nursing homes. *Journal of Gerontological Nursing, 17*(1), 12–15. doi: 10.3928/0098-9134-19910101-05

Gay, P. (1988). *Freud: A life for our time.* New York: W. W. Norton.

Gee, N. R., Church, M. T., and Altobelli, C. L. (2010). Preschoolers make fewer errors on an object categorization task in the presence of a dog. *Anthrozoös, 23*(3), 223–230. doi: 10.2752/175303710X12750451258896

Gee, N. R., Crist, E. N., and Carr, D. N. (2010). Preschool children require fewer instructional prompts to perform a memory task in the presence of a dog. *Anthrozoös, 23*(2), 173–184. doi: 10.2752/175303710X12682332910051

Gee, N. R., Harris, S. L., and Johnson, K. L. (2007). The role of therapy dogs in speed and accuracy to complete motor skills tasks for preschool children. *Anthrozoös, 20*(4), 375–386. doi: 10.2752/089279307X245509

Gee, N. R., Reed, T., Whiting, A., Friedmann, E., Snellgrove, D., and Sloman, K. (2019). Observing life fish improves perceptions of mood, relaxation and anxiety, but does not consistently alter heart rate or heart rate variability. *International Journal of Environmental Research and Public Health*, *16*(*3113*), 1–15. doi: 10.3390/ijerph16173113

Gee, N. R., Rodriguez, K. E., Fine, A. H., and Trammell, J. P. (2021). Dogs supporting human health and well-being: A biopsychosocial approach. *Frontiers in Veterinary Science*, *8*, 1–11. doi: 10.3389/fvets.2021.630465

Gee, N. R., Sherlock, T. R., Bennett, E. A., and Harris, S. L. (2009). Preschoolers' adherence to instructions as a function of presence of a dog and motor skills task. *Anthrozoös*, *22*(3), 267–276. doi: 10.2752/175303709X457603

Geraci, J. R., and Ridgway, S. H. (1991). On disease transmission between cetaceans and humans. *Marine Mammal Science*, *7*(2), 191–194. doi: 10.1111/j.1748-7692.1991.tb00565.x

Ghazal, R. (2014, January 9). It's puppy love at the UAE's new animal therapy center, Sense. *The National*. Retrieved on July 25, 2023: www.thenational.ae/lifestyle/family/its-puppy-love-at-the-uaes-new-animal-therapy-centre-sense

Glasser, W. (1999). *Choice Theory: A new psychology of personal freedom*. New York, NY: Harper Perennial.

Gordon, P. (2013, September 26). Service dogs aid with comfort at Washington Navy Yard. Navy News Service. Retrieved on July 25, 2023: https://www.military.com/daily-news/2013/09/26/service-dogs-offer-comfort-at-navy-yard.html

Gore, T., Gore, P., Giffin, J. M., and Adelman, B. (2008). *Horse Owner's Veterinary Handbook*. Hoboken, NJ: Howell Book House.

Gosling, S., Kwan, V., and John, O. (2003). A dog's got personality: A cross-species comparative approach to personality judgments in dogs and humans. *Journal of Personality and Social Psychology*, *85*(6), 1161–1169. doi: 10.1037/0022-3514.85.6.1161

Grandin, T. (1993). Welfare of livestock in slaughter plants. In T. Grandin (Ed.), *Livestock Handling and Transport* (pp. 289–311). Wallingford, Oxon, UK: CAB International.

Grandin, T., and Smith, G. (2004, November). Animal welfare and humane slaughter. Unpublished paper on Dr. Temple Grandin's webpage. University of Colorado. Retrieved on July 25, 2023: www.grandin.com/references/humane.slaughter.html

Green, J. (2000). Can dogs be trained to detect epileptic seizures? Maybe, experts say. *Working dogs*. Retrieved on September 27, 2016: www.workingdogs.com/vcepilepsy.htm

Green Chimneys. (n.d.). A history of Green Chimneys. Retrieved on July 25, 2023: www.greenchimneys.org/

Greenwald, A. J. (2000). *The Effect of a Therapeutic Horsemanship Program on Emotionally Disturbed Boys*. Unpublished dissertation. Pace University, New York.

Greer, K. L., Pustay, K. A., Zaun, T. C., and Coppens, P. (2001). A comparison of the effects of toys versus live animals on the communication of patients with dementia of the Alzheimer's type. *Clinical Gerontologist*, *24*(3–4), 157–182. doi: 10.1300/J018v24n03_13

Grigore, A. A., and Rusu, A. S. (2014). Interaction with a therapy dog enhances the effects of Social Story method in autistic children. *Society and Animals*, 241–261. doi: 10.1163/15685306-12341326

Grinker, R. R. Sr. (1979). *Fifty Years in Psychiatry: A living history*. Springfield, IL: Charles C. Thomas.

Guralnik, D. (Ed.). (1980). *Webster's New World Dictionary* (2nd college ed.). New York: Simon and Schuster.

HABRI Central (n.d.). About. Retrieved on July 25, 2023: https://habricentral.org/kb/management—oversight/habricentral-faq

Hall, C. (1954). *A Primer of Freudian Psychology*. New York: World Publishing.

Hallberg, L. (2008). *Walking the Way of the Horse: Exploring the power of the horse–human relationship*. Bloomington, IN: iUniverse.

Hallberg, L. (2017a). *The Clinical Practice of Equine-assisted Therapy: Including horses in human healthcare*. New York, NY: Routledge.

Hallberg, L. (2017b). *The Equine-assisted Therapy Workbook: A learning guide for professionals and students*. New York, NY: Routledge.

Hama, H., Yogo, M., and Matsuyama, Y. (1996). Effects of stroking horses on both humans' and horses' heart rate responses. *Japanese Psychological Research*, *38*, 66–73. doi: 10.1111/j.1468-5884.1996.tb00009.x

Hamama, L., Hamama-Raz, Y., Dagan, K., Greenfeld, H., Rubenstein, C., and Menachem, B. (2011). A preliminary study of group intervention along with basic canine training among traumatized teen-agers: A 3-month longitudinal study. *Children and Youth Services Review*, *33*(*10*), 1975–1980. doi: 10.1016/j.childyouth.2011.05.021

Handlin, L., Hydbring-Sandberg, E., Nilsson, A., Ejdebäck, M., Jansson, A., and Uvnäs-Moberg, K. (2011). Short-term interaction between dogs and their owners: Effects on oxytocin, cortisol, insulin, and heart rate—an exploratory study. *Anthrozoös*, *24*(*3*), 301–315. doi: 10.2752/175303711X 13045914865385

Hanselman, J. L. (2002). Coping skills interventions with adolescents in anger management using animals in therapy. *Journal of Child and Adolescent Group Therapy*, *11*(*4*), 159–195. doi: 10.1023/A:1014802324267

Hansen, K., Messinger, C., Baun, M., and Megel, M. (1999). Companion animals alleviating distress in children. *Anthrozoös*, *12*(*3*), 142–148. doi: 10.2752/089279399787000264

Harbolt, T., and Ward, T. H. (2001). Teaming incarcerated youth with shelter dogs for a second chance. *Society and Animals*, *9*(*2*), 177–182. Retrieved on July 25, 2023: https://www.animalsandsociety. org/wp-content/uploads/2015/11/harbolt.pdf

Harper, C. M., Dong, Y., Thornhill, T. S., Wright, J., Ready, J., Brick, G. W., and Dyer, G. (2015). Can therapy dogs improve pain and satisfaction after total joint anthroplasty? A randomized control trial. *Clinical Orthopedics and Related Research*, *473*(*1*), 372–379. doi: 10.1007/s11999-014-3931-0

Hatch, A. (2007). The view from all fours: A look at an animal-assisted activity program from the animal's perspective. *Anthrozoös*, *20*(*1*), 37–50. doi: 10.2752/089279307780216632

Havey, J., Vlasses, F. R., Vlasses, P. H., Ludwig-Beymer, P., and Hackbarth, D. (2015). The effect of animal-assisted therapy on pain medication use after joint replacement. *Anthrozoös*, *27*(*3*), 361–369. doi: 10.2752/175303714X13903827487962

Haynes, M. (1991, August). Pet therapy: Program lifts spirits, reduces violence in institution's mental health unit. *Corrections Today*, *53*(*5*), 120–122. Retrieved on July 25, 2023: https://www.ojp.gov/ ncjrs/virtual-library/abstracts/pet-therapy-program-lifts-spirits-reduces-violence-institutions

HeartMath. (n.d.). Institute of HeartMath. Retrieved on July 25, 2023: www.heartmath.org

HeartMath. (2006, Spring). New meaning to "horse sense." *A Change of Heart*, *5*(*1*), 1, 4.

Hediger, K., Thommen, S., Wagner, C., Gaab, J., and Hund-Georgiadis, M. (2019). Effects of animal-assisted therapy on social behaviour in patients with acquired brain injury: A randomised controlled trial. *Scientific Reports*, *9*(*5831*), 1–8. doi: 10.1038/s41598-019-42280-0

Heindl, B. A. (1996). The effectiveness of pet therapy as an intervention in a community-based children's day treatment program. *Dissertation Abstracts International*, *57*(*4-A*), 1501.

Henry, R. (2007, July 26). Cat predicts deaths in nursing home. Associated Press. *Fort Worth Star Telegram*. Retrieved on September 27, 2016: www.star-telegram.com

Heppner, P. P., Kivlighan, D. M., and Wampold, B. E. (1999). *Research Design in Counseling* (2nd ed.). Belmont, CA: Wadsworth.

Hergovich, A., Monshi, B., Semmler, G., and Zieglmayer, V. (2002). The effects of the presence of a dog in the classroom. *Anthrozoös*, *15*(*1*), 37–50. doi: 10.2752/089279302786992775

Herzog, H. A. (2007). Gender differences in human–animal interactions: A review. *Anthrozoös*, *20*(*1*), 7–21. doi: 10.2752/089279307780216687

Herzog, H. A., Betchart, N. S., and Pittman, R. B. (1991). Gender, sex role orientation, and attitudes toward animals. *Anthrozoös*, *4*(*3*), 184–191. doi: 10.2752/089279391787057170

Hill, C. (2006). *How to Think Like a Horse: The essential handbook for understanding why horses do what they do*. North Adams, MA: Storey.

Hoffman, M. (1999). *Dogspeak: How to understand your dog and help him understand you*. Emmaus, PA: Rodale Press.

Hogan, K. (2008, December 2). Pets on campus? Yes, say many universities. *People Pets*. Retrieved on July 25, 2023: http://people.com/pets/pets-on-campus-yes-say-many-universities/

Holcomb, R., Jendro, C., Weber, B., and Nahan, U. (1997). Use of an aviary to relieve depression in elderly males. *Anthrozoös*, *10*(*1*), 32–36. doi: 10.2752/089279397787001292

Holcomb, R., and Meacham, M. (1989). Effectiveness of an animal-assisted therapy program in an inpatient psychiatric unit. *Anthrozoös*, *2*(*4*), 259–264. doi: 10.2752/089279389787057902

Holder, T. R. N., Gruen, M. E., Roberts, D. L., Somers, T., and Bozkurt, A. (2020a). A systematic literature review of animal-assisted interventions (Part I): Methods and results. *Integrative Cancer Therapies*, *19*, 1–18. doi: 10.1177/1534735420943278

Holder, T. R. N., Gruen, M. E., Roberts, D. L., Somers, T., and Bozkurt, A. (2020b). A systematic literature review of animal-assisted interventions in oncology (Part II): Theoretical mechanisms and frameworks. *Integrative Cancer Therapies*, *19*, 1–18. doi: 10.1177/1534735420943269

Holmes, C., Goodwin-Bond, D., Redhead, E., and Goymour, K. (2011). The benefits of equine-assisted activities: An exploratory study. *Child and Adolescent Social Work Journal, 29(2)*, 111–122. doi: 10.1007/s10560-011-0251-z

Hooker, S., Freeman, L., and Stewart, P. (2002). Pet therapy research: A historical review. *Holistic Nursing Practice, 17(1)*, 17–23. doi: 10.1097/00004650-200210000-00006

Hope Animal-Assisted Crisis Response (HOPE AACR). (n.d.). Retrieved on July 25, 2023: http://hopeaacr.org/

Horowitz, A. (2009). The last word: Inside a dog's world. *The Week*. Retrieved on July 25, 2023: http://theweek.com/article/index/100782/The_last_word_Inside_a_dogs_world

Horse and Man. (2010, August 3). I learned something today ... Inmate gentled mustang adoptions. Retrieved on July 25, 2023: www.horseandman.com/people-and-places/i-learned-something-today-inmate-gentled-mustang-adoptions/08/23/2010/

Hounds of Prison Education (HOPE). (n.d.). *HOPE: Hounds of Prison Education*. Correctional Institute at Camp Hill, Pennsylvania. Retrieved on July 25, 2023: www.hopedogs.org/

Hoyle, R. H. (1999). *Statistical Strategies for Small Sample Research*. Thousand Oaks, CA: Sage.

Huffington Post. (2013, April 22). Comfort dogs help provide emotional support in Boston after marathon bombing. Retrieved on July 25, 2023: www.huffingtonpost.com/2013/04/21/comfort-dogs-boston-marathon_n_3124023.html

Human–Animal Interaction. (n.d.). Retrieved on July 25, 2023: https://www.cabidigitallibrary.org/journal/hai/aims-and-scope

Humphries, T. L. (2003). Effectiveness of dolphin-assisted therapy as a behavioral intervention for young children with disabilities. Research and Training Center on Early Childhood Development, *Bridges, 1(6)*. Retrieved on July 25, 2023: www.waterplanetusa.com/images/Effectiveness_of_Dolphin_Assisted_Therapy.pdf

Iannuzzi, D., and Rowan, A. N. (1991). Ethical issues in animal-assisted therapy programs. *Anthrozoös, 4(3)*, 154–163. doi: 10.2752/089279391787057116

Iikura, Y., Sakamoto, Y., Imai, T., Akai, L., Matsuoka, T., Sugihara, K., et al. (2001). Dolphin-assisted seawater therapy for severe atopic dermatitis: An immunological and psychological study. *International Archives of Allergy and Immunology, 124(1–3)*, 389–390. doi: 10.1159/000053766

Institute for Human–Animal Connection (IHAC). (n.d.). History. Retrieved on July 25, 2023: www.du.edu/humananimalconnection/history.html

International Aid for Korean Animals. (n.d.). Retrieved on July 25, 2023: www.koreananimals.org

International Association of Human–Animal Interaction Organizations (IAHAIO). (n.d.). *About IAHAIO*. Washington: Author. Retrieved on July 25, 2023: www.iahaio.org/new/index.php?display=about

International Association of Human–Animal Interaction Organizations (IAHAIO). (2014). *IAHAIO White Paper 2014: The IAHAIO Definitions for Animal-Assisted Intervention and Guidelines for Wellness of Animals Involved*. Washington: Author. Retrieved on July 25, 2023: https://iahaio.org/best-practice/white-paper-on-animal-assisted-interventions/

International Society for Anthrozoology (ISAZ). (n.d.). Welcome/History. Retrieved on July 25, 2034: https://isaz.net/

Irwin, C., and Weber, B. (2001). *Horses Don't Lie: What horses teach us about our natural capacity for awareness, confidence, courage, and trust*. New York: Marlowe and Company.

Iwahashi, K., Waga, C., and Ohta, M. (2007). Questionnaire on animal-assisted therapy (AAT): The expectation for AAT as a day-care program for Japanese schizophrenic patients. *International Journal of Psychiatry in Clinical Practice, 11(4)*, 291–293. doi: 10.1080/13651500701245973

Jalongo, M. R., Astorino, T., and Bomboy, N. (2004). Canine visitors: The influence of therapy dogs on young children's learning and well-being in classrooms and hospitals. *Early Childhood Education Journal, 32(1)*, 9–16. doi: 10.1023/B:ECEJ.0000039638.60714.5f

Jenkins, E. K., DeChant, M. T., and Perry, E. B. (2018). When the nose doesn't know: Canine olfactory function associated with health, management and potential links to microbiota. *Frontiers in Veterinary Science, 5(56)*, 1–16. doi: 10.3389/fvets.2018.00056

Jewell, E., and Abate, F. (Eds.). (2001). *The New Oxford American Dictionary*. New York: Oxford University Press.

John, O., and Srivastava, S. (1999). The big five trait taxonomy: History, measurement, and theoretical perspectives. In L. A. Pervin and O. P. John (Eds.), *Handbook of Personality: Theory and research* (2nd ed., pp. 102–138). New York: Guilford Press.

Johnson, R. A., and Meadows, R. L. (2002). Older Latinos, pets, and health. *Western Journal of Nursing Research, 24*, 609–620. doi: 10.1177/019394502320555377

Jones, K. (1955). *Lunacy, Law, and Conscience 1744–1845*. London: Routledge and Kegan Paul.

K-9 Comfort Dogs. (n.d.). Retrieved on July 25, 2023: https://www.lutheranchurchcharities.org/k-9-comfort-dogs-about.html

K-9 Disaster Relief. (n.d.). Retrieved on July 25, 2023: www.k-9disasterrelief.org/

Kaiser, L., Spence, L. J., Lavergne, A. G., and Vanden Bosch, K. K. (2004). Can a week of therapeutic riding make a difference?—A pilot study. *Anthrozoös, 17*(1), 63–72. doi: 10.2752/089279304786991918

Kaminski, M., Pellino, T., and Wish, J. (2002). Play and pets: The physical and emotional impact of child-life and pet therapy on hospitalized children. *Children's Health Care, 31*(4), 321–335. doi: 10.1207/S15326888CHC3104_5

Karol, J. (2007). Applying a traditional individual psychotherapy model to equine-facilitated psychotherapy (EF): Theory and method. *Clinical Child Psychology and Psychiatry, 12*(1), 77–90. doi: 10.1177/1359104507071057

Katcher, A. H. (1985). Physiologic and behavioral responses to companion animals. In J. Quackenbush and V. Voith (Eds.), *The Human–Companion Animal Bond. The veterinary clinics of North America: Small animal practice, 15*(2), 403–410.

Katcher, A. H. (2000a). The centaur's lessons: Therapeutic education through care of animals and nature study. In A. Fine (Ed.), *Handbook on Animal-Assisted Therapy: Theoretical foundations and guidelines for practice* (pp. 153–177). San Diego, CA: Academic Press.

Katcher, A. H. (2000b). The future of education and research on the animal–human bond and animal-assisted therapy, Part B: Animal-assisted therapy and the study of human–animal relationships: Discipline or bondage? Context or transitional object? In A. Fine (Ed.), *Handbook on Animal-Assisted Therapy: Theoretical foundations and guidelines for practice* (pp. 461–473). San Diego, CA: Academic Press.

Katcher, A., Beck, A., and Levine, D. (1989). Evaluation of a pet program in prison—the PAL project at Lorton. *Anthrozoös, 2*(3), pp. 175–180. doi: 10.2752/089279389787058037

Katcher, A. H., and Wilkins, G. G. (2002). *The Centaur's Lessons: The companionable zoo method of therapeutic education based upon contact with animals and nature study*. Naperville, IL: People, Animals, Nature, Inc.

Katsinas, R. P. (2000). The use and implications of a canine companion in a therapeutic day program for nursing home residents with dementia. *Activities, Adaptation and Aging, 25*(1), 13–30. doi: 10.1300/J016v25n01_02

Kawamura, N., Niiyama, M., and Niiyama, H. (2009). Animal-assisted activity: Experiences of institutionalized Japanese older adults. *Journal of Psychosocial Nursing, 47*(1), 41–47. doi: 10.3928/02793695-20090101-08

Kay, N. (2011). Who was Dr. Leo Bustad? Spot speaks. Retrieved on July 25, 2023: http://speakingfor-spot.com/blog/2011/07/09/who-was-dr-leo-bustad/

Kazdin, A. E. (2011). Establishing the effectiveness of animal-assisted therapies: Methodological standards, issues, and strategies. In P. McCardle, S. McCune, J. A. Griffin, and V. Maholmes (Eds.), *How Animals Affect Us: Examining the influence of human–animal interaction on child development and human health* (pp. 35–51). Washington, D.C.: American Psychological Association.

Keino, H., Funahashi, A., Keino, H., Miwa, C., Hosokawa, M., Hayashi, Y., and Kawakita, K., (2009). Psycho-educational horseback riding to facilitate communication ability of children with pervasive developmental disorders. *Journal of Equine Science, 20*(4), 79–88. doi: 10.1294/jes.20.79

Kellert, S. R., and Berry, J. K. (1987). Attitudes, knowledge, and behaviors toward wildlife as affected by gender. *Wildlife Society Bulletin, 15*, 363–371.

Kemp, K., Signal, T., Botros, H., Taylor, N., and Prentice, K. (2014). Equine-facilitated therapy with children and adolescents who have been sexually abused: A program evaluation study. *Journal of Child and Family Studies, 23*, 558–566. doi: 10.1007/s10826-013-9718-1

Kendall, E., Maujean, A., Pepping, C., Downes, M., Lakhani, A., Byrne, J., and Macfarlane, K. (2015). A systematic review of the efficacy of equine-assisted interventions on psychological outcomes. *European Journal of Psychotherapy and Counseling, 17*(1), 57–79. doi: 10.1080/13642537.2014.996169

Kern, J. K., Fletcher, C. L., Garver, C. R., Mehta, J. A., Grannemann, B. D., Knox, K. R., Richardson, T. A., and Trivedki, M. H. (2011). Prospective trial of equine-assisted activities in Autism Spectrum Disorder. *Alternative Therapies, 17*(3), 14–20.

Kersten, G., and Thomas, L. (2004). *Equine-Assisted Psychotherapy and Learning: Untraining manual*. Santaquin, UT: Equine Assisted Growth and Learning, Association (EAGALA).

Kesner, A., and Pritzker, S. R. (2008). Therapeutic horseback riding with children placed in the foster care system. *ReVision, 30*(1 and 2), 77–87. doi: 10.4298/REVN.30.1/2.77-87

Kids and Animals: A healing partnership. (2006). Amazon.com: CustomFlix.

Kivlen, C., Winston, K., Mills, D., DiZazzo-Miller, R., Davenport, R., and Binfet, J-T. (2022). Canine-assisted intervention effects on the well-being of health science graduate students: A randomized controlled trial. *American Journal of Occupational Therapy, 76,* 7606205120. doi: 10.5014/ajot.2022.049508

Klontz, B. T., Bivens, A., Leinart, D., and Klontz, T. (2007). The effectiveness of equine-assisted experiential therapy: Results of an open clinical trial. *Society and Animals, 15,* 257–267. doi: 10.1163/156853007X217195

Kluger, J. (2010, August 16). Inside the minds of animals: Science is revealing just how smart other species can be—and raising new questions about how we treat them. *Time,* pp. 36–43. Retrieved on July 25, 2023: https://content.time.com/time/magazine/article/0,9171,2008867,00.html

Kogan, L. R. (2000). Effective animal-intervention for long-term care residents. *Activities, Adaptation and Aging, 25*(1), 31–45. doi: 10.1300/J016v25n01_03

Kogan, L. R., Granger, B. P., Fitchett, J. A., Helmer, K. A., and Young, K. J. (1999). The human–animal team approach for children with emotional disorders: Two case studies. *Child and Youth Care Forum, 28*(2), 105–121. doi: 10.1023/A:1021941205934

Kolander, C., Ballard, D., and Chandler, C. (2005). *Contemporary Women's Health: Issues for today and the future* (2nd ed.). St. Louis, MO: McGraw-Hill.

Konok, V., Nagy, and K., Miklósi, A. (2015). How do humans represent the emotions of dogs? The resemblance between the human representation of the canine and the human affective space. *Applied Animal Behavior Science, 162,* 37–46. doi: 10.1016/j.applanim.2014.11.003

Kotrschal, K., and Ortbauer, B. (2003). Behavioral effects of the presence of a dog in a classroom. *Anthrozoös, 16*(2), 147–159. doi: 10.2752/089279303786992170

Kottman, T. (2003). *Partners in Play: An Adlerian approach to play therapy* (2nd ed.). Alexandria, VA: American Counseling Association.

Kovács, Z., Bulucz, J., Kris, R., and Simon, L. (2006). An exploratory study of the effect of animal-assisted therapy on nonverbal communication of three schizophrenic patients. *Anthrozoös, 19*(4), 353–364. doi: 10.2752/089279306785415475

Kovács, Z., Kis, R., Rózsa, S., and Rózsa, L. (2004). Animal-assisted therapy for middle-aged schizophrenic patients living in a social situation: A pilot study. *Clinical Rehabilitation, 18,* 483–486. doi: 10.1191/0269215504cr765oa

Kraemer, H. C., and Thiemann, S. (1989). A strategy to use soft data effectively in randomized controlled clinical trials. *Journal of Consulting and Clinical Psychology, 57*(1), 148–154. doi: 10.1037/0022-006X.57.1.148

Kramer, S. H., and Rosenthal, R. (1999). Effect sizes and significance levels in small-sample research. In R. H. Hoyle (Ed.), *Statistical Strategies for Small Sample Research* (pp. 59–79). Thousand Oaks, CA: Sage.

Kršková, L., Talarovičová, A., and Olexová, L. (2010). Guinea pigs—the "small great" therapist for autistic children, or: Do guinea pigs have positive effects on autistic child social behavior? *Society and Animals, 18*(2), 139–151.

Künzi, P., Ackert, M., Holtforth, M., Hund-Geogiadis, M., and Hediger, K. (2022). Effects of animal-assisted psychotherapy incorporating mindfulness and self-compassion in neurorehabilitation: a randomized controlled feasibility trial. *Scientific Reports, 12* (10898), 1–13. doi: 10.1038/s41598-022-14584-1

Kutty, A. (2010, November 2). Muslims owning dogs: Permissible? *Islam Online.* Retrieved on July 25, 2023: https://fiqh.islamonline.net/en/muslims-owning-dogs-permissible/

Lambert, M. J., and Ogles, B. (2004). The efficacy and effectiveness of psychotherapy. In M. J. Lambert (Ed.), *Bergin and Garfield's Handbook of Psychotherapy and Behavior Change* (5th ed., pp. 139–193). New York: Wiley.

Landreth, G. (2002). *Play Therapy: The art of the relationship* (2nd ed.). New York: Brunner-Routledge.

Lange, A., Cox, J., Bernert, D., and Jenkins, C. (2007). Is counseling going to the dogs? An exploratory study related to the inclusion of an animal in group counseling with adolescents. *Journal of Creativity in Mental Health, 2*(2), 17–31. doi: 10.1300/J456v02n02_03

Lanning, B., and Krenek, N. (2013). Examining effects of equine-assisted activities to help combat veterans improve quality of life. *Journal of Rehabilitation Research and Development, 50*(8), xv–xxii. doi: 10.1682/JRRD.2013.07.0159

Lanning, B. A., Matyastik Baier, M. E., Ivey-Hatz, J., Krenek, N., and Tubbs, J. D. (2014). Effects of equine-assisted activities on autism spectrum disorder. *Journal of Autism and Developmental Disorders, 44,* 1897–1907. doi: 10.1007/s10803-014-2062-5

Lawrence, E. A. (1995). Cultural perceptions of differences between people and animals: A key to understanding human–animal relationships. *Journal of American Culture, 18*(3), 75–82. doi: 10.1111/J.1542-734X.1995.T01-1-00075.X

Lee, D. R. (1983). Pet therapy—Helping patients through troubled times. *California Veterinarian, 5*, 24–25, 40.

Lee, R., Zeglen, M. E., Ryan, T., and Hines, L. M. (1983). Guidelines: Animals in nursing homes. *California Veterinarian, 3*, 1a–43a.

Lefkowitz, C., Paharia, I., Prout, M., Debiak, D., and Bleiberg, J. (2005). Animal-assisted prolonged exposure: A treatment for survivors of sexual assault suffering post-traumatic stress disorder. *Society and Animals, 13*(4), 275–295. doi: 10.1163/156853005774653654

Lerner, M., Shelton, R., and Crawford, R. (2001). *Acute Traumatic Stress Management*. American Academy of Experts in Traumatic Stress.

Lerner, M., Volpe, J., and Lindell, B. (2004a). *A Practical Guide for Crisis Response in Our Schools* (5th ed.). American Academy of Experts in Traumatic Stress.

Lerner, M., Volpe, J., and Lindell, B. (2004b). *A Practical Guide for University Crisis Response*. American Academy of Experts in Traumatic Stress.

Levinson, B. M. (1962). The dog as a "co-therapist." *Mental Hygiene, 46*, 59–65.

Levinson, B. M. (1969). *Pet-Oriented Child Psychotherapy*. Springfield, IL: Charles C. Thomas.

Limond, J., Bradshaw, J., and Cormack, K. (1997). Behavior of children with learning disabilities interacting with a therapy dog. *Anthrozoös, 10*(2–3), 84–89. doi: 10.2752/089279397787001139

Lipin, T. (2009). Healing connections: One whisker, beak, hoof and cottontail at a time. *Interactions Magazine, 27*(2), 5–7, 24.

Locke, J. (1699). *Some Thoughts Concerning Education*. Reprinted with an introduction by F. W. Garforth (1964). Woodbury, NY: Barron's Educational Series.

Longnecker, E. (2009, June 24). Inmates give shelter cats new lease on life. Retrieved on October 14, 2016: www.wthr.com/Global/story.asp?S=10591589

Looney, A. (2009, April 6). LSU Ag Residential College pilots animal-assisted therapy program. *LSU News, 3*(2), Louisiana State University. Retrieved on October 14, 2016: www.lsu.edu

Lou, J. (2010, June 9). Dogs on campus. *The Bark: Dog is my co-pilot*. Retrieved on October 14, 2016: http://thebark.com/content/dogs-campus

Lucidi, P., Bernabò, N., Panunzi, M., Dalla Villa, P., and Mattioli, M. (2005). Ethotest: A new model to identify (shelter) dogs' skills as service animals or adoptable pets. *Applied Animal Behaviour Science, 95*, 103–122. doi: 10.1016/j.applanim.2005.04.006

Lukina, L. N. (1999). Influence of dolphin-assisted therapy sessions on the functional state of children with psychoneurological symptoms of diseases. *Human Physiology, 25*(6), 676–679.

Lynch, J. J., Fregin, G. F., Mackie, J. B., and Monroe, R. R. Jr. (1974). Heart rate changes in the horse to human contact. *Psychophysiology, 11*(4), 472–478. doi: 10.1111/j.1469-8986.1974.tb00575.x

Maayan, E. (2013). The therapy zoo as a mirror to the psyche. In N. Parish-Plass (Ed.), *Animal-Assisted Psychotherapy: Theory, issues and practice*. Lafayette, IN: Purdue University Press.

Macauley, B. L., and Gutierrez, K. M. (2004). The effectiveness of hippotherapy for children with language-learning disabilities. *Communication Disorders Quarterly, 25*(4), 205–217. doi: 10.1177/15257401040250040501

Macdonald, A. (2007). *Solution-Focused Therapy: Theory, research and practice*. Los Angeles, CA: Sage.

MacGill, M. (2015, September 21). Oxytocin: What is it and what does it do? *Medical News Today*. Retrieved on July 25, 2023: www.medicalnewstoday.com/articles/275795.php

Mackin, T. (2014, April 10). Shelter cats find freedom at Pendleton Prison. Retrieved on July 25, 2023: https://www.wishtv.com/news/shelter-cats-find-freedom-at-pendleton-prison/

Malavasi, R., and Huber, L. (2016). Evidence of heterospecific referential communication from domestic horses (*Equus caballus*) to humans. *Animal Cognition, 19*, 899–909. doi: 10.1007/s10071-016-0987-0

Mallon, G. P. (1994a). Cow as co-therapist: Utilization of farm animals as therapeutic aides with children in residential treatment. *Child and Adolescent Social Work Journal, 11*(6), 455–474. doi: 10.1007/BF01876570

Mallon, G. P. (1994b). Some of our best therapists are dogs. *Child and Youth Care Forum, 23*(2), 89–101. doi: 10.1007/BF02209256

Marcus, D. A. (2013). The science behind animal-assisted therapy. *Current Pain and Headache Reports, 17*, 1–7. doi: 10.1007/s11916-013-0322-2

Marino, L., and Lilienfeld, S. O. (1998). Dolphin-assisted therapy: Flawed data, flawed conclusions. *Anthrozoös, 11*(4), 194–200. doi: 10.2752/089279398787000517

Marino, L., and Lilienfeld, S. O. (2007). Dolphin-assisted therapy: More flawed data and more flawed conclusions. *Anthrozoös, 20*(3), 239–249. doi: 10.2752/089279307X224782

Marmer, L. (1997, October 6). A llama at school: It makes the children laugh and play. *Advance Online for Occupational Therapists.* Retrieved on October 17, 2016: http://occupationaltherapy.advance web.com

Marr, C., French, L., Thompson, D., Drum, L., Greening, G., Mormon, J., et al. (2000). Animal-assisted therapy in psychiatric rehabilitation. *Anthrozoös, 13*(1), 43–47. doi: 10.2752/089279300786999950

Marshall, C., and Rossman, G. B. (1999). *Designing Qualitative Research* (3rd ed.). Thousand Oaks, CA: Sage.

Martens, P., Enders-Slegers, M. J., and Walker, J. (2016). The emotional lives of companion animals: Attachment and subjective claims by owners of cats and dogs. *Anthrozoös, 29*(1), 73–88. doi: 10.1080/08927936.2015.1075299

Martin, F., and Farnum, J. (2002). Animal-assisted therapy for children with pervasive developmental disorders. *Western Journal of Nursing Research, 24*(6), 657–671. doi: 10.1177/019394502320555403

Matuszek, S. (2010). Animal-facilitated therapy in various patient populations. *Holistic Nursing Practice*, July/August, 187–203. doi: 10.1097/HNP.0b013e3181e90197

Maxwell, S. E. (1998). Longitudinal designs in randomized group comparisons: When will intermediate observations increase statistical power? *Psychological Methods, 3*(3), 275–290. doi: 10.1037/1082-989X.3.3.275

McCulloch, M., Jezierski, T., Broffman, M., Hubbard, A., Turner, K., and Janecki, T. (2006). Diagnostic accuracy of canine scent detection in early- and late-stage lung and breast cancers. *Integrative Cancer Therapies, 5*(1), 30–39. doi: 10.1177/1534735405285096.

McCullough, A., Ruehrdanz, A., Jenkins, M., Gilmer, M. J., Olson, J., Pawar, A., Holley, L. Sierra-Rivera, S., Linder, D., Pichette, D., Grossman, N., Hellman, C., Guérin, N. A., and O'Haire, M. E. (2018). Measuring the effects of an animal-assisted intervention for pediatric oncology patients and their parents: A multisite randomized controlled trial. *Journal of Pediatric Oncology Nursing, 35*(3), 159–177. doi: 10.1177/1043454217748586

McDonough, Y. Z. (2009). In the classroom: Why pets are the perfect pals. *Webvet.com.* Retrieved on September 27, 2016: www.webvet.com/main/article/id/2069

McFalls-Steger, C., Patterson, D., and Thompson, P. (2021). Effectiveness of animal-assisted interventions (AAI) in treatment of adults with depressive symptoms: A systematic review. *Human-Animal Interaction Bulletin, 12*(2), 46–64. Retrieved on July 26, 2023: https://www.cabidigital library.org/doi/pdf/10.1079/hai.2021.0007

McGreevy, P. (2012). *Equine Behavior: A guide for veterinarians and equine scientists* (2nd ed.). New York: Saunders.

McKenzie, A. (2003, May 17). Sit, stay, HEAL: Therapist uses pets to lead patients down the road to recovery. *Dallas Morning News*, pp. 3E, 7E.

McMullin, R. E. (1986). *Handbook of Cognitive Therapy Techniques.* New York: W. W. Norton.

McNair, D., Lorr, M., and Droppleman, L. (1992). *Profile of Mood States Manual.* North Tonawanda, NY: Multi-Health Systems.

McVarish, C. A. (1995). The effects of pet-facilitated therapy on depressed institutionalized inpatients. *Dissertation Abstracts International, 55*(7-B), 3019.

Memishevikj, H., and Hodzhikj, S. (2010). The effects of equine-assisted therapy in improving the psychosocial functioning of children with autism. *Journal of Special Education and Rehabilitation, 11*(3–4), 57–67. doi: 10.5281/zenodo.28308

Merriam-Arduini, S. (2000). *Evaluation of an Experimental Program Designed to Have a Positive Effect on Adjudicated, Violent, Incarcerated Male Juveniles Age 12–25 in the State of Oregon.* Unpublished dissertation. Pepperdine University, Malibu, CA.

Merriam-Webster.com. (n.d.). Online dictionary. Retrieved on October 9, 2016: www.merriam-webster.com

Miklósi, A., Polgárdi, R., Topál, J., and Csányi, V. (2000). Intentional behaviour in dog–human communication: An experimental analysis of "showing" behaviour in the dog. *Animal Cognition, 3*(3), 159–166. doi: 10.1007/s100710000072

Miller, J. (Ed.). (2008). *Evaluation of the C.H.A.M.P. Service Dog Training Program at the Women's Eastern Reception, Diagnostic, and Correctional Center.* Research report to the Missouri Department of Corrections and the C.H.A.M.P Assistance Dogs.

Miller, S. C., Kennedy, K., Devoe, D., Hickey, M., Nelson, T., and Kogan, L. (2009). Oxytocin levels in men and women before and after interaction with a bonded dog. *Anthrozoös, 22*(1), 31–42. doi: 10.2752/175303708X390455

Minatrea, N. B., and Wesley, M. C. (2008). Reality therapy goes to the dogs. *International Journal of Reality Therapy*, *28*, 69–77.

Moneymaker, J. M., and Strimple, E. O. (1991). Animals and inmates: A sharing companionship behind bars. *Journal of Offender Rehabilitation*, *16(3–4)*, 133–152. doi: 10.1300/J076v16n03_09

Monfort, M., Benito, A., Haro, G., Fuertes-Saiz, A., Canabate, M., and Baquero, A. (2022). The efficacy of animal-assisted therapy in patients with dual diagnosis: Schizophrenia and addiction. *International Journal of Environment Research and Public Health*, *19(11)*. doi: 10.3390/ijerph19116695

Morell, V. (2014, November 26). Dogs really do listen to us. *Science*. Retrieved on November 29, 2023: https://www.science.org/content/article/dogs-really-do-listen-us?adobe_mc=MCMID%3D884 194276844225100808991483280134650107CMCORGID%3D242B6472541199F70A4C 98A6%2540AdobeOrg%7CTS%3D1677946179

Morris, P. H., Gale, A., and Howe, S. (2002). The factor structure of horse personality. *Anthrozoös*, *15(4)*, 300–322. doi: 10.2752/089279302786992414

Mossello, E., Ridolfi, A., Mello, A. M., Lorenzini, G., Mugnai, F., Piccini, C., Barone, D., Peruzzi, A., Masotti, G., and Marchionni, N. (2011). Animal-assisted activity and emotional status of patients with Alzheimer's disease in day care. *International Psychogeriatrics*, *23(6)*, 899–905. doi: 10.1017/S1041610211000226

Mulcahy, C., and McLaughlin, D. (2013). Is the tail wagging the dog? A review of the evidence for prison animal programs. *Australian Psychologist*, *48*, 369–378. doi: 10.1111/ap.12021

Munro, E. (2004, May/June). Minority report III: Reservation rescues. *Best Friends Magazine*, 14–15.

Nagengast, S. L., Baun, M., Megel, M., and Leibowitz, M. (1997). The effects of the presence of a companion animal on physiological arousal and behavioral distress in children during a physical examination. *Journal of Pediatric Nursing*, *12*, 323–330. doi: 10.1016/s0882-5963(97)80058-9

Nathans-Barel, I., Feldman, P., Berger, B., Modai, I., and Silver, H. (2005). Animal-assisted therapy ameliorates anhedonia in schizophrenic patients. *Psychotherapy and Psychosomatics*, *74(1)*, 31–35. doi: 10.1159/000082024

Nathanson, D. E. (1989). Using Atlantic bottlenose dolphins to increase cognition of mentally retarded children. In P. Lovibond and P. Wilson (Eds.), *Clinical and Abnormal Psychology* (pp. 233–242). North Holland: Elsevier Science Publishers.

Nathanson, D. E. (1998). Long-term effectiveness of dolphin-assisted therapy for children with severe disabilities. *Anthrozoös*, *11(1)*, 22–32. doi: 10.1080/08927936.1998.11425084

Nathanson, D. E., de Castro, D., Friend, H., and McMahon, M. (1997). Effectiveness of short-term dolphin-assisted therapy for children with severe disabilities. *Anthrozoös*, *10(2–3)*, 90–100.

Nathanson, D. E., and de Faria, S. (1993). Cognitive improvement of children in water with and without dolphins. *Anthrozoös*, *6(1)*, 17–29. doi: 10.2752/089279393787002367

National American Pit Bull Terrier Association (NAPBTA). (2000, Spring–Summer). Delta Society award winner. *NAPBTA Bulletin*, 2.

National Association of Social Workers (NASW). (2008). Code of ethics of the National Association of Social Workers. Retrieved on July 26, 2023: https://www.socialworkers.org/About/Ethics/Code-of-Ethics/Code-of-Ethics-English

National Child Traumatic Stress Network and National Center for PTSD. (2006). *Psychological First Aid* (2nd ed.). Retrieved on July 26, 2023: https://www.nctsn.org/resources/all-nctsn-resources

National Organization for Victim Assistance (NOVA). (2004). Community Crisis Response Team Training Manual. Retrieved on July 26, 2023: www.try-nova.org

Nef, N. (2004, October). The cat programme, an animal-assisted therapy at Saxierriet Prison for men: Its effects and results in a correctional establishment. Paper presented at the 10th International Conference on Human–Animal Interactions, People and Animals: A timeless relationship. Glasgow, Scotland.

Nepps, P., Stewart, C. N., and Bruckno, S. R. (2014). Animal-assisted activity: Effects of a complementary intervention program on psychological and physiological variables. *Journal of Evidenced-Based Complementary and Alternative Medicine*, *19*, 211–215. doi: 10.1177/2156587214533570

New Leash on Life Project. (n.d.). Pet therapy. Juvenile Justice Services, Calcasieu Parish, Louisiana. Retrieved on September 27, 2016: www.cppj.net/index.aspx?page=379

Niederberger, M. (2010, November 11). Pet friendly dorm make life pleasant at W and J. *Pittsburgh Post-Gazette*. Retrieved on July 26, 2023: www.post-gazette.com/local/south/2010/11/11/Pet-friendly-dorm-makes-life-pleasant-at-W-amp-J/stories/201011110339

Nightingale, F. (1859). *Notes on Nursing: What it is and what it is not*. London: Harrison of Pall Mall.

Nimer, J., and Lundahl, B. (2007). Animal-assisted therapy: A meta-analysis. *Anthrozoös*, *20(3)*, 225–238. doi: 10.2752/089279307X224773

Nordgren, L., and Engström, G. (2014). Animal-assisted intervention in dementia: Effects on quality of life. *Clinical Nursing Research*, 23(1), 7–19. doi: 10.1177/1054773813492546

North American Riding for the Handicapped Association (NARHA is now PATH International). (n.d.). Retrieved on September 27, 2016: www.narha.org

NYU Langone Medical Center. (2013, December 2). Welcome to Rusk Rehabilitation. Retrieved on July 26, 2023: http://nyulangone.org/locations/rusk-rehabilitation

Obrusnikova, I., Bibik, J., Cavalier, A., and Manley, K. (2012). Integrating therapy dog teams in a physical activity program for children with autism spectrum disorders. *Journal of Physical Education, Recreation and Dance*, 83(6), 37–48. doi: 10.1080/07303084.2012.10598794

O'Callaghan, D. (2008). *Exploratory Study of Animal-Assisted Therapy Interventions Used By Mental Health Professionals*. Unpublished dissertation. University of North Texas, Denton.

O'Callaghan, D. M., and Chandler, C. K. (2011). An exploratory study of animal-assisted interventions utilized by mental health professionals. *Journal of Creativity in Mental Health*, 6(2), 90–104. doi: 10.1080/15401383.2011.579862

O'Connor, C. (2006). The silent therapist: A review of the development of equine-assisted psychotherapy. Retrieved on October 12, 2016: www.catra.net/info/silent.html

Odendaal, J. S. J. (2000). Animal-assisted therapy—magic or medicine? *Journal of Psychosomatic Research*, 49(4), 275–280. doi: 10.1016/S0022-3999(00)00183-5

Odendaal, J. S., and Meintjes, R. A. (2003). Neurophysiological correlates of affiliative behavior between humans and dogs. *The Veterinary Journal*, 165(3), 296–301. doi: 10.1016/s1090-0233(02)00237-x

Orey, C. (2002). An American symbol: From a WWI poster dog to a movie star, bully breeds embody the American spirit. *Popular Dogs Series: Bully Breeds*, 21, 34–39.

Otting, T. (2016). *Human–animal Relational Theory: A constructivist-grounded theory investigation*. Doctoral dissertation. University of North Texas, Denton, TX.

Otting, T. L., and Chandler, C. K. (2023). Credibility of human–animal relational theory. *Journal of Creativity in Mental Health*, 18(3), 318–331 (first published online, 2021). doi: 10.1080/15401383.2021.1987366

Paddock, C. (2010, April 27). Dogs helped kids improve reading fluency. *Medical News Today*. Retrieved on July 26, 2023: www.medicalnewstoday.com/articles/186708.php

Pamer, M., and Manning, S. (2013, February 15). Dogs make fine companions for cheetahs at San Diego Zoo. *NBC Los Angeles*. Retrieved on July 26, 2023: www.nbclosangeles.com/news/local/Dogs-Make-Fine-Companions-for-Cheetahs-at-San-Diego-Zoo-191441321.html

Panksepp, J. (1998). *Affective Neuroscience: The foundations of human and animal emotions*. New York: Oxford University Press.

Panksepp, J. (2005). Affective consciousness: Core emotional feelings in animals and humans. *Consciousness and Cognition*, 14, 30–80. doi: 10.1016/j.concog.2004.10.004

Panzer-Koplow, S. (2000). *Effects of Animal-Assisted Therapy on Depression and Morale Among Nursing Home Residents*. Doctoral dissertation. Rutgers, The State University of New Jersey.

Parish-Plass, N. (2008). Animal-assisted therapy with children suffering from insecure attachment due to abuse and neglect: A method to lower the risk of intergenerational transmission of abuse? *Clinical Child Psychology and Psychiatry*, 13(1), 7–30. doi: 10.1177/1359104507086338

Parish-Plass, N. (2013). *Animal-Assisted Psychotherapy: Theory, issues and practice*. Lafayette, IN: Purdue University Press.

Parshall, D. P. (2003). Research and reflection: Animal-assisted therapy in mental health settings. *Counseling and Values*, 48, 47–56. doi: 10.1002/j.2161-007X.2003.tb00274.x

PBS Deep Look. (2019, February 27). How your dog's nose knows so much. Retrieved on July 30, 2022: https://www.pbs.org/video/how-your-dogs-nose-knows-so-much-keaa4h/

PBS Nature. (2008, June 9). Underdogs: The bloodhound's amazing sense of smell. Retrieved on July 30, 2022: www.pbs.org/wnet/nature/underdogs-the-bloodhounds-amazing-sense-of-smell/350/

Pedersen, I., Nordaunet, T., Martinsen, E. W., Berget, B., and Braastad, B. O. (2011). Farm animal-assisted intervention: Relationship between work and contact with farm animals and change in depression, anxiety, and self-efficacy among persons with clinical depression. *Issues in Mental Health Nursing*, 32, 493–500. doi: 10.3109/01612840.2011.566982

Pelka, F. (1997). *The ABC-CLIO Companion to the Disability Rights Movement*. Santa Barbara, CA: ABC-CLIO.

Pen Pals: A New Leash on Life. (n.d.). Pen Pals Prison Program. Retrieved on July 26, 2023: http://newleashinc.org/what-we-do/pen-pals-prison-program/

Pendry, P., Carr, A., Smith, A., and Roeter, S. (2014). Improving adolescent social competence and behavior: A randomized trial of an 11-week equine-facilitated learning prevention program. *The Journal of Primary Prevention*, 35, 281–293. doi: 10.1007/s10935-014-0350-7

Pendry, P., and Roeter, S. (2012). Experimental trial demonstrates positive effects of equine-facilitated learning on child competence. *Human–Animal Interaction, 1(1)*, 1–19. Retrieved on July 26, 2023: https://www.cabidigitallibrary.org/doi/pdf/10.1079/hai.2013.0004

Pendry, P., Smith, A., and Roeter, S. (2014). Randomized trial examines effects of equine-facilitated learning on adolescents' basal cortisol levels. *Human–Animal Interaction Bulletin, 2(1)*, 80–95. doi: 10.1079/hai.2014.0003

Perelle, I., and Granville, D. (1993). Assessment of the effectiveness of a pet-facilitated therapy program in a nursing home setting. *Society and Animals, 1(1)*, 91–100. doi: 10.1163/156853093X00172

Perls, F. S., Hefferline, R. F., and Goodman, P. (1980). *Gestalt Therapy*. New York: Bantam.

Pet Partners. (2014). *Pet Partners Handler Student Guide: Pet partners therapy animal program for animal-assisted activities and animal-assisted therapy*. Bellevue, WA: Author.

Pet Partners. (2019). *Team Evaluator Policies and Procedures Manual: Pet Partners therapy animal program for animal-assisted interventions*. Bellevue, WA: Author.

Pet Partners. (2023a). Who we are. Retrieved on March 1, 2023: https://petpartners.org/about-us/who-we-are/

Pet Partners. (2023b). About. Retrieved on March 1, 2023: https://petpartners.org/about-us/

Pet Therapy Program. (n.d.). Dogs bring unconditional love to the residents of the detention center. Department of Juvenile Services, Ocean County, New Jersey. Retrieved on October 14, 2016: www.co.ocean.nj.us/ocjs/PetTherapy.aspx

Peters, S. L. (2008, September 9). Pets take the bite out of dorm life. *USA Today*. Retrieved on October 14, 2016: www.usatoday.com/news/education/2008-09-23-dorm-pets_N.htm

Pew Research Center. (2006). *Gauging family intimacy: Dogs edge cats (dads trail both)*. Washington, D.C.: Author. Retrieved on July 26, 2023: www.pewsocialtrends.org/2006/03/07/gauging-family-intimacy/

Pichot, T. (2011). *Animal-Assisted Brief Therapy: A solution-focused approach* (2nd ed.). New York: Routledge.

Pittman, T. (2015, July 16). A quick breakdown of the difference between Hispanic, Latino and Spanish. *Huffington Post*. Retrieved on July 26, 2023: www.huffingtonpost.com/entry/difference-between-hispanic-latino-and-spanish_us_55a7ec20e4b0c5f0322c9e44

Poss, J. E., and Bader, J. O. (2007). Attitudes toward companion animals among Hispanic residents of a Texas border community. *Journal of Applied Animal Welfare Science, 10(3)*, 243–253. doi: 10.1080/10888700701353717

Preziosi, R. J. (1997, Spring). For your consideration: A pet assisted therapist facilitator code of ethics. *Latham Letter*, 5–6. Retrieved on July 26, 2023: www.latham.org/Issues/LL_97_SP.pdf#page=

Pringle, L. P., and Henderson, M. (2004). *Dog of Discovery: A Newfoundland's adventures with Lewis and Clark*. Honesdale, PA: Boyds Mills Press.

Prison Pet Partnership Program. (n.d.). Washington State Correctional Center for Women Prison Pet Partnership Program: Maximum Security Prison. Retrieved on October 6, 2016: http://prisonp.tripod.com/

Prison PUP Program. (n.d.). Massachusetts Department of Corrections North Central Correctional Institution along with NEADS (National Education for Assistance Dog Services) Prison PUP Program. Retrieved on October 6, 2016: http://prisonp.tripod.com/neads.htm

Professional Association for Therapeutic Horsemanship, International (PATH, Intl.). (n.d.a). About PATH, Intl. Retrieved on September 27, 2016: www.pathintl.org

Professional Association for Therapeutic Horsemanship, International (PATH, Intl.). (n.d.b). Center accreditation. Retrieved on September 27, 2016: www.pathintl.org

Professional Association for Therapeutic Horsemanship, International (PATH, Intl.). (n.d.c). Codes of ethics. Retrieved on September 27, 2016: www.pathintl.org

Prothmann, A., Bienert, M., and Ettrich, C. (2006). Dogs in child psychotherapy: Effects on state of mind. *Anthrozoös, 19(3)*, 265–277. doi: 10.2752/089279306785415583

Prothmann, A., Ettrich, C., and Prothmann, S. (2009). Preference for, and responsiveness to, people, dogs and objects in children with autism. *Anthrozoös, 22(2)*, 161–171. doi: 10.2752/175303709X434185

Ptak, A. L., and Howie, A. R. (2004). Healing paws and tails: The case for animal-assisted therapy in hospitals. *Interactions, 22(2)*, 5–9.

Ptak, A. L., and Howie, A. R. (2005). Pet Partners helping hospice patients. *Interactions, 23(1)*, 4–13.

Puppies Behind Bars. (n.d.). *Puppies Behind Bars*. Department of Corrections, New York. Retrieved on July 26, 2023: www.puppiesbehindbars.com

Raat, H., Botterweck, A., Landgraf, J., Hoogeveen, W., and Essink-Bot, M. (2005). Reliability and validity of the short form of the Child Health Questionnaire for parents (CHQ-PF28) in large random school based and general population samples. *Journal of Epidemiology and Community Health, 59,* 75–82. doi: 10.1136/jech.2003.012914

Rabbitt, S., Kazdin, A., and Hong, J. (2014). Acceptability of animal-assisted therapy: Attitudes toward AAT, psychotherapy, and medication for the treatment of child disruptive behavioral problems. *Antrhozoös, 27*(3), 335–350. doi: 10.2752/175303714X13903827487881

Rainbow Days, Inc. (n.d.). Curriculum-based support groups. Retrieved on October 13, 2016: http://rainbowdays.org/about-us/

Rainbow Days, Inc. (1998). *Kids' Connection: A support group curriculum for children, ages 4–12.* Dallas, TX: Author.

Raymond, J. (2016, April 15). Campus therapy dogs offer a helping paw to stressed students. *NBC News.* Retrieved on July 26, 2023: www.nbcnews.com/feature/college-game-plan/campus-therapy-dogs-offer-helping-paw-stressed-students-n556576

Rea, J. L. (2000, July 31). Special therapy dogs learn how to heal. *The Register-Guard,* p. 1D.

Redefer, L. A., and Goodman, J. F. (1989). Brief report: Pet-facilitated therapy with autistic children. *Journal of Autism and Developmental Disorders, 19*(3), 461–467. doi: 10.1007/BF02212943

Reichert, E. (1994). Play and animal-assisted therapy: A group-treatment model for sexually abused girls ages 9–13. *Family Therapy, 21*(1), 55–62.

Reichert, E. (1998). Individual counseling for sexually abused children: A role for animals and story-telling. *Child and Adolescent Social Work Journal, 15*(3), 177–185. doi: 10.1023/A:1022284418096

Reisen, J. (2020, July 21). The nose knows: Is there anything like a dog's nose? Retrieved on July 30, 2022: https://www.akc.org/expert-advice/news/the-nose-knows/

Reynolds, C. R., and Kamphaus, R. W. (1992). *Manual for the Behavior Assessment System for Children.* Circle Pines, MN: American Guidance Service.

Rhoades, R. (2001, Summer). Sentence for salvation: Behind the walls of correctional institutions, inmates find a renewed sense of purpose through working with injured and rescued animals. *ASPCA Animal Watch,* pp. 24–27.

Richard, J. (2004, March/April). Minority report II: The humane movement in the Latino community. *Best Friends Magazine,* 12–15.

Richeson, N. E. (2003). Effects of animal-assisted therapy on agitated behaviors and social interactions of older adults with dementia. *American Journal of Alzheimer's Disease and Other Dementias, 18,* 353–358. doi: 10.1177/153331750301800610

Risley-Curtiss, C., Holley, L. C., Cruickshank, T., Porcelli, J., Rhoads, C., Bacchus, D., and Nyakoe, S. (2006). "She was family": Women of color and their animal–human connections. *AFFILIA: Journal of Women and Social Work, 21,* 433–447. doi: 10.1177/0886109906292314

Risley-Curtiss, C., Holley, L. C., and Wolf, S. (2006). The animal–human bond and ethnic diversity. *Social Work, 51,* 257–268. doi: 10.1093/sw/51.3.257

Rivera, M. A. (2004). *Canines in the Classroom.* New York: Lantern Books.

Rizzolatti, G., Camarda, R., Fogassi, M., Gentilucci, M., Lupino, G., and Matelli, M. (1988). Functional organization of inferior area 6 in the macaque monkey: II. Area 5 and the control of distal movements. *Experimental Brain Research, 71,* 491–507. doi: 10.1007/BF00248742

Rizzolatti, G., Scandolora, C., Matelli, M., and Gentilucci, M. (1981). Afferent properties of periarcuate neurons in macaque monkeys: I. Somatosensory responses. *Behavioural Brain Research, 2*(2), 125–146. doi: 10.1016/0166-4328(81)90052-8

Roberts, M. (2008). *The Man who Listens to Horses: The story of a real-life horse whisperer.* New York: Ballantine.

Robin, M., and ten Bensel, R. (1985). Pets and the socialization of children. *Marriage and Family Therapy, 8*(3–4), 63–78. doi: 10.4324/9781315784656-6

Robinson, I. H. (1999). The human–horse relationship: How much do we know? *Equine Veterinary Journal,* Supplement *28,* 42–45. doi: 10.1111/j.2042-3306.1999.tb05155.x

Rodriguez, K. E., Green, F. L., Binfet, J-T., Townsend, L., and Gee, N. (2023). Complexities and considerations in conducting animal-assisted intervention research: A discussion of randomized controlled trials. *Human–Animal Interactions.* doi: 10.1079/hai.2023.0004

Rodriguez, K. E., Guérin, N. A., Gabriels, R. L., Serpell, J. A., Schreiner, P. J., and O'Haire, M. E. (2018). The state of assessment in human–animal interaction research. *Human–Animal Interaction Bulletin, 6*(special edition), 63–81. doi: 10.1079/hai.2018.0022

Rodriguez, K. E., Herzog, H., and Gee, N. R. (2021). Variability in human–animal interaction research. *Frontiers in Veterinary Science, 7,* 1–9. doi: 10.3389/fvets.2020.619600

Rogers, C. (1963). Psychotherapy to-day or where do we go from here? *American Journal of Psychotherapy, 17,* 5–16. doi: 10.1176/appi.psychotherapy.1963.17.1.5

Rohnke, K., and Butler, S. (1995). *Quicksilver: Adventure games, initiative problems, trust activities and a guide to effective leadership*. Dubuque, IA: Kendall/Hunt Publishing.

Rollin, B. E. (2009). Animal ethics and breed-specific legislation. *Journal of Animal Law*, 5, 1–14. Retrieved on July 26, 2023: https://www.animallaw.info/policy/journal-animal-law-table-contents-volume-5

Rombold Zeigenfuse, M., and Walker, J. (1997). *Dog Tricks: Step by step*. New York: Howell.

Rørvang, M. V., Nielsen, B. L., and McLean, A. N. (2020). Sensory abilities of horses and their importance for equitation science. *Frontiers in Veterinary Science*, 7(633), 1–17. doi: 10.3389/fvets.2020.00633

Ross, S. B. Jr. (2011). *The Extraordinary Sprit of Green Chimneys: Connecting children and animals to create hope*. West Lafayette, IN: Purdue University Press.

Royal Society for the Prevention of Cruelty to Animals (RSPCA). (2005–2006). Canine tail docking. Retrieved on July 26, 2023: www.rspca.org.uk

Rubin, R. (2014, November 17). AIDET® in the medical practice: More important than ever. The Studer Group. Retrieved on March 17, 2016: www.studergroup.com/resources/news-media/healthcare-publications-resources/insights/november-2014/aidet-in-the-medical-practice-more-important-than

Rud, A. G., and Beck, A. M. (2003). Companion animals in Indiana elementary schools. *Anthrozoös*, 16(3), 241–251. doi: 10.2752/089279303786992134

Rugaas, T. (2005). *Calming Signals: What your dog tells you*. Wenatchee, WA: Dogwise Publishing.

Rusk, H. A. (1972). *A World to Care For: The autobiography of Howard A. Rusk M.D.* New York: Random House.

Russell-Martin, L. (2006). *Equine Facilitated Couples Therapy and Solution Focused Couples Therapy: A comparison study*. Unpublished dissertation. Northcentral University, Prescott, AZ.

Ryan, J. (2010, Summer). Learning with the help of horses. *SCAS Journal*, 10–15.

Salgueiro, E., Nunes, L., Barros, A., Maroco, J., Salgueiro, A., and dos Santos, M. (2012). Effects of a dolphin interaction program on children with autism spectrum disorders—an exploratory research. *BMC Research Notes*, 5(199). Retrieved on October 24, 2016: https://bmcresnotes.biomedcentral.com/articles/10.1186/1756-0500-5-199

Salotto, P. (2001). *Pet Assisted Therapy: A loving intervention and an emerging profession: Leading to a friendlier, healthier, and more peaceful world*. Norton, MA: D. J. Publications.

Sams, M. J., Fortney, E. V., and Willenbring, S. (2006). Occupational therapy incorporating animals for children with autism: A pilot investigation. *American Journal of Occupational Therapy*, 60, 268–274. doi: 10.5014/ajot.60.3.268

Samsung. (2003). Creating a better future for all. Unpublished video recording. Office of International Relations, Samsung Everland, Kyounggio-do, South Korea.

Samuels, A., and Spradlin, T. (1995). Quantitative behavioral study of bottlenose dolphins in swim-with-dolphin programs in the United States. *Marine Mammal Science*, 11(4), 520–544. doi: 10.1111/j.1748-7692.1995.tb00675.x

Sanders, C. R. (1993). Understanding dogs: Caretakers' attributions of mindedness in canine–human relationships. *Journal of Contemporary Ethnography*, 22(2), 205–226. doi: 10.1177/089124193022002003

Sanders, C. R., and Arluke, A. (1993). If lions could speak: Investigating the animal–human relationship and the perspectives of nonhuman others. *Sociological Quarterly*, 34(3), 377–390. doi: 10.1111/j.1533-8525.1993.tb00117.x

Schaffer, C. B. (1993). *The Tuskegee Behavior Test for Selecting Therapy Dogs* [motion picture]. Tuskegee, AL: Center for the Study of Human–Animal Interdependent Relationships, School of Veterinary Medicine, Tuskegee University.

Scheck, H., Williamson, L., and Dell, C. A. (2022). Understanding psychiatric patients' experience of virtual animal-assisted therapy sessions during the COVID-19 Pandemic. *People and Animals: The International Journal of Research and Practice*, 5(1, 6), 1–8. doi: https://docs.lib.purdue.edu/paij/vol5/iss1/6

Schneider, M. S., and Pilchak Harley, L. (2006). How dogs influence the evaluation of psychotherapists. *Anthrozoös*, 19(2), 128–142. doi: 10.2752/089279306785593784

Schoenfeld-Tacher, R., Kogan, L., and Wright, M. L. (2010). Comparison of the strength of the human–animal bond between Hispanic and non-Hispanic owners of pet dogs and cats. *Journal of the American Veterinary Medical Association*, 236(5), 529–534. doi: 10.2460/javma.236.5.529

Schuck, S., Emmerson, N., Fine, A., and Lakes, K. (2015). Canine-assisted therapy for children with ADHD: Preliminary findings from the positive assertive cooperative kids study. *Journal of Attention Disorders*, 19(2), 125–137. doi: 10.1177/1087054713502080

Schultz, P. N., Remick-Barlow, A., and Robbins, L. (2007). Equine-assisted psychotherapy: A mental health promotion/intervention modality for children who have experienced intra-family violence. *Health and Social Care in the Community, 15*(3), 265–271. doi: 10.1111/j.1365-2524.2006.00684.x

Schultz, S. (2000, October 30). Pets and their humans. *U.S. News and World Report, 129*(17), 53–55.

Schwartz, J. J., and Freeberg, T. M. (2008). Acoustic interaction in animal groups: Signaling in noisy and social contexts. *Journal of Comparative Psychology, 122*(3), 231–234. doi: 10.1037/0735-7036.122.3.231

Schwarzer, R., and Jerusalem, M. (1995). Generalized Self-Efficacy Scale. In J. Weinman, S. Wright, and M. Johnston (Eds.), *Measures in Health Psychology: A user's portfolio. Causal and control beliefs* (pp. 35–37). Windsor: NFERNELSON.

Science Daily. (2007, December 24). Dolphin "therapy" a dangerous fad, researchers warn. Retrieved on October 14, 2016: http://sciencedaily.com/releases/2007/12/071218101131.htm

Scott, N. (2005). *Special needs, special horses: A guide to the benefits of therapeutic riding.* Denton: University of North Texas Press.

Serpell, J., McCune, S., Gee, N., and Griffin, J. (2017). Current challenges to research on animal-assisted interventions. *Applied Developmental Science.* doi: 10.1080/10888691.2016.1262775

Shane, F. T. (2004, April 14). Canines in crisis: Mitigating traumatic stress through canine crisis intervention. ATSS Workshop. Retrieved on October 12, 2016: www.K9DisasterRelief.org

Sheade, H. E. (2015). *Effectiveness of Relational Equine-Partnered Counseling (REPC) On Reduction of Symptoms of PTSD in Military Veterans: A single-case design.* Doctoral dissertation. University of North Texas, Denton, TX. Retrieved on October 12, 2016: http://digital.library.unt.edu/ark:/67531/metadc804906/m1/1/

Sheade, H. (2020). *Equine-assisted Counselling and Psychotherapy.* New York, NY: Routledge.

Sheade, H. E. (2021). Steps with Horses. Retrieved on July 8, 2023: https://www.stepswithhorses.org/

Sheade, H. E., and Chandler, C. K. (2014). Cultural diversity considerations in animal-assisted counseling. *Ideas and Research You Can Use: VISTAS* (Article 76). Retrieved on October 14, 2016: www.counseling.org/knowledge-center/vistas

Shin, N. (2003, November). Introduction of human–animal bond. Paper presented at the First International Symposium on the Human–Animal Bond, Samsung Everland, South Korea.

Shostrom, E. L. (1974). *Personal Orientation Inventory Manual: An inventory for the measurement of self-actualization.* San Diego, CA: Educational and Industrial Testing Service.

Shubert, J. (2012). Therapy dogs and stress management assistance during disasters. *The Army Medical Journal,* April–June, 74–78.

Siegford, J. M., Walshaw, S. O., Brunner, P., and Zanella, A. J. (2003). Validation of a temperament test for domestic cats. *Anthrozoös, 16*(4), 332–351. doi: 10.2752/089279303786991982

Singletary, M., and Lazarowski, L. (2021). Canine special senses: considerations in olfaction, vision, and audition. *Veterinary Clinics of North America: Small Animal Practice, 51*(4), 839–858. doi: 10.1016/j.cvsm.2021.04.004

Signal, T., Taylor, N., Botros, H., Prentice, K., and Lazarus, K. (2013). Whispering to horses: Childhood sexual abuse, depression and the efficacy of equine-facilitated therapy. *Sexual Abuse in Australia and New Zealand, 5*(1), 24–32.

Silva, K., Correia, R., Lima, M., Magalhaes, A., and deSousa, L. (2011). Can dogs prime autistic children for therapy? Evidence from a single case study. *The Journal of Alternative and Complementary Medicine, 17*(7), 655–659. doi: 10.1089/acm.2010.0436

Singer, J. (1973). *Boundaries of the Soul: The practice of Jung's psychology.* Garden City, NY: Anchor.

Singer, P. (1975). *Animal Liberation: A new ethics for our treatment of animals.* New York: Random House.

Skeen, J. (2011). Predator–prey relationships: What humans can learn from horses about being whole. In C. Blazina, G. Boyraz, and D. Shen-Miller (Eds.), *The Psychology of the Human–Animal Bond.* New York: Springer.

Smith, B. A. (1981). Using dolphins to elicit communication from an autistic child. *School of Public Affairs and Services,* p. 154, Library at Dolphins Plus, FL.

Smith, C. S. (2002, March). The dog wins by a nose. *AKC Gazette,* pp. 44–47.

Smith, R. (2003). "Mary had a little lamb." *Recess,* October 29. Center for Children's Literature and Culture, University of Florida. Retrieved on October 17, 2016: www.recess.ufl.edu/transcripts/2003/1029.shtml

Sobo, E. J., Eng, B., and Kassity-Krich, N. (2006). Canine visitation (pet) therapy: Pilot data on decreases in child pain perception. *Journal of Holistic Nursing, 24*(1), 51–57. doi: 10.1177/0898010105280112

Sockalingam, S., Li, M., Krishnadev, U., Hanson, K., Balaban, K., Pacione, L. R., et al. (2008). Use of animal-assisted therapy in the rehabilitation of an assault victim with a concurrent mood disorder. *Issues in Mental Health Nursing, 29,* 73–84. doi: 10.1080/01612840701748847

Souter, M. A., and Miller, M. D. (2007). Do animal-assisted activities effectively treat depression? A meta-analysis. *Anthrozoös, 20*(2), 167–180. doi: 10.2752/175303707X207954

Spanier, G. B. (1976). Measuring dyadic adjustment: New scales for assessing the quality of marriage and similar dyads. *Journal of Marriage and the Family, 38,* 15–28. doi: 10.2307/350547

Spielberger, C. D. (1970). *State-Trait Anxiety for Children.* Palo Alto, CA: Consulting Psychologists Press.

Spielberger, C. D., Gorsuch, R. I., and Lushene, R. E. (1983). *Manual for the State-Trait Anxiety Inventory.* Palo Alto, CA: Consulting Psychologists Press.

Sprinkle, J. E. (2008). Animals, empathy, and violence: Can animals be used to convey principles of prosocial behavior to children? *Youth Violence and Juvenile Justice, 6*(1), 47–58. doi: 10.1177/1541204007305525

Steed, H. N., and Smith, B. S. (2002). Animal-assisted activities for geriatric patients. *Activities, Adaptation and Aging, 27*(1), 49–61. doi: 10.1300/J016v27n01_04

Stern, C., and Chur-Hansen, A. (2013). Methodological considerations in designing and evaluating animal-assisted interventions. *Animals, 3,* 127–141. doi: 10.3390/ani3010127

Stetson, U. (2010, February 26). Stetson a pet-friendly campus. *i-Visual @ Stetson University.* Retrieved on October 14, 2016: www2.stetson.edu/pr/econnect/?p=456

Stewart, L. A., Chang, C. Y., Parker, L. K., and Grubbs, N. (2016, June 21). Animal-assisted therapy in counseling competencies. *ACAeNews.* Alexandria, VA: American Counseling Association. Retrieved on June 8, 2022: https://www.counseling.org/docs/default-source/competencies/animal-assisted-therapy-competencies-june-2016.pdf?sfvrsn=6

Stewart, L. A., Chang, C. Y., and Rice, R. (2013). Emergent theory and model of practice in animal-assisted therapy in counseling. *Journal of Creativity in Mental Health, 8,* 329–348. doi: 10.1080/15401383.2013.844657

Stoker, P. (2011, October 27). Prison opens facility to care for neglected horses: Inmates believe program will be beneficial. *Gainsvilletimes.com.* Retrieved on October 24, 2016: www.gainesville times.com/archives/58260/

Strimple, E. O. (2003). A history of prison inmate–animal interaction programs. *American Behavioral Scientist, 47*(1), 70–78. doi: 10.1177/000276420325521

Struckus, J. E. (1989). *The Use of Pet-Facilitated Therapy in the Treatment of Depression in the Elderly: A behavioral conceptualization of treatment effects.* Doctoral dissertation. University of Massachusetts.

Studer, Q., Robinson, B. C., and Cook, K. (2010). *The HCAPS Handbook: Hardwire your hospital for pay-for-performance success.* Gulf Breeze, FL: Fire Starter Publishing.

Stumpf, E., and Breitenbach, E. (2014). Dolphin-assisted therapy with parental involvement for children with severe disabilities: Further evidence for a family-centered theory for effectiveness. *Anthrozoös, 27*(1), 95–109. doi: 10.2752/175303714X13837396326495

Tahan, M., Saleem, T., Sadeghifar, A., and Ahangri, E. (2022). Assessing the effectiveness of animal-assisted therapy on alleviation of anxiety in pre-school children: A randomized controlled trial. *Contemporary Clinical Trials Communications, 28,* 1–6. doi: 10.1016/j.conctc.2022.100947

Tangley, L. (2000, October 30). Animal emotions. Sheer joy. Romantic love. The pain of mourning. Scientists say pets and wild creatures have feelings too. *U.S. News and World Report, 129*(17), 48–52.

Tannenbaum, J. (1995). *Veterinary Ethics: Animal welfare, client relations, competition, and collegiality.* St. Louis, MO: Mosby.

Tarrant, D. (2000, January 21). Teacher's pets: Lucy and Dottie are top dogs in the classroom. *Dallas Morning News,* 1C, 3C.

Taunton, S., and Smith, C. (1998). *The Trick Is in the Training: 25 fun tricks to teach your dog.* Hauppauge, NY: Barron's.

Taverna, G., Tidu, L., Grizzi, F., Torri, V., Mandressi, A., Sardella, P., La Torre, G., Cocciolone, G., Seveso, M., Giusti, G., Hurle, R., Santoro, A., and Graziotti, P. (2015). The *Journal of Urology, 93*(4), 1382–1387. doi: 10.1016/j.juro.2014.09.099

Taylor, S. M. (2001). *Equine-facilitated Psychotherapy: An emerging field.* Unpublished master's thesis. Saint Michael's College, Vermont.

Teal, L. (2002). Pet Partners help with the healing process. *Interactions Magazine, 19*(4), 3–5.

Tellington-Jones, L., and Taylor, S. (1995). *The Tellington Touch: A revolutionary natural method to train and care for your favorite animal.* New York: Penguin.

Texas Secretary of State (2016). Texas colonias: A thumbnail sketch of conditions, issues, challenges and opportunities. Texas Border and Mexican Affairs, Austin, TX. Retrieved on October 14, 2016: www.sos.state.tx.us/border/colonias/faqs.shtml

Therapy Dogs International (TDI). (2023a). About TDI. Retrieved on March 1, 2023: www.tdi-dog. org/About.aspx

Therapy Dogs International (TDI). (2023b). Testing guidelines. Retrieved on March 1, 2023: https://www.tdi-dog.org/HowToJoin.aspx?Page=New+TDI+Test

Thomas, W. H. (1994). *The Eden Alternative: Nature, hope, and nursing homes.* Sherburne, NY: Eden Alternative Foundation.

Thompson, B. (2002). "Statistical," "practical," and "clinical": How many kinds of significance do counselors need to consider? *Journal of Counseling and Development, 80,* 64–71. doi: 10.1002/j.1556-6678.2002.tb00167.x

Thornton, K. C. (2002). Famous bully breeds. *Popular Dogs Series: Bully Breeds, 21,* 10. Irvine, CA: Fancy Publications.

Tidmarsh, A., and Tidmarsh, D. (2005). Give and take exercise. Paper presented at the Equine-Assisted Psychotherapy and Learning Association Annual Conference, Las Vegas, NV.

Tournier, I., Vives, M-F., and Postal, V. (2017). Animal-assisted intervention in dementia: Effects on neuropsychiatric symptoms and on caregivers' distress perceptions. *Swiss Journal of Psychology, 76(2),* 51–58. doi: 10.1016/j.ctcp.2022.101574

Trotter, K. S. (2006). *The Efficacy of Equine-Assisted Group Counseling with At-Risk Children and Adolescents.* Unpublished dissertation. Department of Counseling and Higher Education, University of North Texas, Denton.

Trotter, K. S. (Ed.) (2011). *Harnessing the Power of Equine-assisted Counselling.* New York, NY: Routledge.

Trotter, K. S. (2012). Is labeling people really harmless? Using equines to explore labeling stigma. In K. S. Trotter (Ed.), *Harnessing the Power of Equine-Assisted Counseling* (pp. 195–199). New York: Routledge.

Trotter, K. S., and Baggerly, J. (Eds.) (2018a). *Equine-assisted Mental Health Interventions: Harnessing solutions to common problems.* New York, NY: Routledge.

Trotter, K. S., and Baggerly, J. (Eds.) (2018b). *Equine-assisted Mental Health for Healing Trauma.* New York, NY: Routledge.

Trotter, K. S., Chandler, C. K., Goodwin-Bond, D., and Casey, J. (2008). A comparative study of the efficacy of group equine-assisted counseling with at-risk children and adolescents. *Journal of Creativity in Mental Health, 3(3),* 254–284. doi: 10.1080/15401380802356880.

Tsai, C., Friedmann, E., and Thomas, S. A. (2010). The effect of animal-assisted therapy on stress responses in hospitalized children. *Anthrozoös, 23(3),* 245–258. doi: 10.2752/175303710X12750451258977

Tucker, M. (2002). *Visiting Hospitalized Children: A Delta Society handbook for Pet Partners.* Bellevue, WA: Delta Society (name changed to Pet Partners).

Tudor, K., and Worrall, M. (2006). *Person-Centered Therapy: A clinical philosophy.* New York: Routledge.

Turner, K., Stetina, B. U., Burger, E., Lederman Maman, T., Handlos, U., and Kryspin-Exner, I. (2009). Enhancing emotion regulation and recognition among first graders through animal-assisted group training. *Journal of Veterinary Behavior, 4(2),* 93–94. doi: 10.1016/j.jveb.2008.10.018

Tyson, P. (2012, October 3). Dog's dazzling sense of smell. PBS: NOVA: Nature. https://www.pbs.org/wgbh/nova/article/dogs-sense-of-smell/ (archived on August 19, 2021).

U.S. Census Bureau. (2023a). Quick facts. United States. https://www.census.gov/quickfacts/fact/table/US/RHI725222

U.S. Census Bureau. (2023b). 3.5 million reported Middle Eastern and North African descent in 2020. https://www.census.gov/library/stories/2023/09/2020-census-dhc-a-mena-population.html#:~:text=Who%20Identified%20as%20a%20Detailed%20MENA%20Group%3F,population)%20identified%20as%20MENA%20alone.

Uvnäs-Moberg, K. (1998a). Oxytocin may mediate the benefits of positive social interaction and emotions. *Psychoneuroendocrinology, 23(8),* 819–835. doi: 10.1016/S0306-4530(98)00056-0

Uvnäs-Moberg, K. (1998b). Antistress pattern induced by oxytocin. *News in Physiological Science, 13,* 22–26. doi: 10.1152/physiologyonline.1998.13.1.22

Uvnäs-Moberg, K. (2010, July). Coordinating role of oxytocin. Paper presented at the Twelfth International Conference of the International Association of Human–Animal Interaction Organizations

(IAHAIO), Stockholm, Sweden. Proceedings available at: https://iahaio.org/wp/wp-content/uploads/2017/05/past-events-conference2010stockholm.pdf

Uvnäs-Moberg, K., Arn, I., and Magnusson, D. (2005). The psychobiology of emotion: The role of the oxytocinergic system. *International Journal of Behavioral Medicine, 12*(2), 59–65. doi: 10.1207/s15327558ijbm1202_3

VanFleet, R. (2008). *Play Therapy with Kids and Canines: Benefits for children's developmental and psychosocial health.* Sarasota, FL: Professional Resource Press.

VanFleet, R., and Faa-Thompson, T. (2010). The case for using animal-assisted play therapy. *British Journal of Play Therapy, 6,* 4–18.

VanFleet, R., and Faa-Thompson, T. (2017). *Animal Assisted Play Therapy.* Sarasota, FL: Professional Resource Press.

Varni, J. W., Seid, M., and Kurtin, P. S. (2001). PedsQL 4.0: Reliability and validity of the Pediatric Quality of Life Inventory version 4.0 generic core scales in healthy and patient populations. *Medical Care, 8,* 800–812. doi: 10.1097/00005650-200108000-00006

Vidrine, M., Owen-Smith, P., and Faulkner, P. (2002). Equine-facilitated group psychotherapy: Applications for therapeutic vaulting. *Issues in Mental Health Nursing, 23,* 587–603. doi: 10.1080/01612840290052730

Volhard, J., and Volhard, W. (1997). *The Canine Good Citizen: Every dog can be one.* New York: Howell.

Volhard, J., and Volhard, W. (2001). *Dog training for dummies.* Hoboken, NJ: Wiley Publishing.

Volhard, W. (2003). Puppy Aptitude Test. Retrieved on October 3, 2016: www.volhard.com/pages/pat.php

Voorhees, R. (1995). *The Effect of a Unique Stimulus (Swimming with Dolphins) on the Communication Between Parents and Their Children with Disabilities.* Unpublished master's thesis. University of Miami, School of Medicine.

Wall, M. J. (1994). *The Effects of Companion Animal Visitation on Mood State And Level of Speech Activity of Nursing Home Residents.* Doctoral dissertation. California School of Professional Psychology, San Diego.

Wallace, J. (2012). Equine program rehabilitates inmates at Pulaski State Prison. *WALB News.* Retrieved on October 24, 2016: www.walb.com/story/18946234/equine-program-rehabilitates-inmates-at-pulaski-state-prison

Walsh, F. (2009). Human–animal bonds I: The relational significance of companion animals. *Family Process, 48*(4), 462–480. doi: 10.1111/j.1545-5300.2009.01296.x

Walsh, P., and Mertin, P. (1994). The training of pets as therapy dogs in a women's prison: A pilot study. *Anthrozoös, 7*(2), 124–128. doi: 10.2752/089279394787002014

Walsh, P., Mertin, P., Verlander, D., and Pollard, C. (1995). The effects of a "pets as therapy" dog on persons with dementia in a psychiatric ward. *Australian Occupational Therapy Journal, 42,* 161–166. doi: 10.1111/j.1440-1630.1995.tb01331.x

Walters Esteves, S., and Stokes, T. (2008). Social effects of a dog's presence on children with disabilities. *Anthrozoös, 21*(1), 5–15. doi: 10.1080/08927936.2008.11425166

Warm Springs Correctional Center. (n.d.). Wild horse gentling program. *Prison Place.* Retrieved on October 14, 2016: http://prisonplace.com/forums/t/655.aspx

Webb, N. L., and Drummond, P. D. (2001). The effects of swimming with dolphins on human well-being and anxiety. *Anthrozoös, 14*(2), 81–85. doi: 10.2752/089279301786999526

Webber, J., and Mascari, J. B. (2010). *Terrorism, Trauma and Tragedies* (3rd ed.). Alexandria, VA: American Counseling Association.

Weeks, J., and Beck, A. M. (1996). Equine agitation behaviors. *Equine Practice, 18,* 23–24.

Wells, M., and Perrine, R. (2001). Pets go to college: The influence of pets on students' perceptions of faculty and their offices. *Anthrozoös, 14*(3), 161–168. doi: 10.2752/089279301786999472

Wendt, M. (2011). *How Horses Feel and Think: Understanding behaviour, emotions and intelligence.* Richmond, UK: Cadmos.

Wendt, M. (2011). *Trust Instead of Dominance: Working towards a new form of ethical horsemanship.* Richmond, UK: Cadmos.

Wesley, M. C., Minatrea, N. B., and Watson, J. C. (2009). Animal-assisted therapy in the treatment of substance dependence. *Anthrozoös, 22*(2), 137–148. doi: 10.2752/175303709X434167

Wilkes, C. N., Shalko, T. K., and Trahan, M. (1989). Pet Rx: Implications for good health. *Health Education, 20,* 6–9. doi: 10.1080/00970050.1989.10616097

Willett, J. B. (1989). Questions and answers in the measurement of change. In E. Z. Rothkopf (Ed.), *Review of Research in Education* (pp. 345–422). Washington, D.C.: AERA.

Willett, J. B. (1994). Measurement of change. In T. Husen and T. N. Postlethwaite (Eds.), *The International Encyclopedia of Education* (2nd ed., pp. 671–678). Oxford, UK: Pergamon.

Willis, C. M., Church, S. M., Guest, C. M., Cook, W. A., McCarthy, N., Bransbury, A. J., et al. (2004). Olfactory detection of human bladder cancer by dogs: Proof of principle study. *British Medical Journal (BMJ)*, doi: 10.1136/bmj.329.7468.712.

Wilson, D. B., Gottfredson, D. C., and Najaka, S. S. (2001). School-based prevention of problem behaviors: A meta-analysis. *Journal of Quantitative Criminology, 17*, 247–272. doi: 10.1023/A:1011050217296

Wilson, E. O. (1984). *Biophilia.* Cambridge, MA: Harvard University Press.

Winerman, L. (2005, October). The mind's mirror. *Monitor on Psychology, 36*(9), 48. Retrieved on July 26, 2023: https://www.apa.org/monitor/oct05/mirror

Wisconsin Correctional Liberty Dog Program. (n.d.). Wisconsin Correctional Liberty Dog Program: Minimum security prison. Retrieved on October 14, 2016: http://prisonp.tripod.com/men.htm

Wu, A. S., Niedra, R., Pendergast, L., and McCrindle, B. W. (2002). Acceptability and impact of pet visitation on a pediatric cardiology inpatient unit. *Journal of Pediatric Nursing, 17*(5), 354–362. doi: 10.1053/jpdn.2002.127173

Wyoming Honor Farm Inmate/Wild-Horse Program. (n.d.). Retrieved on October 14, 2016: www.cowboyshowcase.com/honorfarm.htm

Yanes-Hoffman, N. (1981). Howard Rusk, MD: An equal chance. *Journal of the American Medical Association, 246*(14), 1503–1510. doi: 10.1001/jama.1981.03320140005002

Yang, J. (2010, September 6). Stephens College allows students to keep their pets in their dorm rooms. *NBC News*. Retrieved on October 14, 2016: www.kshb.com/dpp/news/education/stephens-college-allows-students-to-keep-their-pets-in-their-dorm-rooms

Yeh, M. (2008). Canine animal-assisted therapy model for the autistic children in Taiwan. Presentation at the International Conference on Human–Animal Interactions. Tokyo, Japan.

Yorke, J., Adams, C., and Coady, N. (2008). Therapeutic value of equine-human bonding in recovery from trauma. *Anthrozoös, 21*(1), 17–30. doi: 10.2752/089279308X274038

Young, M. (2005). *Learning the Art of Helping: Building blocks and techniques* (3rd ed.). Upper Saddle River, NJ: Pearson.

Zamir, T. (2006). The moral basis of animal-assisted therapy. *Society and Animals, 14*(2), 179–199. doi: 10.1163/156853006776778770

Zasloff, L. R., Hart, L. A., and Melrod Weiss, J. (2003). Dog training as a violence prevention tool for at-risk adolescents. *Anthrozoös, 16*(4), 353–359. doi: 10.2752/089279303786992044

Zeig, J. K., and Munion, W. M. (1999). *Milton H. Erickson.* Thousand Oaks, CA: Sage.

Zilcha-Mano, S., Mikulincer, M., and Shaver, P. (2011). Pet in the therapy room: An attachment perspective on animal-assisted therapy. *Attachment and Human Development, 13*(6), 541–561. doi: 10.1080/14616734.2011.608987

Appendix A
Recommended Competency Areas and Accompanying Performance Guidelines for the Practice of Animal-Assisted Therapy in Counseling

1. Describe the history, evolution, and current status of AAT applications, training, and credentialing related to counseling. Performance guidelines:

   — Have knowledge of historical and current AAT applications in the mental health field.
   — Stay current with, describe, and critically evaluate quantitative and qualitative counseling-related research on AAT.
   — Have knowledge of the origins or current status of major AAT training and registration/credentialing organizations and institutions.

2. Understand and explain the benefits, role, and function of AAT in counseling. Performance guidelines:

   — Understand and explain the potential benefits of AAT in counseling.
   — Have knowledge regarding the impact on the counseling environment when a therapy animal is present.
   — Have knowledge and awareness of the unique dynamics presented in counseling relationships when a therapy animal is present.
   — Understand the therapy animal's role as a transitional being and therapeutic agent in the counseling process.

3. Integrate AAT in a manner consistent with the counseling process. Performance guidelines:

   — Assess client needs that may be met through AAT interventions.
   — Develop counseling treatment goals and plans that integrate AAT.
   — Have knowledge and skill in the application of AAT interventions (techniques and intentions), and apply them in a manner consistent with the goals of counseling.
   — Be knowledgeable of animal behavior and be able to interpret therapy animal vocal and nonvocal communications during a therapy session, as well as consider how these communications may be beneficial in understanding and assisting a client.
   — Assess the efficacy of AAT interventions in moving a client toward treatment goals.

4. Comply with ethical, legal, and professional standards and guidelines related to AAT applications in counseling. Performance guidelines:

— Follow ethical codes and standards of practice established by animal welfare and AAT organizations.
— Follow ethical codes and standards of practice of professional mental health organizations.
— Follow local, state, and federal guidelines governing the welfare and protection of humans and animals.
— Apply AAT in a manner that is culturally sensitive; consider cultural, racial, ethnic, and other individual differences, especially differences in attitudes toward animals, before and during application of AAT with a particular client and in a particular environment.

5. Work as a team with a therapy animal in a counseling facility, practice, or program. Performance guidelines:

— Evaluate client appropriateness for participation in AAT.
— Evaluate a facility or counseling environment for appropriateness of AAT.
— Network with appropriate facility staff regarding the intent and activities of therapy animals working in a facility or program.
— Follow facility or program policies and procedures regarding the practice of AAT in a particular facility or program; where no policies or procedures exist, establish policies and procedures with the assistance of appropriate facility and program personnel.
— Demonstrate competency in orchestrating a therapy animal to enact appropriate behaviors and comply with appropriate commands under circumstances consistent with the demands of AAT in a counseling environment and in a manner that protects the welfare and safety of all involved, including both humans and animals.

6. Serve as an advocate for the therapy animal. Performance guidelines:

— Establish and maintain a healthy and functional handler relationship with an animal that will be or is participating in the counseling process as a therapy animal.
— Assess an animal's ability to work as a therapy animal.
— Provide a comfortable environment for the therapy animal to participate in AAT. This includes providing a space and allowing time for food, water, rest, exercise, recreation, and so forth as needed.
— Identify and acknowledge when an animal is communicating fatigue, stress, distress, discomfort, or a lack of desire to participate in AAT, and provide for the animal's needs.

Appendix B
Client Screening Form for Animal-Assisted Therapy

Name of potential client: _____ Date: _____

Age of client: _____ Gender of client: _____

Guardian's name: _____

Client's/guardian's address: _____

Client's/guardian's phone number(s): _____

Permission granted to contact via telephone: _____ yes _____ no

Name of intake interviewer: _____

Does the client have any of the following?

_____ Animal allergies (if yes, which animals?) _____

_____ Animal fears or phobias (if yes, which animals?) _____

_____ History of aggression or abuse toward animals

_____ History of aggression or abuse toward people

_____ Hallucinations

_____ Dementia

_____ Emotional problems

_____ Behavioral problems

_____ Severe developmental disorder Describe: _____

Animals the client has had as pets: _____

Any negative experiences with animals: _____

Would this person like to participate in animal-assisted therapy? _____ yes _____ no

Additional information: _____

Based on the available information is this person appropriate for animal-assisted therapy? _____ yes _____no

Appendix C
Psychosocial Session Form

Client's name: _____ Date of session: _____ Session number:_____

Location of session: _____

Estimated length of session (hours/minutes): _____

Session format: Individual: ___ Group: ___ Family: ___ Other (list): _____

Counselor's name(s): _____

Therapy animals: _____

AAT type: Equine: _____ Canine: _____ Feline: _____ Other (list): _____

Rating comparison (check one): The client's behavior ratings are based on:

_____ 1. A comparison of the client with what is considered to be typical, normal, healthy functioning in society (this is the preferred format for each session).

_____ 2. A comparison of the client with self from the previous session, or if this is the first session this is a baseline rating based on (1), (3), or (4).

_____ 3. A comparison of the client with other members of the group.

_____ 4. Other (describe) _____

For evaluation purposes the comparison category checked above should be consistent across all sessions for the client and for clients in the same group. This form is designed to track client progress in a consistent and measurable format. If possible, the same therapists should complete the form for consistency in interpretation of client behaviors. If a treatment team is involved, then as many team members as possible should give their input as to the client's scores on the following various behaviors.

Circle the number that best describes the amount of client behavior that is listed.

	NO/NA[a]	None	Very Low	Low	Medium	High	Very High
Positive Behaviors							
Participation	×	0	1	2	3	4	5
Positive interactions	×	0	1	2	3	4	5
Cooperation	×	0	1	2	3	4	5
Appropriately assertive	×	0	1	2	3	4	5
Attention-to-task, focus	×	0	1	2	3	4	5
Follows directions	×	0	1	2	3	4	5
Respectful	×	0	1	2	3	4	5
Integrity/honesty	×	0	1	2	3	4	5
Leadership	×	0	1	2	3	4	5
Teamwork	×	0	1	2	3	4	5
Eye contact	×	0	1	2	3	4	5
Active listening	×	0	1	2	3	4	5
Open-minded	×	0	1	2	3	4	5
Accepts feedback	×	0	1	2	3	4	5
Positive feelings	×	0	1	2	3	4	5
Positive vocalizations	×	0	1	2	3	4	5
Empathy	×	0	1	2	3	4	5
Sharing	×	0	1	2	3	4	5
Helpful	×	0	1	2	3	4	5
Problem solving	×	0	1	2	3	4	5
Self-confidence	×	0	1	2	3	4	5
Self-esteem	×	0	1	2	3	4	5
Insight about self	×	0	1	2	3	4	5
Insight about others	×	0	1	2	3	4	5
Expression of needs, appropriately	×	0	1	2	3	4	5
Other positive behaviors (list):							
_____	×	0	1	2	3	4	5
_____	×	0	1	2	3	4	5
Negative Behaviors							
Belligerent	×	0	1	2	3	4	5
Resistant	×	0	1	2	3	4	5
Guarded	×	0	1	2	3	4	5
Manipulative	×	0	1	2	3	4	5
Deceptive	×	0	1	2	3	4	5
Negative vocalizations	×	0	1	2	3	4	5
Argumentative	×	0	1	2	3	4	5
Angry or agitated	×	0	1	2	3	4	5
Closed-minded	×	0	1	2	3	4	5
Overly fearful	×	0	1	2	3	4	5
Fidgety or hyperactive	×	0	1	2	3	4	5
Verbally aggressive	×	0	1	2	3	4	5
Physically aggressive	×	0	1	2	3	4	5

	NO/NA[a]	None	Very Low	Low	Medium	High	Very High
Overly passive	×	0	1	2	3	4	5
Overly submissive	×	0	1	2	3	4	5
Sad or depressed	×	0	1	2	3	4	5
Withdrawn	×	0	1	2	3	4	5
Other negative behaviors (list):							
_____	×	0	1	2	3	4	5
_____	×	0	1	2	3	4	5

[a] *NO/NA*: no opportunity to observe or does not apply.

Session Scores and Summary

Do not count the items marked × (no opportunity to observe or does not apply) as scored items.

_____ **Total Positive Behavior Score** (Add scores and divide by number of items scored 0–5.)

An increasing total positive score across sessions indicates an increase in positive behaviors.

_____ **Total Negative Behavior Score** (Add scores and divide by number of items scored 0–5.)

An increasing total negative score across sessions indicates an increase in negative behaviors.

_____ **Total Behavior Score** (Subtract Total Negative Score from Total Positive Score.)

An increasing total behavior score across sessions indicates overall improvement in positive behaviors relative to negative behaviors.

Other Notes

Any indication in the client of (check those that apply; if so, explain):

_____ Suicidal ideation _____ Crisis _____ Self-harm _____ Harm to others

Describe any progress by client toward existing goals:

_____

Describe any new issues presented or new goals established:

_____

Describe any changes or adjustments in conceptualization of client or diagnosis:

_____

Describe primary presenting problem(s) discussed or exhibited by client in this session:

_____

Therapeutic intervention(s) applied: _____

_____

_____

_____

Other comments (continue on an additional page if necessary): _____

_____

_____

_____

_____

Source: Chandler, C. K., Psychosocial Session Form, in C. K. Chandler (2005), *Animal-Assisted Therapy in Counseling*, pp. 181–184. New York: Routledge. The Psychosocial Session Form may be used with proper citation as listed.

Appendix D
Animal-Assisted Therapy Animal Illustrations: Instructions and Activities

PART I ANIMAL BODY PARTS ACTIVITY: INSTRUCTIONS FOR THERAPIST

These therapist's instructions are to be used with the illustrations of a dog, cat, horse, rabbit, and bird (see following pages for a figure of a dog, cat, horse, rabbit, and bird). This activity can be performed in a group or individually with a client. It is appropriate for any age group.

1 Have the client choose which animal illustration of the ones available the client wishes to color, and provide the client with that animal illustration and a copy of Part III (Animal Body Parts Activity: Instructions for Clients).
2. Provide the client with nontoxic and preferably water-soluble color pencils or markers.
3. On Part III (Animal Body Parts Activity: Instructions for Clients), have the client label what colors will represent which feelings the client is experiencing right now. The client can use the suggested colors as a guide or choose different emotions or different colors for each emotion.

Suggested guide: Colors can represent the following feelings: sad = blue, afraid = yellow, happy = orange, relaxed = green, angry = red, frustrated = black, curious = gray, confused = brown, love = pink, like = purple, and hurt = white or no color.

Feelings	Colors
Sad	_____
Afraid	_____
Happy	_____
Relaxed	_____
Angry	_____
Frustrated	_____
Curious	_____
Confused	_____
Love	_____
Like	_____
Hurt	_____
Other feelings	_____

4. On Part III (Animal Body Parts Activity: Instructions for Clients), have the client label the body parts of the animal with certain important persons or situations in the client's life, such as family, friends, school/work, self, and hopes/dreams. The client can use the suggested body part labeling or choose different life areas or different body parts for life areas.

Suggested guide: Body parts can represent the following topics: eyes = spirit, ears = school or work, head = family, neck = (left blank to be filled in by client), body = love, tail = friend(s), legs = fun or hobbies, and feet = myself.

Animal Body Parts	Life Persons or Situations
Eyes	_____
Ears	_____
Head	_____
Neck	_____
Body	_____
Tail	_____
Legs	_____
Feet	_____

5. Now, have the client color in the animal's body parts that represent different persons or situations in the client's life with colors representing the different feelings the client currently has about those persons or situations.
6. Have the client share the results of their artwork and discuss it at length.

PART II ANIMAL FEELINGS ACTIVITY: INSTRUCTIONS FOR THERAPIST

The following instructions are to be used with the illustrations of dog and cat expressions (see illustrations of dogs and cats with expressions on following pages). This activity can follow the activity presented in Part I or can be performed as a separate activity at a different time. This activity can be performed in a group or individually with a client. It is appropriate for any age group.

1. Have the client look at the illustrations of dog or cat expressions and label each animal with an emotion the client thinks the animal is expressing. Five basic emotions are presented in the following order: (for the group of three dogs) dog 1 (*top*), scared; dog 2 (*middle*), angry or aggressive; dog 3 (*bottom*), sad; (for the group of two dogs) dog 4 (*top*), content, calm, and relaxed; dog 5 (*bottom*), happy; (for the group of three cats) cat 1 (*top*), scared; cat 2 (*middle*), sad; cat 3 (*bottom*), angry or aggressive; (for the group of two cats) cat 4 (*top*), happy; and cat 5 (*bottom*), content, calm, and relaxed. The client is allowed to label the animals with other emotions than the suggested five presented. The client can then color each animal expression based on the color the client wants to represent that emotion. Have the client discuss which dog or cat the client most closely identifies with as a primary or dominant emotion in the client's life.

2. Now have the client discuss at what times in the client's life he or she experiences each emotion in each life area based on Part IV (Animal Feelings Activity: Instructions for Clients). You can instruct the client to skip Step 3a on this activity, if the client is too young to have a significant other; and/or skip Step 3f on this activity, if the client is too young to understand spirituality.

PART III ANIMAL BODY PARTS ACTIVITY: INSTRUCTIONS FOR CLIENTS

This exercise is designed to help you get in better touch with your feelings about different areas of your life. Look at the drawing of the animal that has been given to you. You will be coloring this animal's body parts to represent different areas of your life. You will have an opportunity to discuss your animal drawing when you are done.

1. Based on the colors available to you, decide what color you want to represent each emotion, and write it down in the following table. You can use the suggested guide if you prefer.

    Suggested guide: Colors can represent the following feelings: sad = blue, afraid = yellow, happy = orange, relaxed = green, angry = red, frustrated = black, curious = gray, confused = brown, love = pink, like = purple, and hurt = white or no color.

Feelings	Colors
Sad	_____
Afraid	_____
Happy	_____
Relaxed	_____
Angry	_____
Frustrated	_____
Curious	_____
Confused	_____
Love	_____
Like	_____
Hurt	_____
Other feelings	_____

2. Based on the body parts presented in the animal drawing, decide what body parts you want to represent each area of your life, and write them down in the following table. You can use the suggested guide if you prefer.

    Suggested guide: Body parts can represent the following topics: eyes = spirit, ears = school or work, head = family, neck = (left blank to be filled in by client), body = love, tail = friend(s), legs = fun or hobbies, and feet = myself.

Animal Body Parts	Life Persons or Situations
Eyes	_____
Ears	_____
Head	_____
Neck	_____
Body	_____
Tail	_____
Legs	_____
Feet	_____

3. Now color the animal drawing based on the choices you wrote in the tables.

PART IV ANIMAL FEELINGS ACTIVITY: INSTRUCTIONS FOR CLIENTS

1. Look at the expressions of the animals in the drawings that have been given to you. How would you label each emotion that each animal seems to be expressing? (*Suggested guide*: the animals could be expressing five basic emotions of sad, angry, happy, afraid, or relaxed, but you may see something different in the animals' expressions so describe the animals' emotions the way that you see them.) Write the emotion next to that animal. Color each animal based on what color you want to represent that emotion for the animal.

2. What emotion do you feel more than any other emotion right now in your life?

3. List in the following sections at what times in your life and under what circumstances you experience certain emotions in each of your major life areas:

   a. With your significant other (girlfriend/boyfriend, husband/wife, or life partner), or, if you are not in a relationship with a significant other right now, the emotion you have about not being in a relationship currently:

   Sad   _____
   Angry   _____
   Happy   _____
   Afraid   _____
   Content/calm/relaxed   _____
   Other emotion(s)   _____

   b. With members of your family:

   Sad   _____
   Angry   _____
   Happy   _____
   Afraid   _____
   Content/calm/relaxed   _____
   Other emotion(s)   _____

   c. When you are with friends:

   Sad   _____
   Angry   _____
   Happy   _____
   Afraid   _____
   Content/calm/relaxed   _____
   Other emotion(s)   _____

   d. When you are at work or school:

   Sad   _____
   Angry   _____
   Happy   _____
   Afraid   _____
   Content/calm/relaxed   _____
   Other emotion(s)   _____

e. In relation to yourself:

Sad	_____
Angry	_____
Happy	_____
Afraid	_____
Content/calm/relaxed	_____
Other emotion(s)	_____

f. In relation to your spirituality:

Sad	_____
Angry	_____
Happy	_____
Afraid	_____
Content/calm/relaxed	_____
Other emotion(s)	_____

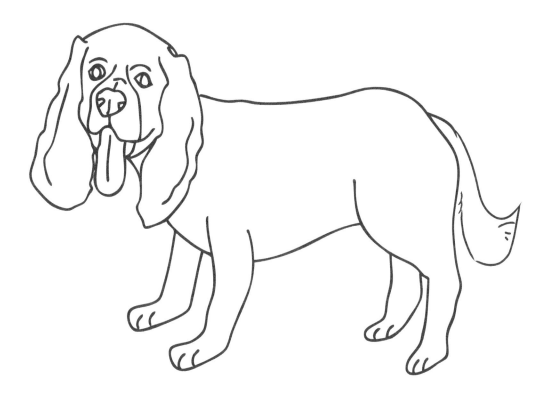

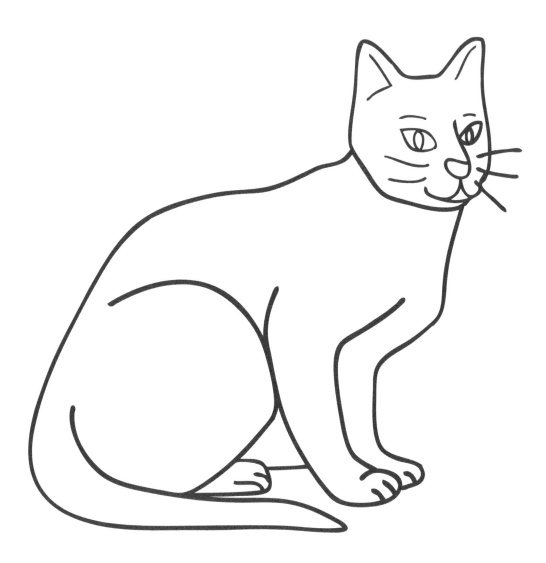

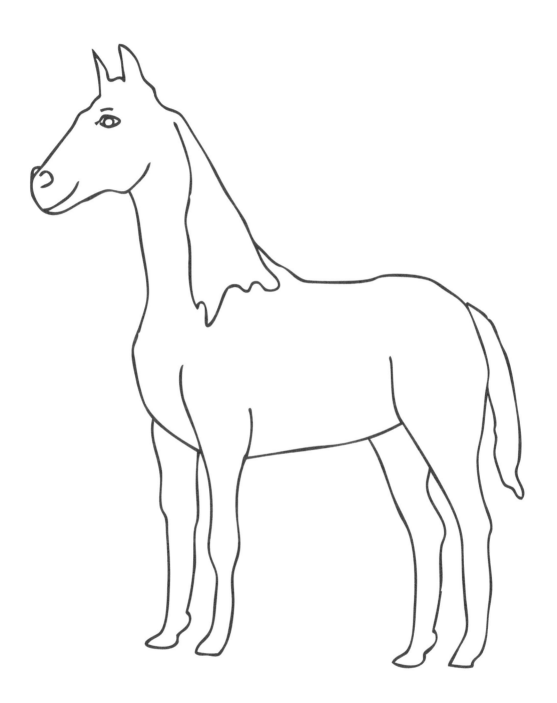

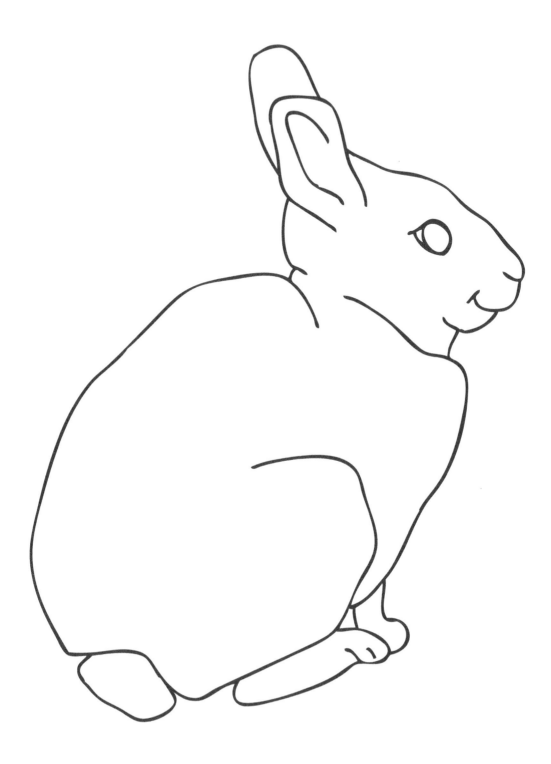

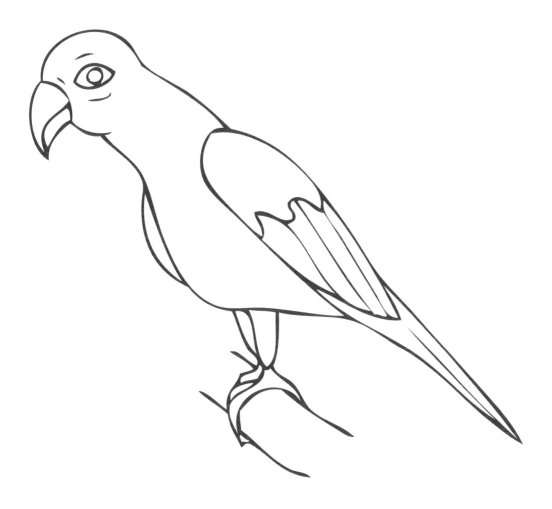

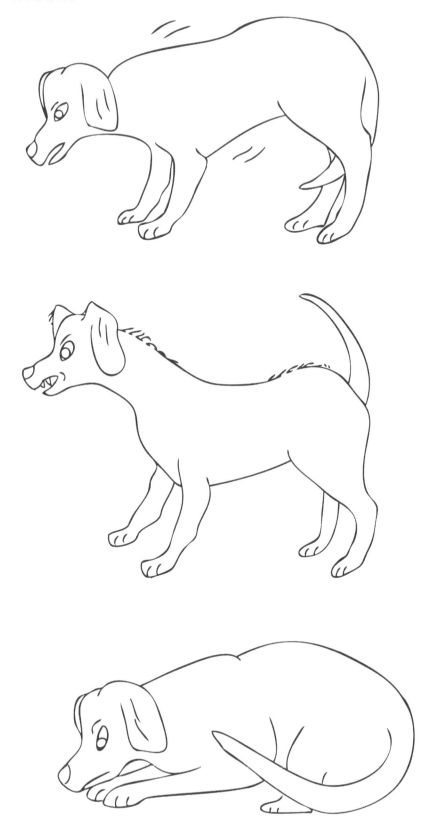

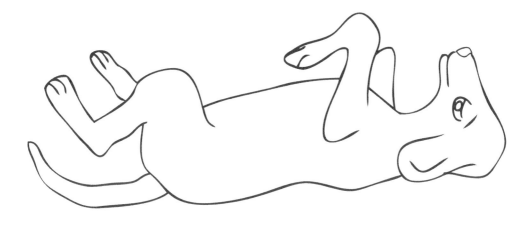

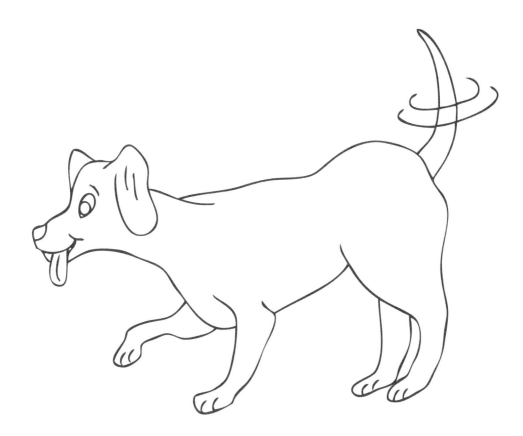

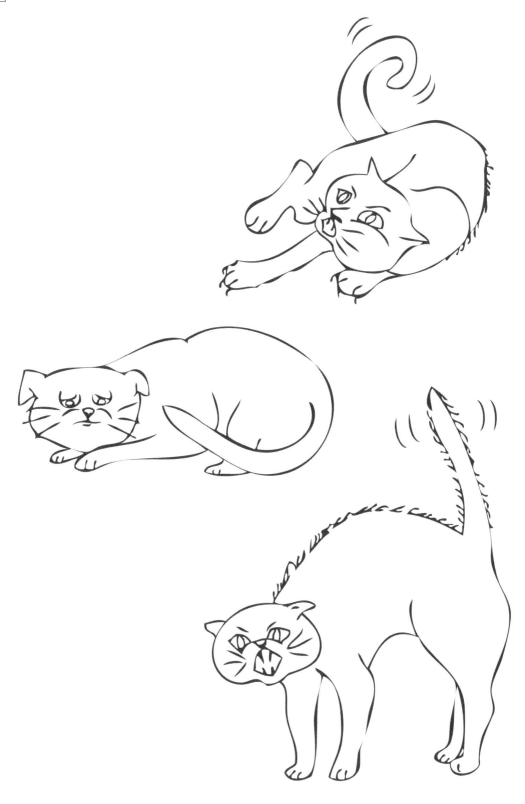

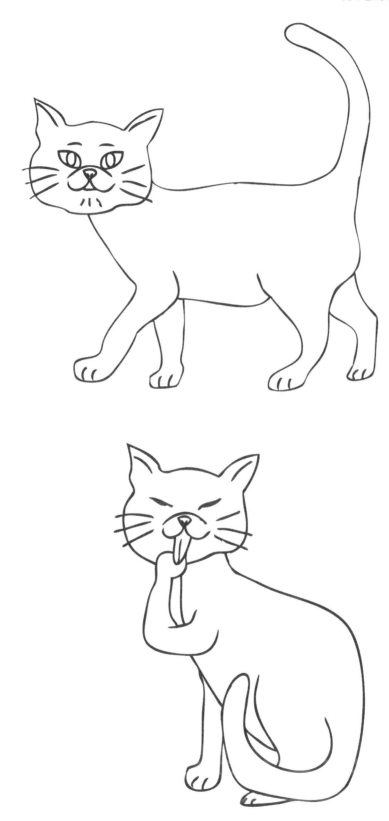

Appendix E
Sample Policy and Procedures for the Practice of Animal-Assisted Therapy in a Counselor Education and Training Program

University policy allows registered therapy animals that are accompanied by a qualified handler into university buildings and classrooms for the purposes of providing clinical and/or educational services. Individual departments and services may impose restrictions for access by therapy animals when deemed appropriate. Students, faculty, and staff must follow all university, college, department, and program policies, procedures, and guidelines related to therapy animals on campus and in campus facilities.

COUNSELOR EDUCATION AND TRAINING PROGRAM POLICY AND PROCEDURES FOR AAT

The following counselor education and training program recognizes the potential value of AAT in the counseling field. To support this recognition, students who are in training to be counselors will be allowed to practice AAT under the provisions listed in the program's policy and procedures for AAT. The counselor education and training program policy and procedures for AAT are provided in Part I and Part II that follow.

Part I AAT—Conditions for Practice in a Counselor Education and Training Program

1. No student may practice AAT in a counseling practicum or internship unless that student has completed a sufficient amount of training in AAT, such as a course in AAT. To clarify, AAT training in a brief (1- or 2-day) workshop format is typically not sufficient training to prepare a student to practice AAT in a counseling practicum or internship.
2. No student may practice AAT in a counseling practicum or internship unless the student and animal have obtained a proper credential, for example, a Pet Partners registration or some similar credential.
3. No student may practice AAT in a counseling practicum or internship without the approval of the instructor for that practicum or internship.
4. No student may practice AAT at an off-campus practicum or internship site without the approval of the site clinic director and the site supervisor for that experience.
5. No student may practice AAT with a client without first obtaining permission from the client (and the client's legal guardian where appropriate). Prior to participation in AAT, all clients must be adequately screened and determined to be appropriate for AAT.

6. No therapy animal is allowed in a program office, classroom, clinic, or other related facility unless the animal is healthy, clean, obedient, nonaggressive, friendly, and very well behaved.

7. No student may bring a therapy animal into a counseling clinic without prior approval of the clinic director and informing the clinic receptionist, as well as other relevant staff, in advance of the therapy animal's visits. In addition, no student may bring a therapy animal into a program classroom without the permission of the instructor, and no student may bring a therapy animal into a program office or other related facility without the permission of the office or facility administrator. *Both parts of this condition do not apply to service/disability-assistance animals.*

8. An animal handler can be required to leave the premises with a pet at any time that a clinic director, site supervisor, instructor, administrator, or other appropriate authority deems it necessary for the safety or welfare of any animal or persons.

9. The type of AAT training a student has received must be approved by the clinic director before the student may practice AAT in that counseling practice clinic.

10. No animal is allowed in a campus counseling practice clinic without the proper credential. Proper credential means that the animal has passed a standardized AAT evaluation and has been registered with a reputable AAT organization, such as Pet Partners. *This condition does not apply to service/disability-assistance animals.*

11. All animal handlers who accompany a therapy animal in a campus counseling practice clinic must have a proper AAT credential from a reputable organization, such as Pet Partners.

12. A therapy animal must be accompanied by a trained handler at all times while in the clinic facility. If necessary, the animal may be properly and safely secured in the staff counselor's office or in a pet crate or cage—in a supervised, low-traffic area—for a short period of time when it is not working but it is required to be quiet and well behaved during this time.

13. No animal should ever be left alone with a client. This same rule applies to any clinic or site where the student practices AAT, on or off campus.

14. No animal may participate in AAT, on or off campus, unless the animal is obedient, friendly, and very well behaved.

15. No animal may participate in AAT, on or off campus, unless that animal is healthy, parasite free, clean, and well groomed (including good breath, clean teeth, and clean ears).

16. A handler who accompanies an animal at an on-campus or off-campus counseling practice facility must always clean up after the animal and properly dispose of waste in receptacles outside of the facility (outdoors).

17. Only faculty and supervisors who have had adequate training and/or experience in AAT should supervise a student's AAT practice.

18. No student shall be allowed to practice counseling skills with a therapy animal before the student has first demonstrated the capacity to adequately practice counseling skills without the presence of a therapy animal.

19. Students who practice AAT must commit to following all policies, procedures, and guidelines of their AAT credentialing organizations, such as Pet Partners, and the following entities: college or university, department or program, and any on- or off-campus counseling practice facility where the student trains or practices AAT with an animal. Also see Part II of this document (AAT: Practice Procedures).

20. The coordinator or director of the department's AAT program, or other qualified program designate, will serve as an ongoing consultant for faculty, supervisors, students, and staff regarding the practice of AAT.

21. Only those animal species that have been approved by this program may participate as therapy animals in this program's facilities. (Designate those species here if
applicable.)

Part II AAT—Practice Procedures for a Counselor Education and Training Program

1. All persons who wish to be involved with the practice of AAT must read and agree to
follow the department or program policy and procedures pertaining to the practice
of AAT (this document).

2. Additional AAT practice procedures (in addition to these) for each clinic in this
counselor training program may be developed by each clinic director.

3. Practicum students and interns who wish to practice AAT must be supervised by a
supervisor with adequate training or experience in AAT. Students who wish to practice AAT in counseling practicum should attempt to take practicum from a faculty
member who has adequate training or experience in AAT practice (certain practicum
course sections will be designated for the practice of AAT). If a student's practicum
or internship site supervisor does not have adequate AAT training or experience, the
student may still be allowed to practice AAT in practicum or internship if the student
receives additional supervision from a supervisor with adequate training or experience in AAT, as long as the student receives permission to follow this route from the
practicum or internship site supervisor and the student's training program.

4. Practicum students and interns who wish to practice AAT with a client are responsible for screening their clients for appropriateness to participate in AAT. Thus, the
therapy animal is not present in the therapy room while the screening takes place or
until it is determined that the client is appropriate for and desires to participate in
AAT; this requires consultation with the student's supervisor or instructor.

5. Practicum students and interns must first demonstrate their counseling skills without the presence of a therapy animal before they may begin practice with a therapy
animal. Thus, some counselors in training may have to delay the incorporation of a
therapy animal into their practice until a time when their supervisor determines it is
appropriate.

6. Before entering a "small-sized" waiting area with a therapy animal, a handler should
check with the occupants in the waiting area to see if they are okay with the handler
entering the area with the therapy animal. If any individual in the small-sized waiting area does not want to interact with the therapy animal, then the therapy animal
should not be taken into that waiting area. In this case, clients should preferably meet
the handler with the therapy animal outside of or away from the small waiting area.
Thus, a handler accompanied by a therapy animal may have to wait at the entryway of
the small waiting area and call a client from the doorway or ask another staff person
to call the client.

7. Since not all clients of a counselor will want to participate in AAT, when a therapy
animal is on site but not participating in a counseling session the therapy animal
should be secured in a proper cage or crate in an area where it can be supervised by
other students, staff, or faculty. An animal that cannot behave when secured and left
by its owner cannot participate in AAT. If a counselor has no clients participating in
AAT on a particular day, the therapy animal should not accompany the counselor to
the practice setting or facility.

8. AAT should be practiced only in therapy rooms designated for AAT practice. All
therapy rooms in which AAT is practiced should be labeled as such for the protection

of clients with animal allergies. Also, a sign should be placed on the outside door of the practice facility informing persons of the presence of certain species of animals inside the facility. Where appropriate or when requested, clients with animal allergies should be provided a therapy room where AAT is not or has not been practiced.

9. It is recommended that all clients wash their hands, or use a hand sanitizer, before and after interacting with a therapy animal. This reduces the instance of contamination and infection that may hurt the animal and that may be transferred from person to person via the animal's coat.

10. Animal handlers should make available to the client a fur-removal brush for clients to remove hair shed from a therapy animal to their clothing.

11. Animal handlers should bring accessories to care for the therapy animal at the worksite, such as food and water bowls, bottled water, appropriate treats or snacks, appropriate client–animal interaction tools (e.g., pet toys), a pet cage or crate, and devices to clean up animal excrement and animal fur.

12. Therapy animals shall be kept on a leash or held in species-appropriate containers at all times, with the following exception. Therapy animals may be allowed off-lead or out of appropriate containers only when in a closed area where the animal cannot escape (e.g., when in a therapy room or classroom with the door closed).

13. It is poor practice to tie a therapy animal to a piece of furniture by a leash since the animal may be able to topple the furniture. Also, risk of accidental strangulation is possible for animals that have been tied up by their leash and left unsupervised.

14. Prior to bringing a therapy animal to a facility, examine the facility for appropriateness and safety of the therapy animal, and, with permission and approval of facility staff, make necessary modifications or accommodations for the benefit of the animal.

15. Prior to working with a therapy animal in a counseling session, bring the approved therapy animal to the facility at least two times so it may become familiar with the environment and the therapy room or area where it will be working.

16. Be aware of people's reactions to the therapy animal. Handlers with a therapy animal should be respectful of individuals who do not want to interact with or come near the therapy animal. Handlers with a therapy animal should be friendly and sociable with persons in the facility who may want to visit briefly with the therapy animal though they may not be the counselor's client. Handlers with a therapy animal should be wary of behaviors of individuals in the facility who may or do show aggression toward the therapy animal and should avoid having those persons make contact with the therapy animal.

Appendix F

Sample Policy and Procedures for the Practice of Animal-Assisted Therapy in an Agency or Private Practice

The following agency (or private practice) recognizes the potential value of AAT in the counseling field. To support this recognition, staff counselors who have been properly trained will be allowed to practice AAT under the provisions listed in Part I and Part II.

Part I AAT—Conditions for Practice in an Agency or Private Practice

1. A staff counselor or intern who wishes to practice AAT in this agency (or private practice) must have completed a sufficient amount of AAT training. The type of AAT training a staff member has received must be approved by the clinic director before the staff member may practice AAT in that counseling clinic.
2. No staff counselor or intern may practice AAT without the approval of the site clinic director.
3. No staff counselor or intern may practice AAT with a client without first obtaining permission from the client (and the client's legal guardian where appropriate). Prior to participation in AAT, all clients must be adequately screened and determined to be appropriate for AAT.
4. No therapy animal is allowed in the counseling clinic unless it is healthy, clean, obedient, nonaggressive, friendly, and very well behaved.
5. No therapy animal may participate in AAT unless it is healthy, parasite free, clean, and well groomed (e.g., good breath, clean teeth, and clean ears).
6. No therapy animal may participate in AAT unless it is obedient, friendly, and very well behaved.
7. No staff member or intern may bring any animal into the counseling clinic without prior approval of the clinic director and informing the clinic receptionist, as well as other relevant staff, in advance of the animal's visits. *This condition does not apply to service/disability assistance animals.*
8. An animal handler can be required to leave the premises with a pet at any time that a clinic director, site supervisor, instructor, administrator, or other appropriate authority deems it necessary for the safety or welfare of any animal or persons.
9. A therapy animal must be accompanied by a trained handler at all times while in the clinic facility. If necessary, the animal may be properly and safely secured in the staff counselor's office or in a pet crate or cage—in a supervised, low-traffic area—for

a short period of time when it is not working but is required to be quiet and well behaved during this time.

10. No therapy animal should ever be left alone with a client.
11. A handler who accompanies an animal must always clean up after the animal and properly dispose of waste in receptacles outside of the facility (outdoors).
12. Only staff counselors and supervisors who have had adequate training or experience in AAT should supervise an intern's AAT practice.
13. At least one staff member should be designated as the coordinator or director of the facility's AAT program.
14. Only animal species that have been approved by this clinical facility director may participate as therapy animals in this clinical facility. (Designate species here if applicable.)

Part II AAT—Practice Procedures for an Agency or Private Practice

1. All persons who wish to be involved with the practice of AAT must read and agree to follow its policy and procedures (this document).
2. Interns who wish to practice AAT must be supervised by a supervisor with adequate training or experience in AAT. If an intern's site supervisor does not have adequate AAT training or experience, an intern may still be allowed to practice AAT if the intern receives additional supervision from a supervisor with adequate training or experience in AAT, as long as the intern receives permission to follow this route from the internship site supervisor and the clinical director.
3. Staff counselors or interns who wish to practice AAT with a client are responsible for screening their clients for appropriateness to participate in AAT. Thus, the therapy animal is not present in the therapy room while the screening takes place or until it is determined that the client is appropriate for and desires to participate in AAT; for interns this requires consultation with the intern's supervisor or instructor.
4. AAT should be practiced only in therapy rooms designated for AAT practice. All therapy rooms in which AAT is practiced should be labeled as such for the protection of clients with animal allergies. Also, a sign must be posted on the outside door of the clinical facility informing persons of the presence of certain species of animals inside the facility. Where appropriate or when requested, clients with animal allergies should be provided a therapy room where AAT is not or has not been practiced.
5. It is recommended that all clients wash their hands, or use a hand sanitizer, before and after interacting with a therapy animal. This reduces the instance of contamination and infection that may hurt the animal and that may be transferred from person to person via the animal's coat.
6. Animal handlers should make available to the client a fur-removal brush for clients to remove hair shed from a therapy animal to their clothing.
7. Animal handlers should bring accessories to care for the therapy animal at the worksite, such as food and water bowls, bottled water, appropriate treats or snacks, appropriate client–animal interaction tools (e.g., pet toys), a pet cage or crate, and devices to clean up animal excrement and animal fur.
8. Therapy animals shall be kept on a leash or held in species-appropriate containers at all times, with the following exception. Therapy animals may be allowed off-lead or out of appropriate containers when in a closed area where the animal cannot escape (e.g., when in a therapy room or classroom with the door closed).

9. It is poor practice to tie a therapy animal to a piece of furniture by a leash since the animal may be able to topple the furniture. Also, risk of accidental strangulation is possible for animals that have been tied up by their leash and left unsupervised.

10. Prior to bringing a therapy animal to this clinical facility, examine the facility for appropriateness and safety of the therapy animal, and, with permission and approval of facility staff, make necessary modifications or accommodations for the benefit of the animal.

11. Prior to working with a therapy animal in a counseling session, animal handlers must bring the approved therapy animal to the facility at least two times so it may become familiar with the environment and the therapy room or area where it will be working.

12. Be aware of people's reactions to the therapy animal. Handlers with a therapy animal should be respectful of individuals who do not want to interact with or come near the therapy animal. Handlers with a therapy animal should be friendly and sociable with persons in the facility who may want to visit briefly with the therapy animal though they may not be the counselor's client. Handlers with a therapy animal should be wary of behaviors of individuals in the facility who may or do show aggression toward the therapy animal and should avoid having those persons make contact with the therapy animal.

Index

Note: Page numbers followed by 'f' refer to figures and followed by 't' refer to tables.

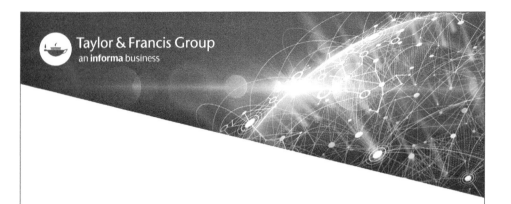
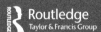
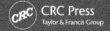